Clinical Cardiology

Clinical Cardiology

Edited by Bernard Tyler

hayle medical
New York

Hayle Medical,
750 Third Avenue, 9th Floor,
New York, NY 10017, USA

Visit us on the World Wide Web at:
www.haylemedical.com

ISBN: 978-1-63241-484-7

The publisher's policy is to use permanent paper from mills that operate a sustainable forestry policy. Furthermore, the publisher ensures that the text paper and cover boards used have met acceptable environmental accreditation standards.

Printed in China.

Cataloging-in-Publication Data

Clinical cardiology / edited by Bernard Tyler.
p. cm.
Includes bibliographical references and index.
ISBN 978-1-63241-484-7
1. Cardiology. 2. Heart--Diseases. I. Tyler, Bernard.
RC667 .C55 2018
616.1--dc23

Table of Contents

Preface

Over the recent decade, advancements and applications have progressed exponentially. This has led to the increased interest in this field and projects are being conducted to enhance knowledge. The main objective of this book is to present some of the critical challenges and provide insights into possible solutions. This book will answer the varied questions that arise in the field and also provide an increased scope for furthering studies.

Cardiology is the science of medicine that deals with disorders of the heart and the circulatory system. This book on clinical cardiology deals with the specialized branches of cardiology and the treatments that are followed in the same. Modern advancements in the field of surgery have allowed for more precise and less invasive surgical procedures for the treatment of cardiovascular disorders. This book on clinical cardiology is a collective contribution of a renowned group of international experts. A number of latest researches have been included to keep the readers up-to-date with the global concepts in this area of study.

I hope that this book, with its visionary approach, will be a valuable addition and will promote interest among readers. Each of the authors has provided their extraordinary competence in their specific fields by providing different perspectives as they come from diverse nations and regions. I thank them for their contributions.

Editor

1

Effects of Candesartan on Electrical Remodeling in the Hearts of Inherited Dilated Cardiomyopathy Model Mice

Fuminori Odagiri[1,2], Hana Inoue[3], Masami Sugihara[1,2], Takeshi Suzuki[1,2], Takashi Murayama[1], Takao Shioya[4], Masato Konishi[3], Yuji Nakazato[2], Hiroyuki Daida[2], Takashi Sakurai[1], Sachio Morimoto[5], Nagomi Kurebayashi[1]*

1 Department of Cellular and Molecular Pharmacology, Juntendo University Graduate School of Medicine, Tokyo, Japan, 2 Department of Cardiovascular Medicine, Juntendo University Graduate School of Medicine, Tokyo, Japan, 3 Department of Physiology, Tokyo Medical University, Tokyo, Japan, 4 Department of Physiology, Faculty of Medicine, Saga University, Saga, Japan, 5 Department of Clinical Pharmacology, Graduate School of Medical Sciences, Kyushu University, Fukuoka, Japan

Abstract

Inherited dilated cardiomyopathy (DCM) is characterized by dilatation and dysfunction of the ventricles, and often results in sudden death or heart failure (HF). Although angiotensin receptor blockers (ARBs) have been used for the treatment of HF, little is known about the effects on postulated electrical remodeling that occurs in inherited DCM. The aim of this study was to examine the effects of candesartan, one of the ARBs, on cardiac function and electrical remodeling in the hearts of inherited DCM model mice (*TNNT2* ΔK210). DCM mice were treated with candesartan in drinking water for 2 months from 1 month of age. Control, non-treated DCM mice showed an enlargement of the heart with prolongation of QRS and QT intervals, and died at $t_{1/2}$ of 70 days. Candesartan dramatically extended the lifespan of DCM mice, suppressed cardiac dilatation, and improved the functional parameters of the myocardium. It also greatly suppressed prolongation of QRS and QT intervals and action potential duration (APD) in the left ventricular myocardium and occurrence of ventricular arrhythmia. Expression analysis revealed that down-regulation of Kv4.2 (I_{to} channel protein), KChIP2 (auxiliary subunit of Kv4.2), and Kv1.5 (I_{Kur} channel protein) in DCM was partially reversed by candesartan administration. Interestingly, non-treated DCM heart had both normal-sized myocytes with moderately decreased I_{to} and I_{Kur} and enlarged cells with greatly reduced K^+ currents (I_{to}, I_{Kur} I_{K1} and I_{ss}). Treatment with candesartan completely abrogated the emergence of the enlarged cells but did not reverse the I_{to}, and I_{Kur} in normal-sized cells in DCM hearts. Our results indicate that candesartan treatment suppresses structural remodeling to prevent severe electrical remodeling in inherited DCM.

Editor: German E. Gonzalez, University of Buenos Aires, Faculty of Medicine. Cardiovascular Pathophysiology Institute, Argentina

Funding: This study was supported by a Grant-in Aid (23136514, S1311011) and the Ministry of Education, Culture, Sports, Science and Technology (MEXT)-supported Program for the Strategic Research Foundation at Private Universities (2011–2015) from the Ministry of Education, Culture, Sports, Science and Technology of Japan. The authors also thank the Vehicle Racing Commemorative Foundation (http://www.vecof.or.jp/index.html) and the Institute of Seizon and Life Sciences (http://seizon.umin.jp/) for financial support. The funders had no role in study design, data collection and analysis, decision to publish, or preparation of the manuscript.

Competing Interests: The authors have declared that no competing interests exist.

* Email: nagomik@juntendo.ac.jp

Introduction

Inherited dilated cardiomyopathy (DCM) is a progressive disease characterized by dilatation and dysfunction of the ventricles, and often results in heart failure (HF) or sudden cardiac death (SCD) from lethal arrhythmia [1–2]. It has recently become clear that gene mutations in various cytoskeletal and sarcomeric proteins lead to weaknesses in the systems involved in force production, which can contribute to the development of DCM [3]. Mortality of DCM patients remains high, and the only treatment for DCM patients with severe HF symptoms is heart transplantation. In addition to HF development, electrical remodeling, which is accompanied by prolongation of the action potential duration (APD), can also be observed in DCM hearts and is thought to be related to increased arrhythmogenicity [4–5].

Recently, angiotensin II receptor blockers (ARBs) have been used for the treatment of HF. A growing body of evidence shows that ARBs inhibit cardiac hypertrophy, structural remodeling and ventricular arrhythmias in HF and thereby reduce cardiac morbidity and mortality [6–9]. However, their effects on inherited DCM are not well known. Because data in humans are confounded by various environmental and genetic factors, investigations with animal models of inherited DCM are required.

Among various gene mutations in inherited DCM, the deletion mutation ΔK210 in cardiac troponin T is a recurrent DCM-causing mutation that has been identified worldwide [10–11]. This mutation causes a lowered Ca^{2+} sensitivity in force generation of cardiac myofilaments [11]. A knock-in mouse model carrying this mutation was created by Morimoto and colleagues [12–14]. These mice closely recapitulate the phenotypes of human DCM, and previous study of this DCM model mouse indicated that down-regulation of various K^+ channels is one of the causes of lethal arrhythmia and SCD [13].

The aim of this study was to examine whether candesartan, one of the ARBs, would have beneficial effects on cardiac function and electrical remodeling in inherited DCM using the ΔK210 knock-in mouse model. Our results indicate that early initiation of candesartan treatment dramatically expands lifespan, preserves cardiac function, suppresses cardiac enlargement as well as cellular enlargement, and attenuate electrical remodeling. Importantly, the suppressive effects of candesartan on electrical remodeling proved to be associated with the preventive effect on structural remodeling.

Materials and Methods

Animal model

All experiments were approved and carried out in accordance with the guidelines of the Committee for Animal Experimentation of Juntendo University (approval number 240001). Knock-in mice with the deletion mutation Lys-210 in their endogenous cardiac troponin T gene (*Tnnt2* ΔK210) were used as DCM model animals [12]. These mice had been backcrossed with the C57BL/6J line for at least 10 generations, and were maintained under specific pathogen-free conditions. Mixed-gender homozygous mutant and wild-type (WT) mice were obtained by crossing heterozygous mutant mice, and were used as DCM and non-DCM models, respectively.

Drug administration

Candesartan cilexetil (TCV116), an ARB, was kindly provided by Takeda Chemical Industries, Ltd (Osaka, Japan). Candesartan was dissolved in drinking water for the mice. DCM mice were treated with candesartan (1 or 3 mg/kg/day) from 1 month of age. DCM mice at 3 months of age (after 2 months of treatment with candesartan, 3 mg/kg/day) and age-matched untreated DCM and WT mice were mainly used in this study. Hydralazine hydrochloride was obtained from Sigma-Aldorich Co. and administered in drinking water at 20 mg/kg/day.

Electrocardiography (ECG), echocardiography, and blood pressure measurements

ECG recording of conscious mice was performed every 2 weeks from 1 month of age using an ECGenie (Mouse Specifics, Inc., Quincy, MA, USA), which non-invasively detected signals from the palmar and plantar aspects of the feet using footplate electrodes [13]. QT, RR, PR, and QRS intervals and heart rate (HR) were quantified. A HR-Corrected QT (QTc) interval was calculated with a modified Bazett correction formula for mice, $QTc = QT/(RR/100)^{1/2}$ [15]. Telemetric ECG recordings were carried out using an implantable telemetry system with ECG transmitters (ETA-F10; Data Sciences International, St. Paul, MN, USA), which was implanted in mice at 2 months of age under isoflurane anesthesia [13]. ECG records were analyzed with ECG Analysis software (AD Instruments Japan, Nagoya, Japan).

The left ventricular end-systolic dimension (LVESD), end-diastolic dimension (LVEDD), fractional shortening (FS) and ejection fraction (EF) were measured by transthoracic echocardiography (Sonos 5500; Philips Electronics Co. Amsterdam, The Netherlands). Blood pressure was measured by a non-invasive tail-cuff system (Softron, Tokyo, Japan).

Determination of wheel running activity

To estimate the extent of HF in DCM mice, physical activity was evaluated by measuring voluntary wheel running activity [13,16]. Mice at 1.5 months or later were housed with free access to a running wheel (6 cm radius; Mini Mitter Co. Inc. OR, USA) for 2 days every 10 days, and their running activities (rounds/day) were measured.

Determination of heart-to-body and lung-to-body weight ratios and plasma angiotensin II (Ang II) levels

Mice were deeply anesthetized with pentobarbital sodium (100 mg/kg i.p.), and their hearts and lungs were excised, rinsed in Krebs solution, and then weighed. Lung weight/body weight (LW/BW) and heart weight/body weight (HW/BW) ratios were calculated. To determine plasma Ang II levels, mice were euthanized and blood samples were obtained from the ventricles. The plasma concentration of Ang II was determined by a double antibody radioimmunoassay at Asuka Pharma Medical Co. Ltd (Tokyo, Japan).

Solutions and reagents used in experiments with myocardium

Normal Krebs solution for myocardial experiments consisted of 120 mM NaCl, 5 mM KCl, 25 mM $NaHCO_3$, 1 mM NaH_2PO_4, 2 mM $CaCl_2$, 1 mM $MgCl_2$ and 10 mM glucose, and was saturated with 95% O_2 and 5% CO_2. High-K^+ Krebs solution used for muscle preparation consisted of 25 mM KCl instead of 5 mM. Di-4-ANEPPS was obtained from Invitrogen/Molecular Probes (Eugene, OR, USA).

Optical determination of APD in isolated myocardium

The APD in myocardium was optically determined as described previously [13,17]. Briefly, muscles of the left ventricle (LV) were loaded with di-4-ANEPPS and mounted in a chamber on the stage of an inverted microscope equipped with a Nipkow disc confocal system (CSU22; Yokogawa, Tokyo, Japan) and W-view/EM-CCD camera system (Model 8509; Hamamatsu Photonics, Hamamatsu, Japan). Myocardium was field stimulated at 0.5 Hz in normal Krebs solution. Di-4-ANEPPS was excited by 488 nm laser light and fluorescence images at 525 and 620 nm were simultaneously captured, and ratio images were then calculated. Membrane potential signals were obtained at 3.67 ms intervals. The APD_{50} (i.e., the time at which the down-stroke of the action potential (AP) had recovered 50% toward the baseline) was obtained as the activation minus the repolarization time points. Experiments were carried out at 25–27°C.

Real-time RT-PCR

Total RNA was isolated from the LV using an RNeasy Fibrous Tissue Mini Kit (Qiagen). First strand cDNA was synthesized using a High-Capacity RNA-to-cDNA kit (Applied Biosystems) [13]. The expression of genes encoding Kv1.5, Kv2.1, Kv4.2, Kir2.1, Kir2.2, and KChIP2 was assessed by quantitative real-time PCR analysis using Fast SYBR Green Master Mix (Applied Biosystems). The primers used for real-time PCR have been described previously [13]. PCR was carried out using an 7500 Fast Real Time PCR System (Applied Biosystems). mRNA expression of each gene was normalized to that of the glyceraldehyde 3-phosphate dehydrogenase (GAPDH) gene.

Western blot analysis

Membrane protein samples were analyzed by western blotting as described elsewhere [13]. The following antibodies were used: rabbit monoclonal IRK1 (Kir2.1) antibody (GTX62777, GeneTex), rabbit polyclonal anti-KCNB1 (Kv2.1) (SAB2101203, Sigma-Aldorich), rabbit polyclonal anti-Kv4.2 (APC-023; Alomone labs), rabbit polyclonal KChIP2 antibody (GTX116483, GeneTex), goat polyclonal anti-Kv1.5 (sc-11679; Santa Cruz Biotechnology), and mouse monoclonal anti-β-actin (ab8226; Abcam). The densities of specific bands were determined by

MultiGauge software (Fujifilm, Tokyo, Japan) and normalized to that of the β-actin band.

Whole-cell clamp recording

Single cells were isolated from the ventricles of mice using an established enzymatic method [18]. After isolation, the cells were whole-cell clamped in the voltage-clamp mode using a patch-clamp amplifier (Axopatch200B; Molecular Devices, Union city, CA, USA). Patch-pipettes (1.7–2.3 MΩ) were pulled from thin-wall glass capillaries (GC150TF-7.5; Harvard Apparatus, Holliston, MA, USA), and series resistance (2.5–5 MΩ) was compensated by 75–80% electronically. Data acquisition and analysis were performed using pClamp 10 software suit and a DigiData 1321A signal interface (Molecular Devices). All voltage data were corrected for a liquid junction potential of −10 mV assumed at the pipette tip. All measurements were carried out at room temperature (24–26°C). Ventricular cells were perfused with a bath solution consisting of 140 mM NaCl, 5.4 mM KCl, 1.8 mM $CaCl_2$, 0.5 mM $MgCl_2$, 0.33 mM NaH_2PO_4, 0.1 mM $CdCl_2$, 11 mM glucose, and 5 mM HEPES-NaOH (pH 7.4). The pipette (intracellular) solution consisted of 110 mM K-aspartate, 30 mM KCl, 5 mM Mg-ATP, 0.1 mM Tris GTP, 4 mM BAPTA, and 20 mM HEPES-KOH (pH 7.2).

To record I_{K1} and I_{ss}, 2 s test pulses were applied to the cells every 4 s from a holding potential of −80 mV. To record I_{to} and I_{Kur}, 1 s test pulses with or without a prepulse (60 ms to −20 mV) were applied every 10 s from the holding potential. We confirmed that I_{Kur} was inhibited by 100 μM 4-aminopyridine (4AP) but not by the inactivating prepulse at 25°C, whereas I_{to} was inactivated by the prepulse but not by 4AP. Detailed procedures for isolation of each K^+ current are described elsewhere [13,19].

Determination of cell length in isolated single myocytes

Isolated single cells on a laminin-coated glass bottom dish were incubated in a Ca^{2+} free Tyrode solution (140 mM NaCl, 5.4 mM KCl, 0.33 mM NaH_2PO_4, 0.5 mM $MgCl_2$, 5.5 mM glucose and 5 mM HEPES, pH 7.4) and quickly fixed with a 4% paraformaldehyde (PFA) in phosphate buffered saline (PBS). Alternatively, concentrated single cells in the Ca^{2+} free Tyrode solution (~50 μL) were fixed by adding ~1 mL of 4% PFA in PBS. Both methods gave the same results. Fixed cells in a glass-bottom dish were observed with an inverted microscope and their images were captured. Cell lengths were measured with the AquaCosmos software (Hamamatsu Photonics, Hamamatsu, Japan). Cells showing contracture, which were distinguishable by collapsed shape or shortened sarcomere length, were omitted from the measurements.

Statistics

Data are presented as the mean ± SEM unless indicated otherwise. Mean values were compared by one-way analysis of variance (ANOVA) followed by the post-hoc Kruskal-Wallis multiple comparison test for three groups. Two-way ANOVA followed by the Bonferroni post-test was used for comparison of multiple groups in a x-y relationship. P-values of <0.05 were considered significant.

Results

Effects of candesartan on survival rate, and cardiac histology and functions

In this study, treatment of DCM mice with candesartan was started at 1 month of age when their death rate was still low [13,16]. Fig. 1A shows the Kaplan-Meier survival curve of DCM mice treated with candesartan (1 or 3 mg/kg/day) and the untreated control. In control DCM mice, $t_{1/2}$ was approximately 70 days after birth (corresponding to 40 days of treatment) as described previously [12–13]. In contrast, the survival rates of candesartan-treated DCM mice were dramatically improved in a dose-dependent manner. Notably, in the group treated with 3 mg/kg/day, about 8% of mice died within 1 month after initiation of the treatment, but thereafter they rarely died until 6 months of age. In the following experiments, we analyzed DCM mice treated with 3 mg/kg/day.

First, we compared blood pressure to confirm the effect of candesartan in DCM mouse. The blood pressure in untreated DCM mice was already significantly lower than that in WT mice, and treatment with candesartan further reduced the blood pressure (Table 1). Plasma levels of Ang II were elevated in untreated DCM mice (Fig. 1B), indicating an increase of Ang II production. Plasma Ang II was also high in candesartan-treated DCM mice, which might be caused by production of plasma renin because of reduced blood pressure [20–21].

Fig. 1C–F and Table 1 show the comparison of the properties of hearts from 3-month-old WT and DCM mice with or without candesartan treatment for 2 months. There were no significant differences in body weights between the three groups (Table 1). Fig. 1C shows the typical gross morphology of hearts (upper panel), and the average HW/BW ratios (lower panel). Untreated control DCM mice had considerably enlarged hearts compared with WT mice, and candesartan strongly suppressed the enlargement of the heart. However, it should be noted that the HW/BW in candesartan-treated mice was still higher ($P<0.05$) than that of WT mice.

Cardiac fibrosis was compared using Azan staining (Fig. 1D). The control DCM group showed advanced interstitial fibrosis, whereas candesartan greatly suppressed the fibrosis. The expression levels of brain natriuretic peptide (BNP) in the left ventricular myocardium, which have been associated with HF in humans and mice, were higher in control DCM mice than that in WT mice. The expression of BNP in the candesartan-treated group was completely reversed to the level in the WT group (Fig. 1E). Physical activity was measured using a voluntary running wheel to detect congestive HF (Fig. 1F) [13,16]. The average wheel-running activity of control DCM mice was low at 3 months of age. In contrast, the candesartan group maintained a high running activity comparable to that of WT mice, suggesting that congestive HF did not developed in these mice. Importantly, candesartan treatment did not decrease daily motility despite the low blood pressure.

Echocardiographic analysis of untreated control DCM mice showed LV dilatation and systolic dysfunction as evidenced by an increased LVEDD and reduced LV EF, respectively (Table 1). Treatment with candesartan significantly decreased the LVEDD and increased the EF compared with those in control DCM mice (Table 1). Because previous report indicated that the decrease in the Ca^{2+} sensitivity of the myofilament in DCM heart was not improved by candesartan [22], above beneficial effects of candesartan are due to suppression of deterioration of heart. In summary, candesartan treatment greatly suppresses cardiac enlargement, fibrosis, and the development of HF in DCM mice without loss of physical activity.

Effects of candesartan on ECG

ECG records were non-invasively obtained from conscious mice every half month from 1 to 3 months of age. Heart rate (HR) and PQ, QRS, QT and QTc intervals in 3 month-old mice were summarized in Table 1. At 3 month-old, HR was significantly

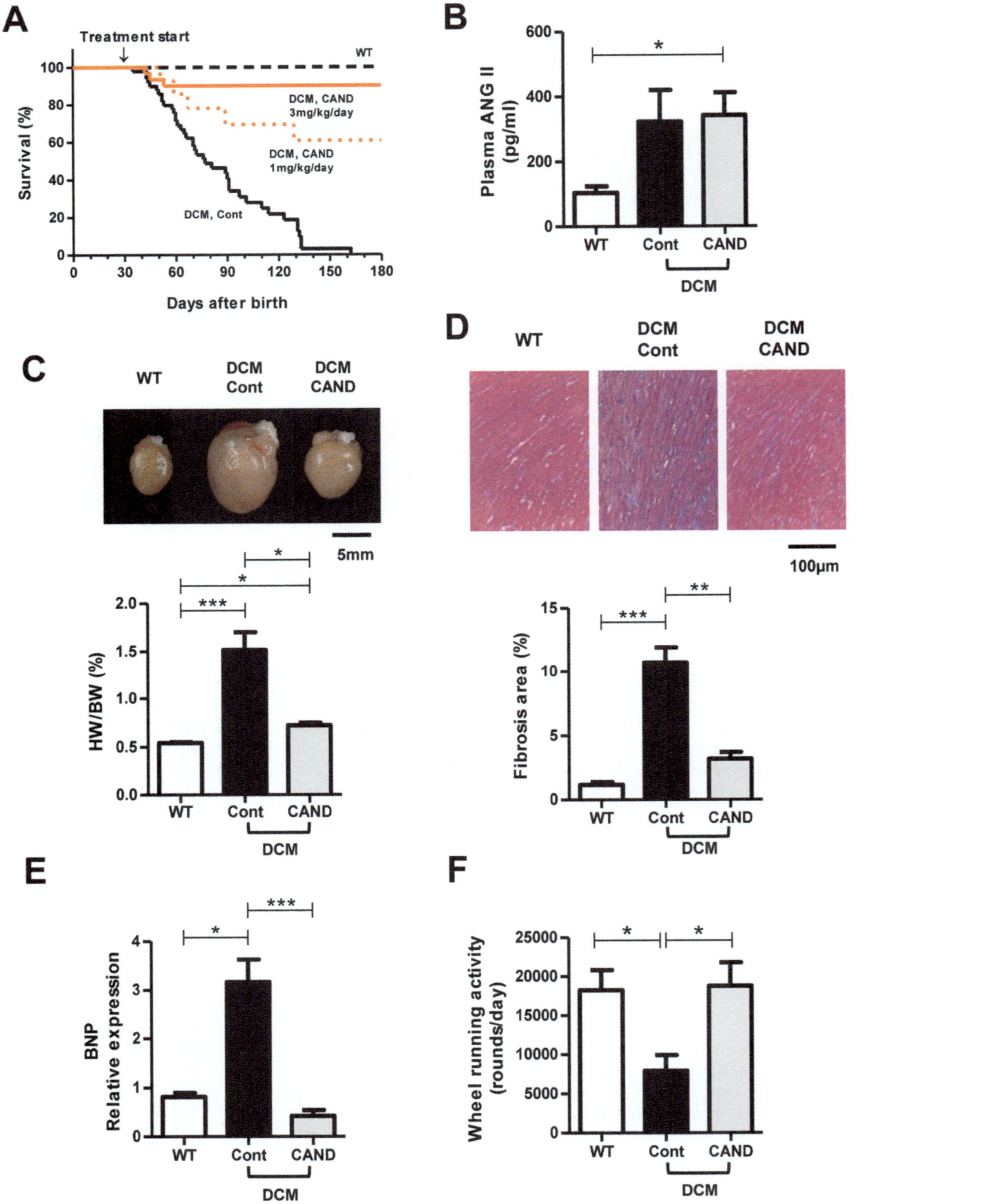

Figure 1. Effects of candesartan on survival rate, and cardiac histology and functions. ***A.*** Survival curves of control DCM (Cont) (n = 49), candesartan-treated DCM (CAND) (1 mg/kg/day: n = 14, 3 mg/kg/day: n = 30) and non-treated WT mice (n = 34). ***B.*** Plasma Ang II level (WT: n = 6, Cont: n = 5, CAND: n = 6). ***C.*** Typical gross morphology of hearts (upper image) and average HW/BW ratio (lower panel) (WT: n = 11, Cont: n = 11, CAND: n = 12). ***D.*** Histology of the LV myocardium. Connective tissues were stained blue with Azan. Upper images: typical images. Lower panel: quantitative analysis of the fibrotic area in the myocardium (three hearts in each group). ***E.*** Gene expression level of BNP in the LV (WT: n = 10, Cont: n = 15, CAND: n = 12). ***F.*** Wheel running activity (WT:n = 11, Cont: n = 10, CAND: n = 10). Data are the mean ± SEM. *P<0.05, **P<0.01, ***P<0.001.

Table 1. In vivo parameters of WT and DCM mice with or without candesartan treatment.

	WT	DCM	
Treatment	-	-	**Candesartan (3 mg/kg/day)**
No. of mice	11	11	12
age, days	90.4±2.3	89.6±3.5	91.1±1.9
BW, g	23.6±1.0	22.4±0.7	23.5±1.1
HW, g	0.13±0.00	0.34±0.04***	0.17±0.01†††
LW, g	0.13±0.00	0.22±0.03**	0.13±0.01††
HW/BW, %	0.54±0.01	1.51±0.19***	0.72±0.02†††
LW/BW, %	0.56±0.02	1.00±0.14**	0.57±0.03†††
Blood pressure			
No. of mice	5	6	4
SBP, mmHg	113±3	99±5***	69±3*†††
DBP, mmHg	74±5	62±5	31±4***††
TTE			
No. of mice	10	11	12
HR, bpm	726.6±9.1	608.0±39.1**	712.5±12.5††
LVESD, mm	1.35±0.04	3.70±0.21***	1.85±0.09*†††
LVEDD, mm	2.82±0.05	4.58±0.22***	3.10±0.05†††
FS, %	52.2±1.6	19.6±1.3***	40.4±2.4***†††
EF, %	84.5±1.3	40.2±2.5***	71.6±3.0*†††
ECG			
No. of mice	11	9	12
HR, bpm	730.5±7.8	591.7±46.6**	715.6±10.9††
PQ, msec	32.0±0.3	35.8±0.8**	32.4±0.8††
QRS, msec	10.2±0.2	18.6±0.9***	12.8±0.1***†††
QT, msec	17.8±0.2	33.4±1.0***	19.5±0.5*†††
QTc, msec	19.3±0.2	27.6±2.2***	21.5±0.2*†††

DCM mice treated with candesartan (3 mg/kg/day) from 1 to 3 months of age and age-matched untreated control DCM and WT mice were used. Blood pressure, surface ECG and trans-thoracic echocardiography (TTE) were measured. Heart weight, lung weight and body weight were measured after sacrifice. BW, body weight; HW, heart weight; LW, lung weight; SBP, systolic blood pressure: DBP, diastolic blood pressure; HR, heart rate; bpm, beat per min; LVESD, LV end-systolic dimension; LVEDD, LV end-diastolic dimension, FS, fractional shortening; EF, ejection fraction.

*P<0.05,

**P<0.01,

***P<0.001 vs WT.

††P<0.01,

†††P<0.001 vs control DCM.

decreased in untreated DCM mice with increased variance; among 9 mice, 2 showed substantial decrease in HR to ~350 beats per min (bpm) whereas others showed much less decrease (620–720 bpm). The HR was reversed to WT level by candesartan treatment (Table 1). Fig. 2B shows QRS and QTc intervals from 1 to 3 months of age. At 1 month of age before treatment with candesartan, QRS and QTc intervals were already significantly longer in DCM mice compared with those in WT mice (Fig. 2A and B). Thereafter, QRS and QTc intervals in control DCM mice were prolonged further. Treatment with candesartan completely suppressed further prolongation (Fig. 2A and B), but did not reverse to the WT level. The prolongation in QRS interval can be explained by an increase in conduction time in the ventricle probably because of cardiac enlargement and fibrosis, whereas the QTc prolongation suggests prolongation of APD.

There arises a question whether the suppressing effects of candesartan on prolongation of QRS and QTc intervals are due to direct inhibition of angiotensin receptor in heart or indirect action via further decreased blood pressure by vasodilation, which may reduce preload and afterload. To examine this, DCM mice were treated with a vasodilator, hydralazine, which lowers blood pressure independently of angiotensin receptor. Similarly to candesartan, hydralazine at 20 mg/kg/day further decreased blood pressure (from 99±5/62±5 mmHg (n = 6) to 74±2/47±3 mmHg (n = 6)) and increased HR (from 592±47 bpm to 722±7 bpm) in DCM mice. However, hydralazine treatment did not suppress the prolongation of QRS and QTc intervals in DCM mice (Figure S1 in File S1). Thus, the suppressive effects of candesartan on prolongation of QRS and QTc could not be attributed to the decreased blood pressure.

We also obtained ECG records using an implantable telemetry system with ECG transmitters with mice at 2–5 months of age until the battery of the transmitter stopped functioning (Fig. 2C). All untreated control DCM mice (n = 6) showed occasional ventricular arrhythmia including premature ventricular contraction (PVC), ventricular tachycardia (VT) (Fig. 2C, middle), and/or

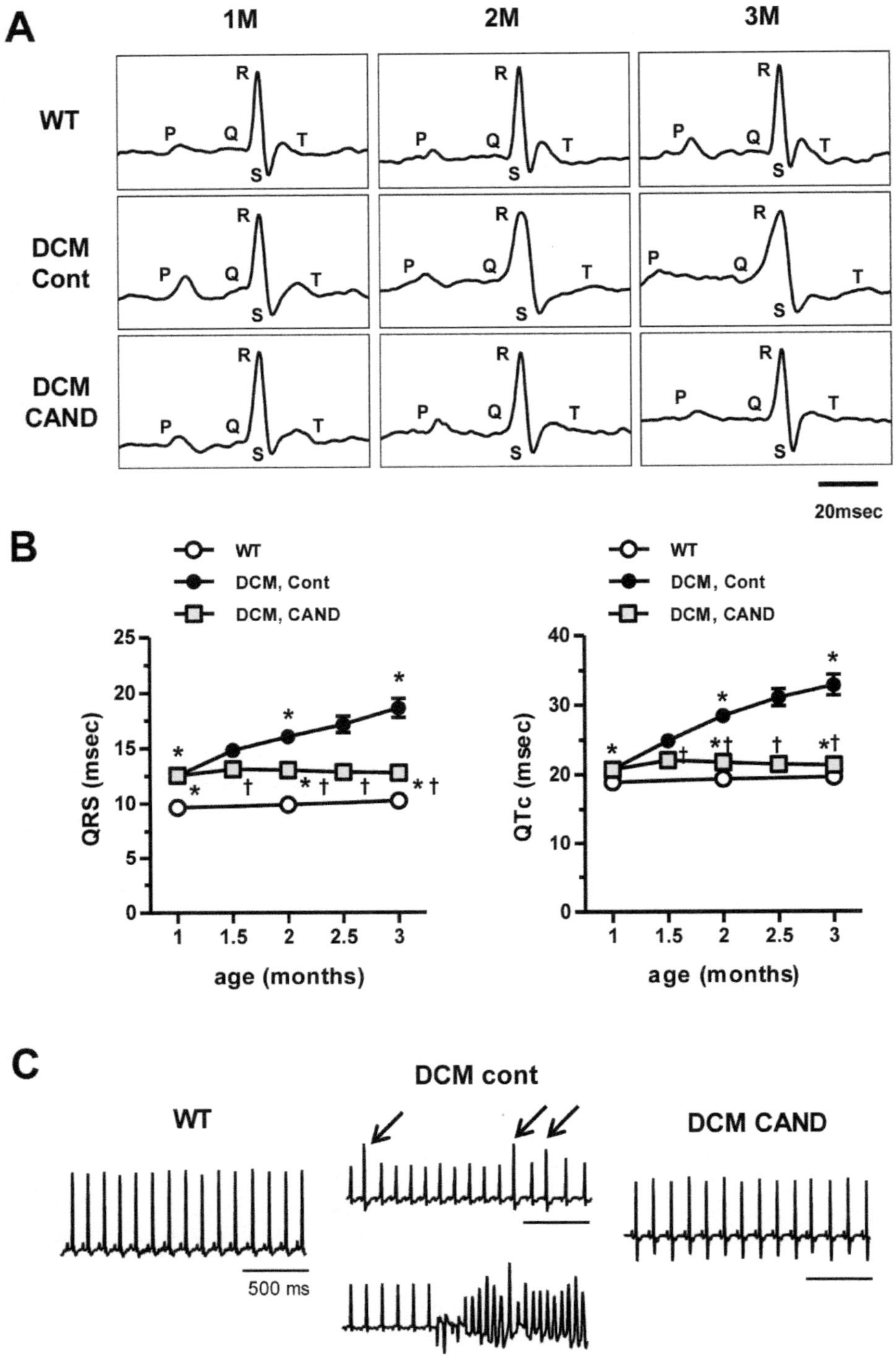

Figure 2. Effects of candesartan on ECG data. *A.* Typical traces of ECG in a time course. *B.* Comparison of QRS and QTc intervals in WT (n = 11), control (n = 11) and candesartan-treated DCM mice (n = 12). *P<0.05 vs WT, †P<0.05 vs control DCM. **C.** Typical ECG records obtained with a telemetric recording system. Left: normal ECG trace from WT mouse. Center: representative traces of PVCs (upper panel, arrows) and VT (lower panel) in control DCM mice. Right: representative normal ECG trace from candesartan-treated DCM mouse.

T wave alternans, and finally died with VT or Torsades des pointes within a ~2.5 months of monitoring period as reported previously [12–13,16]. In contrast, WT (n = 5) and candesartan-treated DCM mice (n = 6) showed no such ventricular arrhythmia and survived far beyond the monitoring period. These results suggest that some changes in electrical properties related to APD and arrhythmia may be suppressed by candesartan treatment. Because the differences in QRS and QTc intervals between DCM control and candesartan-treated mice were most clear after 2 months of treatment (at 3 months of age), comparisons were made at this age in the following experiments.

Effects of candesartan on APD in isolated myocardium

Because QT interval is closely related to APD, AP signals were optically obtained at apical and basal regions of the LV as described previously [13]. APD_{50} (APD at 50% repolarization) values were used because they are relatively stable compared with longer APD measurements such as APD_{90}, which are more variable as they are affected by Na^{+}-Ca^{2+} exchange activity. In the basal region of the WT LV, the average APD_{50} was approximately 20 ms, whereas that in the DCM LV was about 3.2-fold longer (64±4 ms) (Fig. 3A and B). In the candesartan-treated DCM LV, APD_{50} was significantly shorter (31±2 ms) than that in the control DCM. These results were consistent with QTc intervals in the three groups (Fig. 2 and Table 1). Comparison of APD_{50} at the apical region among the three groups gave similar conclusions. The spatial difference between basal and apical regions was largest in control DCM mice, and was much smaller in candesartan-treated DCM mice (Fig. 3B).

Effects of candesartan on the gene and protein expression of K^{+} channels

The shortened APD in the myocardium of candesartan-treated DCM mice can be explained by increased repolarizing currents. APD has been reported to be influenced by I_{to}, I_{Kur}, I_{K1} and I_{ss} [19], and we have previously found that the expression of I_{to}- and I_{Kur}-related molecules is considerably decreased in DCM mice at 2 months [13]. In this study, we analyzed the expression levels of genes encoding the various ion channels that carry I_{K1} (Kir2.1 and Kir2.2), I_{ss} (Kv2.1), I_{to} (Kv4.2 and the accessory subunit KChIP2), and I_{Kur} (Kv1.5) in WT and DCM mice at 3 months.

There was no significant difference in the expression levels of Kir2.1, Kir2.2 and Kv2.1 among the three groups. In contrast, the mRNA levels of Kv4.2, KChIP2, and Kv1.5 were significantly diminished in the untreated control DCM LV to about half or less of the WT level (Fig. 4). These results were consistent with our previous report [13]. Candesartan significantly, but only partially restored the expression of Kv4.2 and Kv1.5, and greatly restored the expression of KChIP2. To know whether the candesartan directly up-regulate these channels, WT mice were also treated with candesartan and gene expression levels were determined. As shown in Figure S2 in File S1, candesartan has no significant effects on any of Kir2.1, Kir2.2, Kv2.1, Kv4.2, KChIP2 and Kv1.5. These results suggest that candesartan does not directly up-regulate these channels but inhibit action of Ang II elevated in DCM mice.

Expression of channel proteins was verified by western blot analysis. Fig. 5 shows typical data (A) and the comparison of the averaged values of each protein level (B). There was no significant difference in the protein levels of Kir2.1 between WT and control DCM LVs, and candesartan moderately up-regulated Kir2.1 protein expression. The expression level of Kv2.1appeared to be reduced in control DCM and restored in candesartan treatment, but without significant difference. In contrast, Kv4.2 and KChIP2 levels were decreased in DCM LVs to ~50% of those in WT LVs, and were considerably restored by candesartan treatment. These results are roughly correlated with the gene expression data. The level of Kv1.5 was also significantly decreased to about half of that in WT LVs, and candesartan had no significant effect on the expression. The reason for the discrepancy between gene and protein expression of Kv1.5 is unclear.

Effects of candesartan treatment on K^{+} currents

We next examined the effects of candesartan treatment on major K^{+} currents (I_{K1}, I_{ss}, I_{to}, and I_{Kur}) in ventricular myocytes

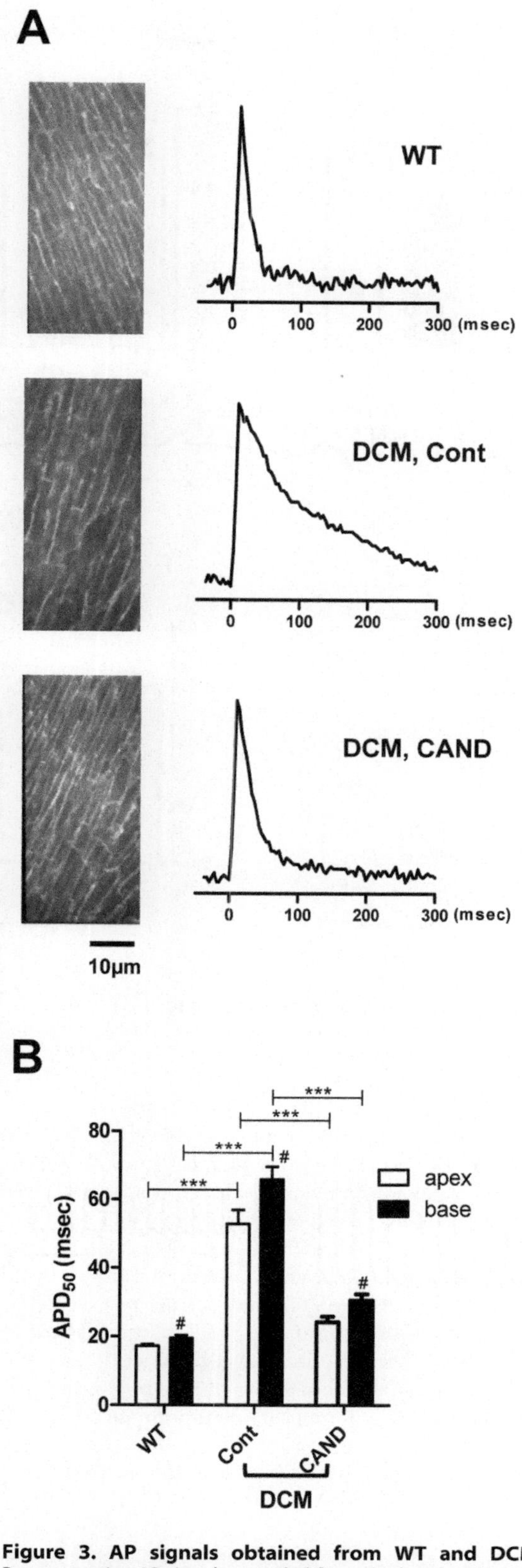

Figure 3. AP signals obtained from WT and DCM LVs. ***A.*** Representative AP signals recorded from the basal region of LVs of WT (top), control DCM (middle) and candesartan-treated DCM (bottom) mice stimulated at 0.5 Hz. ***B.*** Comparison of APD_{50} values in the basal and apical regions of LVs from WT (base: n = 10, apex: n = 12 from five hearts) control DCM (base: n = 31, apex: n = 35 from 6 hearts) and candesartan-treated DCM (base: n = 25, apex: n = 21 from four hearts) mice. ***P<0.001, #P<0.05 vs the apex in the same group.

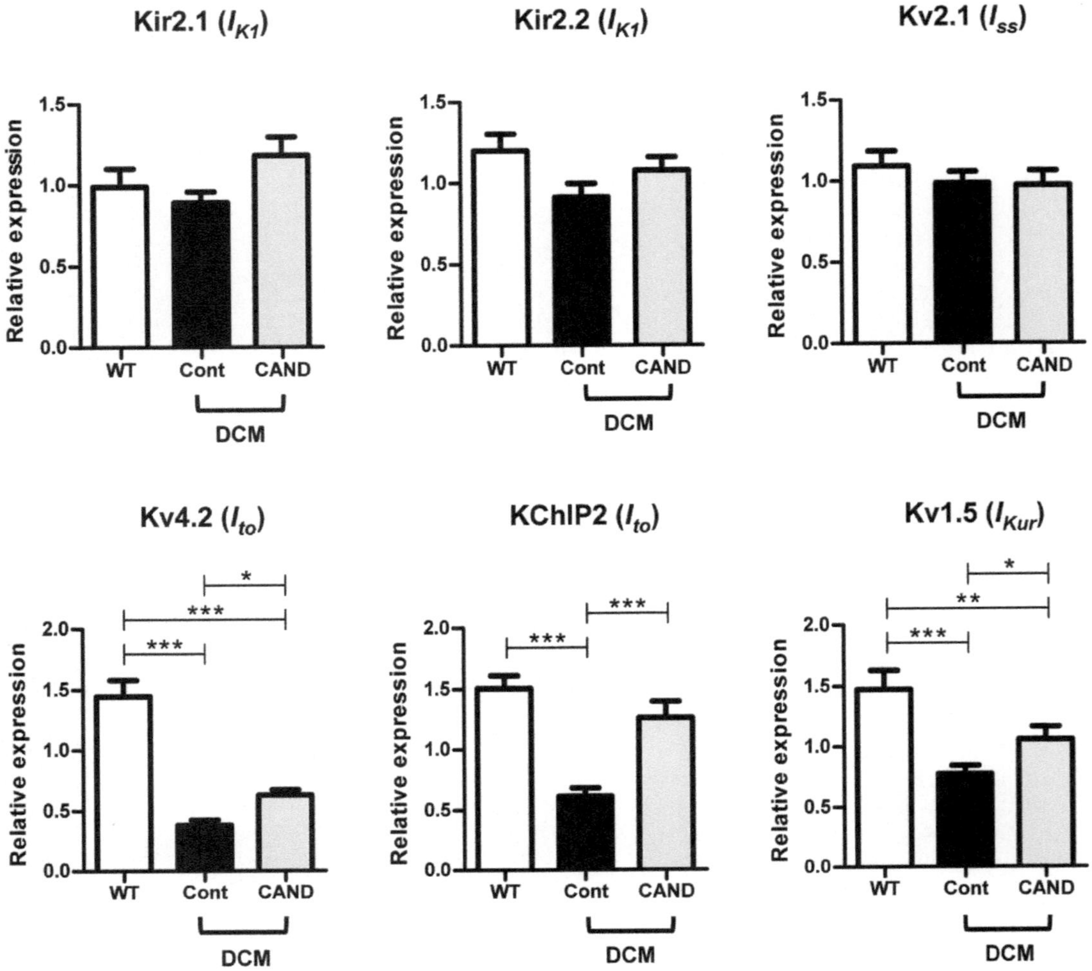

Figure 4. Expression levels of mRNA encoding the K^+ channels and auxiliary subunits that contribute to the repolarizing phase of APs. Quantitative real-time PCR analysis was carried out with LVs from WT (n = 10), control (n = 15) and candesartan-treated DCM (n = 11) mice. The GAPDH gene was used as an internal control. *P<0.05, **P<0.01, ***P<0.001.

[13,19]. As we noticed that the membrane capacitance (Cm) of untreated control DCM myocytes was often large, we carried out current measurements from randomly selected cells that allowed successful patch clamp recording except for cells with a Cm of > 500 pF, which are thought to be difficult to clamp voltage. Fig. 6A-a shows typical whole cell K^+ currents in myocytes activated by 2 s square pulses (−120 to +40 mV) from a holding potential of −80 mV. The amplitude of outward whole-cell current activated by depolarizing pulse was reduced in control DCM cells compared with WT cells, and was considerably restored in cells from candesartan-treated DCM mice, consistent with the results of APD_{50} measurements.

Because there was a large Cm variation in control DCM cells, currents in individual cells at the largest voltage step (−120 mV for I_{K1}, +40 mV for I_{SS}, +50 mV for I_{to} and I_{Kur}) were plotted against their Cm, which reflects the cell surface area (Fig. 6-b, d, g, j). Since the largest Cm for WT myocytes was approximately 250 pF, I–V relationships of control DCM cells were plotted for two groups, cells with normal Cm (Cm<250 pF) and cells with large Cm (300 pF<Cm<500 pF) (Fig. 6-c, e, h, k). Interestingly, no large-Cm cells were detected in population of candesartan-treated myocytes.

The inward rectifier K^+ current (I_{K1}) was measured as a steady-state current activated by hyperpolarizing pulses (Fig. 6A-a). When comparisons were made between normal-Cm cells, I_{K1} was smaller in control DCM cells (67%) compared with that in WT cells (Fig. 6A-c). In large-Cm DCM cells, I_{K1} was further reduced (43%). In contrast, candesartan treatment completely reversed I_{K1} to the level in WT cells (Fig. 6A-c). The I_{ss} was isolated as the steady-state whole-cell current at depolarizing pulse end (Fig. 6A-a). The amplitude of the I_{ss} in normal-Cm control DCM cells was slightly smaller (73%) than that in WT cells, and that in large-Cm cells was further reduced (45%). The amplitude of the I_{ss} in candesartan-treated cells was much closer to the WT level (Fig. 6A-e).

Both I_{to} and I_{Kur} are transient outward currents, but they exhibit different sensitivities to 4 aminopyridine (4AP) and an inactivating prepulse [13,19]. I_{to} was measured as the prepulse-sensitive outward current in the presence of 4AP, while I_{Kur} was measured as the 4AP-sensitive outward current activated by depolarizing test pulses with the prepulse as described previously [13]. I_{to} in control DCM cells with a normal Cm had significantly smaller peak amplitudes (~50%) than those in WT cells (Fig. 6A-f–h). To our surprise, control DCM cells with a large Cm appeared to have much lower current densities (~11%) (Fig. 6A-g, h). The I_{to} in

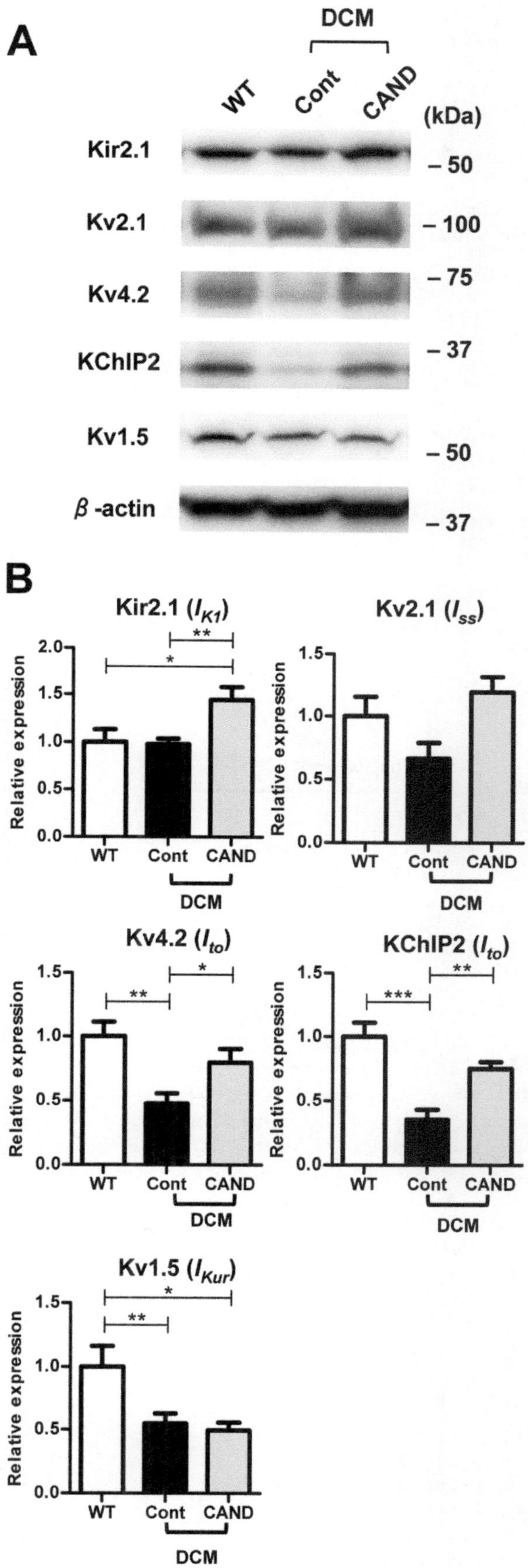

Figure 5. Western blot analysis of the K⁺ channels and auxiliary subunits in the LV. Membrane protein samples (50 μg) of WT (n = 6), control (n = 10) and candesartan-treated DCM (n = 7) LVs were separated by SDS-PAGE and western blot analysis was carried out. See Methods for details. ***A.*** Representative blots of individual experiments. ***B.*** Averaged expression levels. The relative expression levels for each protein were normalized to the average value for WT LVs. *P<0.05, **P<0.01, ***P<0.001.

candesartan-treated cells was approximately 50% of WT level, similar to that in normal-Cm control DCM cells (Fig. 6A-k). I_{Kur} in normal-Cm control DCM cells was also significantly smaller (37%) than that in WT cells (Fig. 6A-j, k). I_{Kur} in large-Cm DCM cells was further reduced (~13%) compared to normal-Cm cells (Fig. 6A-j, k). I_{Kur} in candesartan-treated DCM cells was similar to that in normal-Cm control DCM cells (50% of WT).

Because measurements of current densities for I_{to} and I_{Kur} in large-Cm cells might be less accurate by distortion of the time courses of transient outward currents, we examined current kinetics (time to peak from onset of voltage step and decay time from 100 to 50% of peak) and plotted against Cm (Figure S3 in File S1). Since the time to peak and decay time were similar over Cm range of 80–500 pF, values for these K⁺ currents in large-Cm cells were considered acceptable. In summary, the above current measurements indicate that current densities of all four components decrease in both normal- and large-Cm control DCM cells. Candesartan completely restores I_{K1} and I_{SS} with no significant effect on I_{to} or I_{Kur} in DCM cells with normal Cm. More importantly, however, candesartan suppresses emergence of large-Cm cells, which have very low densities of I_{to} and I_{Kur}.

Effects of candesartan treatment on cell-length distribution of ventricular myocytes in DCM heart

The presence of large-Cm cells with low densities of K⁺ currents may account for the data on mRNA/protein expression, APD and current measurements. However, the fraction of the large-Cm cells appeared to be smaller for successful patch-clamp recordings than that of the *in vivo* population in the DCM myocardium because making the whole-cell configuration with them was difficult by unstable sealing. To determine the actual size distribution of isolated ventricular myocytes, myocytes were fixed with PFA and cell lengths were determined (see Materials and methods, Fig. 6Ba, Figure S4 in File S1). The frequency distributions of longitudinal cell lengths were plotted in Fig. 6B-b. WT myocytes ranged between 52 and 184 μm (mean±SD: 111±25 μm, n = 310), whereas untreated control DCM cells ranged between 59 and 290 μm with a larger standard deviation (161±50 μm, n = 290, P<0.001 vs WT). Thus, the distribution of cell size increased in the control DCM heart, and about 27% of myocytes were out-of-range compared with the WT cell distribution. In contrast, candesartan-treated DCM cells ranged from 64 to 182 μm (119±21 μm, n = 294, P<0.05 vs WT, P<0.001 vs control DCM). Although the mean size of candesartan-treated DCM cells was significantly larger than that of WT cells, we did not detect any enlarged cells (>190 μm). It should be noted that hydralazine treatment did not suppress the emergence of enlarged cells (data not shown). These results confirm that candesartan treatment prevent the emergence of enlarged cells in DCM hearts.

Discussion

The beneficial effects of ARBs on chronic HF have been well established in animal models [6–8], but the effects on electrical remodeling in inherited DCM have not been well known because

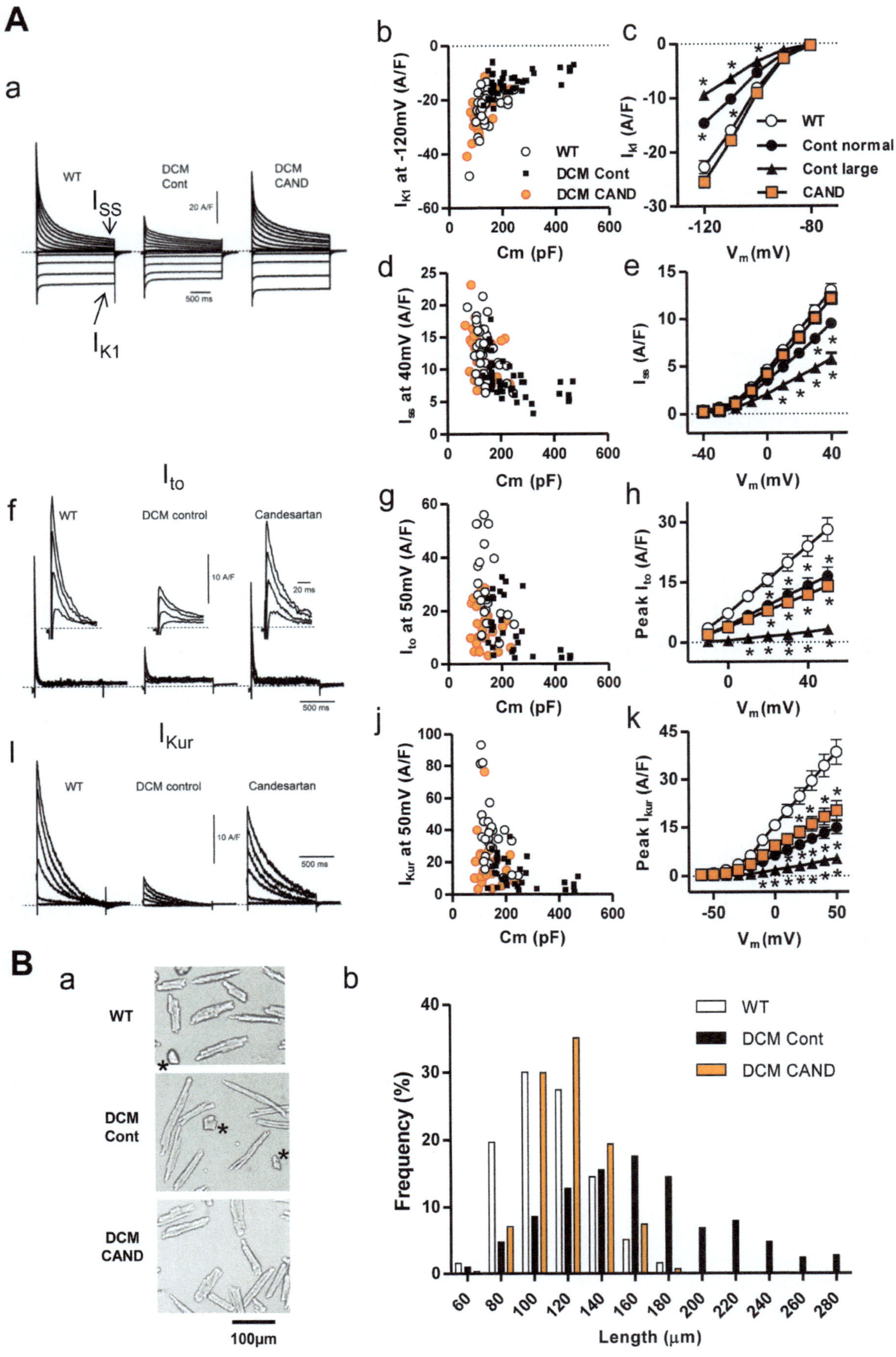
A
a
WT
DCM Cont
DCM CAND
ISS
IK1
20 A/F
500 ms
b
IK1 at -120mV (A/F)
Cm (pF)
WT
DCM Cont
DCM CAND
c
IK1 (A/F)
Vm (mV)
WT
Cont normal
Cont large
CAND
d
Iss at 40mV (A/F)
Cm (pF)
e
Iss (A/F)
Vm (mV)
Ito
f
WT
DCM control
Candesartan
10 A/F
20 ms
500 ms
g
Ito at 50mV (A/F)
Cm (pF)
h
Peak Ito (A/F)
Vm (mV)
IKur
i
WT
DCM control
Candesartan
10 A/F
500 ms
j
IKur at 50mV (A/F)
Cm (pF)
k
Peak IKur (A/F)
Vm (mV)
B
a
WT
DCM Cont
DCM CAND
100µm
b
Frequency (%)
Length (µm)
WT
DCM Cont
DCM CAND

Figure 6. Whole-cell currents of major K^+ channels which contribute to repolarization and the size distribution of ventricular myocytes. ***A.*** I_{K1}, I_{ss} I_{to}, I_{Kur} of WT, control and candesartan-treated DCM cells. ***a.*** Representative current traces of whole cell currents activated by voltage steps (2 s, −120 to +40 mV in 10 mV increments) from a holding potential of −80 mV. I_{K1} and I_{ss} were measured as the steady-state amplitude of the whole-cell current at pulse end. ***b*** and ***d,*** I_{K1} and I_{ss} in individual cells at the largest voltage step (−120 mV and +40 mV, respectively) were plotted against their Cm, which reflects the cell surface area. ***c*** and ***e.*** Current-voltage (IV) relations of I_{K1} and I_{SS}, respectively. ***f.*** Representative current traces of I_{to} activated at −10, +10, +30, and +50 mV (insets expand the peaks on a fast time-base). ***g.*** I_{to} in individual cells at the largest voltage step, 50 mV. ***h.*** IV relations of I_{to}. ***i.*** Representative current traces of I_{Kur} activated at −50, −30, −10, +10, +30, and +50 mV. ***j.*** I_{Kur} in individual cells at the voltage step of 50 mV. ***k.*** IV relations of I_{Kur}. ***b, d, g*** and ***j:*** WT (open circle, n = 25–34 from six hearts), Cont (filled square, n = 33–43 from eight hearts), CAND (orange circle, n = 26–36 from five hearts). ***c, e, h*** and ***k:*** WT (open circle, n = 25–34), normal-Cm control DCM (Cm<250 pF, filled triangle, n = 14–23), large-Cm control DCM, (300 pF<Cm<500 pF, filled circle, n = 6–8), candesartan-treated DCM (orange square, n = 26–36), Dotted lines: zero-current level. *P<0.001 vs WT. ***B.*** Length distributions of ventricular myocytes. ***a.*** Typical pictures of myocytes obtained with 10× objective lens. Images at higher magnifications were shown in Figure S4 in File S1. *Cells showing contracture, which were discernable from shrunken shape and shortened sarcomere length, were excluded from analysis. **b.** Histogram of longitudinal length of ventricular myocytes for WT (n = 310 from five heart), Cont (n = 290 from six heart) and CAND (n = 294 from five hearts).

of the lack of appropriate models. Thus far, only a few studies have revealed the effects of ARBs on DCM using animal models [23], and these studies have not assessed the effects of ARBs on electrical remodeling in inherited DCM. In the present study, we found that candesartan improved the survival rate and cardiac systolic function, and suppressed progression of cardiac dilation and fibrosis using a DCM mouse model with the ΔK210 mutation in *TNNT2*, which closely recapitulates the human phenotype [12–14,16]. In addition to the above effects, candesartan suppressed occurrence of ventricular arrhythmia as well as various changes in the electrical properties in DCM hearts. These effects are probably due to the direct inhibition of angiotensin receptor in heart, but not due to indirect action via decreased blood pressure, because vasodilator hydralazine did not show suppressive effects on cardiac enlargement or prolongation of QT/APD. This is consistent with a previous report that many of β-adrenoreceptor blocker, which reduce mean blood pressure, had no suppressive effects on cardiac enlargement or prolongation of QT [14]. Interestingly, the changes in electrical properties of DCM heart seem to be closely related to the emergence of enlarged cells, and candesartan dramatically prevented the emergence.

Progression of multiple types of electrical remodeling in ΔK210 DCM hearts

Our previous study [13] and this study demonstrated that multiple types of progressive channel remodeling occur at different time points in the hearts of DCM model mice. (1) Some genes are already modulated in DCM heart from neonate when they show no symptoms of HF and very low mortality. For example, the mRNA level of Kv4.2 is significantly reduced in DCM heart in the neonatal period [13]. (2) Then the DCM mice start to display high mortality at around 2 months of age in parallel with prolongation of the QT interval and APD_{50} as well as a reduction in I_{Kur}/Kv1.5 and I_{to}/Kv4.2 and KChIP2. However, most of DCM mice do not develop congestive HF at this age [13,16]. (3) Thereafter, at around 3 months, their hearts enlarge further as they enter the congestive HF stage [13,16]. Expression levels of Kv4.2, Kv1.5, and KChIP2 decrease further together with prolongation of the APD_{50}. In addition, this study revealed that, at 3 months, I_{K1} and I_{SS} decreased without significant changes in mRNA or protein levels, which is probably because of post-translational changes that occurred in later stage of HF [23–25].

A prominent change in DCM heart was the emergence of enlarged cells with very low densities of K^+ currents, which is probably related to cardiac dilation. The longitudinal length distribution of isolated myocytes at 3 months of age indicates that about 27% of myocytes were out-of-range compared with the WT cell distribution. If only longitudinal length increases in DCM heart, the enlarged cells would occupy 40% of total volume because cell volume is proportional to the length in this case. However, volume occupancy of the enlarged cells should be greater than 40% because heart weights of DCM mice were 2∼3 times greater than that of WT mice. Cell width and thickness of DCM cells may also be increased. Actually, enlarged cells with increased length and width were often observed at endocardium side in DCM myocardium (data not shown), although quantitative analysis was difficult at present. Another explanation is that enlarged cells might be lost during preparation of single cells because of their labile property. In addition, non-cardiac cells such as fibroblast might contribute to heart weight. In any event, the enlarged cells with low K^+ currents may greatly contribute to prolonged APD, unstable repolarization and arrhythmia. Although there are differences in K^+ current components between human and mice, similar changes in structural and electrical properties are likely to occur in human inherited DCM hearts.

Effect of candesartan on various types of electrical remodeling

This study showed that many but not all types of electrical remodeling in DCM mice were ameliorated by candesartan treatment. *In vivo* and *in situ* measurements indicated that candesartan substantially suppressed prolongations of the QT interval and APD_{50}. Interestingly, prolongation of these parameters occurred long before onset of congestive HF [13,16] and the suppressive effect of candesartan was already obvious at early age (Fig. 2). Thus, candesartan inhibits effects of Ang II that elevates in DCM mice when their hearts are still compensated.

The most likely explanation for the shortened APD_{50} by candesartan treatment is restoration of the repolarizing K^+ currents (I_{to}, I_{Kur}, I_{K1}, and I_{ss}) [19]. In particular, I_{to} and I_{Kur} underlie the early phase of myocardial AP repolarization, contributing to the APD_{50} and coordinated propagation of activity in the heart. In the hearts of candesartan-treated mice, enlarged cells were virtually absent. Instead, I_{to} and I_{Kur} were moderately lowered (∼50% of WT) in normal sized cells in candesartan-treated DCM heart. As a results, *in vivo* average of I_{to} and I_{Kur} in the candesartan-treated DCM heart can be higher than that in the control DCM heart which have enlarged cells with very low I_{to} and I_{Kur} (∼10∼20% of WT). In summary, suppression of the emergence of the enlarged cells with low K^+ current density is one plausible explanation for the shortened QT interval and APD_{50} in the candesartan-treated DCM heart.

It is interesting that candesartan could not reverse the moderate decrements in I_{to} and I_{Kur} in normal sized DCM cells (∼50% of WT). DCM mice may be safe with such moderate decrease alone. Furthermore, this indicates that other molecules than Ang II also contribute to the down regulation of these channels. A wide range of signaling molecules including, Ang II, catecholamine and glucocorticoids, has been implicated in regulating long-term changes in expression of K^+ channels [26–29]. Further studies are needed to understand the regulatory mechanisms of ion channel expression during progression of DCM disease.

In contrast to partial recovery of I_{to} and I_{Kur}, candesartan completely restored the decrements in I_{K1} and I_{SS}, which was not associated with changes in protein or mRNA levels. Because there were no differences in I_{K1} and I_{SS} between WT and DCM at 2 months [13], candesartan probably suppresses the post-translational reduction that occurs in the later stage of DCM. Thus, treatment of DCM mice with candesartan starting at 1 month completely prevented the reduction of I_{K1} and I_{ss}. These effects may also partially contribute to the suppression of the prolongation of QT intervals and APD_{50}.

In addition to the reduction of K^+ currents, another prominent change in DCM hearts was the pathologic proliferation of fibroblasts. The progression of fibrosis is associated with conduction disorder, arrhythmogenesis and the prolonged APD_{50} in the control DCM heart because fibroblast could electrically couple to cardiomyocytes [30]. Collectively, abrogation of such fibrosis by candesartan treatment also contributes to prevention of conduction disorder, APD prolongation and arrhythmogenicity in DCM mice.

Candesartan-insensitive remodeling

We noticed both candesartan-sensitive and -insensitive remodeling in this model mouse. The candesartan-sensitive remodeling may be attributed to the renin-angiotensin system (RAS) because there was an elevation of the plasma Ang II concentration. A transgenic mouse model over-expressing the Ang II receptor, which shows a reduction of I_{to}, I_{Kur}, I_{K1} and I_{ss} [31], also supports this idea. On the other hand, the candesartan-insensitive electrical remodeling was probably because of mechanisms other than the RAS [24,26]. For example, changes such as basal cardiac enlargement (Fig. 1) and prolongation of QRS and QT intervals (Fig. 2) occurring in the early stage [13], i.e., moderate decrements in Kv4.2 and Kv1.5 in early stage (Figs. 4–6), and an increment in Cav3.1 (data not shown), appear to be unaffected by candesartan. However, an alternative possibility is that the remodeling once developed in the early stage cannot be reversed by ARB treatment. Further studies are required to understand the detailed remodeling processes in the inherited DCM heart.

Conclusion

In this study, we found that inhibition of changes in the later stage of DCM, i.e., cardiac enlargement, fibrosis and various changes in channel expression, contributes to the beneficial effect of ARBs. Our results suggest that the effect of candesartan on electrical remodeling is closely related to the suppressive effect on structural remodeling and that the early initiation of candesartan treatment is highly effective for prevention of disease in inherited DCM. Because candesartan treatment does not suppress voluntary exercise activity and hence preserves the quality of life, ARBs are an excellent candidate drug for treating inherited DCM patients.

Supporting Information

File S1 Figure S1. Effects of hydralazine on ECG data. ***A.*** Typical traces of ECG from WT and Hydralazine treated DCM mice. ***B.*** Comparison of QRS (upper panel) and QTc (lower panel) intervals. Data with WT, untreated control and candesartan-treated DCM mice are same as those in Fig. 2B. n = 7 for hydralazine. $^*P<0.05$ vs WT, $^\dagger P<0.05$ vs control DCM. **Figure S2. Effects of candesartan treatment on expression levels of mRNA encoding K^+ channels and accessory subunit in WT left ventricle.** Quantitative real-time PCR analysis was carried out with LVs from control WT (n = 10) and candesartan-treated WT (n = 8) mice. The GAPDH gene was used as an internal control. **Figure S3. Current kinetics of I_{to} (*A* and *C*) and I_{Kur}(*B* and *D*).** Time to peak (*A* and *B*) and decay time (100 to 50% of peak) (*C* and *D*) are plotted against membrane capacitance. Cm was poorly correlated with current kinetics of I_{to} or I_{Kur}. **Figure S4. Typical images of myocytes obtained with 60× objective lens.** ***A.*** WT, ***B.*** Candesartan treated DCM. ***C.*** Control DCM.

Acknowledgments

The authors are thankful for technical assistance by the staff at the Division of Genome Research, Atopy Research Center, and Laboratory of Molecular and Biochemical Research, Research Support Center, Juntendo University Graduate School of Medicine.

Author Contributions

Conceived and designed the experiments: FO HI MS T. Suzuki TM NK. Performed the experiments: FO HI MS T. Suzuki TM NK. Analyzed the data: FO HI MS T. Suzuki TM T. Shioya MK NK. Contributed reagents/materials/analysis tools: YN HD T. Sakurai SM. Wrote the paper: FO HI TM MK NK.

References

1. Dec GW, Fuster V (1994) Idiopathic dilated cardiomyopathy. N Engl J Med 331: 1564–1575.
2. Kasper EK, Agema WR, Hutchins GM, Deckers JW, Hare JM, et al. (1994) The causes of dilated cardiomyopathy: a clinicopathologic review of 673 consecutive patients. J Am Coll Cardiol 23: 586–590.
3. Arozal W, Watanabe K, Veeraveedu PT, Thandavarayan RA, Harima M, et al. (2010) Beneficial effects of angiotensin II receptor blocker, olmesartan, in limiting the cardiotoxic effect of daunorubicin in rats. Free Radic Res 44: 1369–1377.
4. Yu H, McKinnon D, Dixon JE, Gao J, Wymore R, et al. (1999) Transient outward current, Ito1, is altered in cardiac memory. Circulation 99: 1898–1905.
5. Thuringer D, Deroubaix E, Coulombe A, Coraboeuf E, Mercadier JJ (1996) Ionic basis of the action potential prolongation in ventricular myocytes from Syrian hamsters with dilated cardiomyopathy. Cardiovasc Res 31: 747–757.
6. Pourdjabbar A, Parker TG, Nguyen QT, Desjardins JF, Lapointe N, et al. (2005) Effects of pre-, peri-, and postmyocardial infarction treatment with losartan in rats: effect of dose on survival, ventricular arrhythmias, function, and remodeling. Am J Physiol Heart Circ Physiol 288: H1997–2005.
7. Cohn JN, Tognoni G (2001) A randomized trial of the angiotensin-receptor blocker valsartan in chronic heart failure. N Engl J Med 345: 1667–1675.
8. Pfeffer MA, Swedberg K, Granger CB, Held P, McMurray JJ, et al. (2003) Effects of candesartan on mortality and morbidity in patients with chronic heart failure: the CHARM-Overall programme. Lancet 362: 759–766.
9. Nieminen T, Verrier RL (2010) Usefulness of T-wave alternans in sudden death risk stratification and guiding medical therapy. Ann Noninvasive Electrocardiol 15: 276–288.
10. Otten E, Lekanne Dit Deprez RH, Weiss MM, van Slegtenhorst M, Joosten M, et al. (2010) Recurrent and founder mutations in the Netherlands: mutation p.K217del in troponin T2, causing dilated cardiomyopathy. Neth Heart J 18: 478–485.
11. Morimoto S (2009) Expanded spectrum of gene causing both hypertrophic cardiomyopathy and dilated cardiomyopathy. Circ Res 105: 313–315.
12. Du CK, Morimoto S, Nishii K, Minakami R, Ohta M, et al. (2007) Knock-in mouse model of dilated cardiomyopathy caused by troponin mutation. Circ Res 101: 185–194.
13. Suzuki T, Shioya T, Murayama T, Sugihara M, Odagiri F, et al. (2012) Multistep ion channel remodeling and lethal arrhythmia precede heart failure in a mouse model of inherited dilated cardiomyopathy. PLoS One 7: e35353.

14. Wang YY, Morimoto S, Du CK, Lu QW, Zhan DY, et al. (2010) Up-regulation of type 2 iodothyronine deiodinase in dilated cardiomyopathy. Cardiovasc Res 87: 636–646.
15. Mitchell GF, Jeron A, Koren G (1998) Measurement of heart rate and Q-T interval in the conscious mouse. Am J Physiol 274: H747–751.
16. Sugihara M, Odagiri F, Suzuki T, Murayama T, Nakazato Y, et al. (2013) Usefulness of running wheel for detection of congestive heart failure in dilated cardiomyopathy mouse model. PLoS One 8: e55514.
17. Nishizawa H, Suzuki T, Shioya T, Nakazato Y, Daida H, et al. (2009) Causes of abnormal Ca2+ transients in Guinea pig pathophysiological ventricular muscle revealed by Ca2+ and action potential imaging at cellular level. PLoS One 4: e7069.
18. Shioya T (2007) A simple technique for isolating healthy heart cells from mouse models. J Physiol Sci 57: 327–335.
19. Brouillette J, Clark RB, Giles WR, Fiset C (2004) Functional properties of K+ currents in adult mouse ventricular myocytes. J Physiol 559: 777–798.
20. Goldberg MR, Bradstreet TE, McWilliams EJ, Tanaka WK, Lipert S, et al. (1995) Biochemical effects of losartan, a nonpeptide angiotensin II receptor antagonist, on the renin-angiotensin-aldosterone system in hypertensive patients. Hypertension 25: 37–46.
21. Inada Y, Wada T, Ojima M, Sanada T, Shibouta Y, et al. (1997) Protective effects of candesartan cilexetil (TCV-116) against stroke, kidney dysfunction and cardiac hypertrophy in stroke-prone spontaneously hypertensive rats. Clin Exp Hypertens 19: 1079–1099.
22. Hongo K, Morimoto S, O-Uchi J, Kusakari Y, Komukai K, et al. RENNIN-ANGIOTENSIN SYSTEM PLAYS AN IMPORTANT ROLE IN THE PATHOGENESIS OF DCM IN MOUSE; 2009; Kyoto, Japan. Springer. pp. 24.
23. Qin M, Huang H, Wang T, Hu H, Liu Y, et al. (2012) Absence of Rgs5 prolongs cardiac repolarization and predisposes to ventricular tachyarrhythmia in mice. J Mol Cell Cardiol 53: 880–890.
24. Nattel S, Maguy A, Le Bouter S, Yeh YH (2007) Arrhythmogenic ion-channel remodeling in the heart: heart failure, myocardial infarction, and atrial fibrillation. Physiol Rev 87: 425–456.
25. Janse MJ (2004) Electrophysiological changes in heart failure and their relationship to arrhythmogenesis. Cardiovasc Res 61: 208–217.
26. Rosati B, McKinnon D (2004) Regulation of ion channel expression. Circ Res 94: 874–883.
27. Shimoni Y, Liu XF (2003) Role of PKC in autocrine regulation of rat ventricular K+ currents by angiotensin and endothelin. Am J Physiol Heart Circ Physiol 284: H1168–1181.
28. Bru-Mercier G, Deroubaix E, Capuano V, Ruchon Y, Rucker-Martin C, et al. (2003) Expression of heart K+ channels in adrenalectomized and catecholamine-depleted reserpine-treated rats. J Mol Cell Cardiol 35: 153–163.
29. Takimoto K, Levitan ES (1994) Glucocorticoid induction of Kv1.5 K+ channel gene expression in ventricle of rat heart. Circ Res 75: 1006–1013.
30. Yue L, Xie J, Nattel S (2011) Molecular determinants of cardiac fibroblast electrical function and therapeutic implications for atrial fibrillation. Cardiovasc Res 89: 744–753.
31. Rivard K, Paradis P, Nemer M, Fiset C (2008) Cardiac-specific overexpression of the human type 1 angiotensin II receptor causes delayed repolarization. Cardiovasc Res 78: 53–62.

2

Cardiac-Specific Inhibition of Kinase Activity in Calcium/Calmodulin-Dependent Protein Kinase Kinase-β Leads to Accelerated Left Ventricular Remodeling and Heart Failure after Transverse Aortic Constriction in Mice

Shin Watanabe[1], Takahiro Horie[1], Kazuya Nagao[1], Yasuhide Kuwabara[1], Osamu Baba[1], Hitoo Nishi[1], Naoya Sowa[1], Michiko Narazaki[2], Tetsuya Matsuda[2], Genzou Takemura[3], Hiromichi Wada[4], Koji Hasegawa[4], Takeshi Kimura[1], Koh Ono[1]*

1 Department of Cardiovascular Medicine, Graduate School of Medicine, Kyoto University, Kyoto, Japan, **2** Department of Systems Science, Graduate School of Informatics, Kyoto University, Kyoto, Japan, **3** Department of Internal Medicine, Asahi University, Gifu, Japan, **4** Division of Translational Research, Kyoto Medical Center, National Hospital Organization, Kyoto, Japan

Abstract

Background: The mechanism of cardiac energy production against sustained pressure overload remains to be elucidated.

Methods and Results: We generated cardiac-specific kinase-dead (kd) calcium/calmodulin-dependent protein kinase kinase-β (CaMKKβ) transgenic (α-MHC CaMKKβ^{kd} TG) mice using α-myosin heavy chain (α-MHC) promoter. Although CaMKKβ activity was significantly reduced, these mice had normal cardiac function and morphology at baseline. Here, we show that transverse aortic binding (TAC) in α-MHC CaMKKβ^{kd} TG mice led to accelerated death and left ventricular (LV) dilatation and dysfunction, which was accompanied by significant clinical signs of heart failure. CaMKKβ downstream signaling molecules, including adenosine monophosphate-activated protein kinase (AMPK), were also suppressed in α-MHC CaMKKβ^{kd} TG mice compared with wild-type (WT) mice. The expression levels of peroxisome proliferator-activated receptor-γ coactivator (PGC)-1α, which is a downstream target of both of CaMKKβ and calcium/calmodulin kinases, were also significantly reduced in α-MHC CaMKKβ^{kd} TG mice compared with WT mice after TAC. In accordance with these findings, mitochondrial morphogenesis was damaged and creatine phosphate/β-ATP ratios assessed by magnetic resonance spectroscopy were suppressed in α-MHC CaMKKβ^{kd} TG mice compared with WT mice after TAC.

Conclusions: These data indicate that CaMKKβ exerts protective effects on cardiac adaptive energy pooling against pressure-overload possibly through phosphorylation of AMPK and by upregulation of PGC-1α. Thus, CaMKKβ may be a therapeutic target for the treatment of heart failure.

Editor: Vincenzo Lionetti, Scuola Superiore Sant'Anna, Italy

Funding: This work was supported in part by the Global COE program "Center for Frontier Medicine" and by a Grant-in-Aid for Scientific Research from the Ministry of Education, Culture, Sports, Science and Technology (MEXT) of Japan to K. Ono, K. Hasegawa, T. Kita, and T. Kimura, and in part by the Innovative Techno-Hub for Integrated Medical Bio-imaging of the Project for Developing Innovation Systems, from the Ministry of Education, Culture, Sports, Science and Technology (MEXT) of Japan to M. Narazaki and T. Matsuda. The funders had no role in study design, data collection and analysis, decision to publish, or preparation of the manuscript.

Competing Interests: The authors have declared that no competing interests exist.

* Email: kohono@kuhp.kyoto-u.ac.jp

Introduction

Previous studies determined that a calcium (Ca^{2+})-mediated signaling cascade resulting from mechanical overload or Gq-mediated signaling initiates changes that lead to cardiac hypertrophy through the activation of calcineurin and consequent targeting of nuclear factor of activated T-cells (NFAT) transcription factors. Ca^{2+}/calmodulin kinase (CaMK) II activation and subsequent NFAT3 signaling act in concert to promote pathologic hypertrophic signaling and cardiac growth. However, there is a lack of knowledge whether there is a signaling mechanism to compensate for cardiac energy production against sustained pressure load.

Numerous hormones, growth factors, and physiological processes cause a rise in cytosolic Ca^{2+} concentration, which is translated into cellular responses by interacting with a large number of Ca^{2+}-binding proteins [1]. The Ca^{2+}-binding protein that is most pervasive in mediating these responses is calmodulin (CaM), which acts as a primary receptor for Ca^{2+} in all eukaryotic cells [2]. Upon Ca^{2+} binding, CaM increases its affinity for a large number of CaM-binding proteins, including three multifunctional CaM kinases (CaMKs; CaMKI, CaMKII, and CaMKIV). CaMK kinases (CaMKKs) initiate the signaling cascade by phosphorylation and activation of two CaMKs, CaMKI and CaMKIV, whereas CaMKII can be activated by Ca^{2+}/CaM without the activation of CaMKK [3]. Two CaMKK genes (CaMKKα and CaMKKβ) have been identified in mammals, both of which are strongly expressed in the brain [4,5]. For full activation, CaMKI and CaMKIV require phosphorylation on an activation loop Thr by CaMKKα or CaMKKβ. In addition to its role in these enzymatic cascades, CaMKKβ is also a physiologically relevant upstream activator of adenosine monophosphate (AMP)-activated protein kinase (AMPK); this CaMKKβ-AMPK complex is known to regulate the energy balance by acting in the hypothalamus [6]. We demonstrated previously that CaMKKβ is important for GLUT4 translocation through AMPK activation in cardiomyocytes [7]. Moreover, CaMKKβ was shown to be important for mitochondrial biogenesis and exercise tolerance through its downstream target of peroxisome proliferator-activated receptor-γ coactivator (PGC)-1α by the use of muscle-specific adiponectin-deficient mice [8]. Therefore, it is possible that CaMKKβ in the heart exerts its role to compensate cardiac energy production against Ca^{2+} overload induced by sustained pressure load.

In this study, we focused on CaMKKβ in the control of cardiac function after transverse aortic constriction (TAC). We generated cardiac-specific kinase-dead (kd) CaMKKβ ($CaMKK\beta^{kd}$) transgenic (TG) mice, using an α-myosin heavy chain (α-MHC) promoter to define the structural and functional responses of the left ventricle to pressure-overload stress in the absence of an intact CaMKKβ cascade.

Materials and Methods

1. Mice

Male C57BL/6 mice were purchased from Japan SLC inc. (Shizuoka, Japan) and maintained in a specific pathogen-free facility. The α-MHC promoter drives transgene expression exclusively in cardiac myocytes and has been used extensively in transgenic studies. A kd form of CaMKKβ harboring a mutation of aspartic acid residue 329 to alanine had no effect on its downstream kinases [9] was utilized in our previous experiments [7]. To generate α-MHC $CaMKK\beta^{kd}$ TG mice, we placed an α-MHC promoter and FLAG tag at the 5′ end of a kd form of CaMKKβ. Transgenic DNA was microinjected into zygotes using a standard methodology, as described previously [10]. Transgenic mice and non-transgenic littermates as controls were maintained on a 12-h light/dark cycle, fed a normal laboratory diet *ad libitum*, sacrificed by decapitation under ether anesthesia at the indicated age and analyzed. This investigation conformed to the Guide for the Care and Use of Laboratory Animals published by the US National Institutes of Health (NIH Publication No. 85-23, revised 1996). All animal care, experiments, and methods were approved by the Animal Care and Use Committees of Kyoto University Graduate School of Medicine. We determined humane endpoints beforehand for the survival study. The criteria used to determine when the animals should be humanely sacrificed is rapid or progressive weight loss of more than 20% of the body weight, dehydration determined by an increase in skin tenting, sunken eyes, respiratory symptoms such as labored breathing, nasal discharge, coughing, or cyanosis. The animals were carefully monitored three times a day.

2. Surgery

Constriction of the transverse thoracic aorta was performed on 3-month-old mice as described previously [11]. In brief, mice were anesthetized, intubated, and placed on a respirator. Midline sternotomy was performed, the aorta was visualized, and a 6.0 prolene suture was placed around the aorta distal to the brachiocephalic artery. The suture was tightened around a blunt 26-gauge needle placed adjacent to the aorta. The needle was then removed, and the chest and overlying skin were closed. Sham-operated mice underwent a similar operation in which the aortic arch was isolated and a band was tightened around the aorta but not ligated and was removed subsequently.

3. Transthoracic echocardiography

Echocardiography was performed as described previously [12]. Briefly, mice were anesthetized using an intraperitoneal injection of 2-2-2 tribromoethanol (240 mg/kg, Wako Pure Chemical Industries, Osaka, Japan), and transthoracic echocardiography was performed using a Sonos-5500 echocardiograph (Agilent Technologies, Santa Clara, CA) with a 15-MHz linear transducer. M-mode echocardiograms were obtained at the papillary muscle level. At least two independent M-mode measurements per animal were carried out by an examiner blinded to the genotype of the animals. Fractional shortening was calculated as (LVIDd–LVIDs)/LVIDd*100.

4. Histological analysis

After anesthesia, we injected 0.1 mL of 1% $CdCl_2$ via inferior vena cava to achieve diastolic arrest. Then we perfused and fixed mice with 4% paraformaldehyde at 30 cm H_2O before excising the heart, which was further fixed in 4% paraformaldehyde at 4°C overnight. Paraffin sections were stained with Masson trichrome and Sirius red staining. All photos were taken using a BZ-9000 microscope (Keyence, Osaka, Japan).

5. Transmission electron microscopy

Left ventricular (LV) cardiac tissue was quickly cut into 1 mm cubes, immersion-fixed with 2.5% glutaraldehyde in 0.1 mol/L phosphate buffer (pH 7.4) overnight at 4°C, and postfixed in 1% buffered osmium tetroxide. The specimens were then dehydrated through a graded ethanol series and embedded in epoxy resin. Ultrathin sections (90 nm), double-stained with uranyl acetate and lead citrate, were examined using an electron microscope (H-800, Hitachi, Tokyo, Japan).

6. Mitochondrial DNA analysis

The amount of mitochondrial DNA was quantified using quantitative PCR as described previously [13]. Total DNA was isolated using a QIAmp DNA microkit (Qiagen, Venlo, Netherlands). The levels of cytochrome b (*Cytb*), NADH dehydrogenase subunit 1 (*Nd1*), and cytochrome c oxidase 1 (*Co1*) genes in the mtDNA genome were quantified. Results were normalized to the nuclear housekeeping gene H19. The delta-delta Ct method was used for quantification. Primer sequences are indicated in Table S1.

7. Measurement of superoxide

Superoxide levels were measured using a superoxide-sensitive dye, dihydroethidine (DHE). DHE is cell permeable and, in the presence of superoxide, is converted to fluorescent ethidium bromide (EtBR), which is trapped by intercalating with DNA. 5 μM DHE (Sigma-Aldrich, St. Louis, MO) was applied to heart cross-sections (7 μm) and incubated in a light-protected and

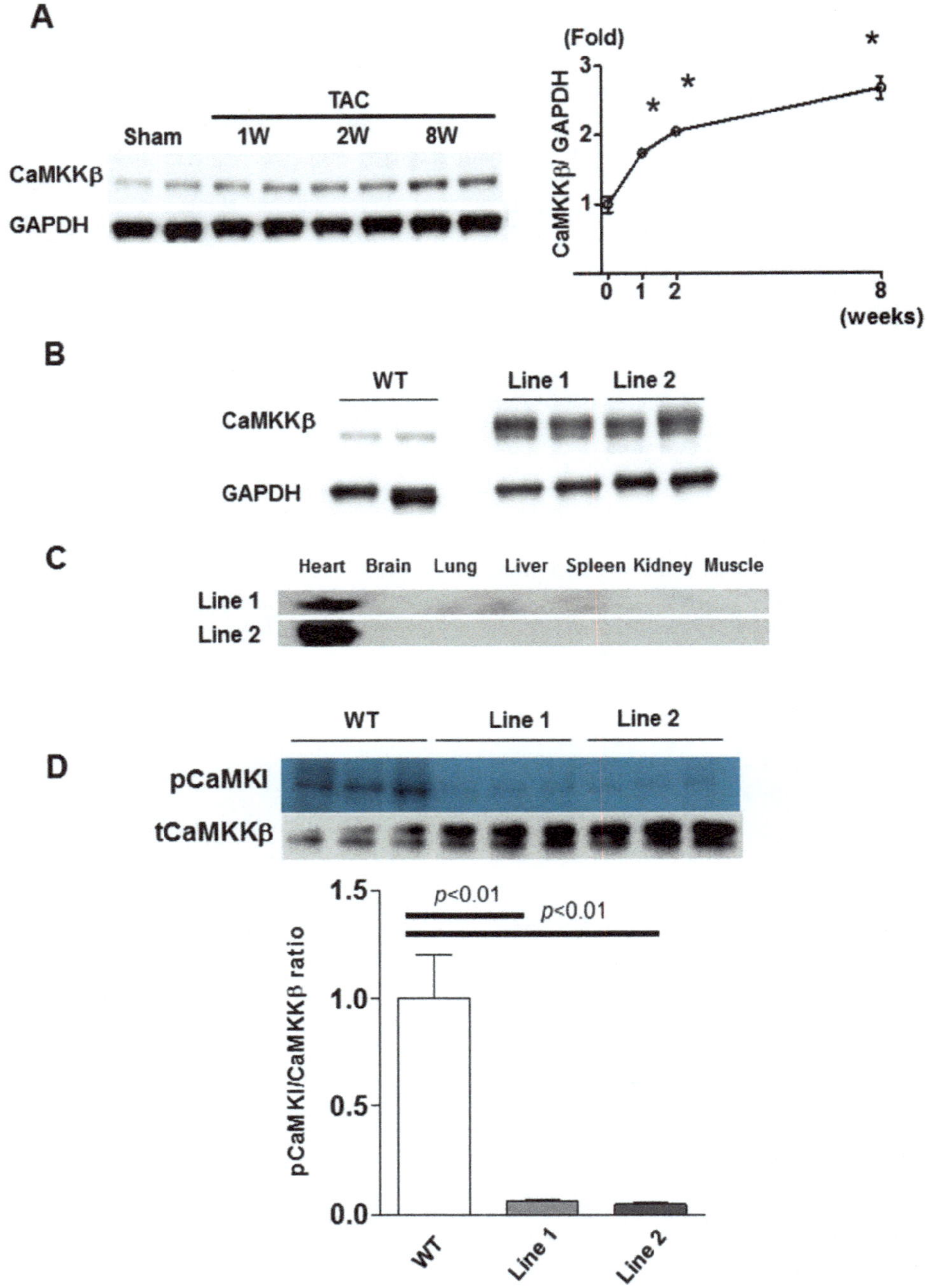

Figure 1. Generation of α-MHC CaMKKβ^{kd} TG mice. A. Immunoblotting and densitometry for calcium/calmodulin-dependent protein kinase kinase-β (CaMKKβ) after transverse aortic binding (TAC) in wild-type (WT) mice. Values are the means ± standard error (S.E.) of four independent experiments (*$p<0.05$ vs 0 week). B. Immunoblotting for CaMKKβ in WT mice and two lines of α-MHC CaMKKβ^{kd} TG mice. C. Immunoblotting for flag tag in two lines of α-MHC CaMKKβ^{kd} TG mice indicating the heart-specific overexpression of the transgene. D. Activities of CaMKKβ in the hearts of two lines of α-MHC CaMKKβ^{kd} TG mice by immunoprecipitate kinase assays.

humidified chamber at 37°C for 30 min. In situ fluorescence was assessed using fluorescence microscopy.

8. Western blotting

Total protein was extracted from frozen hearts, resolved and subjected to sodium dodecylsulfate polyacrylamide gel electrophoresis (SDS-PAGE) followed by standard Western blotting procedures [7]. A total of 20 μg protein was fractionated using NuPAGE 4–12% Bis-Tris (Invitrogen) gels and transferred to a Protran nitrocellulose transfer membrane (Whatman). The antibodies used for Western blotting were as follows: anti-CaMKKβ (H-95) (Santa Cruz Biotechnology, Dallas, TX, USA), 1:500; anti-total-CaMKI (sc-33165) (Santa Cruz Biotechnology), 1:1000; anti-phospho-CaMKIV (sc-28443-R) (Santa Cruz Biotechnology), 1:500; anti-total-CaMKIV (sc-55501) (Santa Cruz Biotechnology), 1:1000; anti-phospho-AMPKα (Cell Signaling Technology, Beverly, MA, USA), 1:500; anti-total-AMPKα (Cell Signaling Technology), 1:1000; and anti-GAPDH (Cell Signaling Technology), 1:2000. Anti-phospho-CaMKI (Thr177) was a kind gift from

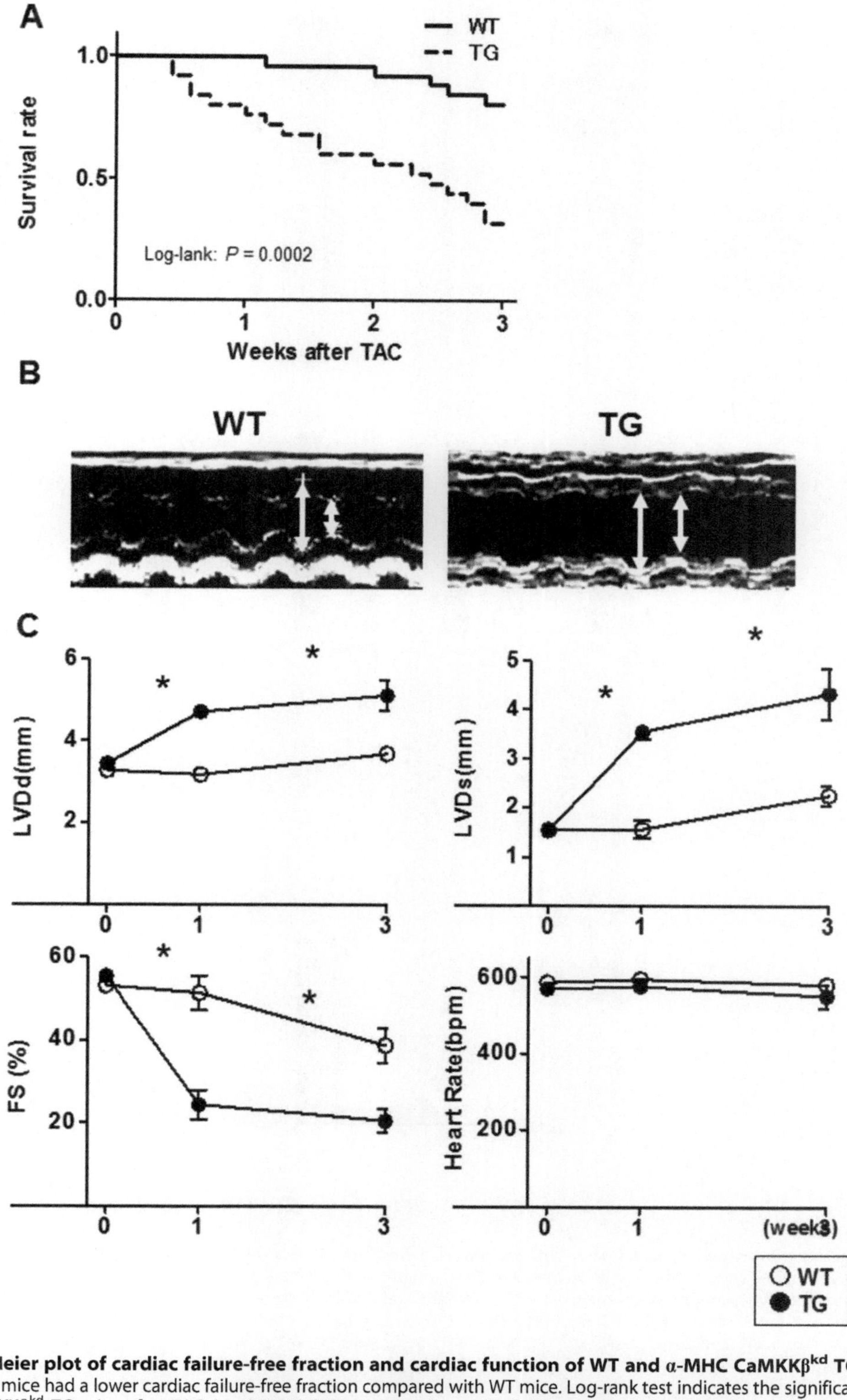

Figure 2. Kaplan-Meier plot of cardiac failure-free fraction and cardiac function of WT and α-MHC CaMKKβ^{kd} TG mice after TAC. A. α-MHC CaMKKβ^{kd} TG mice had a lower cardiac failure-free fraction compared with WT mice. Log-rank test indicates the significant difference between WT and α-MHC CaMKKβ^{kd} TG mice after TAC ($p = 0.0002$) (WT; n = 26, TG; n = 25). B. Representative echocardiograph pictures of WT and α-MHC CaMKKβ^{kd} TG hearts 3 weeks after TAC. Arrows indicate left ventricular cavities of diastolic and systolic phase. C. Serial changes in echocardiographic parameters of WT and α-MHC CaMKKβ^{kd} TG mice after TAC. *$p < 0.05$ vs WT (n = 3–5 for each group).

Dr. Naohito Nozaki (Kanagawa Dental College, Yokosuka, Kanagawa, Japan) and used at the dilution of 1:50. Anti-rabbit IgG (GE Healthcare) and anti-mouse IgG (GE Healthcare) were used as secondary antibodies at a dilution of 1:2000.

9. CaMKKβ activity

Heart tissues were rapidly frozen in liquid nitrogen. The frozen tissue was ground and resuspended in 100 μL homogenization buffer (50 mM Tris/HCl, 0.25 nM mannitol, 50 mM NaF, 5 mM

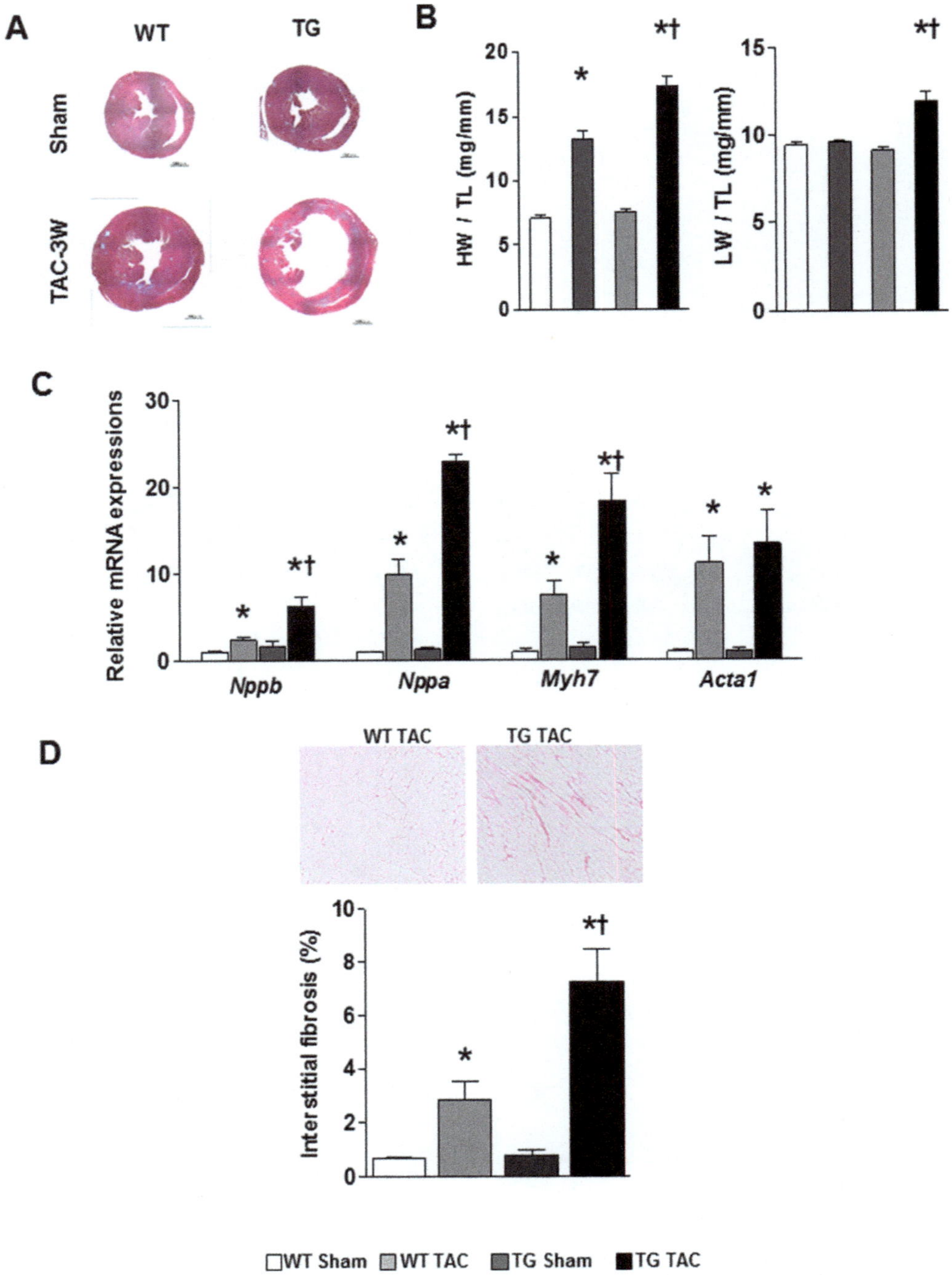

Figure 3. Left ventricular dilatation, hypertrophy, and fibrosis is prominent in α-MHC CaMKKβ^{kd} TG mice compared with WT mice after TAC. A. Low-power magnifications of Masson Trichrome stained images of the left ventricle of WT and α-MHC CaMKKβ^{kd} TG mice with or without TAC. B. Heart weight (HW) and lung weight (LW) of WT and α-MHC CaMKKβ^{kd} TG mice with or without TAC. Each value was normalized to tibial length (TL). Values are the means ± S.E. of 5 mice (*$p<0.05$ vs sham control, †$p<0.05$ vs WT after TAC). C. Relative expression levels of hypertrophy-associated genes in WT and α-MHC CaMKKβ^{kd} TG mice with or without TAC. Values are the means ± S.E. of four mice (*$p<0.05$ vs sham control, †$p<0.05$ vs WT after TAC). D. Picrosirius staining of the left ventricle in WT and α-MHC CaMKKβ^{kd} TG mice with or without TAC and measurement the area of fibrosis. Values are the means ± S.E. of three to five mice (*$p<0.05$ vs sham control, †$p<0.05$ vs WT after TAC).

sodium pyrophosphate, 150 mM NaCl, 5 μg/mL soybean trypsin inhibitor, 0.1 mM PMSF, 1% (v/v) Triton X-100) per 20 mg of tissue and further homogenized using a hand-held motor driven pestle. The samples were left on ice for 30 min, and then cell debris was pelleted by centrifugation. The supernatants were removed and protein concentrations were determined. CaMKKβ was immunoprecipitated from 500 μg of protein for 2 h at 4°C with 10 μl of anti CaMKKβ antibody (H-95, Santa Cruz Biotechnology). The immunoprecipitates were washed and then resuspended in kinase buffer containing 25 μM ATP and 5 μCi of [γ-^{32}P]ATP in the presence of 1 mM calcium and plus 1 μM calmodulin and 0.5 μg of purified recombinant human CAMKI (P01, Abnova Corporation, Taipei, Taiwan) was added and incubated on an orbital shaker at 37°C for 45 min. The reactions

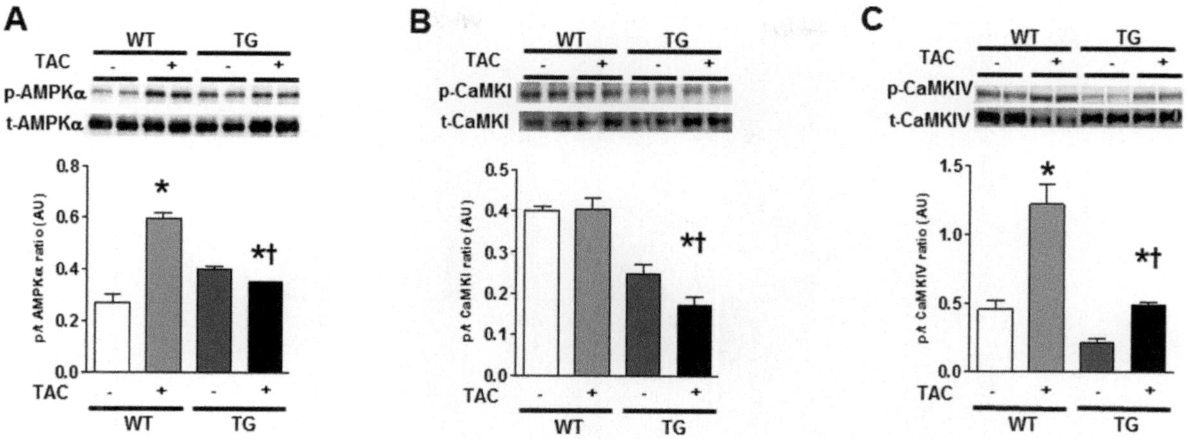

Figure 4. Phosphorylation of downstream targets of CaMKKβ in WT and α-MHC CaMKKβ^{kd} TG mice with or without TAC. Representative pictures of immunoblotting for phosphorylated form and total amount of adenosine monophosphate (AMP)-activated protein kinase (AMPK), calcium/calmodulin-dependent protein kinase (CaMK) I, and CaMKIV (A–C). Results of densitometric analysis are indicated. Values are the means ± S.E. of five mice (*$p<0.05$ vs sham control, †$p<0.05$ vs WT after TAC).

were stopped by addition of sample loading dye. The reaction mixtures were separated by SDS-PAGE and exposed to X-ray film after drying the gel. Total immunoprecipitated CaMKKβ protein were analyzed individually by Western blotting.

10. Quantitative real-time (q-RT) PCR for mRNA

Total RNA was isolated using TRIzol reagent (Invitrogen, Carlsbad, CA). cDNA was synthesized using SuperScript II reverse transcriptase (Invitrogen) and the PCR reaction was performed using SYBR Green PCR master mix (Applied Biosystems, Foster, CA), normalized with GAPDH. Gene-specific primer sequences are indicated in Table S1.

11. Magnetic resonance imaging protocol

Magnetic resonance (MR) imaging experiments were performed as described previously [14]. Briefly, experiments were carried out using a Bruker Biospec MRI/MRS spectrometer (Ettlingen, Germany) equipped with a 7-T/20-cm Oxford magnet and a 12-cm (inner diameter) actively shielded gradient set, as described previously. In vivo MRI/MRS studies were carried out on wild-type (WT) and TG mice before and after TAC. Anesthesia was induced with ~1% isoflurane, as described previously. The probe set was a 20-mm $^{1}H/^{31}P$ MRS coil. Metabolite areas were determined from the integrated peak areas of the creatine phosphate (PCr) and [β-P]ATP resonances from voxels centered on cardiac muscle as identified by high-resolution MR imaging.

12. Statistics

Data are presented as means ± standard error (SE). Statistical comparisons were performed using unpaired two-tailed Student's *t*-tests or one-way analysis of variance with Bonferonni's post hoc test where appropriate. We sat the level for statistical significance at a $p<0.05$.

Results

1. CaMKKβ expression is upregulated by TAC

It is known that mechanical overload evokes a Ca^{2+}-mediated signaling cascade in the heart. Moreover, CaMKK is activated by the elevation of intracellular Ca^{2+} and it may transduce important signals during cardiac hypertrophy. Thus, we first examined the expression of CaMKKβ in the course of cardiac hypertrophy induced by TAC. We found that the mRNA and protein levels of CaMKKβ were significantly increased 1 week after TAC and continued to increase gradually thereafter (Fig. 1A).

2. Generation of α-MHC CaMKKβ^{kd} TG mice

To study the impact of CaMKKβ expression on pressure-loaded heart failure, we generated α-MHC CaMKKβ^{kd} TG mice. A catalytically inactive mutant of CaMKKβ was made by mutating aspartic acid 329 to alanine (D329A) [7,9,15]. The cardiomyocyte-specific α-MHC promoter has a transient burst of activity in embryonic hearts between embryonic day 9.5 and 10.5, and its activity is reactivated during early postnatal life and remains persistently high into adulthood [16]. We obtained three independent transgenic lines. The results from two lines are shown in Fig. 1. Western blotting using anti-FLAG and anti-CaMKKβ antibodies confirmed cardiac overexpression and the levels of CaMKKβ^{kd} transgenes in α-MHC CaMKKβ^{kd} TG mice (Fig. 1B and C). We also determined the activities of CaMKKβ in the hearts of these mice using immunoprecipitate kinase assays (Fig. 1D). CaMKKβ activity was significantly suppressed in the two lines of α-MHC CaMKKβ^{kd} TG mice. These transgenic mice appeared to have normal cardiac development and life span (survival of over 12 months). There was no change in body weight, systolic blood pressure, or heart rate in intermediate and high expression lines of α-MHC CAMKKβ^{kd} TG mice.

3. α-MHC CaMKKβ^{kd} TG mice had higher mortality compared with WT mice

Three-month-old α-MHC CaMKKβ^{kd} TG lines and WT control mice underwent TAC and were followed over the next 8 weeks. According to the humane endpoint rules, mice subjected to TAC had to be sacrificed when the criteria of endpoints were reached. Using such criteria, Kaplan-Meier analysis demonstrated that α-MHC CaMKKβ^{kd} TG mice were significantly more likely to develop this degree after TAC than WT control mice (Fig. 2A). To determine the functional aspects of α-MHC CaMKKβ^{kd} TG hearts, we used an echocardiograph to analyze cardiac structure and function after TAC. Fig. 2B shows representative results of echocardiography of the heart of WT mice and the high expression line of α-MHC CaMKKβ^{kd} TG mice at 3 weeks after

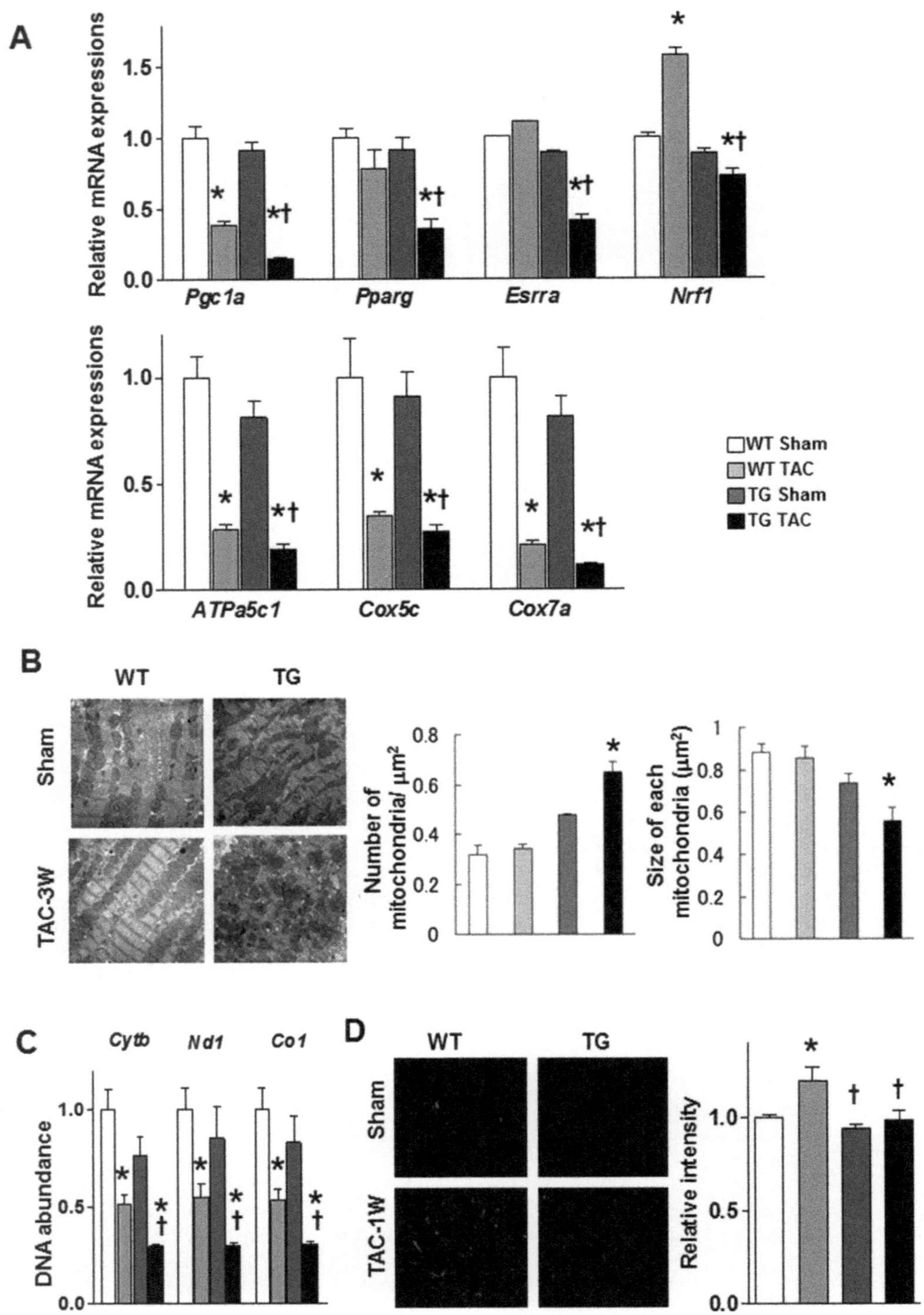

Figure 5. Mitochondrial ultrastructure, DNA abundance, and metabolism-related gene expression levels in WT and α-MHC CaMKKβ^{kd} TG mice with or without TAC. A. Relative mRNA expression levels related to mitochondrial function and biogenesis. Values are the means ± S.E. of six mice (*p<0.05 vs sham control, †p<0.05 vs WT after TAC). B. Abnormal mitochondrial ultrastructure in α-MHC CaMKKβ^{kd} TG hearts after TAC. C. The amount of mitochondrial DNA quantified by quantitative PCR. Cytochrome b (*Cytb*), NADH dehydrogenase subunit 1 (*Nd1*) and cytochrome c oxidase 1 (*Co1*) expression levels relative to nuclear DNA in the ventricles of WT and α-MHC CaMKKβ^{kd} TG mice with or without TAC are shown. Values are the means ± S.E. of three to four mice (*p<0.05 vs sham control, †p<0.05 vs WT after TAC). D. Superoxide levels detected using a superoxide-sensitive dye, dihydroethidine (DHE). Representative pictures are shown on the left. Relative intensities are shown on the right. Values are the means ± S.E. of three to six mice (*p<0.05 vs sham control, †p<0.05 vs WT after TAC).

TAC. The other line of TG mice showed the same results. Fig. 2C demonstrates that α-MHC CaMKKβ^{kd} TG mice had a significant increase in LV end diastolic diameter (LVDd) and LV systolic diameter (LVDs), accompanied by a reduction in contraction

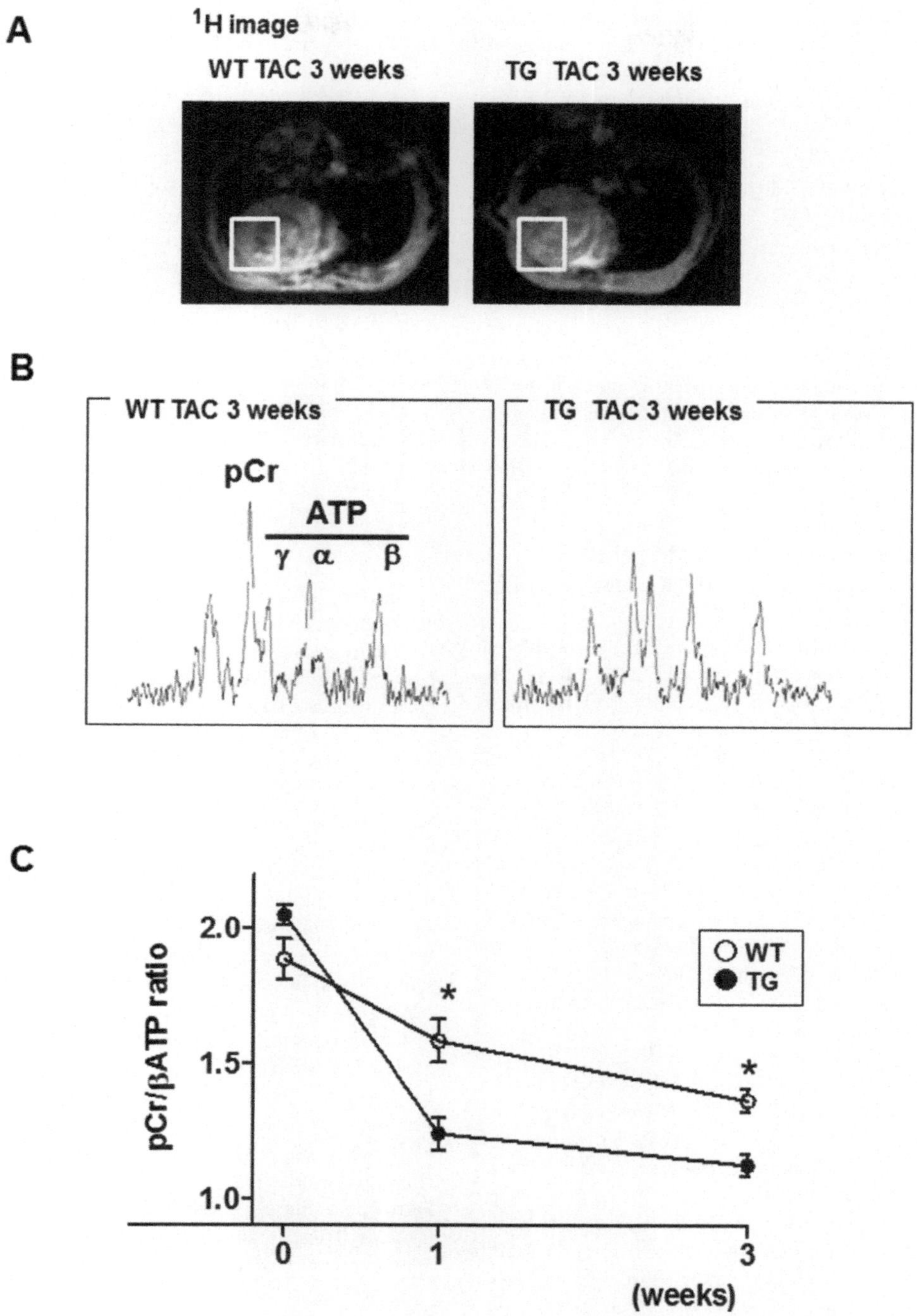

Figure 6. Myocardial energy reserve measured by in situ ^{31}P magnetic resonance (MR) spectroscopy. A. A ^{1}H MR image to define the region of interest to measure a ^{31}P MR spectrum of the left ventricular anterior wall. B. In vivo cardiac ^{31}P MR spectra from WT and α-MHC CaMKKβ^{kd} TG mice 3 weeks after TAC. C. The creatine phosphate/ATP ratio of the left ventricle in WT and α-MHC CaMKKβ^{kd} TG after TAC. Values are mean±standard error of the mean. *$p<0.05$ vs WT at same time point, n = 3–8 for each group.

measured as fractional shortening (FS). Further experiments were carried on the high expression line. Fig. 3A contains low-power magnifications of Masson trichrome staining of the heart, which confirmed that marked dilatation occurred in the hearts of α-MHC CaMKKβ^{kd} TG mice subjected to TAC compared with both WT TAC hearts and α-MHC CaMKKβ^{kd} TG hearts without TAC. Hearts from WT mice subjected to TAC were enlarged and their weight increased twofold compared with those from WT mice without TAC (Fig. 3B), which was consistent with cardiac hypertrophy. In contrast, hearts from α-MHC CaMKKβ^{kd} TG mice almost tripled in weight compared with those from α-MHC CaMKKβ^{kd} TG mice without TAC (Fig. 3B) and the lungs in α-MHC CaMKKβ^{kd} TG mice also increased in weight, probably resulting from extreme congestion, compared with those in WT TAC mice. mRNA expression levels of both atrial and B-type natriuretic factor (*Nppa* and *Nppb*), heavy chain of β myosin (*Myh7*), and α1 actin (*Acta1*), which are markers of cardiac hypertrophy and failure, were increased significantly in WT mice after TAC compared with mice without TAC and in α-MHC CaMKKβ^{kd} TG mice after TAC compared with WT mice after TAC (Fig. 3C). Picrosirius staining indicated that interstitial fibrosis increased significantly in WT mice after TAC compared with mice without TAC, and the levels increased significantly in α-MHC CaMKKβ^{kd} TG mice after TAC compared with WT mice after TAC (Fig. 3D).

4. Altered CaMKKβ-mediated signaling in α-MHC CaMKKβ^{kd} TG hearts after TAC

Next, we measured the phosphorylation levels of the AMPK, CaMKI, and CaMKIV, which are well-established CAMKKβ downstream targets, in the hearts of WT and α-MHC CaMKKβ^{kd} TG mice after sham surgery or TAC. Figs. 4A to C show the results of Western blotting and densitometry analysis of the blots. The phosphorylation levels increased significantly in WT hearts after TAC except for CaMKI; however, the phosphorylation levels of AMPK, CaMKI, and CaMKIV were significantly reduced in α-MHC CaMKKβ^{kd} TG hearts compared with the WT mice after TAC.

5. Abnormal morphology of mitochondria and mitochondrial gene expression in α-MHC CaMKKβ^{kd} TG hearts after TAC

The expression of PGC-1α has been reported to be modulated in several physiological contexts by increased Ca^{2+} signaling via molecules such as CaMK and CREB [17] and by CaMKKβ [8]. Therefore, we measured PGC-1α expression levels in the left ventricles of WT and α-MHC CaMKKβ^{kd} TG mice with or without TAC. As shown in Fig. 5A, *PGC1a* expression levels were the same in sham-operated WT and α-MHC CaMKKβ^{kd} TG mice; however, its expression was significantly reduced in α-MHC CaMKKβ^{kd} TG hearts compared with WT mice after TAC. *Pparg, Esrrsa, and Nrf1* gene expression levels were significantly reduced in α-MHC CaMKKβ^{kd} TG hearts compared with WT mice after TAC. We further measured *ATPa5c1, Cox5c, and Cox7a* gene expression levels. These levels also showed the same pattern as those of *PGC1a*. We then observed changes in mitochondrial morphology using electron microscopy. As shown in Fig. 5B, the mitochondria of α-MHC CaMKKβ^{kd} TG mice were the same as those of WT mice before TAC; however, the size of mitochondria in α-MHC CaMKKβ^{kd} TG mice became smaller than those of WT mice after 3 weeks' TAC. We then measured the amount of mitochondrial DNA by PCR analysis of *Cytb*, *Nd1*, and *Co1* genes. Fig. 5C indicates that the levels of these genes were significantly decreased after TAC in both WT and α-MHC CaMKKβ^{kd} TG mice compared with those mice before TAC, and the levels were further decreased after TAC in α-MHC CaMKKβ^{kd} TG mice compared with WT mice after TAC. Then, we measured superoxide levels using the superoxide-sensitive dye DHE. The density of DHE increased in WT hearts after TAC; however, such an increase was not observed in α-MHC CaMKKβ^{kd} TG hearts after TAC compared with that before TAC. All of these data show an abnormality in mitochondria-related gene expression patterns and their function in α-MHC CaMKKβ^{kd} TG hearts after TAC.

6. Impaired energetics and ATP depletion in α-MHC CaMKKβ^{kd} TG hearts after TAC

We further tried to measure the changes in energy levels in the hearts of WT and α-MHC CaMKKβ^{kd} TG mice in response to pressure load. ^{31}P MR spectrometry offers a unique means to noninvasively quantify the major cardiac high-energy phosphates PCr and ATP, which are critical for normal myocardial contractile function and viability. We used ^{31}P MR spectrometry to quantify the *in vivo* PCr-to-ATP ratio (PCr/ATP) of murine hearts. Fig. 6A shows a ^{1}H MR image to define the region of interest to measure the ^{31}P MR spectrum of the LV anterior wall. Representative cardiac ^{31}P MR spectra from mice are shown in Fig. 6B. As shown in Fig. 6C, the PCr/ATP ratio of α-MHC CaMKKβ^{kd} TG mice was the same as that of WT before TAC. The mean in vivo myocardial PCr/ATP ratios were 2.05 ± 0.04 and 1.88 ± 0.08, respectively, which were consistent with previous reports [18]. TAC significantly reduced mean PCr/ATP ratio to 1.58 ± 0.08 in WT mice; however, the level was significantly lower in α-MHC CaMKKβ^{kd} TG mice (1.24 ± 0.06) as early as 1 week after TAC compared with that of WT mice. The difference between WT and α-MHC CaMKKβ^{kd} TG mice remained unchanged until 3 weeks after TAC.

Discussion

We have reported previously that CaMKKβ can activate AMPK in cardiomyocytes and is involved in GLUT4 translocation, based on the finding that the CaMKK inhibitor STO-609, as well as overexpression of the dominant-negative form of CaMKKβ, inhibited its H_2O_2-mediated translocation [7]. It was also suggested that H_2O_2-mediated increase in the intracellular Ca^{2+} concentration is most likely to play a more important role than increase in AMP:ATP ratio in AMPK activation [19]. In this experiment, we tried to find out the mechanism of cardiac energy production against sustained pressure overload by the use of α-MHC CaMKKβ^{kd} TG mice, because the Ca^{2+}-mediated signaling cascade is important in this situation. The major findings of this study are as follows: (1) CaMKKβ expression was increased in the left ventricle in response to pressure-overload stress by TAC in WT mice; (2) TAC in α-MHC CaMKKβ^{kd} TG mice resulted in a significant inhibition of CaMKKβ downstream signaling molecules, including AMPK, compared with those in WT mice and led to accelerated cardiac dysfunction, which was accompanied by signs of significant clinical heart failure and death; and (3) the expression levels of PGC-1α, which is a downstream target of both of CaMKKβ and CaMKs, were also significantly reduced in α-MHC CaMKKβ^{kd} TG mice compared with WT mice after TAC. In accordance with these findings mitochondrial morphogenesis was damaged and PCr/β-ATP ratios assessed by MR spectroscopy were also suppressed in α-MHC CaMKKβ^{kd} TG mice compared with WT mice after TAC. To the best of our knowledge, these findings provide the first evidence that CaMKKβ exerts an effect on cardiac adaptive energy pooling against pressure-overload-induced ventricular dysfunction.

Heart failure is a multifactorial, progressive, and disabling syndrome leading to a deterioration of the heart characterized by a symptoms resulting from ventricular dysfunction. Contractile dysfunction is often linked to chronic energy deficit. The increased wall stress of the ventricle enhances local oxygen consumption and worsens the energy deficiency and function. As a consequence, the heart enters a vicious cycle. In this context, alternative therapies that could improve the energetic state and disrupt the vicious cycle of the failing heart are of particular interest.

We hypothesized that there may be a signaling mechanism to compensate cardiac energy production against sustained pressure load. Previous studies explain that the Ca^{2+}-mediated signaling cascade induced by mechanical overload or Gq-mediated signaling initiates the changes that lead to cardiac hypertrophy [20]. CaMKKβ may be one such molecule that links Ca^{2+} signaling and cardiac metabolism, because it is involved in regulating many important physiological processes, including energy balance, adiposity, glucose homeostasis, and hematopoiesis [21].

Our results indicated that phosphorylation of AMPK, CaMKI, and CaMKIV was reduced in α-MHC CaMKKβ^{kd} TG mice compared with WT mice after TAC. AMPK plays an important role in regulating energy balance, protein synthesis, and cell growth. AMPK activation enhances fatty acid and glucose metabolism to augment ATP production and attenuates protein synthesis to preserve ATP. We indicated previously that AMPK is important for oxidative stress-mediated GLUT4 translocation in cardiomyocytes [7]. This pathway may be enhanced under mechanical overload with the elevation of oxidative stress [22]. Moreover, because the energy substrate switches from fatty acids to glucose under cardiac hypertrophy/heart failure [23,24,25], the reduction in AMPK phosphorylation may have negatively affected energy supply in α-MHC CaMKKβ^{kd} TG mice compared with WT mice after TAC. This may be one of the reasons why PCr/β-ATP ratios assessed by MR spectroscopy were suppressed in α-MHC CaMKKβ^{kd} TG mice compared with WT mice after TAC.

Previously, Zhang et al. reported that TAC resulted in more hypertrophy and fibrosis in AMPKα2-deficient hearts than in WT hearts, with a greater increase in LV diameter at end systole and a greater decrease in LV ejection fraction [26]. Although there is a difference in LV phenotype between the study by Zhang et al. and the present study, it may be simply because other downstream target of CaMKKβ such as CaMKI and CaMKIV affected LV structure and function in this experiment.

The expression of PGC-1α has been reported to be modulated in several physiological contexts, for example, in skeletal muscle in response to exercise partly by increased Ca^{2+} signaling via molecules such as CaMK and CREB [17]. A recent study indicated that quiescent and noradrenaline-exposed CaMKKβ-null hepatocytes express less mRNA encoding PGC-1α compared with WT hepatocytes [27]. In line with these findings, CaMKKβ was shown to be important for mitochondrial biogenesis and exercise tolerance through the activation of its downstream target PGC-1α by the use of muscle-specific adiponectin-deficient mice [8]. Therefore, we measured PGC-1α levels and found that its level was significantly reduced in α-MHC CaMKKβ^{kd} TG mice compared with WT mice after TAC. Not only PGC-1α, but other mitochondrial biogenesis genes were dysregulated, and morphology and function also deteriorated in α-MHC CaMKKβ^{kd} TG mice compared with WT mice after TAC. It is known that PGC-1α is abundantly expressed in the heart and a number of gain-of-function and loss-of-function assays have shown that PGC-1α activates most genes of mitochondrial biology and stimulates both fatty acid oxidation and oxidative respiration in cardiac tissues [28,29,30,31,32]. The decrease in PGC-1α expression and mitochondrial morphological changes would be another reason for the reduction in energy pooling in the left ventricle of α-MHC CaMKKβ^{kd} TG mice. These data indicate the vital role that PGC-1α plays in maintaining normal cardiac energetics and contractile function, especially in response to physiological stimuli.

Our data clearly indicate that CaMKKβ exerts beneficial effects against pressure-overload-induced heart failure. It is important to note, however, that massive induction of PGC-1α in the heart increased mitochondrial content to such an extent that myofibrils were displaced and resulted in cardiomyopathy [28,31]. Hence, it may be necessary to increase CaMKKβ activity in an appropriate and moderate fashion for the treatment of heart failure.

Supporting Information

Table S1 Primer sequences used for Quantification of mRNA and DNA levels.

Checklist S1 ARRIVE Checklist.

Acknowledgments

Authors would like to thank Naoya Sowa for excellent technical assistance.

Author Contributions

Conceived and designed the experiments: SW TH KO. Performed the experiments: SW TH KN YK OB HN NS MN TM GT HW KH. Analyzed the data: TH TK KO. Contributed reagents/materials/analysis tools: KN. Contributed to the writing of the manuscript: SW KO. Interpreted the data: TH TK KO.

References

1. Clapham DE (2007) Calcium signaling. Cell 131: 1047–1058.
2. Chin D, Means AR (2000) Calmodulin: a prototypical calcium sensor. Trends Cell Biol 10: 322–328.
3. Colbran RJ (2004) Protein phosphatases and calcium/calmodulin-dependent protein kinase II-dependent synaptic plasticity. J Neurosci 24: 8404–8409.
4. Tokumitsu H, Enslen H, Soderling TR (1995) Characterization of a Ca2+/calmodulin-dependent protein kinase cascade. Molecular cloning and expression of calcium/calmodulin-dependent protein kinase kinase. J Biol Chem 270: 19320–19324.
5. Anderson KA, Means RL, Huang QH, Kemp BE, Goldstein EG, et al. (1998) Components of a calmodulin-dependent protein kinase cascade. Molecular cloning, functional characterization and cellular localization of Ca2+/calmodulin-dependent protein kinase kinase beta. J Biol Chem 273: 31880–31889.
6. Anderson KA, Ribar TJ, Lin F, Noeldner PK, Green MF, et al. (2008) Hypothalamic CaMKK2 contributes to the regulation of energy balance. Cell Metab 7: 377–388.
7. Horie T, Ono K, Nagao K, Nishi H, Kinoshita M, et al. (2008) Oxidative stress induces GLUT4 translocation by activation of PI3-K/Akt and dual AMPK kinase in cardiac myocytes. J Cell Physiol 215: 733–742.
8. Iwabu M, Yamauchi T, Okada-Iwabu M, Sato K, Nakagawa T, et al. (2010) Adiponectin and AdipoR1 regulate PGC-1alpha and mitochondria by Ca(2+) and AMPK/SIRT1. Nature 464: 1313–1319.
9. Woods A, Dickerson K, Heath R, Hong SP, Momcilovic M, et al. (2005) Ca2+/calmodulin-dependent protein kinase kinase-beta acts upstream of AMP-activated protein kinase in mammalian cells. Cell Metab 2: 21–33.
10. Cho A, Haruyama N, Kulkarni AB (2009) Generation of transgenic mice. Curr Protoc Cell Biol Chapter 19: Unit 19 11.
11. Date MO, Morita T, Yamashita N, Nishida K, Yamaguchi O, et al. (2002) The antioxidant N-2-mercaptopropionyl glycine attenuates left ventricular hypertrophy in in vivo murine pressure-overload model. J Am Coll Cardiol 39: 907–912.
12. Inuzuka Y, Okuda J, Kawashima T, Kato T, Niizuma S, et al. (2009) Suppression of phosphoinositide 3-kinase prevents cardiac aging in mice. Circulation 120: 1695–1703.
13. Ellis JM, Mentock SM, Depetrillo MA, Koves TR, Sen S, et al. (2011) Mouse cardiac acyl coenzyme a synthetase 1 deficiency impairs Fatty Acid oxidation and induces cardiac hypertrophy. Mol Cell Biol 31: 1252–1262.
14. Kawashima T, Inuzuka Y, Okuda J, Kato T, Niizuma S, et al. (2011) Constitutive SIRT1 overexpression impairs mitochondria and reduces cardiac function in mice. J Mol Cell Cardiol 51: 1026–1036.
15. Tokumitsu H, Iwabu M, Ishikawa Y, Kobayashi R (2001) Differential regulatory mechanism of Ca2+/calmodulin-dependent protein kinase kinase isoforms. Biochemistry 40: 13925–13932.
16. Subramaniam A, Jones WK, Gulick J, Wert S, Neumann J, et al. (1991) Tissue-specific regulation of the alpha-myosin heavy chain gene promoter in transgenic mice. J Biol Chem 266: 24613–24620.
17. Handschin C, Spiegelman BM (2008) The role of exercise and PGC1alpha in inflammation and chronic disease. Nature 454: 463–469.
18. Murakami Y, Zhang Y, Cho YK, Mansoor AM, Chung JK, et al. (1999) Myocardial oxygenation during high work states in hearts with postinfarction remodeling. Circulation 99: 942–948.
19. Sartoretto JL, Kalwa H, Shiroto T, Sartoretto SM, Pluth MD, et al. (2012) Role of Ca2+ in the control of H2O2-modulated phosphorylation pathways leading to eNOS activation in cardiac myocytes. PLoS One 7: e44627.

20. Molkentin JD, Lu JR, Antos CL, Markham B, Richardson J, et al. (1998) A calcineurin-dependent transcriptional pathway for cardiac hypertrophy. Cell 93: 215–228.
21. Racioppi L, Means AR (2012) Calcium/calmodulin-dependent protein kinase kinase 2: roles in signaling and pathophysiology. J Biol Chem 287: 31658–31665.
22. Tsutsui H, Kinugawa S, Matsushima S (2011) Oxidative stress and heart failure. Am J Physiol Heart Circ Physiol 301: H2181–2190.
23. Lopaschuk GD, Rebeyka IM, Allard MF (2002) Metabolic modulation: a means to mend a broken heart. Circulation 105: 140–142.
24. Sambandam N, Lopaschuk GD, Brownsey RW, Allard MF (2002) Energy metabolism in the hypertrophied heart. Heart Fail Rev 7: 161–173.
25. Depre C, Vanoverschelde JL, Taegtmeyer H (1999) Glucose for the heart. Circulation 99: 578–588.
26. Zhang P, Hu X, Xu X, Fassett J, Zhu G, et al. (2008) AMP activated protein kinase-alpha2 deficiency exacerbates pressure-overload-induced left ventricular hypertrophy and dysfunction in mice. Hypertension 52: 918–924.
27. Anderson KA, Lin F, Ribar TJ, Stevens RD, Muehlbauer MJ, et al. (2012) Deletion of CaMKK2 from the liver lowers blood glucose and improves whole-body glucose tolerance in the mouse. Mol Endocrinol 26: 281–291.
28. Lehman JJ, Barger PM, Kovacs A, Saffitz JE, Medeiros DM, et al. (2000) Peroxisome proliferator-activated receptor gamma coactivator-1 promotes cardiac mitochondrial biogenesis. J Clin Invest 106: 847–856.
29. Vega RB, Huss JM, Kelly DP (2000) The coactivator PGC-1 cooperates with peroxisome proliferator-activated receptor alpha in transcriptional control of nuclear genes encoding mitochondrial fatty acid oxidation enzymes. Mol Cell Biol 20: 1868–1876.
30. Huss JM, Kopp RP, Kelly DP (2002) Peroxisome proliferator-activated receptor coactivator-1alpha (PGC-1alpha) coactivates the cardiac-enriched nuclear receptors estrogen-related receptor-alpha and -gamma. Identification of novel leucine-rich interaction motif within PGC-1alpha. J Biol Chem 277: 40265–40274.
31. Russell LK, Mansfield CM, Lehman JJ, Kovacs A, Courtois M, et al. (2004) Cardiac-specific induction of the transcriptional coactivator peroxisome proliferator-activated receptor gamma coactivator-1alpha promotes mitochondrial biogenesis and reversible cardiomyopathy in a developmental stage-dependent manner. Circ Res 94: 525–533.
32. Arany Z, He H, Lin J, Hoyer K, Handschin C, et al. (2005) Transcriptional coactivator PGC-1 alpha controls the energy state and contractile function of cardiac muscle. Cell Metab 1: 259–271.

3

Abnormal Mitochondrial L-Arginine Transport Contributes to the Pathogenesis of Heart Failure and Rexoygenation Injury

David Williams[1], **Kylie M. Venardos[1,2]**, **Melissa Byrne[1]**, **Mandar Joshi[1]**, **Duncan Horlock[1]**, **Nicholas T. Lam[1]**, **Paul Gregorevic[3]**, **Sean L. McGee[4]**, **David M. Kaye[1,2*]**

1 Heart Failure Research Group, Baker IDI Heart & Diabetes Institute, Melbourne, Australia, 2 Department of Medicine, Monash University, Melbourne, Australia, 3 Muscle Research & Therapeutics Laboratory, Baker IDI Heart & Diabetes Institute, Melbourne, Australia, 4 Metabolic Research Unit, Deakin University, Geelong, Australia

Abstract

Background: Impaired mitochondrial function is fundamental feature of heart failure (HF) and myocardial ischemia. In addition to the effects of heightened oxidative stress, altered nitric oxide (NO) metabolism, generated by a mitochondrial NO synthase, has also been proposed to impact upon mitochondrial function. However, the mechanism responsible for arginine transport into mitochondria and the effect of HF on such a process is unknown. We therefore aimed to characterize mitochondrial L-arginine transport and to investigate the hypothesis that impaired mitochondrial L-arginine transport plays a key role in the pathogenesis of heart failure and myocardial injury.

Methods and Results: In mitochondria isolated from failing hearts (sheep rapid pacing model and mouse Mst1 transgenic model) we demonstrated a marked reduction in L-arginine uptake ($p<0.05$ and $p<0.01$ respectively) and expression of the principal L-arginine transporter, CAT-1 ($p<0.001$, $p<0.01$) compared to controls. This was accompanied by significantly lower NO production and higher 3-nitrotyrosine levels (both $p<0.05$). The role of mitochondrial L-arginine transport in modulating cardiac stress responses was examined in cardiomyocytes with mitochondrial specific overexpression of CAT-1 (mtCAT1) exposed to hypoxia-reoxygenation stress. mtCAT1 cardiomyocytes had significantly improved mitochondrial membrane potential, respiration and ATP turnover together with significantly decreased reactive oxygen species production and cell death following mitochondrial stress.

Conclusion: These data provide new insights into the role of L-arginine transport in mitochondrial biology and cardiovascular disease. Augmentation of mitochondrial L-arginine availability may be a novel therapeutic strategy for myocardial disorders involving mitochondrial stress such as heart failure and reperfusion injury.

Editor: Junichi Sadoshima, Rutgers New Jersey Medical School, United States of America

Funding: Funding provided by NHMRC Program Grant 1036352. The funders had no role in study design, data collection and analysis, decision to publish, or preparation of the manuscript.

Competing Interests: The authors have declared that no competing interests exist.

* Email: david.kaye@bakeridi.edu.au

These authors contributed equally to this work.

Introduction

Heightened oxidative stress is a key feature of numerous chronic diseases including cardiovascular disease and neurodegenerative diseases. In particular the generation of reactive oxygen species (ROS) and reactive nitrogen species (RNS) is now considered to be a central contributor to the development and progression of many diseases, via a range of effects including the oxidative and nitrosative damage of proteins, enzymes, lipids, DNA and cellular membranes [1]. Within the heart, elevated oxidative stress has been reported to play a key role in the pathogenesis of heart failure and ischemia reperfusion injury [2–4]. Several sources of cellular ROS production are recognized in the myocardium including the mitochondrial electron transport chain, NADPH oxidase, xanthine oxidase and cytoplasmic NO synthase (NOS) [1], however the relative contribution of each source to overall cellular ROS production has not been clearly defined.

Mitochondrial dysfunction is increasingly understood to be central to the pathophysiology of heart failure and ischemia-reperfusion injury [5,6]. Recent data indicate that oxidative inhibition of complex I or III of the mitochondrial transport can further increase ROS production most likely due to post-translational modifications [7]. In this context, it has been shown that NO may exert a cardioprotective effect by mitigating oxidative damage of components of the electron transport chain by site-specific S-nitrosation [7–9].

Whilst the mechanism underpinning the protective effect of NO within mitochondria is emerging, it remains controversial as to whether NO is derived from mitochondrial or non-mitochondrial sources. In this regard, the presence of a mitochondrial NOS has been reported by several groups as recently reviewed [10]. In this context, some investigators have estimated that a mitochondrial NOS may contribute up to 56% of total cellular production of NO in the heart [11].

Notwithstanding the specific characterization of a mitochondrial NOS, it has been demonstrated that the generation of NO by mitochondria is influenced by the concentration of L-arginine [12]. In this context, it is unclear how L-arginine enters mitochondria and whether this process is altered in cardiovascular disease. Plasmalemmal arginine transport is predominantly mediated by the system y^+ carrier, which is characterized by sodium independent transport of the cationic amino acids. At normal physiological concentrations of L-arginine the cationic amino acid transporter type 1, CAT-1, is the predominant cellular transport system [13]. Previously, we have shown that CAT-1 mediated L-arginine transport is reduced in the setting of heart failure and hypoxia-reperfusion [14–16]. In the current study we aimed to characterize the presence and activity of CAT-1 in cardiac mitochondria and to determine whether altered mitochondrial L-arginine transport contributes to the pathophysiology of heart failure and ischemia reperfusion injury.

Materials and Methods

The research projects were approved by the Department of Primary Industry Animal Ethics Committee, and the Alfred Medical Research and Education Precinct Animal Ethics Committee. The investigations conform to the NHMRC Australian code of practice for the care and use of animals for scientific purpose, and the Guide for the Care and Use of Laboratory Animals published by the National Institutes of Health.

Animal Models of Heart Failure and Isolation of Cardiac Mitochondria

Two animal models of heart failure were employed in the present study. Heart failure was induced in adult sheep by rapid ventricular pacing or tachycardia at 190 beats per minute for four weeks as previously described [17]. In brief, pacemakers were implanted under anesthesia using propofol and isoflurane. At the end of the pacing period, animals were killed by pentobarbitone overdose (100 mg/kg) and hearts were immediately excised and washed in ice-cold PBS prior to mitochondrial isolation. In addition to the sheep model, 16 week old transgenic mice with dilated cardiomyopathy due to cardiac specific overexpression of Mst1 [18] (kindly provided by Dr Julie McMullen, Baker IDI) and littermate controls were also investigated in this study. Mice were killed by pentobarbitone overdose (150 mg/kg i.p.).

Mitochondrial Isolation and Purity

Following cardiac excision, hearts were immediately immersed in ice cold isolation buffer (Mannitol 200 mM, Sucrose 50 mM, KH2PO4 5 mM, EGTA 1 mM, MOPS 5 mM, BSA 0.1%, pH 7.2). For sheep studies, transmural samples of the left ventricle were obtained from the mid-anterior wall. Cardiac tissue was thoroughly minced into ~1 mm pieces and rinsed with isolation buffer. Tissue pieces were transferred to an ice-cold glass homogeniser vessel containing isolation buffer and 1 mg/ml protease (Sigma) and homogenised for 30 seconds using a Teflon homogeniser pestle [19,20]. The tissue homogenate was subsequently transferred to an ice-cold 50 mL homogeniser vessel and diluted 10-fold and homogenised for a further 30 seconds. The tissue homogenate was then centrifuged at 8000 g for 10-minutes. The supernatant was discarded and the pellet was carefully re-suspended and then centrifuged at 700 g for 10 minutes. The supernatant containing the mitochondrial fraction was collected and transferred into fresh isolation buffer without EGTA or BSA and centrifuged at 8000 g for 10 min and the resulting pellet was re-suspended in ice cold isolation buffer without EGTA/BSA and kept on ice until required.

Mitochondrial purity was confirmed by western blotting for a mitochondrial specific protein, 70 kDa subunit of Complex II, together with demonstration of exclusion of the plasmalemmal Na^+K^+ATPase (in mice) or N-cadherin (in sheep). To determine whether the mitochondrial preparations were in a coupled state, mitochondrial respiration (oxygen consumption rates) was measured using a Seahorse XF24 Extracellular Flux Analyser (Seahorse Bioscience, Billerica, USA). Briefly, mitochondria (15 ug) were loaded into XF24 plates in 50 ul basal MAS (Seahorse Bioscience) buffer. Plates were subsequently centrifuged at 2500 g for 20 mins at 4 degrees. Mitochondria were then warmed by the addition of warmed (37°C) MAS buffer containing succinate (10 mM) and rotenone (2 uM). Basal respiration was established after the samples were allowed to equilibrate in the seahorse XF24, followed by injection of ADP (1 mM) to initiate State 3 respiration, then sequential injection of the ATP synthase inhibitor oligomycin, the proton ionophore carbonylcyanide p-trifluoromethoxyphenlhydrazone (FCCP) and the complex III inhibitor antimycin A, (all 1 μM) to allow for calculation of respiratory control ratios (state3/state 4 ratio). Mitochondrial membrane potential was also assessed to confirm the viability of isolated cardiac mitochondria using the fluorescent probe 5,5′, 6,6′,-tetrachloro-1,1,3,3′-tetraethylbenzimidazolylcarbocyanine iodide (1.5 μM JC-1, Molecular Probes, Eugene, OR, USA) [21] in the presence and absence of 2 μM FCCP and 2 μM antimycin A (respiratory chain inhibitor). Green and red fluorescence were measured at 485 nm/535 nm and 485 nm/590 nm (excitation/emission) respectively, and results expressed as a ratio of red/green raw fluorescence units (RFU).

Mitochondrial [^{3}H]-L-Arginine Uptake

Cardiac mitochondrial L-arginine transport was characterised by treating isolated mitochondria with various mitochondrial inhibitors as well as inhibitors or competitors of the y^+ transport system, comprising L-lysine (10 mM), NEM (200 uM) and antimycin (2 uM). Mitochondrial pellets were re-suspended in uptake buffer (220 mM sucrose, 5 mM $MgCl_2$, 20 mM KCl, 10 mM KH_2PO_4, 10 mM HEPES/KOH, 10 mM sodium succinate, pH 7.4) and L-Arginine uptake was measured using radiolabeled [^{3}H]-L-Arginine (specific activity 58 Ci/mmol, Perkin Elmer Life Sciences, Boston, MA, USA). Solutions containing 100 nM [^{3}H]-L-arginine and increasing concentrations of unlabelled L-arginine (0.75–500 μM) were prepared in uptake buffer and incubated for 15 minutes at 37°C. Pellets were washed then resuspended in 0.5% SDS and measurement of radioactivity was made using liquid scintillation spectrometry. CAT1 mediated L-Arginine uptake was calculated as the difference between total uptake and 10 mM L-lysine sensitive uptake. Data is presented as nmol arginine uptake/mg protein.

CAT-1 protein expression in isolated cardiac mitochondria

Mitochondrial protein (20–30 μg) was subjected to SDS-PAGE analysis using 7.5% acrylamide gels. After transfer, membranes were blocked for 1 hour at room temperature in 5% w/v skim milk, then incubated with CAT-1 antibody (1:1000 in 5% w/v BSA, 1X TBS, 0.1% Tween20, polyclonal rabbit anti-CAT-1

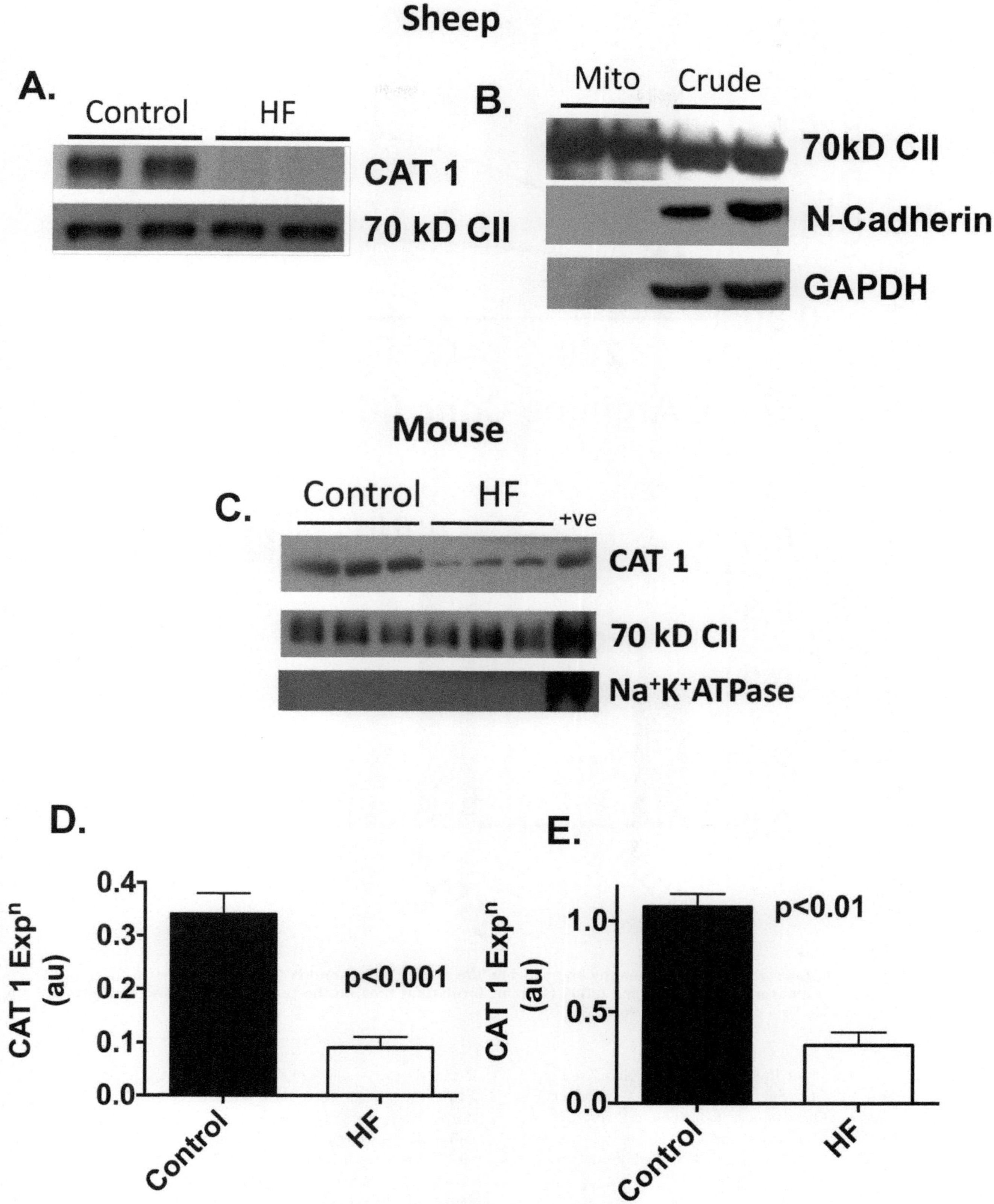

Figure 1. Western blot demonstrating reduced CAT1 expression in failing sheep mitochondria, normalized to expression of the 70 kD subunit of complex II (A). Western blot confirming the absence of contaminating sarcolemmal (N-cadherin) or cytosolic (GAPDH) proteins in mitochondrial preparation (**B**). Western blots showing reduced CAT1 in failing mouse mitochondria (**C**). Sarcolemmal $Na^{+}K^{+}$ATPase is absent from the mitochondrial preparation compared to crude homogenate (+ve). Bar graphs showing CAT1 expression in sheep (**D**) and mice (**E**) (n = 4 per gp).

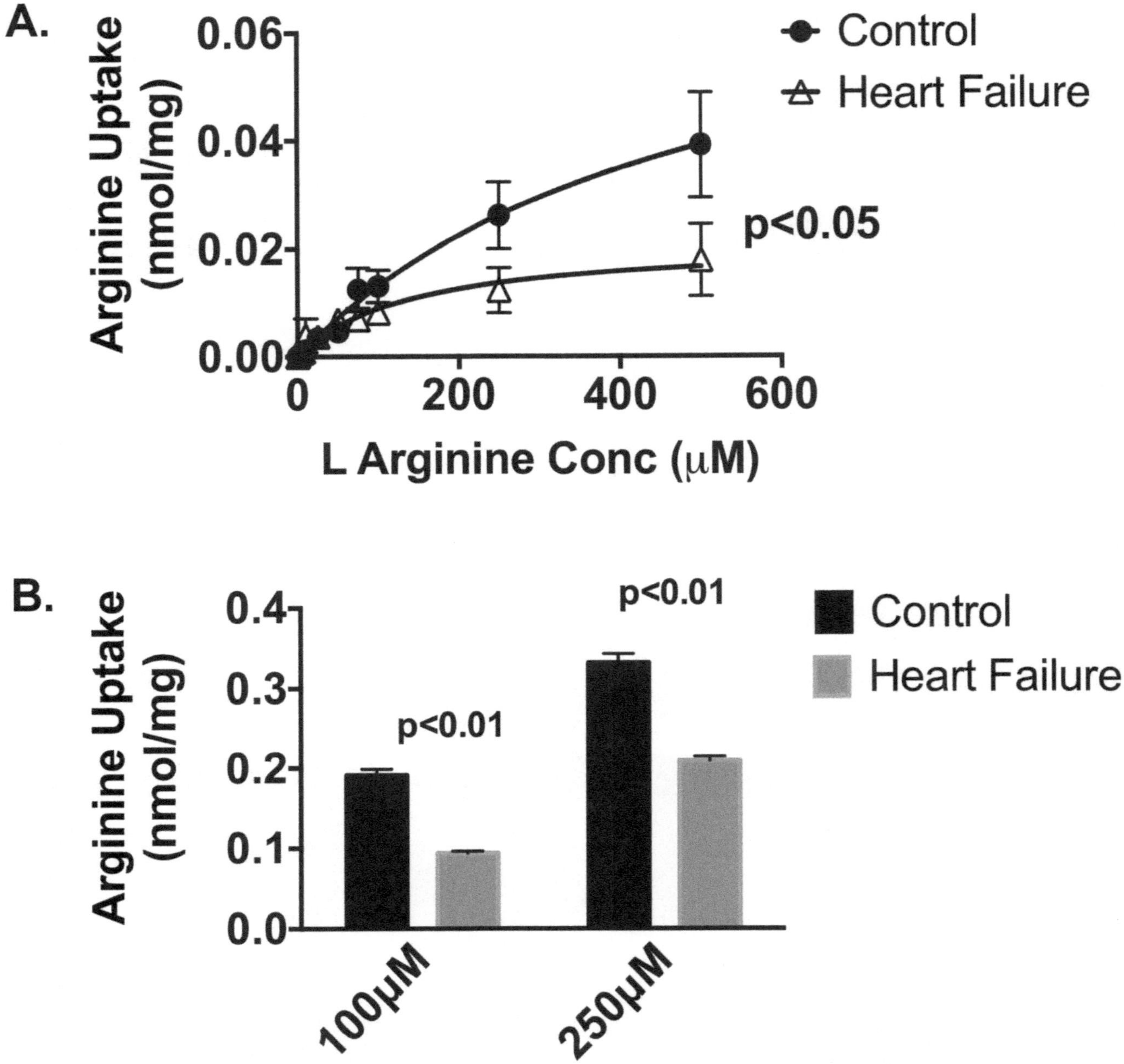

Figure 2. L-Arginine uptake was assessed in healthy and heart failure cardiac mitochondria from A. sheep (n = 5–7 per gp) and B. mice (n = 4 per gp) by measuring [^{3}H]-L-arginine influx (15 mins incubation time) in the presence of varying concentrations of unlabeled L-arginine in. Data is presented as mean ± SEM.

custom made by Rockland Immunochemicals, Gilbertsville, PA, USA) overnight at 4°C. Signal detection was performed by chemiluminescence. Quantitative densitometric analysis was performed (Bio-Rad laboratories) and CAT-1 protein expression levels were indexed to 70 kDa subunit of mitochondrial complex II.

Measurement of nitric oxide (NO) generation by isolated mitochondria and 3-nitrotyrosine as a marker of peroxynitrite formation

NO production in isolated mitochondria (20 μg) from healthy and failing hearts was measured in triplicate using 5 μM 4-amino-5-methylamino-2′,7′-dichlorofluorescein diacetate (DAF-FM, Molecular Probes, Eugene, OR, USA) as previously described [16]. Evidence of nitrosative stress was determined by measuring 3-nitrotyrosine levels in mitochondria isolated from healthy and failing hearts using a OxiSelect Nitrotyrosine competitive ELISA kit (Cell Biolabs Inc; San Diego, CA, USA).

Mitochondrial CAT-1 overexpression in cardiomyocytes

Neonatal rat ventricular cardiomyocytes (NVCMs) were used for all cellular studies. NVMCs from D1-3 neonatal rats were isolated by enzymatic digestion as previously described [16]. Full length mouse CAT-1 was cloned into a vector (pPhi-yellowFP-mito, Evrogen, Moscow, Russia) containing a mitochondrial targeting sequence (MTS) to generate pCAT1-PhiYFP-MTS.

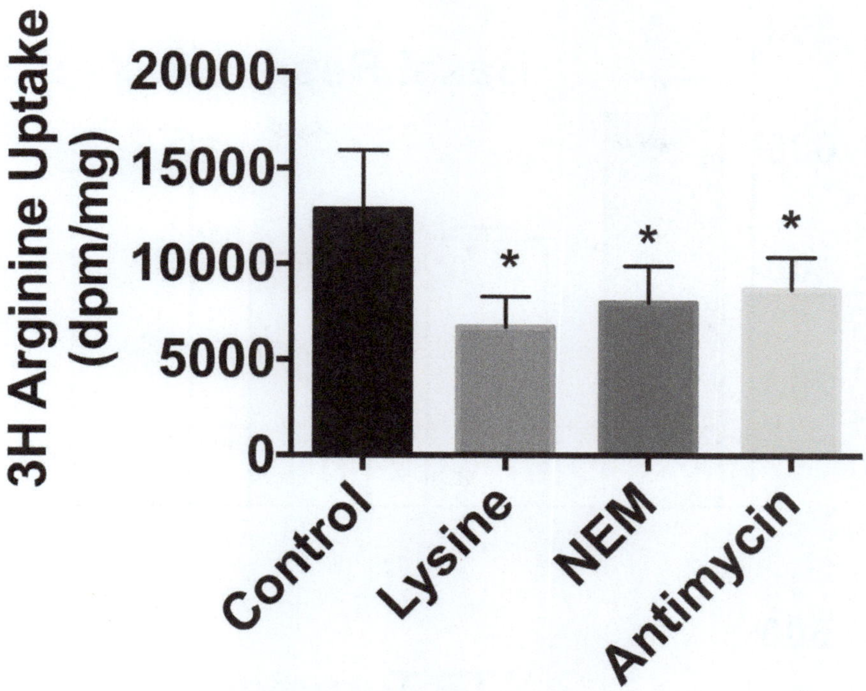

Figure 3. Mitochondrial [^{3}H]-L-arginine uptake was measured in the presence of L-lysine (10 mM), NEM (200 μM) or antimycin (2 μM) (n = 5–7 per gp). Data is presented as mean ± SEM. *$p<0.05$ *vs.* control.

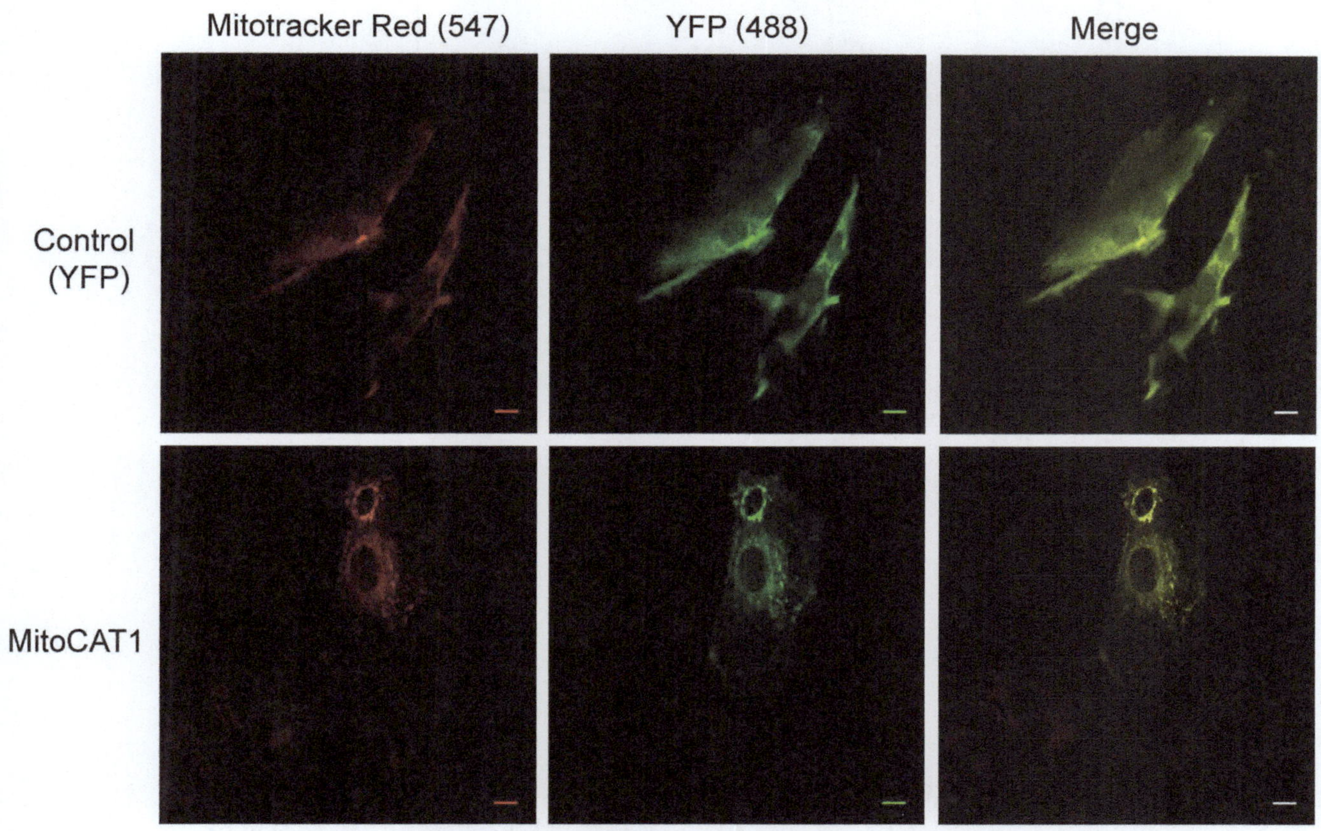

Figure 4. Representative fluorescent confocal images of cardiomyocytes (NVCMs) transfected with control YFP-MTS AAV6 (top panels) or CAT1-YFP-MTS AAV6 (lower panels) incubated with Mitotracker Red. Images confirm mitochondrial targeting in CAT1-YFP-MTS AAV6 transfected cardiomyocytes. Scale bar = 10 μm.

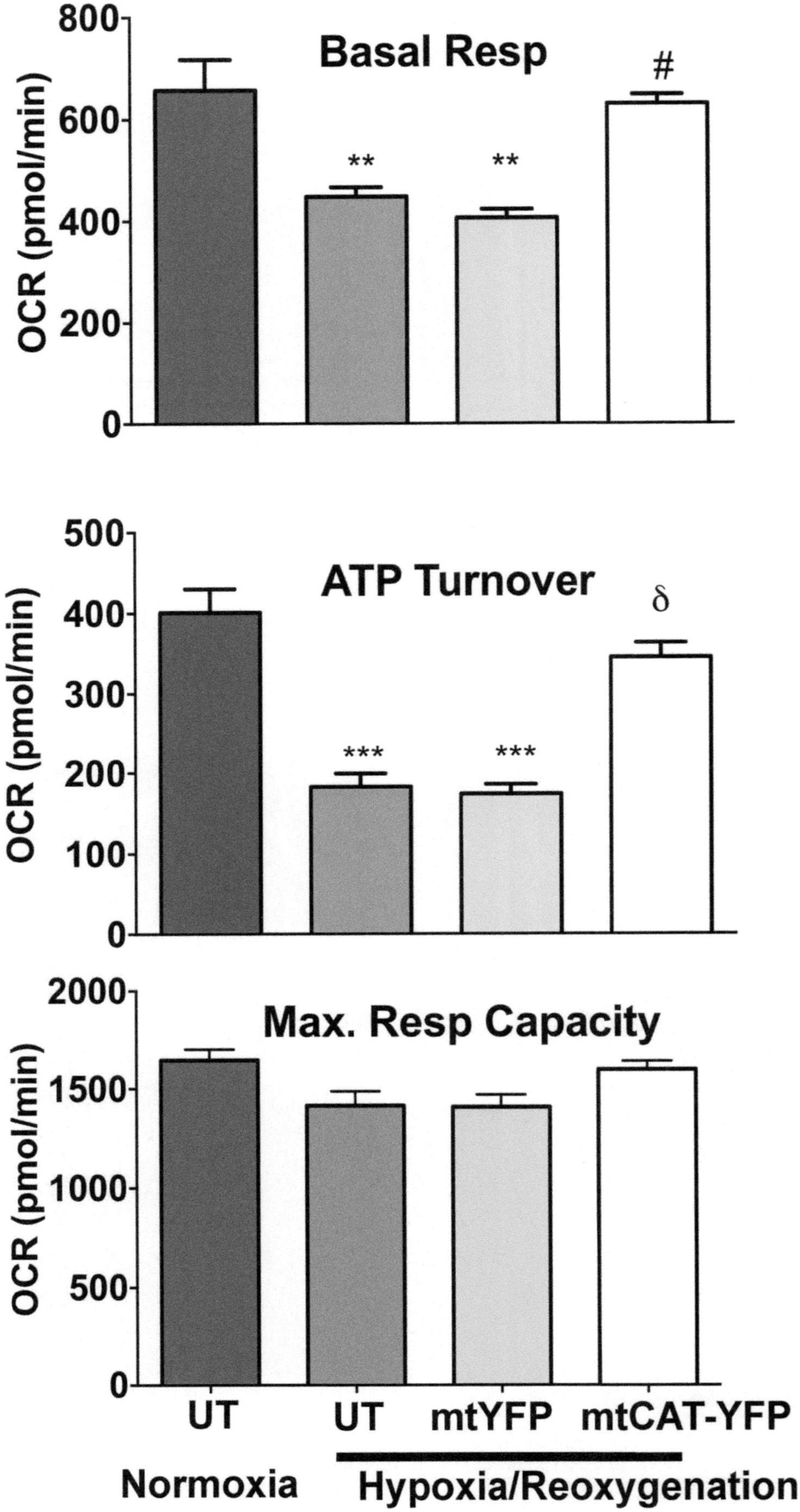
800
600
400
200
0
OCR (pmol/min)
Basal Resp
**
**
#
500
400
300
200
100
0
OCR (pmol/min)
ATP Turnover
***
***
δ
2000
1500
1000
500
0
OCR (pmol/min)
Max. Resp Capacity
UT
UT
mtYFP
mtCAT-YFP
Normoxia
Hypoxia/Reoxygenation

Figure 5. Bar graphs show oxygen consumption rates (OCR) due to basal respiration (top panel), OCR required for ATP turnover (mid panel) and maximal respiratory capacity (lower panel) as evaluated by oxygen consumption rates in isolated cardiomyocytes following hypoxia-reoxygenation. Cells were control untransfected (UT) or transfected with CAT1-YFP-MTS or YFP-MTS AAV6 for 72 hr then subjected to 3 hr hypoxia-2 hr reoxygenation. Data is presented as mean ± SEM. **p<0.01 and ***p<0.001 *vs.* non-transfected normoxic controls; δ p<0.05 and #p<0.01 *vs.* non-transfected hypoxia-reoxygenated NVCMs.

CAT1-PhiYFP-MTS or PhiYFP-MTS were then cloned into the Adeno-Associated Virus (AAV) Vector pAAV-CMV-MCS-SV40pA-deltahPLAP to generate AAV6-CAT1-PhiYFP-MTS or AAV6-PhiYFP-MTS. Transfected cells were then subjected to various mitochondrial stresses including hypoxia/reoxygenation (3 hours hypoxia followed by 2 hours normoxia) [16] or exposure to the mitochondrial respiratory chain inhibitor, antimycin A (0.5 μM) for 5 hours. ROS production, mitochondrial membrane potential, mitochondrial respiration and ATP turnover along with lactate dehydrogenase release were then measured. ROS production was measured with 10 μM 2′,7′-dichlorodihydrofluorescein diacetate (H_2DCF-DA, Molecular Probes) and mitochondrial membrane potential using the fluorescent probe JC-1 both as previously described [16]. Mitochondrial localisation of CAT-1 within cardiomyocytes was investigated by confocal microscopy with 50 nM MitoTracker Red (Molecular Probes Eugene, OR, USA).

Mitochondrial function was also examined in cells transfected with CAT1-YFP-MTS or YFP-MTS AAV following hypoxia/reoxygenation using the Seahorse XF24 Extracellular Flux Analyser. Briefly, NVCMs were plated into 24well Seahorse V7 plates at 6×10^4 cells/well, as described above. Basal energetics were then established through the simultaneous measurement of oxygen consumption rate (OCR) and extracellular acidification rate (ECAR) in the Seahorse XF24, followed by sequential injection of oligomycin, FCCP and antimycin A (all 1 μM) to allow for calculation of basal respiration, OCR attributable to ATP turnover, uncoupled respiration and maximal and spare respiratory capacity. Mitochondria were also isolated from NVCMs as previously described [22]. Studies were performed in triplicate over at least three independent experiments.

Statistical analysis

Data was analysed with by either Student t-tests or by one-way analysis of variance (ANOVA) followed by Bonferonni post-hoc tests for multiple comparisons. All statistical tests were performed using GraphPad Prism program, version 6 (GraphPad Software, San Diego, USA), and $p<0.05$ was considered indicative of statistical significance. All data are presented as mean ± SEM.

Results

Mitochondrial CAT-1 expression in healthy and failing hearts

To investigate the hypothesis that a specific L-arginine transporter is present within cardiac mitochondria, we conducted western blotting on mitochondrial samples to determine the expression of CAT-1. As shown in Figure 1A–C, CAT-1 was readily detected in mitochondria isolated from both sheep and mice. The absence of contaminating sarcolemma was confirmed by the absence of Na^+K^+ATPase in mice and by N-cadherin in sheep. In mitochondrial samples isolated from failing hearts there was a significant reduction in CAT-1 abundance compared with controls in both sheep (73%, $p<0.001$) and mice (70%, $p<0.01$) with heart failure (Figure 1A–E).

To corroborate the demonstration of CAT1 mitochondrial protein, we next evaluated the uptake of [^{3}H] L-arginine in both models of HF. Preliminary L-arginine uptake time course studies over 30 minutes in isolated cardiac mitochondria demonstrated a progressive linear accumulation of [^{3}H] L-arginine over time ranges from 1–25 minutes ($R^2=0.9905$ data not shown) and accordingly an incubation time of 15 minutes was selected. In parallel we investigated mitochondrial respiration using the Seahorse platform. Mitochondrial viability was first confirmed by the presence of respiratory control ratios of ≥4. State 3 respiration, as assessed in the presence of succinate, was however significantly ($p<0.05$) decreased in mitochondria isolated from failing hearts compared to controls (997±117 *vs* 1726±198 pmol O_2/min). As shown in Figure 2, there was a concentration dependent increase in L-arginine uptake in mitochondria isolated from the normal heart. By contrast, L-arginine uptake was significantly reduced in mitochondria from failing sheep and mouse hearts when compared with healthy controls. L-arginine transport by sheep mitochondria from control animals was significantly reduced by the competitive inhibitor L-lysine (48%, $p<0.05$), NEM (37%, $p<0.05$) and antimycin (32%, $p<0.05$) as shown in Figure 3.

Nitric oxide production and nitrosative damage in HF mitochondria

To evaluate whether altered CAT1 expression and L-arginine transport was associated with an alteration in nitric oxide (NO) production we evaluated mitochondrial NO release fluorometrically. Under basal conditions, by DAF fluorescence, NO generation was modestly but significantly reduced in failing sheep mitochondria and compared to control (4404±797 vs 4004±852 rfu, $p<0.05$). In association, protein nitrosation, measured as 3-nitrotyrosine, was significantly ($p<0.05$) higher in mitochondria isolated from failing hearts (327±70 nM) versus mitochondria from healthy controls (109±31 nM).

Effect of mitochondrial L-arginine availability during cardiomyocyte stress

To extend the above observations we next aimed to investigate the potential role of mitochondrial L-arginine transport in the myocardial response to metabolic stress. To address this question we generated an adeno-associated virus (AAV) encoding CAT1-YFP-MTS that incorporates a mitochondrial targeting sequence allowing for CAT-1 overexpression specifically in the mitochondria and transfected isolated ventricular cardiomyocytes. Control transfections were performed using AAV-YFP-MTS. Expression and localisation of CAT-1 was confirmed using confocal microscopy with MitoTracker Red as shown in Figure 4.

To confirm that mitochondria from cardiomyocytes transfected with mitochondrial overexpression of CAT1 possessed an increased capacity for arginine uptake and to generate NO from arginine, we isolated mitochondria from CAT1-YFP-MTS and YFP-MTS AAV transfected cardiomyocytes. Mitochondria isolated from CAT1-YFP-MTS transfected cardiomyocytes had significantly greater capacity for ^{3}H arginine transport compared to mitochondria from YFP-MTS transfected myocytes (1645±211 vs 772±254 dpm/mg protein, $p=0.03$, $n=5$). In conjunction, we determined the ability of 100 uM arginine to yield NO release as assessed by DAF fluorescence. In CAT1 transfected mitochondria,

Table 1. Effect of mitochondrial L-arginine availability on isolated ventricular cardiomyocytes during mitochondrial stress.

	Control	Antimycin A	CAT1-MTS AAV + Antimycin A	YFP-MTS AAV +Antimycin A	Hypoxia-Reox[n]	CAT1-MTS AAV +Hypoxia- Reox[n]	YFP-MTS AAV +Hypoxia- Reox[n]
ROS production (% control)	100	142±4***	120±1†**	155±1.1***	144±2.3***	121±1.6$^{\#}$**	146±2.4***
Mitochondrial membrane potential (% control)	100	68±1.5***	86±1.1††**	65±1.8***	60±1.4***	79±1$^{\$}$**	57±1.7***
LDH release (absorbance units×10^3)	7±0.2	.255±22***	172±5†***	291±9***	200±8***	123±5$^{\$}$***	203±5***

NVCMs were either untreated, or infected with either CAT1-YFP-MTS AAV6 or YFP-MTS AAV6. Cells were then subjected to 3 hr hypoxia-2 hr reoxygenation or treated with antimycin A for 5 hr. ROS generation and mitochondrial membrane potential were measured in these cells using the fluorescent probes H_2DCF-DA and JC-1 respectively. LDH release was also measured as a marker of cell death (n = 3 individual experiments with 4 replicates per experiment for fluorescent probes, or n = 3 for LDH). Data represents mean ± SEM (*$p<0.05$, **$p<0.01$ and ***$p<0.001$ *vs.* normoxic untreated controls; $^{\dagger}p<0.01$ and $^{\dagger\dagger}p<0.001$ *vs.* antimycin A; and $^{\#}p<0.01$ and $^{\$}p<0.001$ *vs.* untreated cells after 3 hr hypoxia-2 hr reoxygenation).

arginine caused a 1.72±0.16 vs 1.28±0.06 ($p<0.05$) fold rise in NO production.

Basal respiration (Fig. 5A) was significantly decreased in NVCMs following hypoxia-reoxygenation (447±18 *versus* 657±60 pmol O_2/min in normoxic cells, $p<0.01$). By contrast, NVCMs transfected with CAT1-YFP-MTS AAV were completely protected and exhibit significantly improved basal OCR compared with non-transfected cells following hypoxia-reoxygenation (630±18 pmol O_2/min, $p<0.05$ versus non-transfected hypoxia-reoxygenation). Hypoxia-reoxygenation significantly decreased oxidative ATP turnover ($p<0.001$ *versus* normoxic controls, Fig. 5B), which was also significantly restored in CAT1-YFP-MTS AAV NVCMs ($p<0.01$ compared with non-transfected hypoxia-reoxygenated NVCMs, Fig. 5B). There were no significant changes in maximal respiratory capacity following hypoxia-reoxygenation (Fig. 5C). There were no significant differences in OCR or ATP turnover after hypoxia-reoxygenation in NVCMs transfected with the control AAV (YFP-MTS AAV) compared with non-transfected hypoxia-reoxygenated NVCMs (Fig. 5). CAT1-YFP-MTS transfection had no effect on basal respiratory rate (631±53 pmol O_2/min), ATP turnover (361±37 pmol O_2/min) or maximal respiratory capacity (1680±84 pmol O_2/min) in normoxic NVCM.

Exposure of NVCMs to hypoxia with reoxygenation significantly reduced mitochondrial membrane potential (60±1.4% of normoxic controls, $p<0.001$) and significantly increased ROS production (144±2.3% of normoxic controls, $p<0.001$) as shown in Table 1. NVCMs treated with antimycin A also exhibited significantly decreased mitochondrial membrane potential (68±1.5% of untreated controls, $p<0.001$) and significantly increased ROS generation (142±4% of untreated controls, $p<0.001$, Table 1). In conjunction, LDH release, a marker of cell death or necrosis, significantly increased during both hypoxia-reoxygenation and with antimycin A treatment (200±8 and 255±23 *versus* control, 7±0.2 arbitrary units x10^3, both $p<0.001$, Table 1).

By contrast, NVCMs transfected with CAT1-YFP-MTS AAV exhibit significantly reduced ROS generation and significantly improved mitochondrial membrane potentials following both hypoxia-reoxygenation or antimycin A treatment when compared with their non-transfected controls (Table 1). ROS production during hypoxia-reoxygenation was limited to 121±1.6% in CAT1-YFP-MTS AAV NVCMs *versus* 144±2.3% in non-transfected cells ($p<0.01$), whilst mitochondrial membrane potential depolarized to 79±1% in CAT1-YFP-MTS AAV cells compared with 60±1.4% in non-transfected cells ($p<0.001$). ROS production following antimycin A treatment was significantly lower in CAT1-YFP-MTS AAV NVCMs than in non-transfected cells (120±1% *versus* 142±4%, $p<0.01$) and mitochondrial membrane potential was significantly higher in CAT1-YFP-MTS AAV cells (86±1.1% compared with 68±1.5% in non-transfected controls, $p<0.001$). Furthermore, CAT1-YFP-MTS NVCMs had significantly decreased LDH release following hypoxia-reoxygenation and antimycin A treatment ($p<0.001$ and $p<0.01$ respectively compared with non-transfected control, Table 1). There were no significant differences in ROS generation, mitochondrial membrane potential or LDH release after 2 hrs reoxygenation or with antimycin A treatment in NVCMs transfected with the control AAV (YFP-MTS AAV) compared with relevant non-transfected cells (Table 1). There was also no significant difference in LDH release in normoxic cells transfected with either CAT1-YFP-MTS or YFP-MTS AAV when compared with non-transfected normoxic controls.

Discussion

In the present study we aimed to determine whether mitochondria possess a specific transport system for the translocation of L-arginine from the cytoplasm and to investigate its role in the pathophysiology of cardiovascular disease states associated with heightened oxidative stress, specifically heart failure and hypoxia-reoxygenation stress. Our study was predicated upon emerging evidence that NO plays an important role in the regulation of several mitochondrial processes and that mitochondria may contain enzymatic systems including NOS which generate NO [10].

We demonstrated evidence for the concentration dependent accumulation of L-arginine in the mitochondria of both mice and sheep. The plasmalemmal transport of L-arginine in many cell types including cardiomyocytes is predominantly mediated by the biochemical system y^+ carrier, which is principally represented by the CAT-1 transporter [23]. The presence of such a transporter in the mitochondria has previously remained unclear in mammalian cells. Further evaluation by western blotting on isolated cardiac mitochondria and confocal microscopy of isolated cardiomyocytes confirmed the presence of CAT-1 in mitochondria, thus providing new insights into the mechanism responsible for the transport of L-arginine into mitochondria. Previously studies have reported the presence of a mitochondrial ornithine transporter in yeast, which exhibited some capacity for L-arginine transport with a relatively low Km [24]. Additionally a mitochondrial arginase has also been described [25], together suggesting the presence of a complex system for the regulation of intra-mitochondrial L-arginine content. In our study we showed that the mitochondrial transport of L-arginine was significantly reduced by the cationic amino acid L-lysine consistent with a y^+ system mediated transport system. The present study did not investigate the precise localization of the mitochondrial CAT1 transporter. Furthermore we did not establish the relationship between transporter kinetics and the influence of various mitochondrial substrates.

Having established the presence of a mitochondrial CAT-1 L-arginine, we aimed to determine whether mitochondrial CAT1 expression was altered in heart failure. We found that both mitochondrial L-arginine uptake and mitochondrial expression of the CAT-1 L-arginine transporter were significantly reduced in the failing heart, in both models of heart failure. These data are consistent with our previous findings that depressed vascular and myocardial L-arginine transport plays a key role in the pathophysiology of a range of cardiovascular disorders such as hypertension and heart failure [15,26,27]. In the context of heart failure, most previous studies of arginine transport have been conducted in relation to the concomitant decrease in endothelial function, by virtue of its influence on NO production[26]. Similarly, it has been proposed that diminished endothelial arginine transport could contribute to the impairment of endothelial function in hypertension [28,29]. Mechanistically, previous studies of CAT1 activity and expression demonstrated negative effects of angiotensin II and particularly protein kinase C, of which both have pathophysiologic relevance to heart failure [30]. In the context of the present study, a concomitant decrease in plasmalemmal arginine transport would be expected to further magnify the effects of a decrease in mitochondrial arginine transport on mitochondrial function. In relation to the present study, we did not specifically study the mechanism responsible for the regulation of mitochondrial CAT1 expression.

In the current study we also found that mitochondria isolated from failing hearts have significantly lower NO production and significantly higher levels of 3-nitrotyrosine, indicative of increased oxidative/nitrosative stress. 3-nitrotyrosine, a widely used marker of oxidative and nitrosative damage in human and animal disease states, is formed when peroxynitrite attacks tyrosine residues in proteins. Peroxynitrite is known to cause irreversible inhibition of many mitochondrial components including the respiratory chain (specifically complex I and cytochrome c oxidase), the Kreb's cycle enzyme aconitase and Mn-superoxide dismutase [31].

To further investigate the notion that altered mitochondrial L-arginine transport may influence the overall cellular response to oxidative stress we examined whether augmented mitochondrial L-arginine would provide cellular protection during hypoxia-reoxygenation stress. Ventricular cardiomyocytes with mitochondrial overexpression of CAT1 showed a significant decrease in ROS production, perseveration of mitochondrial membrane potential together with evidence of significantly less cellular injury following either hypoxia-reoxygenation or antimycin A exposure. Furthermore, the deleterious effects of hypoxia-reoxygenation on mitochondrial respiration and ATP turnover were attenuated by enhanced mitochondrial CAT1 expression. Although we did not examine the effects of increased mitochondrial CAT1 expression in an experimental model of heart failure, we hypothesise that it would be beneficial given that heart failure is associated with elevated oxidative stress and that mitochondrial arginine transport is reduced as demonstrated above.

Our findings of a cellular protective effect of increased mitochondrial L-arginine transport and NO production are entirely consistent with the findings of Chouchani and colleagues who demonstrated that S-nitrosation of complex I, using a mitochondrial selective NO donor, provided cardioprotection by reducing oxidative damage [7]. Similarly, S-nitrosation of complex I by nitrite has also been shown to be cardioprotective [32]. As such, S-nitrosation of key cysteine residues could protective effects during ischemic injury by preventing the irreversible effects of exposure to peroxynitrite. For example, peroxynitrite can cause direct permeabilisation of mitochondrial membranes leading to the formation of mitochondrial permeability transition pore (MPTP) with subsequent inhibition of ATP synthesis which can lead to cellular necrosis [33]. High concentrations of NO may transiently modify mitochondrial oxygen consumption by interacting with cytochrome *c* oxidase [34]. Nitric oxide has also been reported to exert other aspects of mitochondrial function including the prevention of mitochondrial calcium accumulation, activating expression of a number of mitochondrial proteins including PGC-1α, increasing the production of mitochondrial DNA or inhibiting the pathway of apoptosis [34–37]. Other studies suggest that reduced mitochondrial NO availability impairs mitochondrial biogenesis and decreased myocardial NO levels induce a switch from fatty acid metabolism to glycolytic metabolism [38].

In the present study we did not aim to specifically determine the source of mitochondrial NO. The presence of a constitutively expressed mitochondrial NOS enzyme has been proposed based on the demonstration of mitochondrial NO generation using a range of techniques including electroparamagnetic spin trapping, radiometry, chemiluminescence and fluorescence microscopy [10], however this remains controversial. A mitochondrial NOS has been proposed to be a component of the inner membrane and which generates NO in a calcium-dependent manner [39–46]. The identity of a putative mitochondrial NOS also remains speculative, with some evidence for a neuronal isoform NOS based upon proteomic analysis of mitochondrial extracts and the absence of mitochondrial NO production in nNOS knockout mice [47,48]. The mechanism by which a putative mtNOS localises to the mitochondria is unknown, but may include post-translational modifications or interactions with other proteins [35]. Whilst our observations are consistent with a paradigm in which the mitochondrial L-arginine transporter plays a key role in providing substrate to a mitochondrial NOS which in turn generates NO to regulate mitochondrial function and to provide protection during cellular stress, it is possible that the mitochondrial L-arginine transporter influences mitochondrial function in other ways. For example the generation of ornithine via arginase could participate in other mitochondrial bioenergetic activities.

Conclusion

Our study provides the first evidence for the presence of a CAT-1 isoform L-arginine transporter in mammalian cardiac mitochondria. We demonstrated a significant reduction in L-arginine uptake and NO production in mitochondria obtained from the failing heart and this was accompanied by evidence of nitrosative modification of the mitochondrial membrane. Increasing mitochondrial L-arginine availability by transfection of a mitochondrially targeted CAT-1 significantly improved cardiomyocyte responses to mitochondrial stresses, reducing oxidative stress and improving survival. Taken together, these data provide new insights into the nature of myocardial mitochondrial L-arginine transport, its role in mitochondrial biology and the pathogenesis of cardiovascular disease.

Author Contributions

Conceived and designed the experiments: DW KV MB SM DK. Performed the experiments: DW KV MB MJ DH NL PG SM DK. Analyzed the data: DW KV MJ SM DK. Contributed reagents/materials/analysis tools: PG SM DK. Contributed to the writing of the manuscript: DW KV MB MJ DH NL PG SM DK.

References

1. Venardos KM, Perkins A, Headrick J, Kaye DM (2007) Myocardial ischemia-reperfusion injury, antioxidant enzyme systems, and selenium: a review. Curr Med Chem 14: 1539–1549.
2. Huss JM, Kelly DP (2005) Mitochondrial energy metabolism in heart failure: a question of balance. J Clin Invest 115: 547–555.
3. Ide T, Tsutsui H, Kinugawa S, Utsumi H, Kang D, et al. (1999) Mitochondrial electron transport complex I is a potential source of oxygen free radicals in the failing myocardium. Circ Res 85: 357–363.
4. Sawyer DB, Colucci WS (2000) Mitochondrial oxidative stress in heart failure: "oxygen wastage" revisited. Circ Res 86: 119–120.
5. Duranski MR, Greer JJM, Dejam A, Jaganmohan S, Hogg N, et al. (2005) Cytoprotective effects of nitrite during in vivo ischemia-reperfusion of the heart and liver. Journal of Clinical Investigation 115: 1232–1240.
6. Yellon DM, Hausenloy DJ (2007) Myocardial reperfusion injury. New England Journal of Medicine 357: 1121–1135+1074.
7. Chouchani ET, Methner C, Nadtochiy SM, Logan A, Pell VR, et al. (2013) Cardioprotection by S-nitrosation of a cysteine switch on mitochondrial complex I. Nat Med 19: 753–759.
8. Prime TA, Blaikie FH, Evans C, Nadtochiy SM, James AM, et al. (2009) A mitochondria-targeted S-nitrosothiol modulates respiration, nitrosates thiols, and protects against ischemia-reperfusion injury. Proceedings of the National Academy of Sciences of the United States of America 106: 10764–10769.
9. Sun J, Aponte AM, Kohr MJ, Tong G, Steenbergen C, et al. (2013) Essential role of nitric oxide in acute ischemic preconditioning: S-Nitros(yl)ation versus sGC/cGMP/PKG signaling? Free Radical Biology and Medicine 54: 105–112.
10. Zaobornyj T, Ghafourifar P (2012) Strategic localization of heart mitochondrial NOS: a review of the evidence. Am J Physiol Heart Circ Physiol 303: H1283–1293.
11. Boveris A, Valdez LB, Zaobornyj T, Bustamante J (2006) Mitochondrial metabolic states regulate nitric oxide and hydrogen peroxide diffusion to the cytosol. Biochimica et Biophysica Acta - Bioenergetics 1757: 535–542.
12. Valdez LB, Zaobornyj T, Boveris A (2006) Mitochondrial metabolic states and membrane potential modulate mtNOS activity. Biochimica et Biophysica Acta - Bioenergetics 1757: 166–172.
13. Closs EI, Simon A, Vekony N, Rotmann A (2004) Plasma membrane transporters for arginine. J Nutr 134: 2752S–2759S; discussion 2765S–2767S.
14. Kaye DM, Ahlers BA, Autelitano DJ, Chin-Dusting JP (2000) In vivo and in vitro evidence for impaired arginine transport in human heart failure. Circulation 102: 2707–2712.
15. Kaye DM, Parnell MM, Ahlers BA (2002) Reduced myocardial and systemic L-arginine uptake in heart failure. Circ Res 91: 1198–1203.
16. Venardos KM, Zatta AJ, Marshall T, Ritchie R, Kaye DM (2009) Reduced L-arginine transport contributes to the pathogenesis of myocardial ischemia-reperfusion injury. J Cell Biochem 108: 156–168.
17. Byrne M, Kaye DM, Power J (2008) The synergism between atrial fibrillation and heart failure. J Card Fail 14: 320–326.
18. Yamamoto S, Yang G, Zablocki D, Liu J, Hong C, et al. (2003) Activation of Mst1 causes dilated cardiomyopathy by stimulating apoptosis without compensatory ventricular myocyte hypertrophy. J Clin Invest 111: 1463–1474.
19. Riess ML, Costa AD, Carlson R Jr, Garlid KD, Heinen A, et al. (2008) Differential increase of mitochondrial matrix volume by sevoflurane in isolated cardiac mitochondria. Anesth Analg 106: 1049–1055, table of contents.
20. Mootha VK, Arai AE, Balaban RS (1997) Maximum oxidative phosphorylation capacity of the mammalian heart. Am J Physiol 272: H769–775.
21. Reers M, Smith TW, Chen LB (1991) J-aggregate formation of a carbocyanine as a quantitative fluorescent indicator of membrane potential. Biochemistry 30: 4480–4486.
22. Frezza C, Cipolat S, Scorrano L (2007) Organelle isolation: functional mitochondria from mouse liver, muscle and cultured fibroblasts. Nat Protoc 2: 287–295.
23. Krotova KY, Zharikov SI, Block ER (2003) Classical isoforms of PKC as regulators of CAT-1 transporter activity in pulmonary artery endothelial cells. Am J Physiol Lung Cell Mol Physiol 284: L1037–1044.
24. Soetens O, Crabeel M, El Moualij B, Duyckaerts C, Sluse F (1998) Transport of arginine and ornithine into isolated mitochondria of Saccharomyces cerevisiae. Eur J Biochem 258: 702–709.
25. Steppan J, Ryoo S, Schuleri KH, Gregg C, Hasan RK, et al. (2006) Arginase modulates myocardial contractility by a nitric oxide synthase 1-dependent mechanism. Proceedings of the National Academy of Sciences of the United States of America 103: 4759–4764.
26. Kaye DM, Ahlers BA, Autelitano DJ, Chin-Dusting JP (2000) In vivo and in vitro evidence for impaired arginine transport in human heart failure. Circulation 102: 2707–2712.
27. Yang Z, Venardos K, Jones E, Morris BJ, Chin-Dusting J, et al. (2007) Identification of a novel polymorphism in the 3'UTR of the L-arginine transporter gene SLC7A1: contribution to hypertension and endothelial dysfunction. Circulation 115: 1269–1274.
28. Schlaich MP, Parnell MM, Ahlers BA, Finch S, Marshall T, et al. (2004) Impaired L-arginine transport and endothelial function in hypertensive and genetically predisposed normotensive subjects. Circulation 110: 3680–3686.
29. Schlaich MP, Ahlers BA, Parnell MM, Kaye DM (2004) beta-Adrenoceptor-mediated, nitric-oxide-dependent vasodilatation is abnormal in early hypertension: restoration by L-arginine. J Hypertens 22: 1917–1925.
30. Venardos K, Enriquez C, Marshall T, Chin-Dusting JP, Ahlers B, et al. (2009) Protein kinase C mediated inhibition of endothelial L-arginine transport is mediated by MARCKS protein. J Mol Cell Cardiol 46: 86–92.
31. Han D, Canali R, Garcia J, Aguilera R, Gallaher TK, et al. (2005) Sites and mechanisms of aconitase inactivation by peroxynitrite: modulation by citrate and glutathione. Biochemistry 44: 11986–11996.
32. Shiva S, Sack MN, Greer JJ, Duranski M, Ringwood LA, et al. (2007) Nitrite augments tolerance to ischemia/reperfusion injury via the modulation of mitochondrial electron transfer. Journal of Experimental Medicine 204: 2089–2102.
33. Borutaite V, Brown GC (2006) S-nitrosothiol inhibition of mitochondrial complex I causes a reversible increase in mitochondrial hydrogen peroxide production. Biochimica et Biophysica Acta - Bioenergetics 1757: 562–566.
34. Brown GC, Borutaite V (2007) Nitric oxide and mitochondrial respiration in the heart. Cardiovasc Res 75: 283–290.
35. Davidson SM, Duchen MR (2006) Effects of NO on mitochondrial function in cardiomyocytes: Pathophysiological relevance. Cardiovasc Res 71: 10–21.
36. Razavi HM, Hamilton JA, Feng Q (2005) Modulation of apoptosis by nitric oxide: implications in myocardial ischemia and heart failure. Pharmacol Ther 106: 147–162.
37. Nisoli E, Tonello C, Cardile A, Cozzi V, Bracale R, et al. (2005) Calorie restriction promotes mitochondrial biogenesis by inducing the expression of eNOS. Science 310: 314–317.
38. Loke KE, Forfia PR, Recchia FA, Xu X, Osorio JC, et al. (2000) Bovine polymerized hemoglobin increases cardiac oxygen consumption and alters myocardial substrate metabolism in conscious dogs: role of nitric oxide. J Cardiovasc Pharmacol 35: 84–92.
39. Ghafourifar P, Cadenas E (2005) Mitochondrial nitric oxide synthase. Trends Pharmacol Sci 26: 190–195.
40. Valerio A, D'Antona G, Nisoli E (2011) Branched-chain amino acids, mitochondrial biogenesis, and healthspan: an evolutionary perspective. Aging (Albany NY) 3: 464–478.
41. Nisoli E, Cozzi V, Carruba MO (2008) Amino acids and mitochondrial biogenesis. Am J Cardiol 101: 22E–25E.
42. Dedkova EN, Blatter LA (2005) Modulation of mitochondrial Ca2+ by nitric oxide in cultured bovine vascular endothelial cells. Am J Physiol Cell Physiol 289: C836–845.

43. Lacza Z, Puskar M, Figueroa JP, Zhang J, Rajapakse N, et al. (2001) Mitochondrial nitric oxide synthase is constitutively active and is functionally upregulated in hypoxia. Free Radic Biol Med 31: 1609–1615.
44. Zanella B, Giordano E, Muscari C, Zini M, Guarnieri C (2004) Nitric oxide synthase activity in rat cardiac mitochondria. Basic Res Cardiol 99: 159–164.
45. Persichini T, Mazzone V, Polticelli F, Moreno S, Venturini G, et al. (2005) Mitochondrial type I nitric oxide synthase physically interacts with cytochrome c oxidase. Neurosci Lett 384: 254–259.
46. Lacza Z, Pankotai E, Busija DW (2009) Mitochondrial nitric oxide synthase: current concepts and controversies. Front Biosci (Landmark Ed) 14: 4436–4443.
47. Elfering SL, Sarkela TM, Giulivi C (2002) Biochemistry of mitochondrial nitric-oxide synthase. Journal of Biological Chemistry 277: 38079–38086.
48. Kanai AJ, Pearce LL, Clemens PR, Birder LA, VanBibber MM, et al. (2001) Identification of a neuronal nitric oxide synthase in isolated cardiac mitochondria using electrochemical detection. Proceedings of the National Academy of Sciences of the United States of America 98: 14126–14131.

Heart Failure Re-Admission: Measuring the Ever Shortening Gap between Repeat Heart Failure Hospitalizations

Jeffrey A. Bakal[1,2], Finlay A. McAlister[1,2], Wei Liu[3], Justin A. Ezekowitz[3]*

1 Patient Health Outcomes Research and Clinical Effectiveness Unit, University of Alberta, Edmonton, Alberta, Canada, 2 Division of General Internal Medicine, University of Alberta, Edmonton, Alberta, Canada, 3 Division of Cardiology, University of Alberta, Edmonton, Alberta, Canada

Abstract

Many quality-of-care and risk prediction metrics rely on time to first rehospitalization even though heart failure (HF) patients may undergo several repeat hospitalizations. The aim of this study is to compare repeat hospitalization models. Using a population-based cohort of 40,667 patients, we examined both HF and all cause re-hospitalizations using up to five years of follow-up. Two models were examined: the gap-time model which estimates the adjusted time between hospitalizations and a multistate model which considered patients to be in one of four states; community-dwelling, in hospital for HF, in hospital for any reason, or dead. The transition probabilities and times were then modeled using patient characteristics and number of repeat hospitalizations. We found that during the five years of follow-up roughly half of the patients returned for a subsequent hospitalization for each repeat hospitalization. Additionally, we noted that the unadjusted time between hospitalizations was reduced ~40% between each successive hospitalization. After adjustment each additional hospitalization was associated with a 28 day (95% CI: 22-35) reduction in time spent out of hospital. A similar pattern was seen when considering the four state model. A large proportion of patients had multiple repeat hospitalizations. Extending the gap between hospitalizations should be an important goal of treatment evaluation.

Editor: Wolfgang Rudolf Bauer, University Hospital of Würzburg, Germany

Funding: The study was supported by in-kind funding from Alberta Health Services - Data Integration, Management, and Reporting. The funders had no role in study design, data analysis, decision to publish, or preparation of the manuscript.

Competing Interests: The authors have declared that no competing interests exist.

* Email: jae2@ualberta.ca

Introduction

Heart Failure (HF) is a common disease with a high morbidity and mortality. Each year in the United States, 5.1 million individuals with heart failure undergo ~1 million hospitalizations, 668,000 emergency department visits and ~3 million physician outpatient visits resulting in an overall cost of approximately $40 billion per year [1]. Given this public health issue, understanding the patterns of recurrent hospitalizations related to HF is important in order to design therapy or management strategies that can help reduce this burden for individual patients and the system.

The 30 day rehospitalization rates for patients with HF remain high in clinical trials (6.0%) [2], registries (24.5%) and in population health studies (18%) [3]. However, the modeling of rehospitalization remains challenging even using models incorporating a large number of patient characteristics [4]. Most analyses attempting to model re-hospitalizations utilize only the first re-hospitalization and fail to incorporate for the repetitive nature or trajectory of re–hospitalizations in patients with HF. A recent study in Olmstead county showed that while 83% of HF patients were hospitalized at least once, 43% were hospitalized four or more times within five years of diagnosis [5]. Several repeated events methods have been considered for these data and have seen limited uptake in part due to the assumptions required for each model [6].

The temporal trends in these data have been explored previously [7] however to this point in time, few studies examining rehospitalization risk have explored the amount of time between hospitalizations (the "gap-time") [8], which may play a role in identifying patients at increased risk for morbid events. Conceivably, while two patients may exhibit a similar risk of at least one hospitalization, a sicker patient may be re-admitted to hospital more than once and/or with a shorter duration between hospitalizations.

The objective of this study was to describe the gap-time and transitions in a cohort of patients who were hospitalized more than once with heart failure, and explore the patient and system level features associated with the gap-time. We developed a model to examine the timing and risk of both HF-specific and all-cause

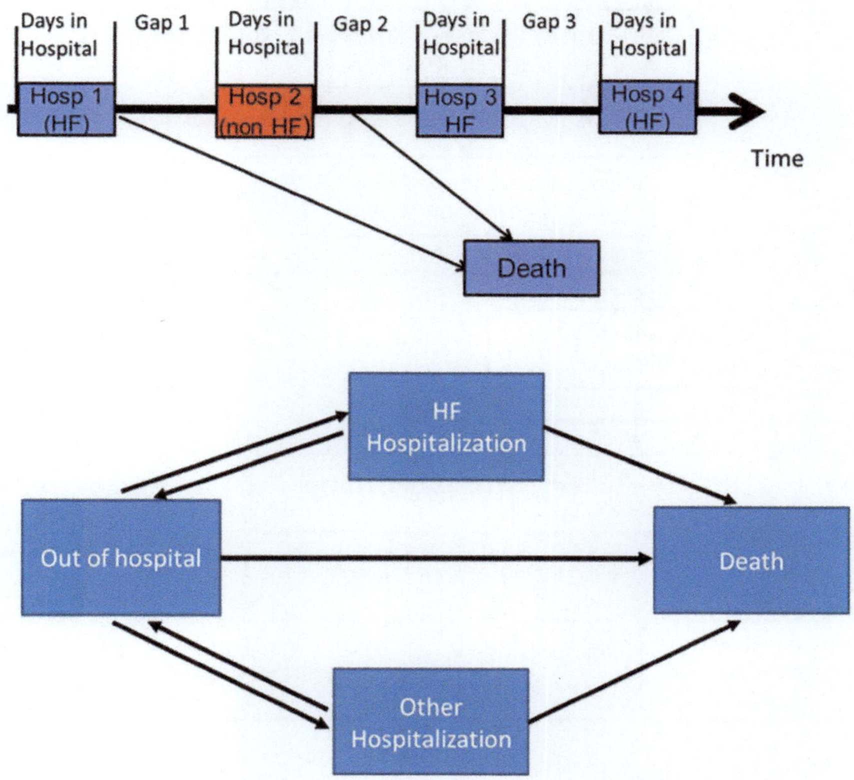

Figure 1. Schematic of timeline for HF patients indicating hospitalizations and Gap times (a); States and transitions for multistate model. Arrows indicate modeled transformations(b).

hospitalization while simultaneously considering the competing risks of all-cause hospitalization and mortality in HF patients, allowing combined modeling of parameters. An improved understanding of the trajectory of heart failure patients is important for determining changes in health state and planning resources.

Methods

Ethics statement

The study was approved by the Health Research Ethics Board at the University of Alberta. Patient consent was not obtained; therefore patient records/information were anonymized and de-identified prior to analysis.

Databases

The province of Alberta has a single payer, government funded health care system, Alberta Health that provides universal access to its 3.7 million residents. Using the data linked from four administrative databases, a cohort was created that identified patients by identifying their first visit with an inpatient diagnosis of heart failure between January 1, 1999, and December 1, 2008.

The four linked databases include: i) the Discharge Abstract Database (DAD), which records dates for all admissions to acute care facilities with the most responsible and up to 25 other diagnoses or comorbidities; ii) the Ambulatory Care Database (which tracks visits to the Emergency Departments and hospital-based clinics and allows for coding of up to 10 conditions; iii) the physician claims database (which tracks all physician claims for outpatient services and includes up to three diagnoses per encounter); and iv) the registry which contains the birth, death and immigration information for all Alberta residents.

Hospitalizations

HF hospitalizations were identified as those hospitalizations with a main diagnosis of HF using ICD-9-CM code 428.x (1999–2002) and ICD-10 code I50.x (2002–2008). The accuracy of these ICD codes for HF has been previously validated against chart audit in Alberta and elsewhere [9–11]. Other (non-HF) hospitalizations were those associated with any acute hospitalization for any other main diagnosis. Due to differences in care patterns for patients with hospitalizations in non-acute facilities, patients entering from or discharged to long term care were censored and removed from further analysis.

The cohort was separated into three groups: patients with a single HF hospitalization; patients with two HF hospitalizations in the five years of follow-up; and patients with three or more HF hospitalizations. Patients were followed for up to five years from their index visit (median: 952 days; IQR: 188–1826).

Statistical analysis

Patient characteristics are presented as numbers and percentages for categorical variables and means and standard deviations or medians and IQRs where relevant. Baseline characteristics were compared according to those with a single hospitalization against those with two and three or more hospitalizations.

Comorbidities were evaluated at every hospitalization so that as patients moved through the maximum five years of follow-up, new diagnoses recorded in hospital, an outpatient clinic or an emergency department could be added. Additionally, at each transition outlined below, the total number of emergency

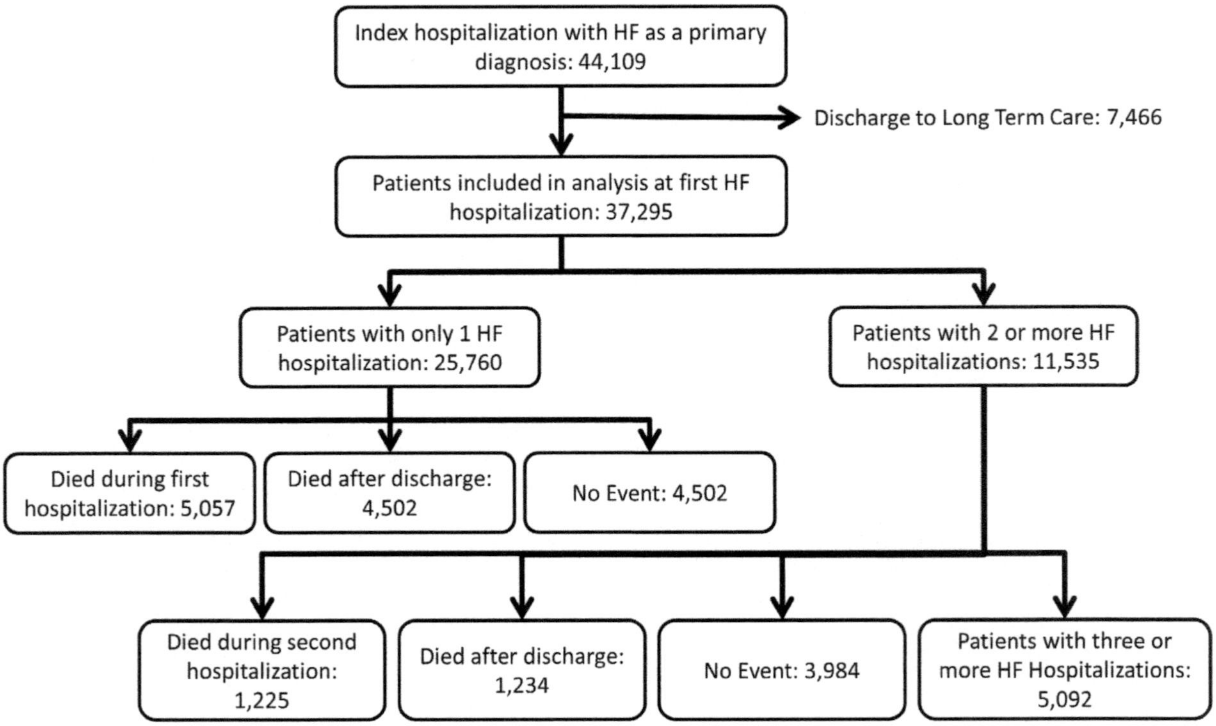

Figure 2. Cohort derivation chart. First two hospitalizations shown

department visits where patients were directly discharged without admission ("treat and release") and physician office visits were counted.

Multivariable models

A series of models were generated adjusted for age, sex, length of stay, acuity of admission, Charlson index, which provides a weighted score based on the number and type of comorbidities, and number of emergency department visits in the six months prior, consistent with the LACE index, which includes the length of stay at the last hospitalization(L), the acuity of the admission (A), the patient's Charlson score (C), and the number of Emergency Department visits in the last six months (E) [12]. Patients were followed for up to five years from their initial HF hospitalization (Figure 1a) to explore changes in gap times as well as the length of stay for each hospitalization. The first set of models utilized a Generalized Estimating Equation (GEE) [8], [13] for the time between hospitalizations. The standard GEE framework examines a single gap-time without consideration for censoring. As such, in the GEE model, we considered the gap-time to be the number of days between discharge from one HF hospitalization until the start of the next hospitalization. Using the GEE approach suggest by Clement, there are limited assumptions about the total number and distribution of events. The GEE model provides a baseline for subsequent model development.

The second model used was a multi-state model [14], [15] where patients are assumed to be in one of four states: 1) Community dwelling (i.e., out of hospital); 2) In hospital with HF as a main diagnosis; 3) In hospital for another reason; or 4) Dead. A multistate model was developed based on both the transitions and time spent in each state; the seven permitted transitions are depicted in Figure 1b. This model considers each non-absorbing state (1 to 3) as a competing risk regression on each available transition, conditional on the patients who have arrived at that state. For example a patient not in hospital is eligible to be hospitalized with HF, hospitalized for another reason, or die as available transitions. This type of model allows for the adjustment of patient factors comorbidities and repeat hospitalizations with a primary diagnosis of HF conditional on the current state. The adjusted times estimates are calculated by comparing the fitted sojourn time (time spent in a given state) between the indicated levels of the target covariate with the other covariates set at the mean level to give an estimate of the effect of changing each variable individually. The index hospitalization is considered to be their first hospitalization with a most responsible diagnosis of HF.

The hospitalizations are considered as episodes of care so that if there are multiple hospitalization records within 24 hours they are treated as a single episode of care. We categorized an episode that had at least one admission with HF as the most responsible diagnosis as an "HF hospitalization" (HFH) while any episode with another main diagnosis as an "Other hospitalization". The model estimates a fitted hazard ratio for the transitions based on the number of hospitalizations, comorbid conditions and outpatient clinic, physician office and emergency department use in the 180 days prior to the hospitalization. From this model, the sojourn time, i.e., the time spent in a given state, was estimated. Two variants of this model are considered: 1) include the number of times that a patient had a HFH to assess the adjusted change in time for repeat hospitalizations; and 2) exclude this information to account only for independent predictors of transition. As a sensitivity analysis we consider the days alive and out of hospital in the year following the discharge from the index episode. In this model we examine the number of days each patient is both alive and not in acute care as a continuous variable during the subsequent year in a multivariable linear regression framework [2].

All Analyses were complete in SAS v. 9.4 (Cary, NC) and R 2.15.2 (Vienna, Austria) using the "msm" package [14].

Table 1. Baseline Cohort Demographics.

Variable	Patients with only one HF Hospitalization	Patients with two HF Hospitalizations	Patients with three or more HF Hospitalizations	*p-value*
N (%)	25760 (69.1)	6443 (17.3)	5092 (13.7)	
Median Follow-up days (IQR)	766 (69,1826)	1117 (391,1826)	1368 (696, 1826)	<0.0001
Median Follow-up days: survivors (IQR)	1580 (679, 1826)	1826 (1004, 1826)	1826 (1391, 1826)	<0.0001
Male	13763 (53.4)	3426 (53.2)	2704 (53.1)	0.88
Age mean (SD)	73.4 (13.6)	74.9 (12.5)	75.4 (11.6)	<0.0001
Ischemic Heart disease	14639 (56.8)	3720 (57.7)	3137 (61.6)	<0.0001
Hypertension	16057 (62.3)	4154 (64.5)	3378 (66.3)	<0.0001
Cerebrovascular disease	4734 (18.4)	1179 (18.3)	930 (18.3)	0.98
Atrial fibrillation	8135 (31.6)	2309 (35.8)	1903 (37.4)	<0.0001
Diabetes	7446 (28.9)	2066 (32.1)	1865 (36.6)	<0.0001
Peripheral Vascular disease	3781 (14.7)	1023 (15.88)	893 (17.5)	<0.0001
Renal disease	3638 (14.1)	966 (15.0)	712 (14.0)	0.17
Chronic Obstructive Pulmonary disease	10182 (39.5)	2866 (44.5)	2432 (47.8)	<0.0001
Dementia	2334 (9.1)	415 (7.0)	232 (4.6)	<0.0001
Cancer	4330 (16.8)	916 (14.2)	671 (13.2)	<0.0001
Charlson Score, mean (SD)	4.88 (2.5)	4.77 (2.3)	4.84 (2.2)	0.004
Visits to emergency department during previous 6 months (mean, SD)	0.74 (1.9)	0.83 (1.9)	1.00 (2.6)	<0.0001
Length of Stay at index hospitalization (mean, SD)	10.2 (7.3)	9.7 (6.9)	9.3 (6.6)	<0.0001
LACE score (mean, SD)	12.7 (2.4)	12.7 (2.4)	12.8 (2.3)	0.0002

The models allowed patient comorbidities to change at later visits, but this table provides only the values from the first HF hospitalization.

Results

We identified 40,667 patients with a first HFH between January 1, 1999 and December 1, 2008 who were not discharged to long term care (Figure 2). During five years of follow-up, this cohort accounted for 127,927 emergency department visits with discharge ("treat and release" visits), 93,924 total hospitalizations, 794,004 total days in hospital, 59,591 HFH and 14,235 deaths (of which 53% [n = 7,590] occurred during a HF hospitalization. Nearly half of the cohort had no further HFH (27,106) during the median follow-up of 2.6 years. The cohort was split into three groups based on whether or not they had one, two or ≥ three HF hospitalizations. Patients hospitalized more often for HF were older and were more likely to have virtually all comorbidities such as diabetes, peripheral arterial disease and COPD but not dementia or cancer (Table 1).

Although approximately half of the patients were not re-hospitalized for HF after each subsequent hospitalization, as the number of successive HF hospitalizations increased, the number of days between both HF specific and all cause hospitalizations dropped (Figure 3, Table 2). The median and IQR days between the first and second hospitalization for patients was 168 (41–533) and then 126 (35–378), 103 (28–280), 80 (23–235) for the 2nd 3rd and fourth gap between hospitalizations. The distribution of patient events (censored alive, re-hospitalized or died) by time groups are given in Figure 4.

For each additional point on the Charlson score at baseline, patients exhibited 13.2 (95% CI: 11.2 to 15.1) fewer days between HF hospitalizations and 14.6 (95% CI: 13.6 to 15.7) fewer days between any hospitalizations (Table 2). Similarly, for each additional year of age there were 2.1 (95% CI: 1.6 to 2.5) fewer days between HF hospitalizations and 1.7 (95% CI: 1.4 to 1.9) fewer days between any hospitalizations. The time between HF hospitalizations was on average reduced by approximately one month (mean 28.6 days; 95%CI 22.4 to 34.8) for each subsequent HF hospitalization. With the exception of gender, the direction and relative magnitude of each covariate was similar between HF and non HF hospitalizations. As a sensitivity analysis, we explored adjusted days alive and out of hospital in the year following the index HF hospitalization and found that the relevant variables in Table 2 exhibited similar associations with this outcome (although length of stay could not be included as it was in the adjusted model; data available on request). We found that the time to first event analysis and the gap time models display similar coefficients; however we note that the precision and thus statistical significance of each parameter is less in the time to first event model. The gap time and the days alive and out of hospital model were similar with the exception of the impact of number of visits to the Emergency Department in the six months prior. This difference is likely due to the insensitivity of the days alive and out of hospital model to differentiate between long hospitalizations, multiple short hospitalizations and deaths. As a sensitivity analysis we re-examined the data using only patients who were alive at the end of the follow-up time and the results were similar (data available on request).

The competing risk hazards for each transition in the multi-state model are presented in Table 3. For example, for each additional

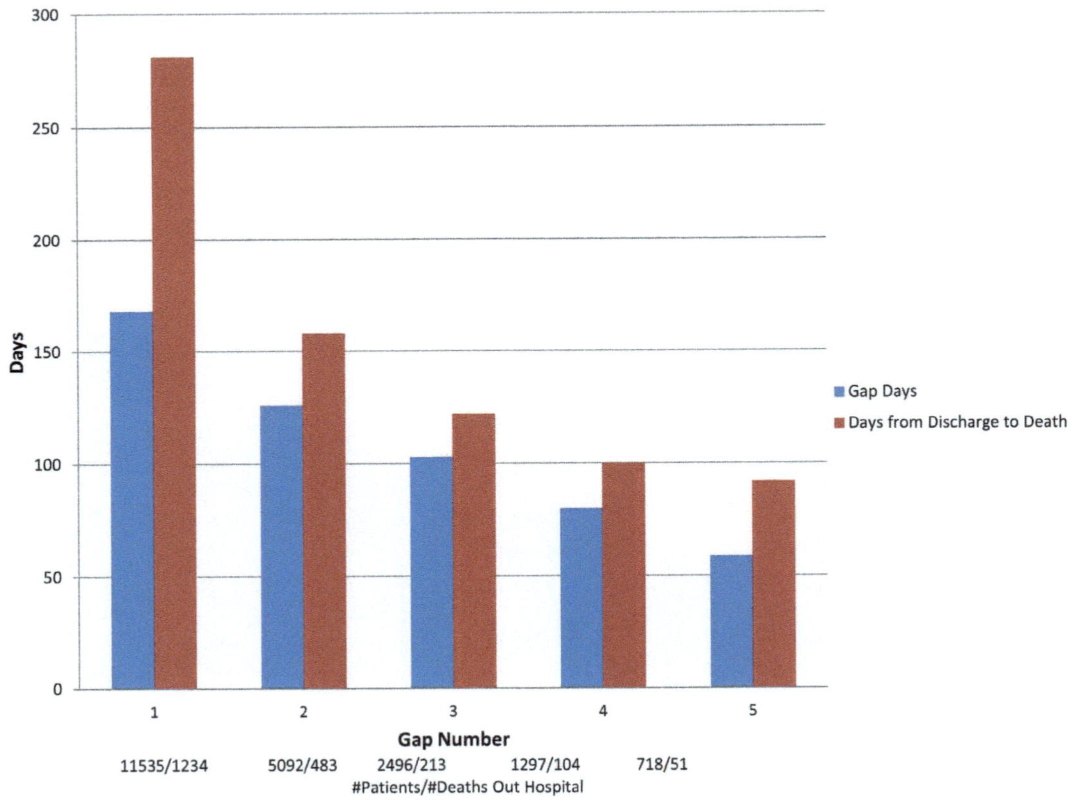

Figure 3. Unadjusted mean times between HF hospitalizations and times to death for HF patients with at least two hospitalizations (1 gap).

point on the Charlson scale, a patient currently out of hospital has a 4% (95% CI 4% to 5%) higher risk of another HF hospitalization, an 7% higher risk (95%CI 7% to 8%) of being hospitalized for another reason, and a 10% (95%CI 8% to 11%) increased risk of out of hospital death. If the number of prior HF hospitalizations is also considered as a factor in the model, a patient with two prior HFH currently out of hospital has a 28% (95% CI 23% to 33%) higher risk of another HF hospitalization, a 4% higher risk (95%CI 1% to 7%) of being hospitalized for another reason, and a 23% (95%CI 13% to 34%) increased risk if they have already had 3 or more HF hospitalizations.

The multistate model extends the days alive and out of hospital model as it allows the estimation of the covariate adjusted time spent in each state (Table 4), as there is no pre-specified or fixed amount of follow-up time. For example, the LOS gives the expected length of stay for a given hospitalization for a patient with the specified demographic/comorbidity level. Each row in the table gives the estimate for that covariate with the other covariates set at their mean values. For example, males spend approximately 5% less time out of hospital despite the fact their length of stay is 10% shorter than female patients (Table 4) – this is because they are more likely to have repeat hospitalizations (Table 3). The time spent out of hospital is reduced with increasing

Table 2. Adjusted 'Gap-time' between hospitalizations in days in GEE model.

Variable	Adjusted time to first event	Adjusted Change in Number of Days between HF hospitalizations	Adjusted Change in Number of Days between all cause hospitalizations	Adjusted Change in Days Alive and out of hospital in the year following index admission
Gap Number	NA	−28.61 (−34.81, −22.41)	−13.62 (−15.39, −11.86)	NA
Male	−0.24 (−10.87, 10.39)	−5.75 (−15.26, −3.76)	2.94 (−2.71, 8.60)	−7.89 (−10.64, −5.14)
Age (per additional year)	−1.98 (−2.40, −1.56)	−2.05 (−2.48, −1.62)	−1.69 (−1.94, −1.44)	−1.90 (−2.00, −1.79)
Length of Stay (per day)	−1.09 (−1.85, −0.33)	−1.13 (−1.85, −0.41)	−0.41 (−0.82, 0.01)	NA
Charlson Score	−18.60 (−20.91, −16.29)	−13.15 (−15.10, −11.20)	−14.62 (−15.69, −13.55)	−13.62 (−14.19, −13.05)
ED visits 180 days prior	−15.99 (−18.18, −13.80)	−8.60 (−10.85, −6.34)	−9.27 (−11.15, −7.38)	−0.97 (−1.39, −0.04)

Negative numbers indicate fewer days between hospitalizations. For example, for any given patient, for each additional year of age, there will be 1.98 fewer days between hospitalizations.

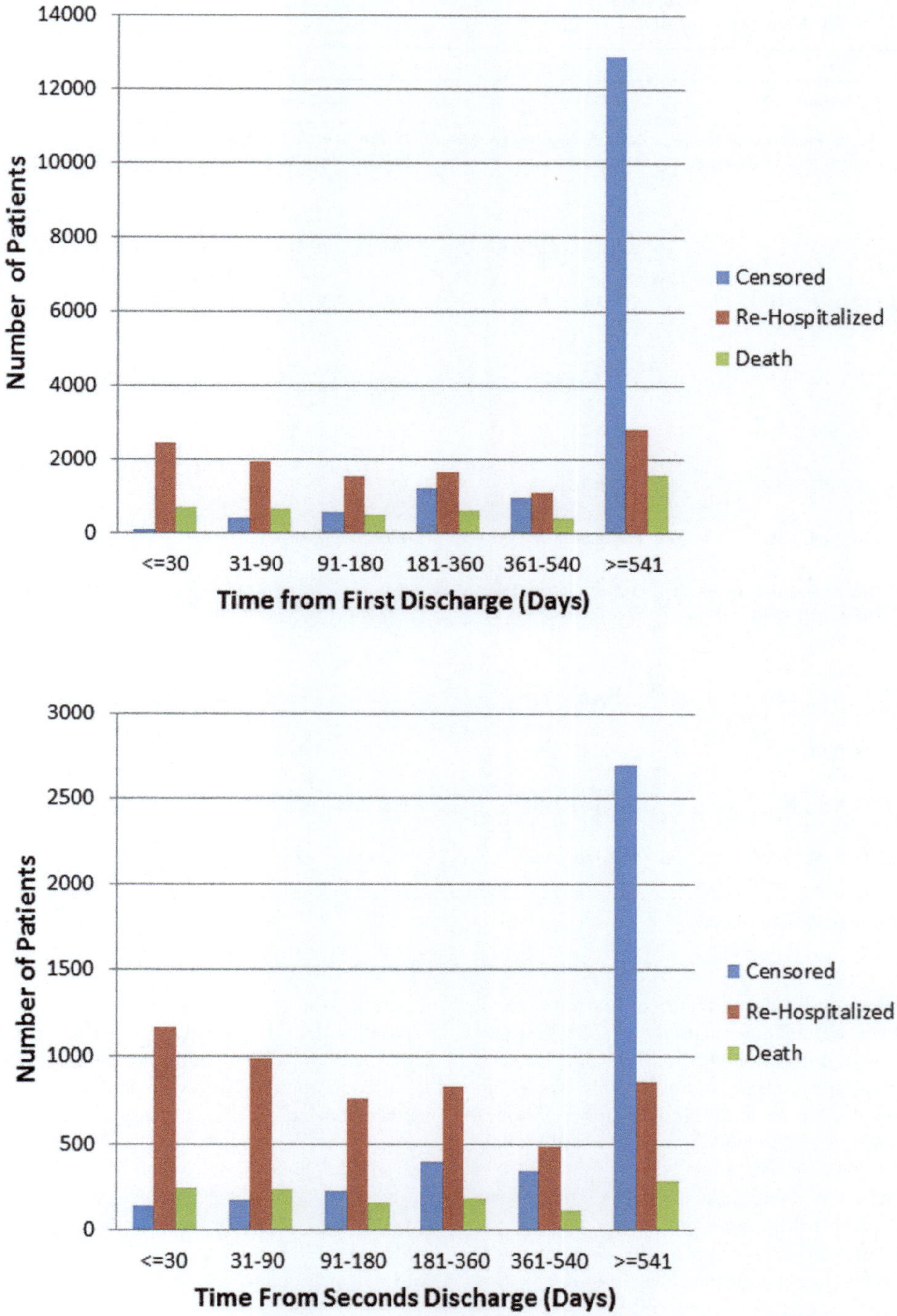

Figure 4. Distribution and times of patients next event following first hospitalization (a); Distribution and times of patients next event following second hospitalization(b).

comorbidity load. Increasing age did not appear to affect the time spent in hospital with HF.

Discussion

Our study demonstrates that the gap-time decreases between each successive hospitalization and this pattern is consistent in both models after adjusting for key prognostic variables such as age, number of Emergency Department visits, and Charlson score. Reporting gap times represent an alternative means of understanding the patient experience that traditional outcomes such as time to first event or proportion of patients who have that event in a defined time frame cannot.

There are a variety of other proportional hazards based repeated events models that have been proposed in the literature [6], these models have the advantage of providing additional information with respect to the models. The Andersen-Gill modifies the proportional hazards model by allowing patients to

Table 3. Hazard Rates for Multistate models.

	Transition				
	Out of Hospital to Heart Failure Hospitalization	**Out of Hospital to Other Hospitalization**	**Death in Hospital Heart Failure Hospitalization**	**Death in Hospital Other Hospitalization**	**Death out of Hospital**
Including Number of Prior HFH					
2 HF Hosp vs 1	1.28 (1.23, 1.33)	1.04 (1.01, 1.07)	0.80 (0.75, 0.85)	0.36 (0.32, 0.42)	0.96 (0.89, 1.03)
3 or more HF Hosp vs 1	3.32 (3.21, 3.43)	1.13 (1.10, 1.17)	0.72 (0.67, 0.78)	1.37 (1.25, 1.51)	1.23 (1.13, 1.34)
Age/5 year	1.03 (1.02, 1.03)	1.03 (1.02, 1.03)	1.09 (1.07, 1.10)	1.00 (0.99, 1.02)	1.15 (1.14, 1.17)
Male vs Female	1.05 (1.02, 1.08)	1.05 (1.02, 1.08)	1.12 (1.06, 1.17)	1.39 (1.30, 1.50)	1.02 (0.96, 1.08)
Number of ED visits 6 months prior	1.00 (0.99, 1.00)	1.00 (0.99, 1.00)	0.99 (0.98, 1.00)	0.95 (0.94, 0.97)	0.95 (0.93, 0.97)
Charlson score	1.04 (1.04, 1.05)	1.07 (1.07, 1.07)	1.05 (1.05, 1.06)	1.06 (1.05, 1.08)	1.10 (1.08, 1.11)
	Out of Hospital to Heart Failure Hospitalization	**Out of Hospital to Other Hospitalization**	**Death in Hospital Heart Failure Hospitalization**	**Death in Hospital Other Hospitalization**	**Death out of Hospital**
Excluding number of Prior HFH					
Age/5 year	1.02 (1.02, 1.03)	1.00 (1.00, 1.01)	1.08 (1.07, 1.09)	1.16 (1.15, 1.18)	1.13 (1.12, 1.15)
Male vs Female	1.04 (1.01, 1.06)	0.97 (0.95, 0.99)	1.11 (1.06, 1.15)	0.94 (0.88, 1.01)	0.98 (0.92, 1.04)
Number of ED visits 6 months prior	0.99 (0.99, 1.00)	1.03 (1.02, 1.03)	0.93 (0.92, 0.95)	1.03 (1.03, 1.04)	1.00 (0.99, 1.02)
Charlson Score	1.04 (1.04, 1.05)	1.06 (1.05, 1.06)	1.11 (1.10, 1.12)	1.01 (1.00, 1.03)	1.12 (1.11, 1.14)

Values are hazard rates (95% confidence intervals).

remain a risk even after the event has occurred, and assumes all events are equal. Other formulations consider stratification and ordering of the events, and do not directly model the time between events. There are important considerations in these models in terms of understanding if there are limits on the number of events and the distribution expected time between events, as well as how to consider the end of follow-up [13].

The use of gap time for evaluating the impact of interventions allows insight beyond simple proportion of patients with mortality/re-hospitalization (after all, if follow-up is sufficiently long then this rate approaches 100% for all patients). This is possible by first separating the re-hospitalizations from the mortality events, then separating the HF hospitalizations from the other hospitalizations, and finally considering both the changing risk and the time spent in the community between multiple hospitalizations. Future studies can utilize this framework to increase the information included in the models. Indeed, there are increasing calls to consider multiple events when evaluating interventions for HF patients but it is important to remember that improved survival outcomes may create multiple re-hospitalizations [16,17].

The gap time concept is similar in concept to the "days alive and out of hospital" which has been reported in several clinical

Table 4. Expected Changes in Adjusted times spent in each state prior to transition with all other covariates set to the mean level.

Comparison	**Alive and out of Hospital Mean Change in Days (95%CI)**	**Length of stay HF Hospitalization Mean Change in Days (95%CI)**	**Length of stay Non HF Hospitalization Mean Change in Days (95%CI)**
Two HF Hospitalizations vs one	−25.47 (−35.22, −16.40)	0.13 (−0.17, 0.42)	−0.21 (−0.44, 0.01)
Three or more HF Hospitalizations vs 2	−94.52 (−97.26, −91.46)	−0.17 (−0.46, 0.13)	−0.29 (−0.48, −0.09)
80 years of age vs 70	−2.88 (−2.89, −2.87)	0.10 (0.09, 0.10)	0.30 (0.29, 0.31)
Male vs Female	2.17 (2.05, 2.29)	0.08 (0.07, 0.09)	0.34 (0.32, 0.36)
1 ED visit in the prior 6 months vs none	−2.06 (−2.17, −1.95)	−0.10 (−0.10, −0.09)	0.09 (0.08, 0.10)
1 point above average on Charlson score	−15.71 (−16.58, −14.88)	0.09 (0.08, 0.10)	0.17 (0.16, 0.18)

trials [2], [18], [19]. As an outcome measurement, "days alive and out of hospital" has the advantage of being a simple metric, but it cannot provide information on how the time was distributed *between* hospitalizations nor does it differentiate if an intervention reduced in-hospital time, death, or both.

There have been numerous attempts to develop prediction scores for HF patients (CMS, LACE etc.) [4], [20], [21]. These models, typically based on 30 day outcomes have not been highly predictive with c-indices between 0.5 and 0.7 [4]. There are three principal reasons that these models do not achieve higher predictive accuracy. First, some (e.g., LACE, LaCE) combine the death and rehospitalization endpoints resulting in a lack of differentiation between those risk factors related to dying and those associated with being re-hospitalized. Secondly, 30 day follow-up windows have no direct physiological implication (i.e., a patient having an event on day 31 is likely similar to one having an event on day 30). Third, these scores typically predict time to first event rather than consideration of total number of events over a longer duration of time. The gap-time method allows the incorporation of the factors related to the multiple events, and additionally provides an indication of whether that gap is increasing or decreasing in length between events. Given the high rate of events and observational data our ability to observe and identify repeat events provides a large cohort on which to model the event patterns. We have used data from an administrative database which, while providing a census of HF hospitalizations in the province of Alberta, does not contain other important indicators of clinical significance. Additional data such as ejection fraction or degree of cardiac remodeling may improve the prediction of our models.

One limitation of the multistate methods is that the outcome states need to be defined and each additional state increases the model complexity exponentially. As such there is still a requirement to create reasonably "simple" groupings and it is difficult to consider every possibility. The multi-state strategy does allow for the important comparison of competing risk conditional on the current state of the patient. For example, a patient with advanced age has a slightly increased risk of another HF hospitalization but is at much higher risk of death out of hospital; if in hospital, for any reason, the hazard ratio of death is smaller. The reasons for the differences in hazard ratio may lie in which patients are healthy enough to be re-hospitalized, are more aware of their condition and seek treatment sooner or some other feature worthy of further investigation. Additionally it is important to consider the impact of each state, a patient in hospital can be discharged home (another transient state) or have a death even in hospital (an "absorbing" state, meaning that the patient does not leave). The inclusion of a treatment strategy could be included as a factor in the model which would allow the identification of which transitions are impacted and to what degree. This type of model could form the foundation for a Markov model (which typically requires the transition probabilities to be pre-specified rather than estimated) and may be clinically useful if deployed in an electronic health record in order to deploy appropriate resources for individual patients flagged as being at above average risk for adverse outcomes. For example, a targeted outpatient intervention may be possible for patients at a high risk of re-hospitalization. We were unable to include medications in our study but this would be next step if it were to include drug type and dose or other interventions into the model.

The development of multi-state models is complex and would benefit from longer term follow-up data and registry/population level data to populate the transitions between states. In the current era of quality metrics, monitoring of these data is becoming increasingly common.

We described the 'gap-time' for patients with heart failure and demonstrated the importance of separating the sources of competing risk for HF patients during follow-up. The gap-time decreased between successive HF hospitalizations, even after accounting for mortality. The use of information such as the gap time provides additional insight into patient experiences (and a potential other outcome for comparative effectiveness studies) beyond the occurrence of short term composite endpoints or time to first even analyses, and is particularly important for chronic diseases like heart failure.

Author Contributions

Analyzed the data: WL. Contributed to the writing of the manuscript: JAB FAM WL JAE.

References

1. Go AS, Mozaffarian D, Roger VL, Benjamin EJ, Berry JD, et al. (2013) Heart disease and stroke statistics–2013 update: A report from the American Heart Association. Circulation 127(1):e6–e245.
2. O'Connor CM, Starling RC, Hernandez AF, Armstrong PW, Dickstein K, et al. (2011) Effect of nesiritide in patients with acute decompensated heart failure. N Engl J Med 365(1): 32–43.
3. McAlister FA, Bakal JA, Kaul P, Quan H, Blackadar R, et al. (2013) Changes in heart failure outcomes after a province-wide change in health service provision a natural experiment in Alberta, Canada. Circ Heart Fail 6(1): 76–82.
4. Au AG, McAlister FA, Bakal JA, Ezekowitz J, Kaul P, et al. (2012) Predicting the risk of unplanned readmission or death within 30 days of discharge after a heart failure hospitalization. Am Heart J 164(3): 365–372.
5. Dunlay SM, Redfield MM, Weston SA, Therneau TM, Hall Long K, et al. (2009) Hospitalizations after heart failure diagnosis a community perspective. J Am Coll Cardiol 54(18): 1695–1702.
6. Kelly PJ, Lim LL (2000) Survival analysis for recurrent event data: An application to childhood infectious diseases. Stat Med 19(1): 13–33.
7. Ezekowitz JA, Kaul P, Bakal JA, Quan H, McAlister FA (2011) Trends in heart failure care: has the incident diagnosis of heart failure shifted from the hospital to the emergency department and outpatient clinics? Eur J Heart Fail. 13(2): 142–147.
8. Hardin J, Hilbe J (2003) Generalized estimating equations. Vol 68(2). London: Chapman and Hall/CRC: 373–379.
9. Lee DS, Donovan L, Austin PC, Gong Y, Liu PP, et al. (2005) Comparison of coding of heart failure and comorbidities in administrative and clinical data for use in outcomes research. Med Care 43(2): 182–188.
10. Quan H, Sundararajan V, Halfon P, Fong A, Burnand B, et al. (2005) Coding algorithms for defining comorbidities in ICD-9-CM and ICD-10 administrative data. Med Care 43(11): 1130–1139.
11. Goff DC Jr, Pandey DK, Chan FA, Ortiz C, Nichaman MZ (2000) Congestive heart failure in the united states: Is there more than meets the I(CD code)? the corpus christi heart project. Arch Intern Med 160(2): 197–202.
12. van Walraven C, Dhalla IA, Bell C, Etchells E, Stiell IG, et al. (2010) Derivation and validation of an index to predict early death or unplanned readmission after discharge from hospital to the community. CMAJ 182(6): 551–557.
13. Clement D, Strawderman R (2009) Conditional GEE for gap times. Biostatistics 10(3): 451–467.
14. Jackson CH (2011) Multi-state models for panel data: The msm package for R. Journal of Statistical Software 38(8): 1–29.
15. Putter H, Fiocco M, Geskus RB (2007) Tutorial in biostatistics: Competing risks and multi-state models. Stat Med 26(11): 2389–2430.
16. Anker SD, McMurray JJ (2012) Time to move on from 'time-to-first': Should all events be included in the analysis of clinical trials? Eur Heart J 33(22): 2764–2765.
17. Claggett B, Wei LJ, Pfeffer MA (2013) Moving beyond our comfort zone. Eur Heart J 34(12): 869–871.
18. Cuffe MS, Califf RM, Adams KF Jr, Benza R, Bourge R, et al. (2002) Short-term intravenous milrinone for acute exacerbation of chronic heart failure: A randomized controlled trial. JAMA 287(12): 1541–1547.
19. Teerlink JR, Cotter G, Davison BA, Felker GM, Filippatos G, et al. (2013) Serelaxin, recombinant human relaxin-2, for treatment of acute heart failure (RELAX-AHF): A randomised, placebo-controlled trial. Lancet 381(9860): 29–39.

20. Keenan PS, Normand SL, Lin Z, Drye EE, Bhat KR, et al. (2008) An administrative claims measure suitable for profiling hospital performance on the basis of 30-day all-cause readmission rates among patients with heart failure. Circ Cardiovasc Qual Outcomes 1(1): 29–37.

21. van Walraven C, Dhalla IA, Bell C, Etchells E, Stiell IG, et al. (2010) Derivation and validation of an index to predict early death or unplanned readmission after discharge from hospital to the community. CMAJ 182(7): 798–803.

5

Excretion of Urinary Orosomucoid 1 Protein Is Elevated in Patients with Chronic Heart Failure

Li-na Hou[1,2]✉, Fei Li[3]✉, Qing-chun Zeng[1], Liang Su[1], Ping-an Chen[1], Zhi-hao Xu[1], Din-ji Zhu[1], Chang-hua Liu[1], Ding-li Xu[1]*

1 State Key Laboratory of Organ Failure Research, Department of Cardiology, Nanfang Hospital, Southern Medical University, Guangzhou, Guangdong, P.R.China, **2** Department of healthy management, Nanfang Hospital, Southern Medical University, Guangzhou, Guangdong, P.R.China, **3** Department of Urology, Nanfang Hospital, Southern Medical University, Guangzhou, Guangdong, P.R.China

Abstract

Easily screening markers for early detection of chronic heart failure (CHF) are lacking. We identified twenty differently expressed proteins including orosomucoid 1(ORM1) in urine between patients with CHF and normal controls by proteomic methods. Bioinformatics analyses suggested ORM1 could be used for further analysis. After verification by western blotting, the urinary levels of ORM1 were quantified with enzyme-linked immunosorbent assay (ELISA) by correcting for creatinine expression. The ORM1-Cr was significantly elevated in CHF patients than normal controls (6498.83 ± 4300.21 versus 2102.26 ± 1069.24 ng/mg). Furthermore, a Spearman analysis indicated that the urinary ORM1 levels had a high positive correlation with the classification of CHF, and the multivariate analysis suggested that the urinary ORM1 content was associated with the plasma amino-terminal pro- brain natriuretic peptide (NT-proBNP) (OR: 2.106, 95% CI: 1.213–3.524, $P = 0.002$) and the New York Heart Association (NYHA) classification (OR: 3.019, 95% CI: 1.329–4.721, $P < 0.001$). In addition, receiving operating curve (ROC) analyses suggested that an optimum cut-off value of 2484.98 ng/mg with 90.91% sensitivity and 85.48% specificity, respectively, could be used for the diagnosis of CHF. To sum up, our findings indicate that ORM1 could be a potential novel urinary biomarker for the early detection of CHF.

Editor: Antonio Paolo Beltrami, University of Udine, Italy

Funding: The authors have no support or funding to report.

Competing Interests: The authors have declared that no competing interests exist.

* Email: dinglixu@fimmu.com

✉ These authors contributed equally to this work.

Introduction

Chronic heart failure (CHF), a clinical syndrome of left ventricular systolic and/or diastolic dysfunction, remains a major threat to public health [1]. It has been estimated that there are currently over 5 million CHF patients, and more than 550,000 new patients diagnosed yearly in the USA [2]. With the ageing of the global population, the CHF populations are increasing. Recent studies have indicated that approximately 20% of people in the world will suffer CHF at some point through their lifetime [3]. Many CHF patients do not receive accurate diagnoses or optimum pharmacological treatments, therefore, resulting in substantial mortality and morbidity.

Although great progress has been made in diagnostic intensity and treatment, the long-term prognosis for CHF is still poor. In addition, the rising incidence of CHF is a cause for concern, and there is currently no gold standard for its diagnosis [4]. Early diagnosis and treatment are extremely important in this disease. Therefore, the development of a reliable, non-invasive biomarker is of considerable clinical importance, aiming at increasing the early detection rate of heart failure and/or predicting the progression of the disease in time.

Proteomic approaches, which could simultaneously analyze thousands of proteins and peptides, can be used to search for novel biomarkers for the early detection of the disease, their development and prognostic assessment, and the selection and monitoring of proper treatment modalities [5]. Proteomic patterns in body fluids present new opportunities for identification of novel, highly-sensitive specific markers for early detection of disease [6]. Obviously, urine samples are derived from minimally invasive procedures in clinical analysis, and recent advances in urinary proteomics have generated interest into new potential biomarkers for various systemic diseases such as various cancers and cardiovascular diseases [7,8]. However, to date, easily applicable screening biomarkers for the early detection of CHF based on urine samples are lacking.

In our study, we applied two-dimensional differential gel electrophoresis (2D-DIGE) proteomic technologies to identify differentially expressed proteins in urinary protein extracts of CHF patients and healthy donors. Furthermore, we suggest that orosomucoid 1 (ORM1) is a potential novel urinary biomarker for the early detection of CHF.

Material and Methods

a) Urinary samples collection and preparation

All subjects in this study were recruited from the Chinese Han population at Nanfang Hospital (Guangzhou, China) from May 2011 to August 2012. The study protocol was approved by the Nanfang Hospital Ethics Committee. All subjects were informed about the purpose of the study and gave their written consent. In all, 197 patients with CHF were confirmed according to the Framingham Heart Study (FHS) diagnostic criteria of CHF [9]. The diagnosis of CHF was based on a complete clinical evaluation, laboratory testing, echocardiography, chest X-ray, and coronary angiography, coupled with plasma amino-terminal pro-brain natriuretic peptide (NT-proBNP) content ≥1000 pg/ml. The diagnosis was conducted independently by two experienced clinicians in Nanfang Hospital, Southern Medical University. Cardiac function for each CHF patient was divided into class II, class III, and class IV according to the Cardiac Function Standard of the New York Heart Association (NYHA). The main exclusion criteria were as follows: unconscious patients; other systemic diseases such as cancer, lung disease, liver cirrhosis, bleeding disorders, severe acute infectious and metabolic disorders. 83 healthy volunteers with no evidence of disease were used as control.

The second voided clean-catch urine samples form subjects were collected in the early morning. Each urine sample (20 ml) was directly collected into a sterile plastic tube and then immediately centrifuged at 2500×g for 10 min at 4°C to remove cell debris and particulate matter. The supernatant was stored at −80°C for further analysis. Repeated freeze-thaw cycles were avoided. All the clinical data of those subjects were collected as well.

b) Proteomic analysis

Equal volume urine specimens from 15 CHF patients and 15 controls were pooled respectively for 2D-DIGE analysis. Of these CHF patients, there were five cases in each NYHA class (II, III and IV). For processing, samples were first thawed on ice with the addition of protease inhibitors, 1 mmol/L phenylmethylsulfonyl fluoride, 5 mmol/L phenanthroline, and 5 mmol/L benzamidine (Sigma, St. Louis, Missouri, USA), and then centrifuged using Centricon Plus-20, 10,000 MWCO devices (Millipore, Bedford, MA, USA). Following extraction, other interfering components in the concentrated urine were removed using a 2D Clean-Up Kit (GE Healthcare, Piscataway, New Jersey, USA) according to the manufacturer's instructions. Protein concentration was measured with the 2D Quant Kit (GE Healtcare, Uppsala, Sweden).

Protein extracts obtained from the pooled urine samples were labeled with Cy2, Cy3 and Cy5 dyes (CyDye DIGE Fluor minimal dyes, GE Healthcare) according to the Ettan two-dimensional difference gel electrophoresis (DIGE) protocol. Briefly, 50 µg of urine protein samples from CHF patients and control group were minimally labeled with 400 pmol of Cy5 and Cy3 fluorescent dyes respectively. An internal pool was labeled with Cy2 and used to assess the reproducibility and statistical inferences. It was generated by combining equal amounts of extracts from all CHF and healthy control samples included in the study. All the labeled reactions were incubated for 30 min on ice protected from light, and then stopped by adding 1 ml of 10 mM lysine for 10 min [10]. Following the labeling reaction, all the three labeled samples were mixed and resolved in one gel.

An immobilized pH gradient (IPG) strip (24 cm, pH 3–10, nonlinear, GE Healthcare) was used for isoelectric focusing. For rehydration, samples were brought to 450 µl with rehydration buffer and 1 ml of mineral oil was added to avoid evaporation. The IPG strips were passively rehydrated overnight at room temperature. Isoelectric focusing was performed according to the protocol provided by the manufacturer (GE Healthcare) as follows: 1 h at 500 V, 1 h at 1000 V, 1 h at 5000 V, 1 h at 8000 V, then maintaining at 8000 V until a total of 60 kVh. After focusing, the strips were prepared for the second dimension gels by incubation for 15 min in equilibrium buffers I and II, respectively. Standard continuous SDS-PAGE electrophoresis for the second dimension (12%) was carried out using an Ettan DALT twelve system (GE Healthcare) until the dye front reached the bottom of the gels. Following SDS-PAGE, image scans were performed immediately using a Typhoon 9410 scanner (GE Healthcare) at the excitation emission of 488/520 nm (Cy2), 532/580 nm (Cy3) and 633/670 nm (Cy5), respectively. In addition, another strip with 1000 mg of proteins loaded was performed in parallel as a preparative gel for spots picking as marked in 2D-DIGE. The gel was stained with Coomassie Brilliant Blue [11]. Identical samples were run in three times.

After scanning, the gel images were analyzed using the DeCyder 5.01 software (GE Healthcare). Its differential in-gel analysis (DIA) module was used for pairwise comparisons of each sample with the internal standard within each gel by calculating the normalized spot volumes. The spot volumes were calculated by the background intensities combined with the borders of the spots. Spot volumes were normalized by dividing each Cy3 or Cy5 spot volume with the corresponding internal standard (Cy2). The average abundance changes for each spot across the different spot maps were calculated with the DeCyder biological variation analysis (BVA) module. The spots whose ratios of Cy5/Cy2 and Cy3/Cy2 changed by 1.5-fold or greater were regarded as differently up- or down- regulated expressed spots and were considered for further protein identification.

As described in our previous studies [12,13], the protein spots were identified by matrix-assisted laser desorption time-of-flight mass spectrometry (MALDI-TOF/TOF-MS). Shortly, the differentially expressed protein spots were excised from the Coomassie-stained gels with an Ettan Spot Picker (GE Healthcare), and then subjected to trypsin digestion, peptide extraction and desalting. The peptide mixtures were analyzed using an ABI Voyager DE-STR mass spectrometer (ABI 4700 Proteomic Analyzer, Applied Biosystems, Foster City, CA, USA). A trypsin- fragment peak was served as an internal standard for mass calibration. A list of the corrected mass peaks was the peptide mass fingerprinting (PMF).

Protein identification using peptide mass fingerprinting was performed using the MASCOT search engine (http://www.matrixscience.com/, Matrix Science Ltd, London, UK) against the MSDB protein database. The search was defined as the Homo sapiens subsets of the sequences in the Swiss–Prot and NCBI nonredundant protein sequence databases. The following search parameters were used during the searche: tolerance of one missed trypsin cleavages, the errors in peptide mass were within 25 ppm for both the precursor mass tolerance and the fragments mass. Carbamidomethylation of cysteine and oxidation of methionine as fixed and variable modifications, respectively, were taken into account for database searching. The proteins matched more than four peptides and with a MASCOT score higher than 63 were considered statistically significant ($P<0.05$). The identification results were filtered by peakErazor software (Lighthouse Data, Odense, Denmark). All matched sequences were manually validated [12,13].

c) Bioinformatic analysis

The interaction network of differentially expressed proteins was performed automatically by STRING (Search Tool for the Retrieval of Interacting Genes/Proteins; version 8.3; http://string.embl.de/) with following analysis parameters[14]: species — Homo sapiens, confidence level — 0.400, active prediction methods — all. The PubGene Analysis tool (http://www.pubgene.org/) was used to search for literature bio-association analysis of these proteins [15]. The bio-associations had the following categories in Pubgene: Process, Function and Component. The key bio-processes related to the identified proteins were retrieved for further analysis.

d) Western blotting analysis

For western blot analyses, the samples involved six CHF patients (n = 2 in each class II, III and IV of NYHA), and six healthy controls. A total of 30 μg prepared urine proteins were separated by 12% SDS-PAGE. The gels were then transferred onto Polyvinylidene Xuoride (PVDF) (Millipore) membranes. The membranes were blocked in a solution of TBS containing 5% nonfat milk powder and 0.1% Tween-20 for 1 h at room temperature and then incubated overnight at 4°C with the monoclonal antibody against the human ORM1 protein (diluted 1:500; Abcam, UK). After three 10-min washes in TBS-T, the membranes were incubated with horseradish peroxidase horseradish (HRP) conjugate of goat anti-rabbit IgG (Bioworld Technology, Louis Park, MN, USA) at a 1:5000 dilution at room temperature for 1 h. The proteins were detected using an enhanced chemiluminescence (ECL, Pierce, Rockford, IL, USA) detection system. Relative intensities were documented and analyzed by densitometry.

e) Enzyme-linked immunosorbent assay (ELISA) analysis

The concentration of ORM1 protein in urine samples was measured with a commercially available ELISA kit (R&D Systems, Minneapolis, USA) according to the manufacturer's instructions. The assay has a minimum detectable dose of ORM1 at 0.538 ng/ml, exhibiting linearity between 3.12 and 200 ng/ml. The standard curve was created using the suppliers' lyophilized human ORM1. The levels of urinary ORM1 were corrected by urinary creatinine (Cr) concentrations to avoid the influence of urine volume. Thereby, the results were expressed as ORM1 -to-Cr ratio (ORM1/Cr nanograms per miligrams of creatinine). Urine creatinine (Cr) levels were measured at the Department of Clinical Laboratory of Nanfang Hospital (Guangzhou, China).

f) Statistical methods

All data were collected and used for statistical analyses with SPSS software 13.0 (SPSS, Chicago, IL, USA). Values were presented as mean ± standard deviation (SD). The difference among two groups or three groups was compared with Student's t test or one-way ANOVA. A Spearman analysis was performed to explore the relationship between urinary ORM1-Cr and the clinical characteristics of subjects where appropriate. Univariate (nonparametric rank sum test) and multivariate (logistic regression) analyses were conducted to evaluate the relationship between urinary ORM1 expression and clinical parameters of CHF, including age, sex, diabetes, hypertension, coronary heart disease, cardiomyopathy, renal dysfunction, left ventricular ejection fraction (LVEF), NT-proBNP and NYHA classification. Receiving operating curve (ROC) analyses were used to define the most optimal diagnostic cutoff as well as the diagnostic performance given by the area under the curve (AUC), estimating the sensitivity versus its false-positive rate at optimal cutoffs. The best statistical cut-off value of ORM1-Cr was defined, which means the point at which the sum of sensitivity and specificity is more than other points. The results were considered statistically significant at P-value <0.05.

Results

a) Clinical characteristics of subjects

Table 1 has list the clinical characteristics of all subjects in our study. There was no statistical difference in clinical characteristics (e.g. age, sex, serum creatinine and urinary creatinine). The urine samples form 15 CHF patients and 15 controls were randomly selected for 2D-DIGE analysis. Among the 15 CHF patients, there were five cases in each class II, III and IV of NYHA. Furthermore, there were 176 CHF patients and 62 healthy volunteers recruited for ELISA quantitative analysis. Of these 176 subjects with CHF, the CHF cases belonging to class II, III and IV numbered 34, 87 and 55 respectively.

b) 2D-DIGE analysis and twenty differently expressed proteins were identified by MALDI-FOF/TOF-MS

Figure 1 has shown a representative 2D-DIGE image from proteomic profiling of urine samples from patients with CHF and healthy controls. After quantitative and statistical analysis, the 28 differential protein spots with volumes changed by 1.5-fold or more were selected for further identification by MALDI-FOF/TOF-MS. These 28 differently expressed protein spots corresponded to twenty different protein accession numbers (Fig. 1). Seven proteins were significantly up-regulated in CHF and the other thirteen were down- regulated. The up-regulated proteins were Cadherin-1 (CDH1), Zinc-alpha-2-glycoprotein (AZGP1), Alpha-1-acid glycoprotein 1 (ORM1), Protein AMBP (AMBP), Ig kappa chain C region (IGKC), Ig lambda-1 chain C regions (IGLC1),Ganglioside GM2 activator (GM2A). The down-regulated proteins involved Uromodulin (UMOD), Kininogen-1 (KNG1), Alpha-amylase 1 (AMY1A), Vitamin D-binding protein (GC), Pancreatic alpha-amylase (AMY2A), Serum albumin (ALB), Leukocyte elastase inhibitor (SERPINB1), Inter-alpha-trypsin inhibitor heavy chain H4 (ITIH4), Prothrombin (F2), Calbindin (CALB1), Basement membrane-specific heparan sulfate proteoglycan core protein (HSPG2), Mannan-binding lectin serine protease 2 (MASP2), CD59 glycoprotein (CD59). Information about these protein spots concerning access numbers, gene names, molecular weight, PI, total ion scores, fold changes of spots volumes and overall trends is presented in Table 2.

c) ORM1 was indicated for further investigation based on bioinformatics analysis

Pubgene analysis of the twenty identified proteins was performed to search for the associated bio-processes. As a result, this analysis predicted 1,600 different bio-processes to be associated with identified proteins. The top 15 closely related bio-processes included growth, induction, signal transduction, pathogenesis, secretion, catabolic process, digestion, localization, translation, coagulation, death, RNA splicing, apoptosis, phosphorylation and complement activation. Noticeably, ORM1 was predicted to play important roles in many of these 15 bio-processes such as growth, induction, signal transduction, pathogenesis, catabolic process, coagulation and phosphorylation (Table 3). Furthermore, we observed tight connections between ORM1 and other identified proteins such as ALB, AMBP and ITIH4 from the Network based on co-occurrence in articles, which was consistent with the result by STRING 9.0 program. Those findings suggested that ORM1 was a key function partner with ALB, AMBP and ITIH4 (Fig. 2B), which play vital roles in the development of acute-phase reaction and inflammation indicated by Pubgene (not shown).

Table 1. Clinical data for subjects in the study.

	Samples for 2D-DIGE		Samples for ELISA	
	Controls	CHF	Controls	CHF
Number	15	15	62	176
Gender (Male/Female)	8/7	6/9	30/32	99/78
Age (years)	58.67±14.89	61.73±13.82	59.82±13.17	62.62±14.59
Urine creatinine (mg/dl)	97.91±46.03	113.29±63.08	97.91±46.03	113.29±63.08
Serum creatinine (umol/L)	99.72±46.57	115.47±68.94	100.63±49.29	118.45±70.57
NT-proBNP (pg/ml)	/	6852.12±7816.69	/	7703.96±8695.85

d) Verification of higher urinary ORM1 levels in patients with CHF

To further verify our proteomic findings, we used western blotting analysis to study the expression of urinary ORM1 in individual samples from patients with CHF and control groups. The results clearly demonstrated that urinary ORM1 was significantly up-regulated in CHF cases in comparison to controls. These variations in urinary ORM1 expression were consistent with our DIGE results (Fig. 3).

e) Quantification of urinary ORM1 by ELISA

ELISA was used to quantify urinary ORM1 levels in 176 patients with CHF and 62 healthy controls. After normalization by creatinine level, the urinary ORM1 was markedly elevated in patients with CHF compared to controls (6498.83±4300.21 versus 2102.26±1069.24 ng/mg, $P<0.0001$) (Fig. 4A). When the CHF patients were stratified by NYHA classification, the urinary ORM1 concentrations were 3086.24±1474.91, 6284.97±4088.02 and 8946.71±4298.05 ng/mg for CHF patients with class II, III and IV, respectively. The expression level of urinary ORM1 was positively associated with the class of CHF classification

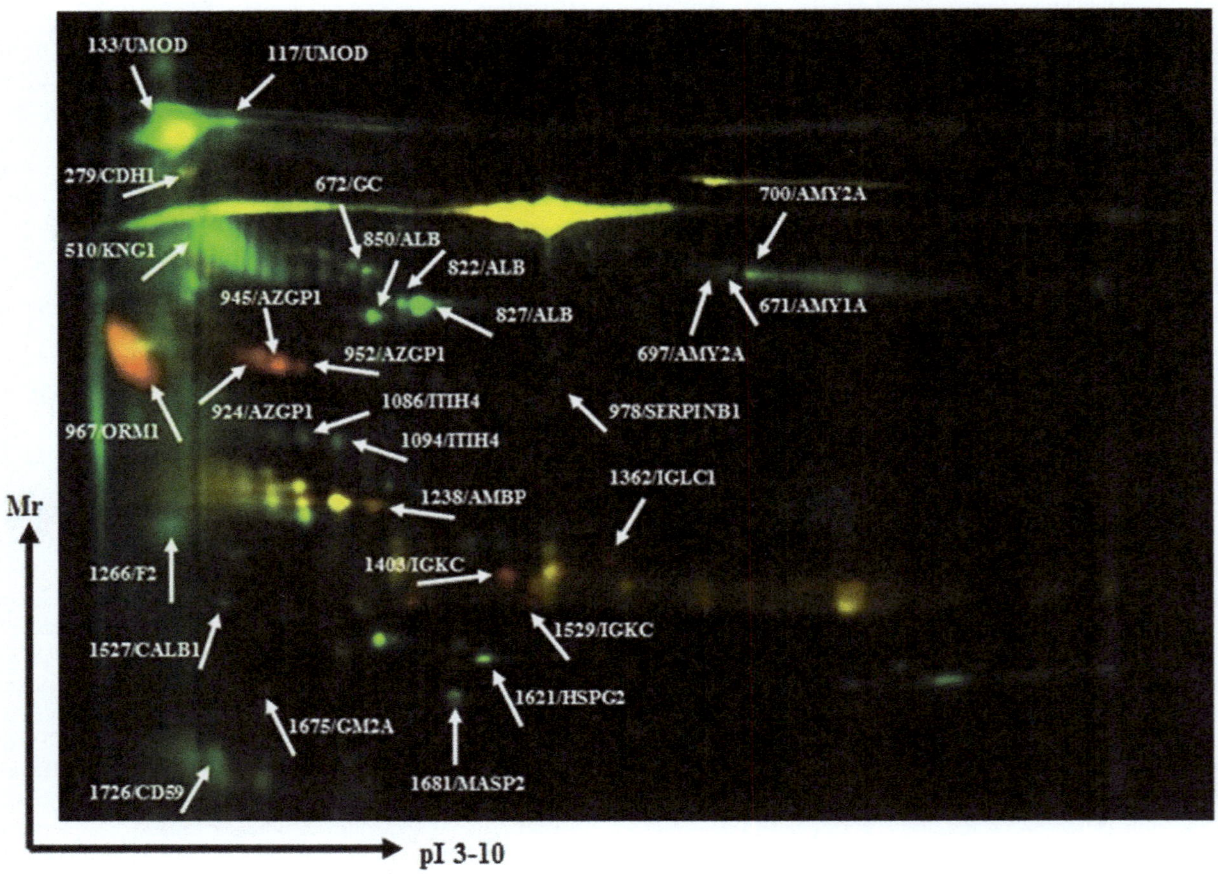

Figure 1. Distribution of all 28 differentially expressed protein spots in a representative two- dimensional fluorescent differential gel electrophoresis (2D-DIGE) image from proteomic profiling of urine samples from patients with CHF and healthy controls. Further identified protein spots are indicated by spot ID. Protein spots, protein name and spot ID are indicated (arrows).

Table 2. Identification of differentially expressed proteins in urine from chronic heart failure and normal control.

Master number	Accession No.	Gene Name	Protein molecular weight	Protein PI	Pep. Count[a]	Total ion score	Fold changes[b]	Overall trend[c]
117	P07911	UMOD	72451.4	5.05	9	518	-12.77 ± 3.46	down
133	P07911	UMOD	72451.4	5.05	9	323	-10.37 ± 3.18	down
279	P12830	CDH1	97852	4.58	3	212	3.15 ± 0.29	up
510	P01042	KNG1	72995.6	6.34	7	263	-2.54 ± 0.33	down
671	P04745	AMY1A	58415.2	6.47	7	213	-3.05 ± 2.19	down
672	P02774	GC	54525.6	5.4	3	134	-3.33 ± 1.26	down
697	P04746	AMY2A	58354.3	6.6	8	106	-2.45 ± 1.06	down
700	P04746	AMY2A	58354.3	6.6	8	215	-2.33 ± 0.52	down
822	P02768	ALB	71317.2	5.92	8	208	-4.33 ± 0.51	down
827	P02768	ALB	71317.2	5.92	9	229	-6.31 ± 1.21	down
850	P02768	ALB	71317.2	5.92	7	163	-6.24 ± 0.89	down
924	P25311	AZGP1	34079	5.57	5	265	7.31 ± 1.54	up
945	P25311	AZGP1	34079	5.57	4	245	7.55 ± 1.89	up
952	P25311	AZGP1	34079	5.57	6	349	7.46 ± 2.27	up
967	P02763	ORM1	23724.8	4.93	3	302	14.81 ± 3.49	up
978	P30740	SERPINB1	42828.7	5.9	5	233	-3.96 ± 1.12	down
1086	Q14624	ITIH4	103521.1	6.51	4	189	-3.96 ± 1.23	down
1094	Q14624	ITIH4	103521.1	6.51	5	212	-2.89 ± 0.63	down
1238	P02760	AMBP	39886.3	5.95	4	298	5.63 ± 2.03	up
1266	P00734	F2	71474.7	5.64	3	167	-4.55 ± 1.96	down
1362	P01842	IGLC1	11400.6	6.92	1	32	-11.72 ± 3.69	up
1403	P01834	IGKC	11772.7	5.58	1	94	17.63 ± 5.67	up
1527	P05937	CALB1	30291.1	4.7	3	77	-4.09 ± 0.86	down
1529	P01834	IGKC	11772.7	5.58	1	50	4.43 ± 1.49	up
1621	P98160	HSPG2	479220.5	6.06	6	253	-2.89 ± 1.34	down
1675	P17900	GM2A	21280.9	5.17	2	152	6.31 ± 3.63	up
1681	O00187	MASP2	77224.2	5.47	7	351	-3.15 ± 1.74	down
1726	P13987	CD59	14795	6.02	1	59	2.99 ± 1.36	down

[a] Calculated by amino acid count.
[b] Fold changes of spot intensities represented as mean ± SD.
[c] up: up-regulated in the heart failure group. down: down-regulated in the heart failure group.

Table 3. Top 15 of total 1600 bio-process for the twenty identified proteins in Pubgene.

Description	Associated Terms	Article (p-value)
Growth	ALB, AMBP, AMY1A, AMY2A, AZGP1, CALB1, CD59, CDH1, F2, GC, GM2A, HSPG2, IGKC ITIH4 KNG1, MASP2, ORM1, SERPINB1, UMOD	7.96
Induction	ALB, AMBP, AMY1A, AMY2A, AZGP1, CALB1, CD59, CDH1, F2, GC, GM2A, HSPG2, IGKC, ITIH4, KNG1, MASP2, ORM1, SERPINB1, UMOD	3.97
Signal transduction	ALB, AMBP, AMY1A, AMY2A, AZGP1, CALB1, CD59, CDH1, F2, GC, GM2A, HSPG2, IGKC, ITIH4, KNG1, MASP2, ORM1, SERPINB1, UMOD	3.93
Pathogenesis	ALB, AMBP, AMY1A, AMY2A, AZGP1, CALB1, CD59, CDH1, F2, GC, GM2A, HSPG2, IGKC, ITIH4, KNG1, MASP2, ORM1, SERPINB1, UMOD	3.76
Secretion	ALB, AMBP, AMY1A, AMY2A, CALB1, CD59, CDH1, F2, GC, GM2A, HSPG2, ITIH4, KNG1, SERPINB1, UMOD	3.15
Catabolic process	ALB, AMY1A, AMY2A, AZGP1, CALB1, CD59, CDH1, F2, GC, GM2A, HSPG2, IGKC, ITIH4, KNG1, ORM1, SERPINB1, UMOD	3.1
Digestion	ALB, AMY1A, AMY2A, AZGP1, CALB1, CD59, CDH1, F2, GC, GM2A, HSPG2, IGKC, ITIH4, KNG1, MASP2, SERPINB1, UMOD	2.49
Localization	ALB, AMY1A, AMY2A, AZGP1, CALB1, CD59, CDH1, F2, GC, GM2A, HSPG2, IGKC, ITIH4, KNG1, MASP2, SERPINB1, UMOD	2.44
Translation	ALB, AMBP, AMY1A, AMY2A, AZGP1, CALB1, CD59, CDH1, F2, GC, GM2A, HSPG2, IGKC, ITIH4, KNG1, MASP2, SERPINB1, UMOD	1.95
Coagulation	ALB, AMY1A, AMY2A, CD59, CDH1, F2, GC, HSPG2, ITIH4, KNG1, MASP2, ORM1, SERPINB1, UMOD	1.53
Death	ALB, AMY1A, AMY2A, AZGP1, CALB1, CD59, CDH1, F2, GC, GM2A, HSPG2, IGKC, ITIH4, KNG1, MASP2, SERPINB1, UMOD	1.33
RNA splicing	ALB, CDH1, IGKC, IGLC1	1.1
Apoptosis	ALB, AMBP, AMY1A, AMY2A, CALB1, CD59, CDH1, F2, GC, HSPG2, ITIH4, KNG1, SERPINB1, UMOD	1.04
phosphorylation	ALB, AMY1A, AMY2A, CALB1, CD59, CDH1, F2, GC, HSPG2, IGKC, ITIH4, KNG1, ORM1, UMOD	1
complement activation	ALB, CD59, CDH1, ITIH4, KNG1, MASP2	0.982

P= term/total (number of records of terms according to a specific function divided by their total number of records in the MEDLINE).

(P<0.0001). The correlation indicated by the Spearman test is 0.499, suggesting that the level of ORM1 was markedly elevated in urine as heart failure worsened. In addition, the relationship between urinary ORM1 levels and the clinical characteristics of patients with CHF is presented in Table 4. There was no significant association between the urinary ORM1 expression and other clinical features of CHF such as age, sex, diabetes, hypertension, coronary heart disease, cardiomyopathy, renal dysfunction and left ventricular ejection fraction (LVEF) except for NT-proBNP and the classification of CHF. Furthermore, the multivariate analysis suggested that the urinary ORM1 content was associated with the NT-proBNP (OR: 2.106, 95% CI: 1.213–3.524, $P = 0.002$) and the NYHA classification of CHF (OR: 3.019, 95% CI: 1.329–4.721, P<0.001) (Table 5).

f) Evaluation of urinary ORM1 as a potential biomarker for CHF

After quantitative measurement of ORM1 in 238 urine samples by ELISA, we applied ROC curves to assess the potential utility of urinary ORM1 in diagnosing and monitoring CHF. ROC analyses rendered an optimum cut-off value of 2484.98 ng/mg corresponding to 90.91% sensitivity and 85.48% specificity. The area under the ROC curve (AUC) of ORM1-Cr for diagnosis of CHF was 0.892 (95% confidence interval (CI) 0.848–0.936).

Discussion

The exact incidence and prevalence of CHF remain probably underestimated due to the difficulties in accurate diagnosis [16]. Easily applicable screening markers for the early detection of the

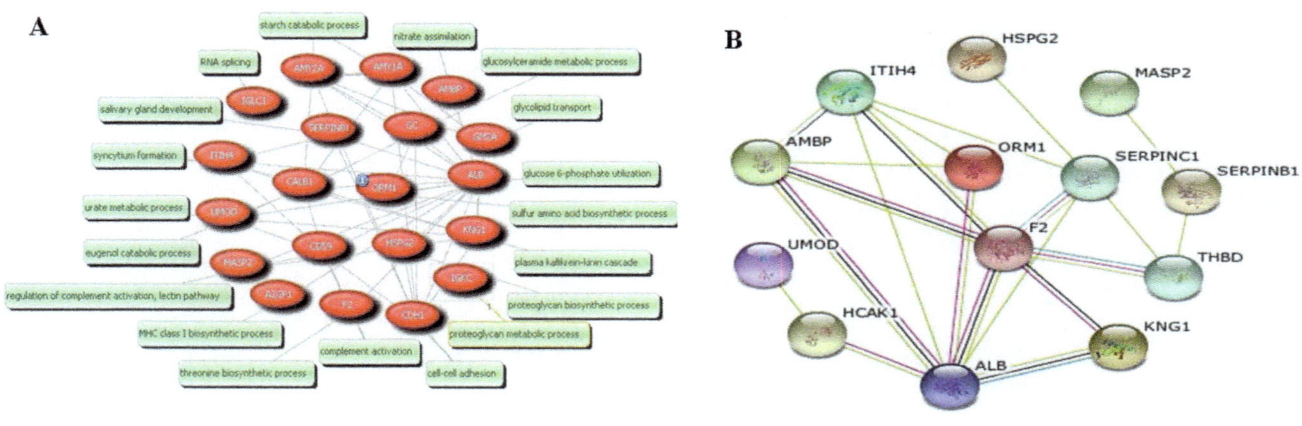

Figure 2. Bioinformatic analysis of bio-association network by Pubgene and String programs. (A) Bio-process associated with the twenty identified proteins was indicated by Pubgene. (B)The ORM1 protein function partner network was indicated by String analysis.

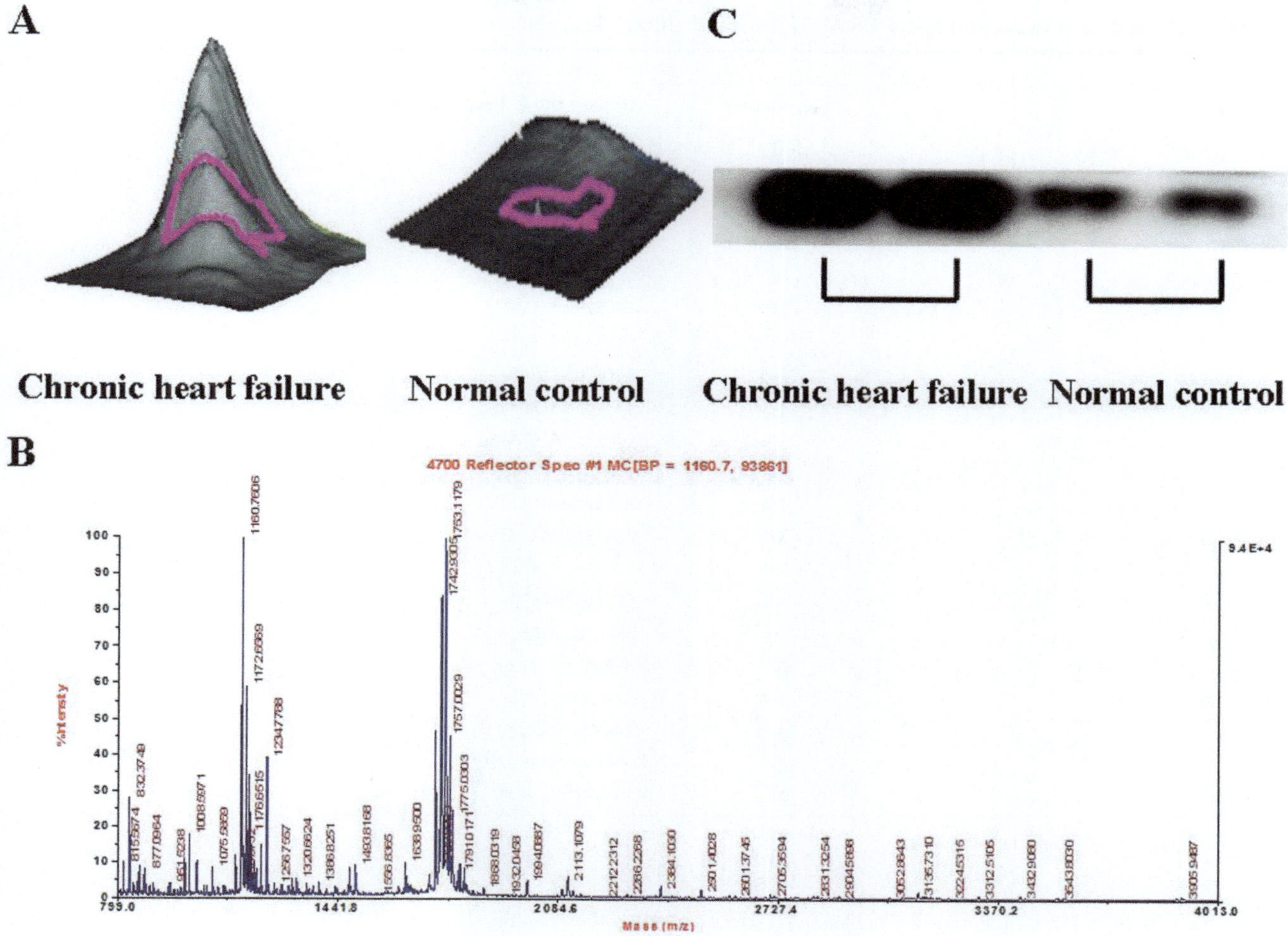

Figure 3. Verification of ORM1 protein expression in urine samples form patients with CHF and normal controls. (A) A 3-D view of ORM1 protein was to show the higher expression of ORM1 protein in urine of patients with CHF compared with normal controls. (B) Verification of ORM1 expression in individual urine samples of patients with CHF and normal controls by western blotting. (C) MS of in-gel trypsin digests of the protein and analysis of the depicted peptide spectrum resulted in the identification of ORM1.

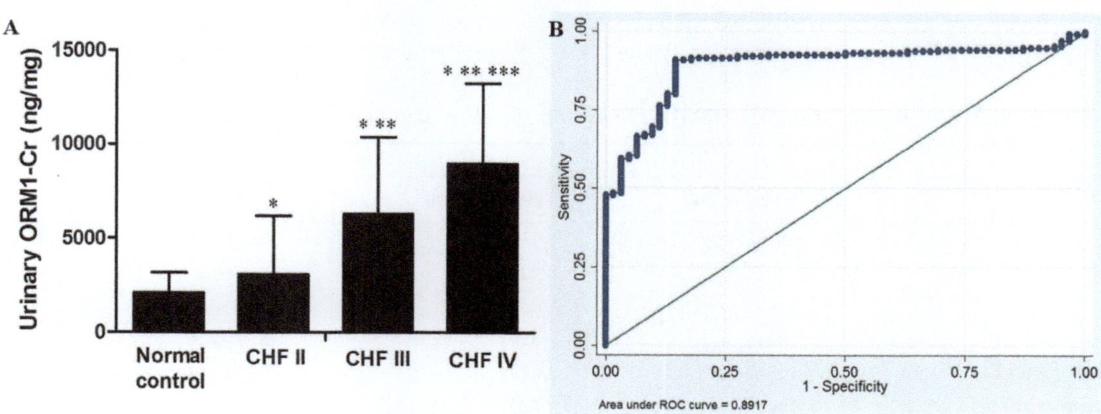

Figure 4. Urinary ORM1 as a potential biomarker for CHF. (A) ELISA was used to quantify urinary ORM1 levels in 176 patients with CHF and 62 healthy controls. The expression level of ORM1 in different NYHA functional classification of CHF. *$P < 0.05$ compared with control group; **$P < 0.05$ compared with CHF I; ***$P < 0.05$ compared with CHF III. (B) ROC curve of urinary ORM1 as a detection marker for CHF was based on a series of 238 urine samples. The optimal cut off was 2484.98 ng/mg, and the area under the ROC curve (AUC) for diagnosis of CHF was 0.892 (95% confidence interval (CI) 0.848–0.936).

Table 4. Relationship between urinary ORM1/Cr level and chronic heart failure.

Clinical features	Number	Urinary ORM1 levels (ng/mg)	*P*
age≥65 years	83	6608.92±4207.72	0.750
age<65 years	93	6400.57±4401.53	
Male	108	6254.27±4292.88	0.343
Female	68	6887.25±4314.96	
With diabetes	28	6284.09±4181.24	0.664
Without diabetes	148	6437.29±4333.47	
With hypertension	68	5894.90±3791.18	0.140
Without hypertension	108	6879.08±4567.93	
With coronary heart disease	62	6885.65±4416.60	0.380
Without coronary heart disease	114	6288.45±4240.41	
With cardiomyopathy	42	6033.04±3915.83	0.423
Without cardiomyopathy	134	6644.82±4417.51	
With renal dysfunction	31	7503.97±4472.75	0.152
Without renal dysfunction	145	6283.94±4247.46	
LVEF<50%	136	6922.04±4432.13	0.153
LVEF≥50%	40	5990.78±4106.26	
NT-proBNP≥7704* pg/ml	62	8344.42±4719.76	<0.001
NT-proBNP<7704 pg/ml	114	5495.09±3705.04	
NYHA II	34	3086.24±1474.91	<0.001
NYHA III	87	6284.97±4088.02	
NYHA IV	55	8946.71±4298.05	

* The mean value of NT-proBNP in CHF patients.

clinical course of CHF are currently lacking. A number of published studies have used proteomic methods to identify novel biomarkers for a variety of diseases. Notably, urinary proteomic biomarker models have recently been developed and shown potential for the accurate identification of several different disorders including ischaemic heart disease [17], endometriosis [18], diabetic nephropathy [19] and some cancers [20,21].

In our present study, we focused on the urinary proteome, because urine is easy to collect relatively large quantities using non-invasive procedures compared with other body fluids. Moreover, the clinical importance of some urinary proteins has been demonstrated not only in urogenital diseases, but also in other systemic diseases [22–24]. Here, we conducted a 2D-DIGE analysis, which is an accurate quantitative comparison proteomic method, to compare the different protein expression profiles in the urine proteomes between CHF patients and healthy controls. Twenty differentially expressed proteins were identified as candidate biomarkers correlated with CHF. We further identified ORM1 as a novel CHF-related biomarker, which was significantly up-regulated in CHF patients, by bioinformatic analysis, western blotting and ELISA analyses.

Our bioinformatic analyses indicated that ORM1 played important roles in many bio-processes such as growth, induction, signal transduction, pathogenesis, catabolic process, coagulation

Table 5. The multivariate analysis of urinary ORM1/Cr level and clinical parameters.

Parameter	*p*-value(uni)	*p*-value(multi)	95% CI	OR
Age	0.815	0.637	0.563–1.426	1.012
Sex	0.567	0.346	0.852–1.639	1.156
Diabetes	0.342	0.266	0.899–1.963	1.818
Hypertension	0.459	0.501	0.603–2.507	1.962
Coronary heart disease	0.147	0.193	0.786–3.722	2.321
Cardiomyopathy	0.861	0.632	0.479–1.892	1.523
Renal dysfunction	0.201	0.153	0.463–1.557	0.678
LVEF	0.747	0.518	0.902–1.010	0.998
NT-proBNP	<0.001	0.002	1.213–3.524	2.106
NYHA classification	<0.001	<0.001	1.329–4.721	3.019

and phosphorylation. ORM1 was also suggested to be a key function partner with ALB, AMBP and ITIH4 (Fig. 2B). Furthermore, inflammation was demonstrated to be associated with the pathophysiology of CHF [25]. ORM1 is a prominent component of the temporary proteinuria, which could be associated with exercise and acute inflammation [26]. To date, a study regarding the association between urinary ORM1 and CHF has not been reported. Thus, ORM1 was selected for further investigation in our study.

ORM1 (Orosomucoid-1, α1-acid glycoprotein 1), a single-chain polypeptide with a high carbohydrate moiety (42%) and a strong negative charge (isoelectric point, 2.7), functions as a transport protein in the bloodstream [27,28]. It binds various ligands in the interior of its beta-barrel domain, and also binds synthetic drugs and influences their distribution and availability in the body. Human liver cells are normally the site of ORM1 production, but it can also be produced in endothelial cells and some tumor cells [29]. Some studies have demonstrated that ORM1 could be also synthesized by lymphocytes, macrophages, monocytes and granulocytes [26,30]. ORM1, a member of immunocalins family, has a regulatory dampening effect on the inflammatory cascade, thereby protecting against tissue damage from excessive inflammation [28,31]. Some studies have demonstrated that the concentrations of ORM1 in plasma and urine are usually much lower than albumin, but increased in urine to concentrations equal to or higher than albumin in conditions of acute inflammation and tissue repair [32–34].

To the best of our knowledge, this study is the first time that ORM1 has been identified in urine from patients with CHF by 2D-DIGE proteomic means. Our urinary proteome findings showed that the expression of ORM1 was significantly increased 14.81-fold in the CHF group compared with healthy controls. Meanwhile, the expression of elevated ORM1 in urine from CHF patients was further confirmed by western blotting. After quantitative ELISA analysis of urinary ORM1 in 238 individual samples, we observed that the levels of urinary ORM1 were elevated in CHF patients than controls, with significant difference found. Furthermore, the Spearman analysis showed that urinary ORM1 had a high positive correlation with the NYHA functional classification of CHF, indicating that the increased level of urinary ORM1 was associated with the CHF worsened, and the multivariate analysis indicated that the urinary ORM1 expression correlated with the plasma NT-proBNP ($P = 0.002$) and NYHA classification ($P<0.001$). In addition, ROC curves suggested at an optimum cut-off value of 2484.98 ng/mg with 90.91% sensitivity and 85.48% specificity respectively could be used for the diagnosis of CHF. Thus, all those results demonstrate the urinary ORM1 protein has potential value for the early diagnosis of CHF.

However, the pathophysiologic mechanisms responsible for those findings are unclear. One possible explanation could be that the increased ORM1 may be correlated with the inflammatory activation in patients with CHF. Previous studies have provided solid evidence to support a pivotal role of inflammation in the underlying pathophysiology of CHF through both animal and human research [35,36]. Cytokines are mainly produced by activated monocytes and macrophages, and these inflammatory proteins have formed the basis of the CHF inflammatory paradigm. Notably, monocyte activation, which plays a core role in the inflammatory pathophysiology of CHF, results in the subsequent release of inflammatory cytokines, their migration to the myocardium, adhesion to the endothelial wall, and other complex processes of the immune system [36,37]. It has been demonstrated that C-reactive protein levels are increased in patients with CHF and could activate monocytes and then stimulate their production of inflammatory cytokines in a dose-dependent manner. Moreover, this cytokine production is significantly enhanced in those patients with ongoing myocardial damage than in those without [37,38]. Thereby, we suppose that the levels of urinary ORM1, similar to the C-reactive protein, may be closely related to inflammatory condition of CHF. Further studies are needed to confirm the reasons leading to the exaggerated excretion of urinary ORM1 in CHF patients.

Most studies have investigated the levels of ORM in serum. Only recently have some studies begun to look at changes in ORM levels in the urine of patients with certain diseases. Christiansen *et al.* [39] reported that levels of ORM were found to be significantly elevated in the urine of patients with type 2 diabetes, even in normoalbuminuric patients. Furthermore, they suggested that the increased excretion of urinary ORM could be an independent, powerful predictor of cardiovascular mortality in patients with type 2 diabetes, as determined through five years of follow-up [30]. Their explanation was that the elevated urinary ORM is associated with cardiovascular risk factors such as inflammation, impaired left ventricular function and endothelial dysfunction [40]. Exaggerated excretion of urinary ORM was also found to predict preeclampsia in pregnant women with pregestational type 1 diabetes, which was probably caused by an increased local renal inflammatory response [41]. The enhanced urinary ORM concentrations were also detected in hypertensive subjects, along with other proteins such as albumin, a-1-antitrypsin, transferrin and retinol binding proteins [42]. In addition, Irmak S *et al.* [43] identified that ORM is significantly increased in urine samples from bladder cancer patients, particularly in those with invasive tumor stages.

Several limitations of the current study, especially about the specificity of this potential biomarker, are needed to be considered when contemplating the potential value of urinary ORM1 in early diagnosis of CHF. First, all the participants were recruited from Chinese Han populations in the same hospital. As a result, our sample must be regarded as a homogeneous cohort that may not represent the overall CHF population. Second, although we did not detect an association between urinary ORM1 levels and other clinical characteristics of CHF such as age, sex, diabetes, hypertension, coronary heart disease, cardiomyopathy, renal dysfunction and LVEF, we could not exclude the possibility that other unknown factors may affect the urinary ORM1 expression. Another point that needs to be addressed is the control group. Inflammation could lead to an elevated level of ORM, and healthy controls made up the only control group in our study, probably resulting in an overestimation of the specificity of ORM1. Therefore, our preliminary findings require further exploration through larger-scale studies with adequate control groups, in particular controls that include subjects with inflammation.

Above all, this study firstly reports the identification and validation of the significantly up-regulated protein of urinary ORM1 in CHF. The elevated urinary ORM1 levels were detected in patients with CHF than healthy controls. Moreover, urinary ORM1 expression had a high positive correlation with the NYHA functional classification of CHF. Thus, our findings suggest that urinary ORM1 could be a potential biomarker for detecting CHF. Further research is warranted to investigate the possible role of urinary ORM1 in the pathogenesis of CHF.

Author Contributions

Conceived and designed the experiments: DLX. Performed the experiments: LNH FL. Analyzed the data: QCZ LS PAC ZHX. Contributed reagents/materials/analysis tools: DJZ CHL. Wrote the paper: DLX LNH FL.

References

1. Remme WJ, Swedberg K (2001) The Task Force for the Diagnosis and Treatment of Chronic Heart Failure of the European Society of Cardiology. Guidelines for the diagnosis and treatment of chronic heart failure. Eur Heart J 22: 1527–1560.
2. Lloyd-Jones D, Adams RJ, Brown TM, Carnethon M, Dai S, et al. (2010) Executive summary: heart disease and stroke statistics: 2010 update: a report from the American Heart Association. Circulation 121: 948–954.
3. Lloyd-Jones DM, Larson MG, Leip EP, Beiser A, D'Agostino RB, et al. (2002) Lifetime risk for developing chronic heart failure: the Framingham Heart Study. Circulation. 106: 3068–3072.
4. Schocken DD (2008) American Society for Preventive Cardiology. Prev Cardiol 11: 127–128.
5. Dawson J, Walters M, Delles C, Mischak H, Mullen W (2012) Urinary proteomics to support diagnosis of stroke. PLoS One 7: e35879.
6. Kaiser T, Wittke S, Just I, Krebs R, Bartel S, et al. (2004) Capillary electrophoresis coupled to mass spectrometer for automated and robust polypeptide determination in body fluids for clinical use. Electrophoresis 25: 2044–2055.
7. Ye B, Skates S, Mok SC, Horick NK, Rosenberg HF, et al. (2006) Proteomic-based discovery and characterization of glycosylated eosinophil-derived neurotoxin and COOH-terminal osteopontin fragments for ovarian cancer in urine. Clin Cancer Res 12: 432–441.
8. Zimmerli LU, Schiffer E, Zurbig P, Good DM, Kellmann M, et al. (2008) Urinary proteomic biomarkers in coronary artery disease. Mol Cell Proteomics 7: 290–298.
9. Hunt SA, Abraham WT, Chin MH, Feldman AM, Francis GS, et al. (2005) ACC/AHA 2005 guideline update for the diagnosis and management of chronic heart failure in the adult. A report of the American College of Cardiology/ American Heart Association Task Force on practical guidelines. Circulation 112: e154–e235.
10. Jiang H, Guan G, Zhang R, Liu G, Cheng J, et al. (2009) Identification of urinary soluble E-cadherin as a novel biomarker for diabetic nephropathy. Diabetes Metab Res Rev 25: 232–41.
11. Zhao L, Wang H, Liu C, Liu Y, Wang X, et al. (2010) Promotion of colorectal cancer growth and metastasis by the LIM and SH3 domain protein 1. Gut 59: 1226–35.
12. Li J, Guo W, Li F, He J, Yu Q, et al. (2012) HnRNPL as a key factor in spermatogenesis: Lesson from functional proteomic studies of azoospermia patients with sertoli cell only syndrome. J Proteomics 75: 2879–91.
13. Li F, Chen DN, He CW, Zhou Y, Olkkonen VM, et al. (2012) Identification of urinary Gc-globulin as a novel biomarker for bladder cancer by two-dimensional fluorescent differential gel electrophoresis (2D-DIGE). J Proteomics 77: 225–36.
14. Jenssen TK, Laegreid A, Komorowski J, Hovig E (2001) A literature network of human genes for high-throughput analysis of gene expression. Nat Genet 28: 21–8.
15. Jensen LJ, Kuhn M, Stark M, Chaffron S, Creevey C, et al. (2009) STRING 8 — a global view on proteins and their functional interactions in 630 organisms. Nucleic Acids Res 37: D412–6.
16. Guha K, McDonagh T (2013) Heart failure epidemiology: European perspective. Curr Cardiol Rev 9: 123–7.
17. Delles C, Schiffer E, von Zur Muhlen C, Peter K, Rossing P, et al. (2010) Urinary proteomic diagnosis of coronary artery disease: identification and clinical validation in 623 individuals. Journal of Hypertension 28: 2316–22.
18. Cho S, Choi YS, Yim SY, Yang HI, Jeon YE, et al. (2012) Urinary vitamin D-binding protein is elevated in patients with endometriosis. Hum Reprod 27: 515–22.
19. Snell-Bergeon JK, Maahs DM, Ogden LG, Kinney GL, Hokanson JE, et al. (2009) Evaluation of urinary biomarkers for coronary artery disease, diabetes, and diabetic kidney disease. Diabetes Technol Ther 11: 1–9.
20. Ye B, Skates S, Mok SC, Horick NK, Rosenberg HF, et al. (2006) Proteomic-based discovery and characterization of glycosylated eosinophil-derived neurotoxin and COOH-terminal osteopontin fragments for ovarian cancer in urine. Clin Cancer Res 12: 432–441.
21. Jou YJ, Lin CD, Lai CH, Chen CH, Kao JY, et al. (2010) Proteomic identification of salivary transferring as a biomarker for early detection of oral cancer. Anal Chim Acta 681: 41–48.
22. Smith ER, Zurakowski D, Saad A, Scott RM, Moses MA (2008) Urinary biomarkers predict brain tumor presence and response to therapy. Clin Cancer Res 14: 2378–2386.
23. Cho SH, Oh YJ, Nam A, Kim HY, Park JH, et al. (2007) Evaluation of serum and urinary angiogenic factors in patients with endometriosis. Am J Reprod Immunol 58: 497–504.
24. Buhimschi CS, Norwitz ER, Funai E, Richman S, Guller S, et al. (2005) Urinary angiogenic factors cluster hypertensive disorders and identify women with severe preeclampsia. Am J Obstet Gynecol 192: 734–741.
25. Bozkurt B, Mann DL, Deswal A (2010) Biomarkers of inflammation in heart failure. Heart Failure Review 15: 331–341.
26. Andersson LC, Gahmberg CG (1979) Surface glycoproteins of resting and activated human T lymphocytes. Mol Cell Biochem 27: 117–131.
27. Ito S, Tsuda A, Momotsu T, Igarashi K, Kasahara S, et al. (1989) Urinary orosomucoid excretion rate in patients with non-insulin-dependent diabetes mellitus. Acta Endocrinol (Copenh) 120: 584–590.
28. Christiansen MS, Hommel E, Friberg L, Mølvig J, Magid E, et al. (2010) Increased urinary orosomucoid excretion is not related to impaired renal function in patients with type 2 diabetes. J Diabetes Complications 24: 28–36.
29. Sorensson J, Matejka GL, Ohlson M, Haraldsson B (1999) Human endothelial cells produce orosomucoid, an important component of the capillary barrier. Am J Physiol 276: H530–534.
30. Gahmberg CG, Andersson LC (1978) Leukocyte surface origin of human alpha1- acid glycoprotein (orosomucoid). J Exp Med 148: 507–521.
31. Christiansen MS, Hommel E, Magid E, Feldt-Rasmussen B (2005) Orosomucoid in urine is a powerful predictor of cardiovascular mortality in normoalbuminuric patients with type 2 diabetes at five years of follow-up. Diabetologia 48: 386–393.
32. Kuller LH, Tracy RP, Shaten J, Meilahn EN (1996) Relation of C-reactive protein and coronary heart disease in the MRFIT nested case-control study. Multiple Risk Factor Intervention Trial. Am J Epidemiol 144: 537–547.
33. Fournier T, Medjoubi N, Porquet D (2000) Alpha-1-acid glycoprotein. Biochim Biophys Acta 1482: 157–171.
34. Logdberg L, Wester L (2000) Immunocalins: a lipocalin subfamily that modulates immune and inflammatory responses. Biochim Biophys Acta 1482: 284–297.
35. Maekawa Y, Anzai T, Yoshikawa T, Asakura Y, Takahashi T, et al. (2002) Prognostic significance of peripheral monocytosis after reperfused acute myocardial infarction: a possible role for left ventricular remodeling. J Am Coll Cardiol 39: 241–246.
36. Wrigley BJ, Lip GY, Shantsila E (2011) The role of monocytes and inflammation in the pathophysiology of heart failure. Eur J Heart Fail 13: 1161–71.
37. Yin WH, Chen JW, Jen HL, Chiang MC, Huang WP, et al. (2004) Independent prognostic value of elevated high-sensitivity C-reactive protein in chronic heart failure. Am Heart J 147: 931–938.
38. Nakagomi A, Seino Y, Endoh Y, Kusama Y, Atarashi H, et al. (2010) Upregulation of monocyte proinflammatory cytokine production by C-reactive protein is significantly related to ongoing myocardial damage and future cardiac events in patients with chronic heart failure. J Card Fail 16: 562–571.
39. Christiansen MS, Hommel E, Magid E, Feldt-Rasmussen B (2002) Orosomucoid in urine predicts cardiovascular and over-all mortality in patients with Type II diabetes. Diabetologia 45: 115–120.
40. Christiansen MS, Iversen K, Larsen CT, Goetze JP, Hommel E, et al. (2009) Increased urinary orosomucoid excretion: a proposed marker for inflammation and endothelial dysfunction in patients with type 2 diabetes. Scand J Clin Lab Invest 69: 272–81.
41. Christiansen MS, Hesse D, Ekbom P, Hesse U, Damm P, et al. (2010) Increased urinary orosomucoid excretion predicts preeclampsia in pregnant women with pregestational type 1 diabetes. Diabetes Res Clin Pract 9: 16–21.
42. Lisowska-Myjak B, Krych A, Kołodziejczyk A, Pachecka J, Gaciong Z (2011) Urinary proteins, N-acetyl-β-D-glucosaminidase activity and estimated glomerular filtration rate in hypertensive patients with normoalbuminuria and microalbuminuria. Nephrology (Carlton) 16: 403–9.
43. Irmak S, Tilki D, Heukeshoven J, Oliveira-Ferrer L, Friedrich M, et al. (2005) Stage-dependent increase of orosomucoid and zinc-alpha2-glycoprotein in urinary bladder cancer. Proteomics 5: 4296–304.

BNP but Not s-cTnIn Is Associated with Cardioembolic Aetiology and Predicts Short and Long Term Prognosis after Cerebrovascular Events

Nicole Nigro[1,6*], Karin Wildi[2,6], Christian Mueller[2,6], Philipp Schuetz[3,6], Beat Mueller[3,6], Felix Fluri[5,6], Mirjam Christ-Crain[1,6⁋¶], Mira Katan[1,4,6⁋¶]

1 Department of Endocrinology, University Hospital Basel, Basel, Switzerland, **2** Department of Cardiology, University Hospital Basel, Basel, Switzerland, **3** Medical University Clinic and Division of Endocrinology, Diabetology and Metabolism, Kantonsspital Aarau, Aarau, Switzerland, **4** Department of Neurology, University Hospital Zurich, Zurich, Switzerland, **5** Department of Neurology, University Hospital Basel, Basel, Switzerland, **6** Department of Clinical Research, University Hospital Basel, Basel, Switzerland

Abstract

Background: We analyzed the prognostic value of b-type natriuretic peptide (BNP) and sensitive cardiac Troponin (s-cTnI) in patients with ischemic stroke or transient ischemic attack (TIA) and their significance in predicting stroke aetiology.

Methods: In a prospectively enrolled cohort we measured BNP and s-cTnI levels upon admission. Primary endpoints were mortality, unfavorable functional outcome and stroke recurrence after 90 days and after 12 months. Secondary endpoint was cardioembolic aetiology.

Results: In 441 patients BNP but not s-cTnI remained an independent predictor for death with an adjusted HR of 1.2 (95% CI 1.1–1.4) after 90 days and 1.2 (95% CI 1.0–1.3) after one year. The comparison of the Area under Receiver Operating Characteristic (AUROC) of model A (age, NIHSS) and model B (age, NIHSS, BNP) showed an improvement in the prediction of mortality (0.85 (95% CI 0.79–0.90) vs. 0.86 (95% CI 0.81–0.92), Log Rank $p = 0.004$). Furthermore the category free net reclassification improvement (cfNRI) when adding BNP to the multivariate model was 57.5%, $p < 0.0001$. For the prediction of functional outcome or stroke recurrence both markers provided no incremental value. Adding BNP to a model including age, atrial fibrillation and heart failure lead to a higher discriminatory accuracy for identification of cardioembolic stroke than the model without BNP (AUC 0.75 (95% CI 0.70–0.80) vs. AUC 0.79, (95% CI 0.75–0.84), $p = 0.008$).

Conclusion: BNP is an independent prognostic maker for overall mortality in patients with ischemic stroke or TIA and may improve the diagnostic accuracy to identify cardioembolic aetiology.

Trial Registration: ClinicalTrials.gov NCT00390962

Editor: Terence J. Quinn, University of Glasgow, United Kingdom

Funding: This study was supported by an unrestricted research grant from Abbott. However Abbott was not involved in data collection, management, analysis and interpretation of the data. As well as grants from the Department of Endocrinology and Metabolism from the University Hospital of Basel. MCC was supported by a grant from the Swiss National Science Foundation (PP00P3_123346). MK was supported by a transatlantic career development award from the foundation Leduqc and a grant from the Swiss National Science Foundation (PZ00P3_142422). All supporting funders had no role in study design, data collection, management, analysis, interpretation of the data, the preparation or approval of the manuscript.

Competing Interests: This study was supported by an unrestricted research grant from Abbott. However Abbott was not involved in data collection, management, analysis and interpretation of the data. CM served as consultant for Abbott and received speaker honoraria. All other authors have no other potential competing interests to declare.

* Email: Nicole.Nigro@usb.ch

⁋ These authors contributed equally to this work.

¶ These authors are last authors on this work.

Introduction

Several prognostic [1] and some aetiological biomarkers have been evaluated in ischemic stroke but so far most failed to show incremental information. Aetiological classification of ischemic stroke and TIA is critical to discern the best treatment for specific secondary prevention. In a European population-based study the highest recurrence rate after stroke or TIA was found among patient with cardioembolic aetiology when compared to all other types of aetiology [2]. Therefore, early identification of cardioembolic aetiology of stroke is crucial.

B-type natriuretic peptide (BNP) is a neurohormone secreted predominantly from the myocardium in response to wall stretch or increased intracardiac pressure [3–6]. High BNP levels have been shown to predict atrial fibrillation within the general population as well as in stroke patients [7]. BNP levels were associated with cardioembolic stroke aetiology [8,9]. Furthermore, high plasma levels of BNP were an independent predictor of short and long-term mortality [10,11] and of functional outcome at 6 months after ischemic stroke [12,13]. New published data show that BNP levels are associated with TIA recurrence after a TIA [14]. However, these data base on a small group of patients and need to be verified in a larger cohort. Recently, a meta-analysis found that BNP levels were associated with all cause mortality but not with functional outcome. The incremental prognostic value concerning overall mortality, however, was limited. The authors of this meta-analysis concluded with the remark that further well designed cohort studies are needed to assess the predictive value of BNP in stroke patients [15].

Troponin is a highly sensitive and specific marker of myocardial necrosis and has an important role in the diagnosis of myocardial infarction [16]. Similar to BNP, also elevated s-cTnI has been suggested as marker for increased risk of mortality after an acute stroke [17–19]. However data on Troponin in the setting of stroke are more spars. To our knowledge, there are no data on the association of s-cTnI levels and stroke recurrence.

The purpose of this study was, first, to further validate BNP and s-cTnI as prognostic markers after stroke and TIA and, second, to evaluate their ability to identify cardioembolic aetiology.

Material and Methods

Study design and setting

The study design of this prospective cohort study has been described in detail elsewhere (ClinicalTrials. gov number, NCT00390962) [20]. Briefly, between November 2006 and November 2007, all consecutive patients (n = 605) presenting at the emergency department of the University Hospital Basel, Switzerland, a 660–bed tertiary care hospital, with a suspected cerebrovascular event were evaluated. All patients presenting with an ischemic stroke or a TIA were included after obtained written informed consent from the patient or the patients' next of kin. We defined initial ischemic stroke according to the World Health Organization criteria as an acute focal neurological deficit lasting longer than 24 hours [21]. TIA was defined accordingly as a transient episode of neurological dysfunction caused by focal brain ischemia with symptoms lasting 24 hours or less. Exclusion criteria were missing informed consent or any diagnosis different from ischemic stroke or TIA (i.e. stroke/TIA mimics)

The Ethics Committee of Basel, Switzerland, approved the trial protocol; informed consent was obtained from all patients.

The protocol for this trial and supporting STROBE Checklist are available as supporting information (see Checklist S1 and Protocol S1).

Clinical variables

On admission, the following data were collected with a standardized bed-side interview and complete chart review: vital signs, co-morbidities as assessed by the Charlson Comorbidity Index (CCI) adjusted for stroke, medication prior to ischemic stroke or TIA and cardiovascular risk factors (i.e. age, gender, smoking habits, history of hypercholesterolemia, hypertension, diabetes mellitus, previous TIA or stroke, positive family history for myocardial infarction, stroke or TIA and history of coronary heart disease).

Severity of stroke was prospectively assessed on admission by a neurologist certified in the use of the National Institute of Health Stroke Scale (NIHSS) [22]. Risk stratification for patients with a TIA was performed according to the ABCD2-score [23].

Stroke aetiology was determined according to the criteria of the TOAST classification [24], which distinguishes large-artery atherosclerosis, cardioembolism, small-artery occlusion, other aetiology and undetermined aetiology. All patients underwent the necessary diagnostic work-up to classify aetiology according to the TOAST criteria [24] such as standard 12-lead electrocardiography and at least 24-hour electrocardiography, echocardiography and neurosonographic study of the extra- and intracranial arteries as well as routine laboratory testing.

The 90 days and the 12 months follow-up was performed using structured telephone interviews from a blinded stroke physician to assess mortality from any cause, functional outcome using the modified Rankin Scale (mRS) and recurrent cerebrovascular events.

Blood sampling

In all patients blood samples were obtained on admission within 72 hours from symptom onset. BNP and sensitive cardiac Troponin T were measured in a batch analysis blinded to clinicians. After centrifugation, samples were frozen at −70°C until they were assayed in a blinded fashion in a dedicated core laboratory. S-cTnI was measured in EDTA-plasma using the recently refined s-cTnI assay (Abbott-Architect, Abbott Laboratories, Abbott Park, IL, USA) [25–27]. For this test, a limit of detection (LoD) of 0.01 μg/L, a 99th-percentile cut-off of 0.028 μg/L and a coefficient of variation (CV) of $<10\%$ of 0.032 μg/L have been reported by the manufacturer. Three s-cTnI strata were predefined: below the limit of detection ($<$ 0.01 μg/L, undetectable), detectable but still in the normal range (0.01–0.027 μg/L), and increased ($\geq$0.028 μg/L, above the 99th percentile of healthy individuals). The concentration of BNP was measured in EDTA-plasma using the Architect BNP assay (Abbott Laboratories, Abbott Park, IL, USA). The analytical range as reported by the manufacturer extends from 15 to 20'000 pg/ml for the AxSYM assay.

Endpoints

The primary endpoints of this analysis were a) mortality within 90 days and 1 year in stroke as well as TIA patients b), functional outcome after 90 days and at 1 year in stroke patients, c) stroke or TIA recurrence within 90 days.

Patients and or their caregivers were questioned by structured telephone interviews from blinded stroke physicians at 3 months and 1 year after the index event to assess mortality from any cause, functional outcome using the modified Rankin Scale (mRS) and recurrent cerebrovascular events. Poor outcome was defined as mRS>2 points. A recurrent cerebrovascular event was defined as an as an acute ischemic lesion in the brain not attributed to infection, tumor, demyelination or a degenerative neurologic disease but due to an occlusive vascular disorder. Further criteria were rapid onset of a focal neurological deficit occurring for at least 24 hours in conjunction with brain imaging consistent with acute ischemic stroke. The CT or MRI may either show a new infarct or no change from the study performed at entry, i.e. the diagnosis is clinical and does not require CT/MRI confirmation.

The secondary endpoint was cardioembolic aetiology of stroke diagnosed during hospitalization according to TOAST criteria [24] by stroke physicians, which were blinded to BNP and Troponin measurements.

Neuroimaging

CCT was performed in all patients on admission mainly to exclude intracranial hemorrhage. Additionally MRI was per-

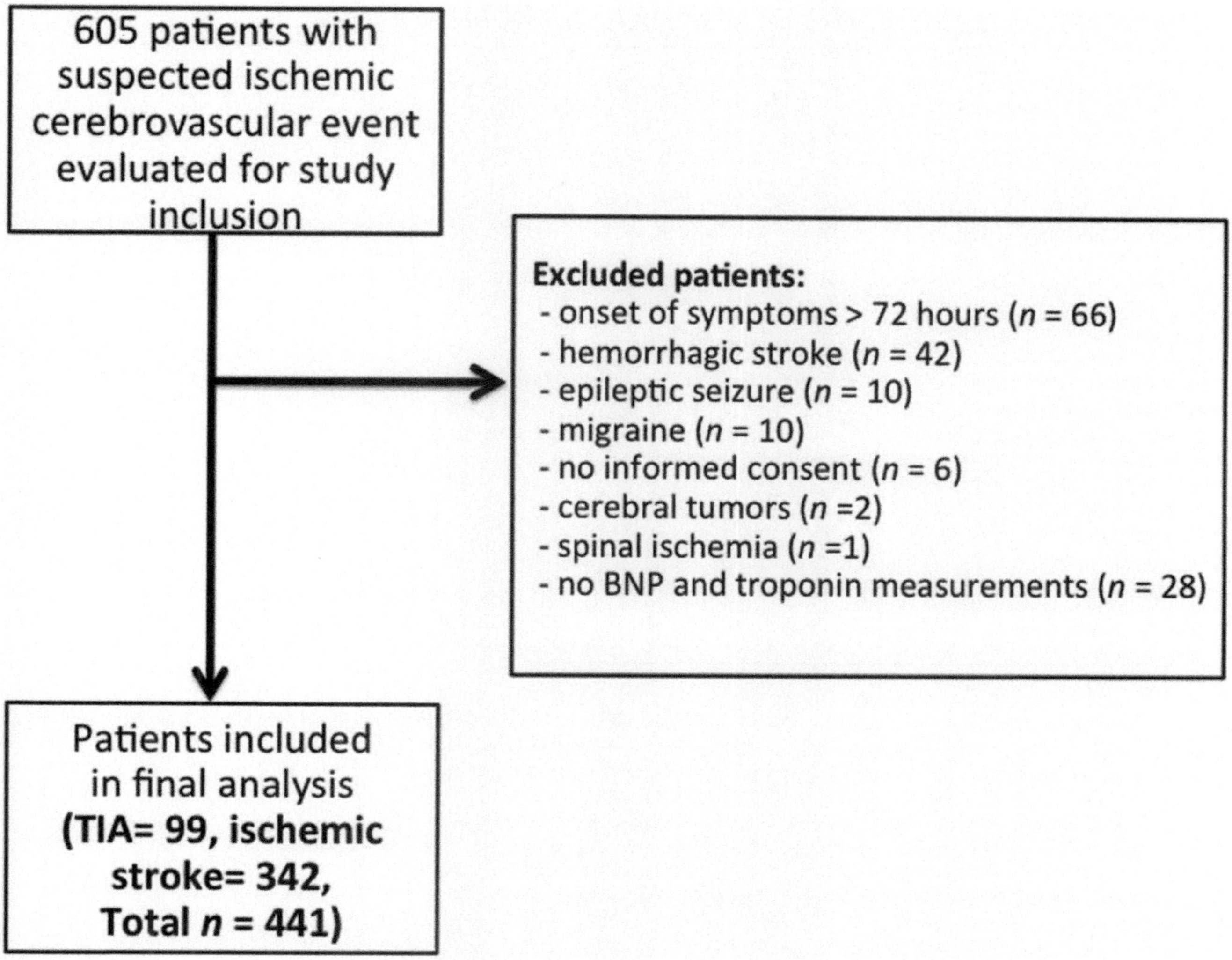

Figure 1. Study flow chart.

formed in 197 (45%) patients on a clinical 1.5 T MR Avant system (SIEMENS, Erlangen, Germany) using a stroke protocol, including T1-, T2-, and diffusion-weighted (DWI) sequences, as well as apparent diffusion coefficient (ADC) maps and a MR angiography. Lesions were ranked into three sizes to represent typical stroke patterns: (1) small lesion with a volume of less than 10 ml, (2) medium lesion of 10 to 100 ml and (3) large lesion with a volume of more than 100 ml [28].

Statistical analysis

Discrete variables are expressed as frequency (percentage), continuous Gaussian variables as means with standard deviation SD and non-Gaussian variables as medians with interquartile ranges [IQR]. Comparisons between groups were made using chi-square test, Mann-Whitney U test and Kruskal-Wallis test as appropriate.

Univariate Cox Proportional Hazard Analysis was utilized to compute hazard ratios and 95% confidence intervals (CI) for potential predictors of death during the follow-up period. All significant variables with a p-value <0.001 (i.e. BNP levels, age, NIHSS, and lesion size) were tested in a multivariate model using the Forward Stepwise Method to avoid over fitting of the model.

To estimate association of BNP and Troponin with functional outcome and re-events, we used logistic regression models. In this analysis we tested all significant variables in the multivariate analysis with a p-value <0.05 (i.e. BNP levels, age, NIHSS, Charlson Comorbidity Index, CRP, heart failure, atrial fibrillation and lesion size). Due to a greater number of endpoints the risk of over fitting was minimal. Receiver operating characteristic (ROC) curves were constructed for different models to assess the discriminative value in terms of sensitivity and specificity for mortality, outcome and aetiology. Comparison was made using the DeLong test [29] and likelihood ratios for nested models as appropriate. Furthermore we calculated the continuous (category free) net reclassification improvement (NRI) [30] for the primary endpoint, i.e. mortality to assess the incremental value of BNP over the multivariate prognostic model, which included the following variables: age and NIHSS. For the secondary endpoint, i.e. cardioembolic aetiology, the NRI was calculated to assess the incremental value of BNP over the multivariate model including age, atrial fibrillation and heart failure. Analyses were performed using SPSS (SPSS 21, Chicago, IL, USA) and MedCalc (MedCalc 10.4, Mariakerke, Belgium), p-values less than 0.05 were considered to indicate statistical significance.

Table 1. Baseline characteristics of patients with ischemic stroke and transient ischemic attack.

Baseline characteristics (n = 441)	
Demographic findings:	
Cerebrovascular re-events, n (%)	27 (6.1)
Death from any cause, n (%)	67 (15.2)
Age, in years	74.6 (62.6–81.9)
Female sex, n (%)	185 (42)
NIHSS at admission, points	5 (2–10)
Charlson score at admission, points	1 (0–2)
ABCD2 score for TIA severity	4 (3–5)
Clinical findings:	
Heart rate, in bpm	76 (67–88)
Systolic blood pressure, in mmHg	161 (±29)
Diastolic blood pressure, in mmHg	90 (80–100)
Body temperature, in °C	37.0 (±0.7)
Laboratory findings:	
BNP, in pg/ml	81.9 (35.0–203.3)
Troponin I, in ug/l	0.003 (0.000–0.012)
Glucose, in mmol/L	6.1 (5.3–7.3)
Stroke aetiology, n (%):	
Small vessel occlusive	81 (18.4)
Large vessel occlusive	79 (17.9)
Cardioembolic	143 (32.4)
Other	19 (4.3)
Undetermined aetiology	119 (27.0)
Cardiovascular risk factors, n (%):	
Hypertension	332 (75.3)
Atrial fibrillation	83 (18.8)
Heart failure	60 (13.6)
Smoking history	154 (34.9)
Dyslipidemia	121 (27.4)
Diabetes mellitus	81 (18.4)
Coronary heart disease	104 (23.6)
Prior TIA or stroke	114 (25.9)
Family history of AMI or stroke	140 (31.7)
Functional outcome (only for stroke patients, n = 344), n (%):	
Bad outcome after 90 days	138 (31.3)
Bad outcome after 1 year	141 (32.0)
Clinical stroke syndrome, n (%):	
TACS	38 (8.6)
PACS	155 (35.1)
LACS	68 (15.4)
POCS	80 (18.1)

Discrete variables are expressed as frequency (percentage) and continuous Gaussian variables as means with SD and non-Gaussian variables as medians with interquartile ranges [IQR].
NIHSS = National Institutes of Health Stroke Scale; AMI = acute myocardial infarction; TACS = total anterior circulation syndrome; PACS = partial anterior circulation syndrome; LACS = lacunar syndrome; POCS = posterior circulation syndrome.

Results

Patients

From 605 screened patients, 469 patients were eligible for our study and 466 completed follow up after 90 days or one year, respectively. In 362 of the 469 patients ischemic stroke was diagnosed, while 107 out of the 469 had a TIA. 28 patients were excluded from the final analysis because BNP and s-cTnI levels were missing (**Figure 1**).

Table 2. Cox regression analysis for mortality after 90 days for all patients (n = 441).

Variables	Univariate Analysis Hazard ratio (95% CI)	p-value	Multivariate Analysis Hazard ratio (95% CI)	p-value
BNP (per 100 pg/ml)	1.2 (1.1–1.2)	<0.001	1.2 (1.1–1.4)	0.007
Troponin I at presentation (per 100 μg/l)	1.0 (1.0–1.0)	0.086		
Age (per 10 years)	2.2 (1.5–3.3)	<0.001	3.2 (1.4–7.6)	0.007
Female sex	1.0 (0.5–1.9)	0.965		
Systolic blood pressure (per 10 mmHg)	0.9 (0.8–1.0)	0.045		
Temperature (per °C)	0.7 (0.4–1.2)	0.23		
CRP (per 10 mg/dl)	1.1 (1.0–1.1)	0.001		
Glucose (per mmol/l)	1.1 (0.9–1.2)	0.48		
NIHSS	1.1 (1.1–1.2)	<0.001	1.1 (1.0–1.2)	0.2
Charlson Score	1.2 (1.0–1.4)	0.02		
History of				
- Hypertension	1.3 (0.6–2.9)	0.47		
- Coronary heart disease	2.0 (1.1–3.9)	0.03		
- Heart failure	2.7 (1.3–5.3)	0.006		
- Atrial fibrillation	3.0 (1.6–5.7)	0.001		
- Dyslipidemia	1.1 (0.6–2.2)	0.75		
- Family history of stroke and/or AMI	0.8 (0.4–1.6)	0.49		
- Diabetes mellitus	1.3 (0.6–2.7)	0.51		
- Smoking	0.9 (0.4–1.7)	0.65		
- Prior stroke	0.7 (0.3–1.5)	0.39		
Cardioembolic aetiology	1.5 (0.8–2.9)	0.2		
Lesion size (per 10 ml)	1.2 (1.1–1.2)	<0.001	1.2 (1.0–1.3)	0.01

CI = confidence interval; CRP = C-reactive protein; NIHSS = National Institutes of Health Stroke Scale; AMI = acute myocardial infarction.

Baseline demographic and cardiovascular risk factors including NIHSS and lesion size were not different when comparing patients with and without available measurements.

Baseline characteristics

The median age was 74.6 (IQR 62.6–81.9) years and 42% were women. On admission, the median NIHSS in stroke patients was 5 points (IQR 2–10) and median ABCD2 Score in TIA patients was 3 (IQR 3–5). After 90 days, overall 42 patients had died and the mortality rate was thus 9.5%. After the one-year follow-up, 67 patients had died and the mortality rate was 15.2%. After 90 days 138 (31.3%) of patients with ischemic stroke had an unfavorable outcome after one year 141 patients (32.0%) of 336 patients with a completed follow up had an unfavorable outcome (mRS>2). Re-events were identified in 27 (6.1%) patients with ischemic stroke or TIA.

The principal baseline characteristics of all patients are provided in **Table 1**. There were no significant differences between stroke and TIA patients concerning demographic and risk factor variables besides the etiologies. In patients with TIA we found more undetermined etiologies (50.1%) than in patients with an ischemic stroke (24.0%) (P<0.0001) and in patients with an ischemic stroke we found more patients with a cardioembolic source (37.4%) than in patients with a TIA (8%) (p<0.0001).

Main results

Cardiac biomarkers and mortality

Median BNP levels in patients with ischemic stroke or TIA were 81.9 (IQR 35.0–203.3) pg/ml. BNP levels were higher in patients who died (n = 46) as compared to patients who survived (n = 395) (309.9 [IQR 162.2–575.8] vs. 69.6 [IQR 31.4–165.3] pg/ml, p< 0.0001) after 90 days. These results were similar for death after one year (279.0 [IQR 98.4–493.4] vs. 67.8 [IQR 331.4–153.8] pg/ml, p<0.0001).

Median s-cTnI levels in patients with ischemic stroke or TIA were 0.003 (IQR 0.000–0.012) μg/L. 310 patients had s-cTnI level below the detection limit (<0.01 μg/L), 65 patients in the normal range (0.01–0.027 μg/L), and 66 patients had an increased s-cTnI level (≥0.028 μg/L). Similarly as for BNP, patients who died showed higher s-cTnI levels as compared to patients who survived after 90 days and one year (0.015 [IQR 0.0045–0.076] vs. 0.0030 [IQR 0.000–0.0100] μg/L, p<0.0001) and (0.011 [IQR 0.003–0.055] vs. 0.003 [IQR 0.000–0.010] μg/L, p<0.0001).

In multivariate cox regression analysis BNP but not s-cTnI remained an independent predictor for death within 90 days with a hazard ratio (per 100pg/ml unit's increase) of 1.2 (95% CI 1.1–1.4). The other independent predictors for death after 90 days were age and lesion size (see **Table 2**). Also for long term mortality (within 1 year) only BNP levels (HR 1.2 (95% CI 1.0–1.3), age (per 10 years increase) (HR 3.43 (95% CI 1.6–7.3) and lesion size (HR 1.2 (95% CI 1.0–1.3) remained independent predictors (see **Table 3**). In a multivariate analysis including coronary heart disease, atrial fibrillation and heart failure instead of the CCI, the hazard ratio of BNP remained similar for 90 days and for one year (HR 1.2 (95% CI 1.0–1.3) and (HR 1.2 (95% CI 1.0–1.3), respectively) while the other parameters did not remain significant in the multivariate model.

Table 3. Cox regression analysis for mortality after one year for all patients (n = 441).

	Univariate Analysis		Multivariate Analysis	
Variables	**Hazard ratio (95% CI)**	**p-value**	**Hazard ratio (95% CI)**	**p-value**
BNP (per 100 pg/ml)	1.2 (1.1–1.2)	<0.001	1.2 (1.0–1.3)	0.02
Troponin I at presentation (per 100 µg/l)	1.0 (1.0–1.0)	0.19		
Age (per 10 years)	2.3 (1.4–3.0)	<0.001	3.4 (1.6–7.3)	0.001
Female sex	1.3 (0.8–2.1)	0.39		
Systolic blood pressure (per 10 mmHg)	0.9 (0.6–1.0)	0.12		
Temperature (per °C)	0.8 (0.5–1.2)	0.25		
CRP (per 10 mg/dl)	1.1 (1.0–1.1)	0.023		
Glucose (per mmol/l)	1.1 (1.0–1.2)	0.18		
NIHSS (per point)	1.1 (1.1–1.2)	<0.001	1.1 (1.0–1.2)	0.2
Charlson Score (per point)	1.3 (1.1–1.4)	<0.001	1.0 (0.8–1.6)	0.6
History of				
- Hypertension	1.1 (0.6–2.0)	0.71		
- Coronary heart disease	1.6 (0.9–2.8)	0.12		
- Heart failure	2.6 (1.5–4.5)	0.001		
- Atrial fibrillation	3.3 (2.0–5.5)	<0.001		
- Dyslipidemia	0.9 (0.5–1.6)	0.79		
- Family history of stroke and/or AMI	0.80(0.5–1.4)	0.42		
- Diabetes mellitus	1.0 (0.5–1.9)	0.95		
- Smoking	0.6 (0.3–1.0)	0.063		
- Prior stroke	0.9 (0.5–1.7)	0.8		
Cardioembolic aetiology	1.6 (0.9–2.6)	0.1		
Lesion size (per 10 ml)	1.2 (1.1–1.2)	<0.001	1.2 (1.0–1.3)	0.01

CI = confidence interval; CRP = C-reactive protein; NIHSS = National Institutes of Health Stroke Scale; AMI = acute myocardial infarction.

BNP was predictive also across all subgroups stratified by presence of atrial fibrillation (HR of BNP among pat with AF 1.16, p = 0.01 after 90 days and HR 1.14, p = 0.005 after one year respectively, without AF 1.19, p<0.001 after 90 days and HR 1.18, p<0.001 after one year respectively) or heart insufficiency (HR of BNP in patients with heart insufficiency 1.12, p<0.001 after 90 days and HR 1.12, p<0.001 after one year respectively, HR of BNP in patients without heart insufficiency 1.24, p<0.001 after 90 days and HR 1.16, p<0.001 after one year respectively), thus we found no relevant effect modification.

Moreover the AUC of BNP to predict mortality after 90 days was 0.81 (95% CI 0.74–0.83) and 0.75 (95% CI 0.68–0.81) after one year respectively. The comparison of ROC curves of model A (i.e. the validated prognostic model of Koenig et al [31] including age and the NIHSS) and model B (age, NIHSS, BNP) revealed an improvement in the prediction of mortality (AUC 0.85 (95% CI 0.79–0.90) vs. AUC 0.86 (95% CI 0.81–0.92), p = 0.004). The category free net reclassification improvement (cfNRI) when adding BNP to the best prognostic model was 57.5%, p<0.0001.

Cardiac biomarkers and functional outcome

For functional outcome only patients with an ischemic stroke (n = 344) were considered. BNP levels in patients with an unfavorable outcome after 90 days and after one year were significantly higher than those in patients with a favorable outcome (150.0 [IQR 57.3–346.5] vs. 59.9 [IQR 30.2–145.2] pg/ml, (p<0.0001) for 90 days and 154.1 [IQR 61.5–346.5] vs.59.9 [IQR 30.2–145.2] pg/mL, (p<0.0001) for one year). S-cTnI levels were higher in patients with an unfavorable outcome as compared to patients with a good outcome (0.008 [IQR 0.001–0.0265] vs. 0.003 [IQR 0.000–0.008] µg/L, (p<0.0001) for 90 days (see **Table 4**) and 0.008 [IQR 0.001–0.0285] vs. 0.003 [IQR 0.000–0.0105] µg/L, (p = 0.0008) for 1 year) (see **Table 5**). However, after adjustment for all other significant outcome predictors, the only independent outcome predictors were the NIHSS, age and lesion size (see **Table 4** and **Table 5**).

Cardiac biomarkers and cerebrovascular recurrence

BNP levels in patients with a cerebrovascular re-event were similar as compared to patients without a re-event (123.3 [IQR 29.4–207.3] vs. 70.4 [IQR 32.9–165.3] pg/ml, p = 0.499).

The same was true for s-cTnI levels (patients with re-event: 0.003 [IQR 0.000–0.010] vs. patients without re-event: 0.004 [IQR 0.000–0.013] µg/L, p = 0.705).

Cardiac biomarkers and cardioembolic aetiology

The aetiology for ischemic stroke or TIA was undetermined in 144 patients (33%), 144 patients (33%) had cardioembolic aetiology, 76 patients (17%) had large arteriosclerosis, 61 patients (14%) had a small arteriocclusion and 16 patients (4%) had other etiologies.

Median BNP levels were higher in patients with a cardioembolic stroke or TIA compared to other etiologies (179.5 [IQR 72.5–367.2] vs. 57.2 [IQR 27.5–128.2] pg/ml, p<0.0001). BNP levels showed an AUC of 0.73 (95% CI 0.68–0.78) to predict a cardioembolic source of ischemic stroke or a TIA and thus had a

Table 4. Logistic regression analysis for functional outcome after 90 days for ischemic stroke patients (n = 342).

	Univariate Analysis		Multivariate Analysis	
Variables	OR (95% CI)	p-value	OR (95% CI)	p-value
BNP (per 100 pg/ml)	1.2 (1.1–1.3)	<0.001	1.1 (0.9–1.3)	0.26
Troponin I at presentation (per 10 ug/l)	1.0 (1.0–1.0)	0.79		
Age	1.1 (1.0–1.1)	<0.001	1.0 (1.0–1.1)	0.07
Female sex	1.6 (1.1–2.5)	0.029	1.0 (0.4–1.1)	0.95
NIHSS (per point)	1.2 (1.1–1.2)	<0.001	1.1 (1.0–1.5)	0.046
Charlson Score (per point)	1.3 (1.1–1.6)	<0.001	1.2 (0.8–1.6)	0.34
Systolic blood pressure (per 10 mmHg)	1.0 (0.9–1.0)	0.29		
Temperature (per °C)	0.8 (0.6–1.2)	0.33		
Heart beat (per 10/min)	1.1 (1.0–1.3)	0.22		
CRP (per 10 mg/dl)	1.1 (1.0–1.2)	0.02	1.0 (0.9–1-2)	0.58
Glucose (per mmol/l)	1.1 (1.0–1.2)	0.21		
History of				
- Hypertension	1.5 (0.9–2.6)	0.11		
- Coronary heart disease	1.3 (0.8–2.1)	0.37		
- Heart failure	2.8 (1.5–5.2)	0.001	1.5 (0.4–5.7)	0.56
- Atrial fibrillation	1.9 (1.1–3.2)	0.02	1.1 (0.4–3.0)	0.82
- Dyslipidemia	0.8 (0.5–1.4)	0.43		
- Family history of stroke and/or AMI	0.8 (0.5–1.3)	0.29		
- Diabetes mellitus	1.2 (0.7–2.0)	0.62		
- Smoking	0.8 (0.5–1.2)	0.22		
Lesion size (per 10 ml)	1.2 (1.1–1.3)	<0.001	1.2 (1.0–1.3)	0.02

OR = odds ratio; CI = confidence interval; CRP = C-reactive protein; NIHSS = National Institutes of Health Stroke Scale; AMI = acute myocardial infarction.

higher predictive value as compared with age (AUC 0.57 (95% CI 0.51–0.62), p<0.001). The combination of BNP with age, the history of or newly detected atrial fibrillation and heart failure in comparison of a nested model had a higher discriminatory accuracy than age, atrial fibrillation and heart failure alone (AUC 0.79, (95%CI 0.75–0.84) vs. AUC 0.75 (95% CI 0.70–0.80, p = 0.008 for comparison). The combination of BNP with the multivariate model led to a category-free net reclassification improvement (cfNRI) of 48.5% (p<0.001) for cardioembolic aetiology.

Patients with a cardioembolic source of ischemic stroke had the highest s-cTnI levels compared to the other etiologies (0.007 [IQR 0.001–0.030] vs. 0.002 [IQR 0.000–0.008] μg/L, p<0.0001). The AUC of s-cTnI to predict a cardioembolic source was 0.62 (95% CI 0.56–0.68).

Discussion

In this prospective study we evaluated both, BNP and s-cTnI levels, in a large cohort of ischemic stroke and TIA patients for prediction of mortality, functional outcome and re-events after 90 days and 1 year as well as for stroke aetiology.

Our data show the following main findings: First, BNP and s-cTnI levels on admission were elevated in patients with ischemic stroke or TIA who had died or had an unfavorable outcome 90 days and one year after the event. After adjustment for other risk factors BNP but not s-cTnI was an independent predictor of death but not of functional outcome or recurrence. Second, BNP improved the identification of patients with cardioembolic strokes or TIAs when compared to clinical information on admission alone (i.e. age, CHF and the history of atrial fibrillation).

Our data showing an independent association of BNP with mortality is mostly in line with findings in the literature. Studies reported high levels of natriuretic peptides and an association with mortality in acute stroke patients at admission [11], during hospitalization [10] and within 6 months [13] after stroke and a recent meta-analysis concluded that natriuretic peptides are independent predictors for all cause mortality after stroke [15]. However a recent study found no incremental value of BNP for the prediction of mortality compared to clinical variables such as age and NIHSS [11]. This discrepant finding might be due to methodological differences. The cohort included hemorrhages and the primary endpoint was mortality or neurological worsening in the stroke unit, thus within the first days after stroke. There was no assessment of several potentially influencing medical comorbidities or of stroke aetiology. In contrast, in our study we assessed only ischemic stroke and TIA patients and the primary endpoint was mortality within 90 days and 1 year. Our data contained more moderate strokes and thus our cohort had a lower level of NIHSS at admission. We took into account stroke aetiology and several medical comorbidities which are known to affect mortality and functional outcome in stroke patients [32]. Importantly, we adjusted for renal insufficiency (within the CCI), which is known to affect BNP levels [33].

Data regarding the predictive value of BNP for functional outcome in patients after a cerebrovascular event are more controversial. Some studies found an association with functional outcome [13,34], other studies showed that especially after

Table 5. Logistic regression analysis for functional outcome after one year for ischemic stroke patients (n = 342).

	Univariate Analysis		Multivariate Analysis	
	OR (95% CI)	p-value	OR (95% CI)	p-value
BNP (per 100 pg/ml)	1.2 (1.1–1.4)	<0.001	1.1 (1.0–1.3)	0.14
Troponin I at presentation (per 10 ug/l)	1.0 (1.0–1.0)	0.88		
Age	1.1 (1.1–1.1)	<0.001	1.1 (1.0–1.1)	0.01
Female sex	1.6 (1.0–2.4)	0.05		
NIHSS (per point)	1.1 (1.1–1.2)	<0.001	1.1 (1.0–1.2)	0.01
Charlson Score (per point)	1.4 (1.2–1.6)	<0.001	1.2 (0.9–1.5)	0.29
Systolic blood pressure (per 10 mmHg)	1.0 (0.9–1.0)	0.21		
Temperature (per °C)	0.9 (0.6–1.3)	0.44		
Heart beat (per 10/min)	1.1 (1.0–1.3)	0.14		
CRP (per 10 mg/dl)	1.0 (1.0–1.0)	0.39		
Glucose (per mmol/l)	1.0 (0.9–1.1)	0.86		
History of				
- Hypertension	1.2 (0.7–2.0)	0.46		
- Coronary heart disease	1.2 (0.7–2.0)	0.5		
- Heart failure	2.5 (1.3–4.7)	0.004	1.7 (0.5–5.6)	0.41
- Atrial fibrillation	2.0 (1.2–3.4)	0.012	1.1 (0.4–2.7)	0.9
- Dyslipidemia	0.7 (0.4–1.2)	0.21		
- Family history of stroke and/or AMI	0.5 (0.3–0.9)	0.11		
- Diabetes mellitus	1.4 (0.8–2.4)	0.27		
- Smoking	0.7 (0.4–1.0)	0.07		
Lesion size (per 10 ml)	1.2 (1.1–1.4)	<0.001	1.2 (1.1–1.4)	0.002

OR = odds ratio; CI = confidence interval; CRP = C-reactive protein; NIHSS = National Institutes of Health Stroke Scale; AMI = acute myocardial infarction.

adjustment in multivariate analyses BNP did not remain an independent prognostic marker for functional outcome [11,35]. This is in line with our results. It is biologically plausible since functional outcome is probably more prominently influenced by other factors such as brain plasticity. On the other hand, hemodynamic changes and underlying cardiac disease are major contributors to mortality after stroke [36].

Data supporting the association of natriuretic peptides with cardioembolic stroke cumulate. Elevated BNP levels in acute cerebral infarction were associated with cardioembolic aetiology in several studies [8,37]. However, the incremental value of BNP when added to clinical variables, which are known to be associated with cardioembolic events such as age, has not been evaluated in these studies. Our data show that the combination of BNP with age and atrial fibrillation (i.e. history of or a newly diagnosed atrial fibrillation) had a higher discriminatory accuracy in comparison to the same model without BNP. BNP may therefore have a role in risk stratification predicting mortality on one hand and may support early specific implementation of secondary prevention such as oral anticoagulants on the other hand.

Midregional proANP (MR-proANP), another natriuretic peptide, was assessed for its predictive role concerning mortality, functional outcome and cardioembolic aetiology in patients with an ischemic stroke but not TIA [38]. As BNP, MR- proANP was an independent predictor of mortality after 90 days and improved the prognostic value of the NIHSS. Moreover it was also associated with cardioembolic aetiology improving the diagnostic accuracy of already known clinical information, such as age, known heart failure, and known AF on admission. However, BNP compared to MRproANP is more widely available and clinically established in most countries and physicians are already familiar with it. In this study we evaluated BNP with further statistical methods such as the cfNRI and found a significant improvement in the prediction even if added to models including not only the NIHSS but all significant predictors. However a direct comparison is needed in the future to establish which natriuretic peptide is better for risk classification and identification of cardioembolic strokes. In our cohort, s-cTnI was not an independent marker for all three endpoints. Recently higher Troponin T levels were found in older patients with a more severe ischemic stroke and with comorbidities such as heart failure and/or renal insufficiency [39]. Another study showed that elevated levels of high sensitive Troponin T are frequently present in patients with acute ischemic stroke but, in accordance to our results, did not provide additional prognostic information in these subjects [40]. Interestingly s-cTnI did also not provide additional information for the identification of cardioembolic aetiology in our study. It may be that s-cTnI is too specific for myocardial infarction; it is therefore possible that by measuring s-cTnI levels patients with underlying cardiac disease not directly due to myocardial damage are missed.

To our knowledge, this is the first study that assesses BNP and s-cTnI for prediction of stroke recurrence. Our results show that neither BNP nor Troponin levels were associated with a re-event after ischemic stroke or TIA. Possibly, these markers have no role in stroke recurrence. Alternatively, our study was underpowered to find a significant association with recurrence. Nevertheless our findings suggest that even if there is an association it is of rather moderate clinical relevance.

The following limitations of our study must be taken into account. First, this was a single center study and further evaluation and validation in a larger cohort of patients should be performed. Second, etiological classification is difficult and a large proportion of patients (especially in the TIA group) remained in the undetermined category, however no patient was classified in to this category due to incomplete diagnostic evaluation. Moreover misclassification might have occurred since at the time of patient recruitment we performed mainly 24 hours ECG monitoring but more recent data suggest that longer monitoring increases the identification of intermittent atrial fibrillation substantially [41,42]. It is therefore possible that we missed some cardioembolic stroke patients. However, this potential misclassification would lead rather to a bias towards the null thus underestimating the positive association. Third, biomarker measurement was performed within a rather large time frame (i.e. within 72 hours after the event). However in 398 patients (90%) blood was drawn within 24 hours of the event, thus it is unlikely that the observed association is only driven by later measurements. Moreover the predictive value remained similar when analyzing BNP levels stratified by time since symptom onset (i.e. 0–3 h, 3–12 h, 12–24 h and 24–72 h) (data not shown). Finally, the lack of association of cardiac biomarkers with stroke recurrence may be due to the relative small number of re-events and thus limited power to find a significant association.

In conclusion BNP but not s-cTnI is an independent marker with incremental value for overall mortality prediction but not for the prediction of functional outcome and re-events in patients with ischemic stroke or TIA. Furthermore BNP levels contribute additional information to prior used clinical variables in identifying cardioembolic stroke aetiology. BNP may therefore be helpful for risk assessment and earlier identification of patients, which may benefit from oral anticoagulation compared to antiplatelet therapy. However, further studies are needed to specifically validate the magnitude of the additional prognostic information, and to evaluate if this information ultimately leads to an improved patient care.

Supporting Information

Checklist S1 STROBE checklist.

Protocol S1 Trial protocol.

Author Contributions

Conceived and designed the experiments: CM PS BM FF MCC MK. Performed the experiments: MK FF. Analyzed the data: NN KW MK. Contributed reagents/materials/analysis tools: CM. Wrote the paper: NN KW MK. Revised the manuscript: NN KW CM PS BM FF MCC MK.

References

1. Katan M, Elkind MS (2011) Inflammatory and neuroendocrine biomarkers of prognosis after ischemic stroke. Expert Rev Neurother 11: 225–239.
2. Kolominsky-Rabas PL, Weber M, Gefeller O, Neundoerfer B, Heuschmann PU (2001) Epidemiology of ischemic stroke subtypes according to TOAST criteria: incidence, recurrence, and long-term survival in ischemic stroke subtypes: a population-based study. Stroke 32: 2735–2740.
3. Davis M, Espiner E, Richards G, Billings J, Town I, et al. (1994) Plasma brain natriuretic peptide in assessment of acute dyspnoea. Lancet 343: 440–444.
4. Maisel AS, Krishnaswamy P, Nowak RM, McCord J, Hollander JE, et al. (2002) Rapid measurement of B-type natriuretic peptide in the emergency diagnosis of heart failure. N Engl J Med 347: 161–167.
5. Lainchbury JG, Campbell E, Frampton CM, Yandle TG, Nicholls MG, et al. (2003) Brain natriuretic peptide and n-terminal brain natriuretic peptide in the diagnosis of heart failure in patients with acute shortness of breath. J Am Coll Cardiol 42: 728–735.
6. Wright SP, Doughty RN, Pearl A, Gamble GD, Whalley GA, et al. (2003) Plasma amino-terminal pro-brain natriuretic peptide and accuracy of heart-failure diagnosis in primary care: a randomized, controlled trial. J Am Coll Cardiol 42: 1793–1800.
7. Schnabel RB, Larson MG, Yamamoto JF, Sullivan LM, Pencina MJ, et al. (2010) Relations of biomarkers of distinct pathophysiological pathways and atrial fibrillation incidence in the community. Circulation 121: 200–207.
8. Montaner J, Perea-Gainza M, Delgado P, Ribo M, Chacon P, et al. (2008) Etiologic diagnosis of ischemic stroke subtypes with plasma biomarkers. Stroke 39: 2280–2287.
9. Shibazaki K, Kimura K, Iguchi Y, Okada Y, Inoue T (2009) Plasma brain natriuretic peptide can be a biological marker to distinguish cardioembolic stroke from other stroke types in acute ischemic stroke. Intern Med 48: 259–264.
10. Shibazaki K, Kimura K, Iguchi Y, Aoki J, Sakai K, et al. (2011) Plasma brain natriuretic peptide predicts death during hospitalization in acute ischaemic stroke and transient ischaemic attack patients with atrial fibrillation. Eur J Neurol 18: 165–169.
11. Montaner J, Garcia-Berrocoso T, Mendioroz M, Palacios M, Perea-Gainza M, et al. (2012) Brain natriuretic peptide is associated with worsening and mortality in acute stroke patients but adds no prognostic value to clinical predictors of outcome. Cerebrovasc Dis 34: 240–245.
12. Shibazaki K, Kimura K, Okada Y, Iguchi Y, Uemura J, et al. (2009) Plasma brain natriuretic peptide as an independent predictor of in-hospital mortality after acute ischemic stroke. Intern Med 48: 1601–1606.
13. Rost NS, Biffi A, Cloonan L, Chorba J, Kelly P, et al. (2012) Brain natriuretic peptide predicts functional outcome in ischemic stroke. Stroke 43: 441–445.
14. Mortezabeigi HR, Taghizadeh A, Talebi M, Amini K, Goldust M (2013) ABCD2 score and BNP level in patients with TIA and cerebral stroke. Pak J Biol Sci 16: 1393–1397.
15. Garcia-Berrocoso T, Giralt D, Bustamante A, Etgen T, Jensen JK, et al. (2013) B-type natriuretic peptides and mortality after stroke: a systematic review and meta-analysis. Neurology 81: 1976–1985.
16. Reiter M, Twerenbold R, Reichlin T, Benz B, Haaf P, et al. (2012) Early diagnosis of acute myocardial infarction in patients with pre-existing coronary artery disease using more sensitive cardiac troponin assays. Eur Heart J 33: 988–997.
17. Christensen H, Johannesen HH, Christensen AF, Bendtzen K, Boysen G (2004) Serum cardiac troponin I in acute stroke is related to serum cortisol and TNF-alpha. Cerebrovasc Dis 18: 194–199.
18. Di Angelantonio E, Fiorelli M, Toni D, Sacchetti ML, Lorenzano S, et al. (2005) Prognostic significance of admission levels of troponin I in patients with acute ischaemic stroke. J Neurol Neurosurg Psychiatry 76: 76–81.
19. Faiz KW, Thommessen B, Einvik G, Brekke PH, Omland T, et al. (2014) Determinants of high sensitivity cardiac troponin T elevation in acute ischemic stroke. BMC Neurol 14: 96.
20. Katan M, Fluri F, Morgenthaler NG, Schuetz P, Zweifel C, et al. (2009) Copeptin: a novel, independent prognostic marker in patients with ischemic stroke. Ann Neurol 66: 799–808.
21. Hatano S (1976) Experience from a multicentre stroke register: a preliminary report. Bull World Health Organ 54: 541–553.
22. Brott T, Adams HP, Jr., Olinger CP, Marler JR, Barsan WG, et al. (1989) Measurements of acute cerebral infarction: a clinical examination scale. Stroke 20: 864–870.
23. Johnston SC, Rothwell PM, Nguyen-Huynh MN, Giles MF, Elkins JS, et al. (2007) Validation and refinement of scores to predict very early stroke risk after transient ischaemic attack. Lancet 369: 283–292.
24. Adams HP, Jr., Bendixen BH, Kappelle LJ, Biller J, Love BB, et al. (1993) Classification of subtype of acute ischemic stroke. Definitions for use in a multicenter clinical trial. TOAST. Trial of Org 10172 in Acute Stroke Treatment. Stroke 24: 35–41.
25. Tang WH, Wu Y, Nicholls SJ, Brennan DM, Pepoy M, et al. Subclinical myocardial necrosis and cardiovascular risk in stable patients undergoing elective cardiac evaluation. Arterioscler Thromb Vasc Biol 30: 634–640.
26. Mingels A, Jacobs L, Michielsen E, Swaanenburg J, Wodzig W, et al. (2009) Reference population and marathon runner sera assessed by highly sensitive cardiac troponin T and commercial cardiac troponin T and I assays. Clin Chem 55: 101–108.
27. Reichlin T, Hochholzer W, Bassetti S, Steuer S, Stelzig C, et al. (2009) Early diagnosis of myocardial infarction with sensitive cardiac troponin assays. N Engl J Med 361: 858–867.
28. Szabo K, Kern R, Gass A, Hirsch J, Hennerici M (2001) Acute stroke patterns in patients with internal carotid artery disease: a diffusion-weighted magnetic resonance imaging study. Stroke 32: 1323–1329.
29. DeLong ER, DeLong DM, Clarke-Pearson DL (1988) Comparing the areas under two or more correlated receiver operating characteristic curves: a nonparametric approach. Biometrics 44: 837–845.
30. Pencina MJ, D'Agostino RB, Sr., Steyerberg EW (2011) Extensions of net reclassification improvement calculations to measure usefulness of new biomarkers. Stat Med 30: 11–21.

31. Konig IR, Ziegler A, Bluhmki E, Hacke W, Bath PM, et al. (2008) Predicting long-term outcome after acute ischemic stroke: a simple index works in patients from controlled clinical trials. Stroke 39: 1821–1826.
32. Jimenez Caballero PE, Lopez Espuela F, Portilla Cuenca JC, Ramirez Moreno JM, Pedrera Zamorano JD, et al. (2013) Charlson comorbidity index in ischemic stroke and intracerebral hemorrhage as predictor of mortality and functional outcome after 6 months. J Stroke Cerebrovasc Dis 22: e214–218.
33. Codognotto M, Piccoli A, Zaninotto M, Mion M, Plebani M, et al. (2007) Renal dysfunction is a confounder for plasma natriuretic peptides in detecting heart dysfunction in uremic and idiopathic dilated cardiomyopathies. Clin Chem 53: 2097–2104.
34. Idris I, Hill R, Ross I, Sharma JC (2010) N-terminal probrain natriuretic peptide predicts 1-year mortality following acute stroke: possible evidence of occult cardiac dysfunction among patients with acute stroke. Age Ageing 39: 752–755.
35. Etgen T, Baum H, Sander K, Sander D (2005) Cardiac troponins and N-terminal pro-brain natriuretic peptide in acute ischemic stroke do not relate to clinical prognosis. Stroke 36: 270–275.
36. Makikallio AM, Makikallio TH, Korpelainen JT, Vuolteenaho O, Tapanainen JM, et al. (2005) Natriuretic peptides and mortality after stroke. Stroke 36: 1016–1020.
37. Foerch C, Montaner J, Furie KL, Ning MM, Lo EH (2009) Invited article: searching for oracles? Blood biomarkers in acute stroke. Neurology 73: 393–399.
38. Katan M, Fluri F, Schuetz P, Morgenthaler NG, Zweifel C, et al. (2010) Midregional pro-atrial natriuretic peptide and outcome in patients with acute ischemic stroke. J Am Coll Cardiol 56: 1045–1053.
39. Jensen JK, Kristensen SR, Bak S, Atar D, Hoilund-Carlsen PF, et al. (2007) Frequency and significance of troponin T elevation in acute ischemic stroke. Am J Cardiol 99: 108–112.
40. Jensen JK, Ueland T, Aukrust P, Antonsen L, Kristensen SR, et al. (2012) Highly sensitive troponin T in patients with acute ischemic stroke. Eur Neurol 68: 287–293.
41. Rizos T, Guntner J, Jenetzky E, Marquardt L, Reichardt C, et al. (2012) Continuous stroke unit electrocardiographic monitoring versus 24-hour Holter electrocardiography for detection of paroxysmal atrial fibrillation after stroke. Stroke 43: 2689–2694.
42. Hendrikx T, Hornsten R, Rosenqvist M, Sandstrom H (2013) Screening for atrial fibrillation with baseline and intermittent ECG recording in an out-of-hospital population. BMC Cardiovasc Disord 13: 41.

7

Abnormal Calcium Handling and Exaggerated Cardiac Dysfunction in Mice with Defective Vitamin D Signaling

Sangita Choudhury[1], Soochan Bae[1], Qingen Ke[1], Ji Yoo Lee[1], Sylvia S. Singh[1], René St-Arnaud[2], Federica del Monte[1], Peter M. Kang[1]*

1 Cardiovascular Institute, Beth Israel Deaconess Medical Center and Harvard Medical School, Boston, Massachusetts, United States of America, **2** Shriners Hospital and Departments of Surgery and Human Genetics, McGill University, Montreal, Canada

Abstract

Aim: Altered vitamin D signaling is associated with cardiac dysfunction, but the pathogenic mechanism is not clearly understood. We examine the mechanism and the role of vitamin D signaling in the development of cardiac dysfunction.

Methods and Results: We analyzed 1α-hydroxylase (1α-OHase) knockout (1α-OHase$^{-/-}$) mice, which lack 1α-OH enzymes that convert the inactive form to hormonally active form of vitamin D. 1α-OHase$^{-/-}$ mice showed modest cardiac hypertrophy at baseline. Induction of pressure overload by transverse aortic constriction (TAC) demonstrated exaggerated cardiac dysfunction in 1α-OHase$^{-/-}$ mice compared to their WT littermates with a significant increase in fibrosis and expression of inflammatory cytokines. Analysis of calcium (Ca^{2+}) transient demonstrated profound Ca^{2+} handling abnormalities in 1α-OHase$^{-/-}$ mouse cardiomyocytes (CMs), and treatment with paricalcitol (PC), an activated vitamin D_3 analog, significantly attenuated defective Ca^{2+} handling in 1α-OHase$^{-/-}$ CMs. We further delineated the effect of vitamin D deficiency condition to TAC by first correcting the vitamin D deficiency in 1α-OHase$^{-/-}$ mice, followed then by either a daily maintenance dose of vitamin D or vehicle (to achieve vitamin D deficiency) at the time of sham or TAC. In mice treated with vitamin D, there was a significant attenuation of TAC-induced cardiac hypertrophy, interstitial fibrosis, inflammatory markers, Ca^{2+} handling abnormalities and cardiac function compared to the vehicle treated animals.

Conclusions: Our results provide insight into the mechanism of cardiac dysfunction, which is associated with severely defective Ca^{2+} handling and defective vitamin D signaling in 1α-OHase$^{-/-}$ mice.

Editor: Sudhiranjan Gupta, Texas A & M University Health Science Center, United States of America

Funding: This work was supported in part by NIH Grants R01 HL65742 (P.M.K.) and the World Class University program (R31-20029) from the Ministry of Education, Science and Technology, South Korea (P.M.K.). Support for generating the 1α-OHase -/- mice was provided by a grant from Shriners Hospitals for Children, Canada (R.St-A.). The funders had no role in study design, data collection and analysis, decision to publish, or preparation of the manuscript.

Competing Interests: The authors have declared that no competing interests exist.

* Email: pkang@bidmc.harvard.edu

Introduction

Cardiovascular disease (CVD) is the most common cause of mortality and morbidity in the United States and other developed nations. Clinical and epidemiological studies suggest an association between vitamin D deficiency and various cardiovascular disorders [1,2], and vitamin D therapy has been shown to improve cardiovascular function [3]. Particularly, in patients with chronic renal failure (CRF), vitamin D deficiency is uniformly present because the critical conversion of nutritional vitamin D_3 ($25(OH)D_3$) to the hormonally active form of vitamin D_3 ($1,25(OH)_2D_3$) occurs primarily in the kidney by 1α-hydroxylase (1α-OHase)[4]. CRF has been shown to be an independent risk factor for CVD, with 10–20 times greater incidence of cardiovascular disease in CRF patients [5]. Clinical studies have also demonstrated that there is an association between improved survival and decreased cardiovascular mortality in hemodialysis patients treated with an activated vitamin D analog, paricalcitol (PC) [6,7]. In fact, similar to CRF patients, 1α-OHase knockout (1α-OHase$^{-/-}$) mice show baseline hypertension, cardiac hypertrophy, and impaired cardiac function [8]. Despite these associations between vitamin D deficiency and cardiac dysfunction, the pathogenic mechanism of cardiac dysfunction associated with vitamin D deficiency is not fully elucidated.

Cardiomyocyte (CM) contractility is regulated by Ca^{2+} handling contractile proteins via regulation of intracellular levels of Ca^{2+} [9]. Thus, abnormalities in Ca^{2+} homeostasis, as seen in vitamin D deficiency, may lead to a chronic defect in E–C coupling, which may in turn lead to cardiac dysfunction. Delays in Ca^{2+} transients, for example, have been observed in myocardial tissue obtained from failing hearts [10]. Although it might not be surprising to find abnormal Ca^{2+} handling in a vitamin D deficiency state, the exact mechanism of vitamin D deficiency affecting the Ca^{2+} handling in CMs, however, is poorly understood. In this study, we examined whether abnormal Ca^{2+} homeostasis and Ca^{2+} handling may mediate structural and functional cardiac abnormalities and examined the relationship between vitamin D deficiency and the development of cardiac hypertrophy in 1α-OHase$^{-/-}$ mice. We hypothesize that restoration of vitamin D signaling improves cardiac functions by restoring Ca^{2+} homeostasis.

Methods

Animal care

Experiments were conducted using 8–10-week old male 1α-OH$^{-/-}$ mice and their littermates in a C57BL/6 background. 1α-OHase$^{+/-}$ and 1α-OHase$^{-/-}$ mice were produced from 1α-OHase$^{+/-}$ [11]. All mice, breeders and offspring were housed at the Animal Research Facility at Beth Israel Deaconess Medical Center (BIDMC) under pathogen-free conditions with a reverse daily 12:12 h light: dark cycle. Euthanasia was performed by CO_2 via a gas cylinder. All experimental procedures were approved by the Institutional Animal Care and Use Committee of BIDMC.

Animal surgery and hemodynamic measurement

TAC was performed in 8–10 week old male C57BL/6 mice and in 1α-OHase$^{-/-}$ [12,13] mice. Cardiac function was analyzed using echocardiography (for baseline cardiac function) and left ventricular (LV) pressure-volume loop measurement (after TAC) as described previously [14,15]. Detailed method is provided in Text S1.

Morphometric analysis of isolated CMs

CMs were enzymatically dissociated from 12 weeks old male mouse hearts according to previously described protocol [16,17]. Detailed method is provided in Text S1.

Serum Ca^{2+} and vitamin D metabolite analysis

Serum 1, 25$(OH)_2$ D_3 (n = 8–10 replicates per group) was analyzed via enzyme immunoassays using commercial kits (Immunodiagnostic Systems). Serum Ca^{2+} (n = 8–10) was analyzed via a quantitative Calcium Colorimetric Detection Kit (Bio Vision).

Serum PTH analysis

Serum PTH (n = 8–10 replicates per group) was analyzed via enzyme immunoassays using commercial kits (Immunooptics Inc.)

Ca^{2+} transients and cell shortening measurements of isolated CMs

Measurement of Ca^{2+} transient and cell shortening in isolated CMs [18]. Briefly, CMs were isolated and contraction parameters and Ca^{2+} transient $[Ca^{2+}]$ i were measured in response to electrical stimulation. Caffeine induced $[Ca^{2+}]$ i release was measured after a 10-second pause following steady-state stimulation at increasing rates. Detailed methods are described in Text S1.

Histology and Western Blots

Hearts were fixed in 10% formalin and paraffin-embedded. Sections were stained with hematoxylin and eosin and Masson Trichrome (MT) at the Histology Core facility at BIDMC [14,15]. Quantification of fibrosis was performed as described previously [16]. To compare the levels of the major proteins involved in Ca^{2+} handling, Western blot analysis was performed on total protein from WT and 1α-OHase$^{-/-}$ mice as described previously [14,15].

Statistical Analysis

Data are reported as mean SEM. Statistical significance was determined by one-way or two-way ANOVA and Student-Newman-Keuls post hoc test. Values of $p<0.05$ were considered significant.

Results

Exaggerated hypertrophic responses after transverse aortic constriction (TAC) in 1α-OHase$^{-/-}$ mice

At baseline, 1α-OHase$^{-/-}$ mice demonstrated a modest 5% increase in heart weight compared to their WT littermates at 12 weeks of age (**Fig. 1A**). Corresponding isolated adult CMs also demonstrated modest increase in surface areas of 1α-OHase$^{-/-}$ mice compared to the age and gender matched WT mice (**Fig. 1B and 1C**). Cross sectional area of the CMs further confirmed these findings (**Fig. 1D and 1E**). We also observed that baseline systolic cardiac function was modestly reduced in 1α-OHase$^{-/-}$ mice compared with the WT mice (**Fig. 1F**). In addition, the mean arterial pressure (MAP) of 1α-OHase$^{-/-}$ was significantly higher than that of WT littermate mice (**Fig. 1G**). These findings suggested that there is baseline mild cardiac hypertrophy and cardiac dysfunction in 1α-OHase$^{-/-}$ mice compared to the WT mice.

To elucidate the effect of defective vitamin D signaling under pathological conditions, we imposed pressure overload on the heart using TAC. Morphometric analysis demonstrated significant increases in heart weight/body weight (HW/BW) ratio in both 1α-OHase$^{-/-}$ and WT mice compared with the corresponding sham-operated groups after 4 weeks of TAC (**Fig. 2A and 2B**). However, there were exaggerated hypertrophic responses to TAC in 1α-OHase$^{-/-}$ mice heart compared to the WT mice. Cardiac functional analysis using pressure-volume (PV) loop measurement revealed that 1α-OHase$^{-/-}$ mice demonstrated significantly greater cardiac dysfunction after TAC, as observed by reduction in stroke volume and cardiac output, compared to their WT littermates (**Fig. 2C and 2D**).

We further analyzed these hearts for the presence of interstitial fibrosis using Masson-Trichrome staining We found that both WT and 1α-OHase$^{-/-}$ mice showed presence of fibrosis after TAC, (**Fig. 2E**) which was significantly increased in 1α-OHase$^{-/-}$ mice compared with those in WT mice (WT = 11.9±1.5% vs. 1α-OHase$^{-/-}$ = 21.5±1.2%; $p<0.05$). These findings demonstrated that there were exaggerated pathological responses to TAC in 1α-OHase$^{-/-}$ mice that are associated with greater decreased cardiac function and more aggressive development of cardiac fibrosis.

Increased fetal gene activation and inflammatory responses after TAC in 1α-OHase$^{-/-}$ mice

We determined the biochemical markers for cardiac hypertrophy and heart failure by measuring the level of "fetal" genes, such as atrial natriuretic factor (ANF) and brain natriuretic peptide (BNP). Ventricular ANF was significantly expressed in all TAC groups. However, there was a 8-fold greater increase in ANF mRNA levels after TAC in 1α-OHase$^{-/-}$ mice compared to the WT littermates (**Fig. 3A**). Similarly, there was also a greater increase in BNP expression in 1α-OHase$^{-/-}$ mice compared to the WT mice hearts after TAC (**Fig. 3B**). Another marker for cardiac hypertrophy, the ratio of ß-MHC to total MHC mRNA expression, was also increased after TAC in both groups. Yet, there were again dramatic and exaggerated increases observed in 1α-OHase$^{-/-}$ mice compared to the WT mice after TAC (**Fig. 3C**).

It's known that vitamin D, a steroid hormone, affects immune regulation by preventing excessive expression of inflammatory cytokines and increasing the 'oxidative burst' potential of macrophages [19]. Interestingly, we observed a reduction in

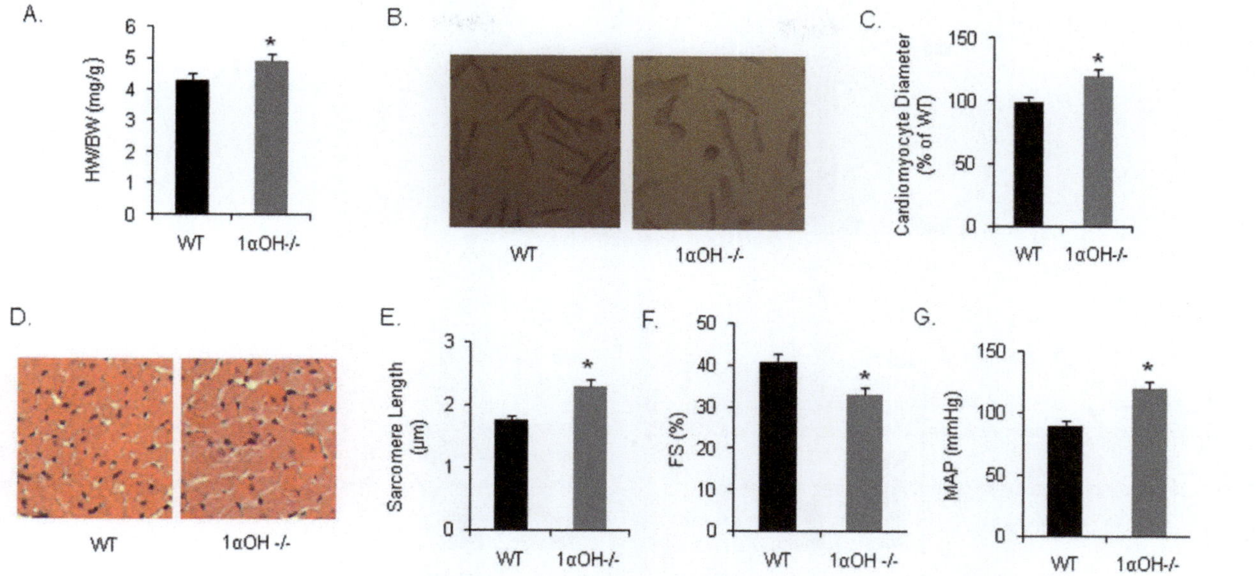

Figure 1. Physiological, echocardiographic, and hemodynamic parameters in 1αOHase−/− mice at baseline: (A) Baseline HW/BW of 1α-OHase −/− mice. *, $p<0.05$ compared to WT. N = 8–10. (B and C) Isolated adult CMs from 1α-OHase$^{-/-}$ mice showing increased surface area compared to WT CMs. *, $p<0.05$ compared to WT. N = 8–10. (D) Cross sectional area of mice heart showing CM surface area. (E) Resting sarcomere length of 1α-OHase$^{-/-}$ and WT CMs. *, $p<0.05$ compared to WT. N = 8–10. (F) Baseline fractional shortening (FS) of WT and KO mice. *, $p<0.05$ compared to WT. N = 8–10. (G) MAP of WT and 1α-OHase−/− mice at baseline. *, $p<0.05$ compared to WT. N = 8–10.

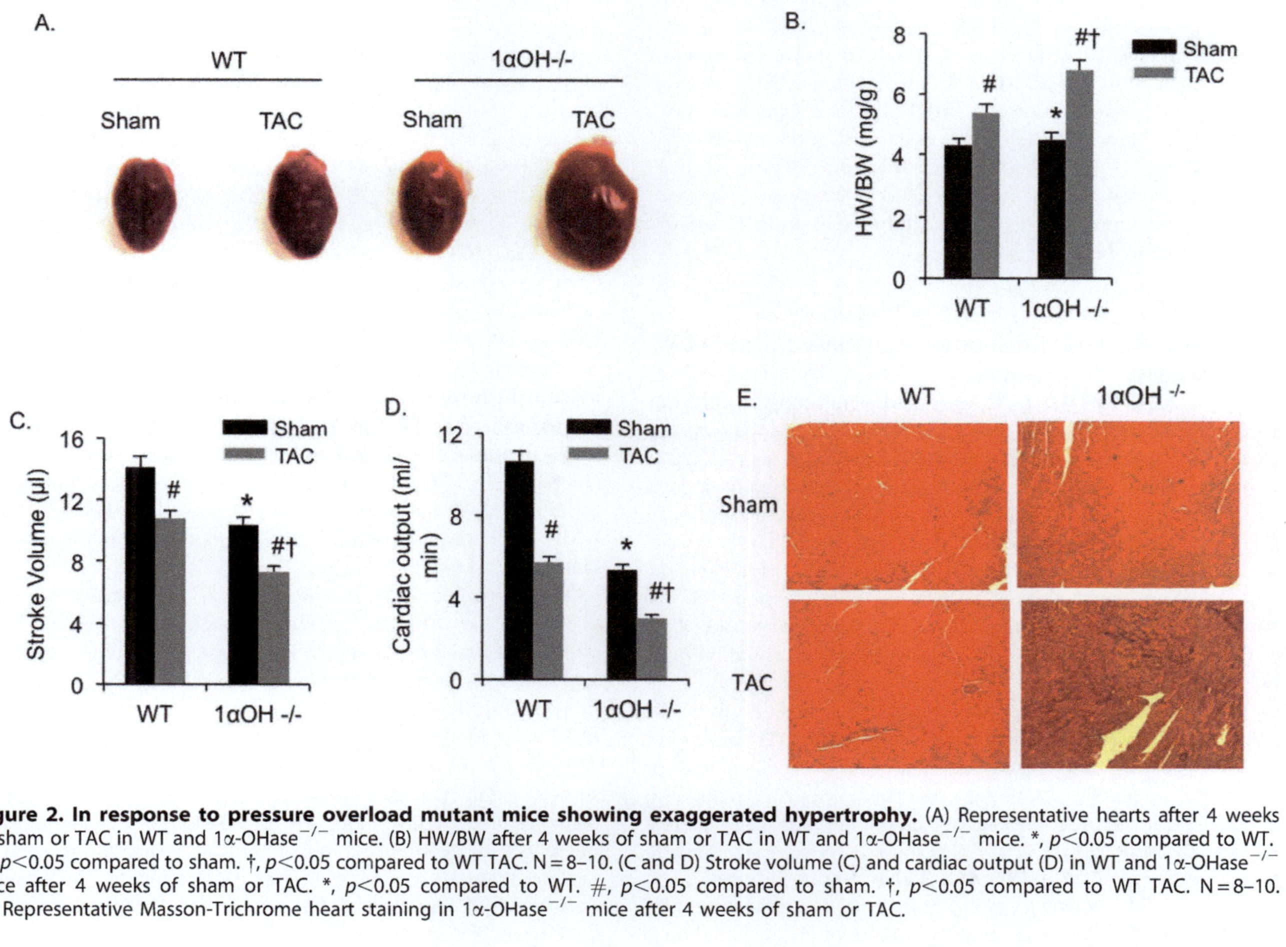

Figure 2. In response to pressure overload mutant mice showing exaggerated hypertrophy. (A) Representative hearts after 4 weeks of sham or TAC in WT and 1α-OHase$^{-/-}$ mice. (B) HW/BW after 4 weeks of sham or TAC in WT and 1α-OHase$^{-/-}$ mice. *, $p<0.05$ compared to WT. #, $p<0.05$ compared to sham. †, $p<0.05$ compared to WT TAC. N = 8–10. (C and D) Stroke volume (C) and cardiac output (D) in WT and 1α-OHase$^{-/-}$ mice after 4 weeks of sham or TAC. *, $p<0.05$ compared to WT. #, $p<0.05$ compared to sham. †, $p<0.05$ compared to WT TAC. N = 8–10. (E) Representative Masson-Trichrome heart staining in 1α-OHase$^{-/-}$ mice after 4 weeks of sham or TAC.

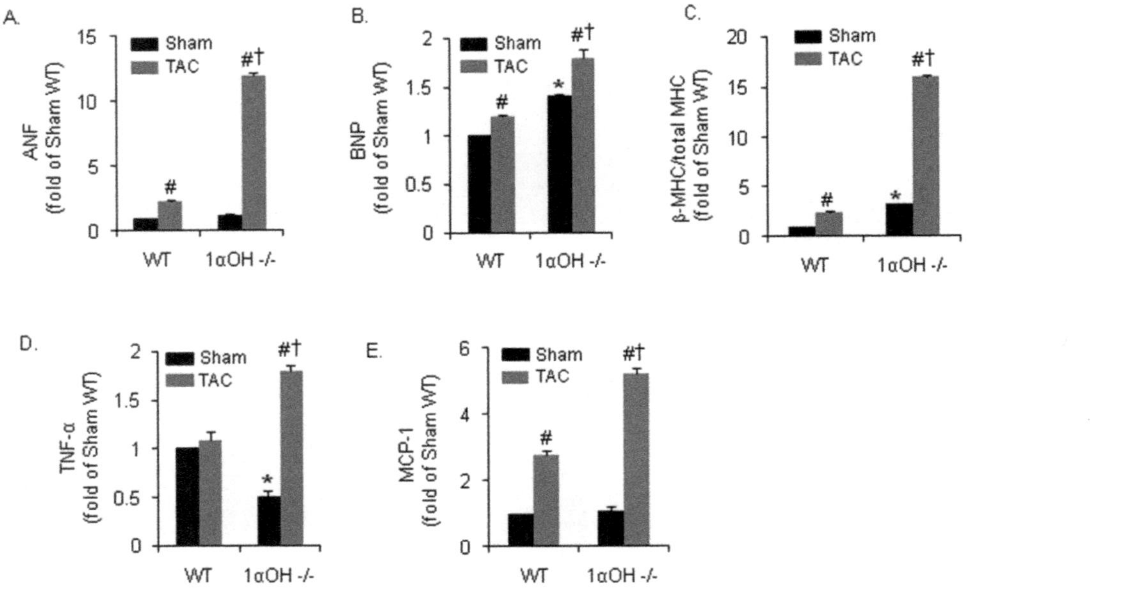

Figure 3. Biochemical findings after 4 weeks of Pressure overload in 1αOHase$^{-/-}$ mice. (A–C) Real-time PCR mRNA expression of ANF (A), BNP (B) and of ß-MHC to total MHC ratio (C) in WT and 1α-OHase$^{-/-}$ mice after 4 weeks of sham or TAC. *, $p<0.05$ compared to WT. #, $p<0.05$ compared to sham. †, $p<0.05$ compared to WT TAC. N = 8–10. (D and E) Real-time PCR mRNA expression of inflammatory cytokines TNF-α (D) and MCP-1 (E) in WT and 1α-OHase -/- mice after 4 weeks of sham or TAC. *, $p<0.05$ compared to WT. #, $p<0.05$ compared to sham. †, $p<0.05$ compared to WT TAC. N = 8–10.

tumor necrosis factor-α (TNF-α) expression at baseline in 1α-OHase$^{-/-}$ mice compared to WT mice. Although no significant differences were observed in TNF-α expression after TAC in WT mice, 1α-OHase$^{-/-}$ mice hearts showed enhanced activation of TNF-α after TAC (**Fig. 3D**). Another inflammatory marker, monocyte chemotactic protein-1 (MCP-1), was activated by TAC in both mice, but with significantly greater activation was observed in 1α-OHase$^{-/-}$ mice after TAC (**Fig. 3E**). These findings demonstrated that there is an exaggerated biochemical evidence of cardiac dysfunction and uncontrolled immune response associated with TAC in 1α-OHase$^{-/-}$ mice.

Defective Ca^{2+} handling and modulation of Ca^{2+} regulatory protein expressions in 1α-OHase$^{-/-}$ mice CMs

We found that the circulating 1, 25(OH) vitamin D_3 level was undetectable in 1α-OHase$^{-/-}$ mice and significantly reduced in heterozygous 1α-OHase$^{+/-}$ littermates (**Fig. 4A**), which coincide with previous findings [20,21]. Without vitamin D supplementation, 1α-OHase$^{-/-}$ mice at 12 weeks showed severe hypocalcemia with plasma Ca^{2+} concentrations as low as 1.2 mmol/L in contrast to the WT littermates, which exhibited normal plasma Ca^{2+} concentrations (WT = 2.5 mmol/L vs. 1α-OHase$^{-/-}$ = 1.2 mmol/L; $P<0.05$). Supplementation of vitamin D using injection of PC (200 ng/kg), an activated vitamin D_3 analog, starting at 4 weeks after birth normalized the plasma Ca^{2+} concentration in 1α-OHase mice by 12 weeks (**Fig. 4B**).

To examine the effect of the vitamin D deficiency in CMs, contraction parameters of individual isolated CM from 1α-OHase$^{-/-}$ mice and their WT littermates were studied by measuring sarcomere shortening (contraction) and relengthening (relaxation) in response to electrical stimulation (**see Text S1 for detail**). Baseline 1α-OHase$^{-/-}$ CM sarcomeres were significantly larger compared to WT (**Fig. 4C, Table S1**). Additionally, 1α-OHase$^{-/-}$ CMs showed a significant decrease in peak shortening, as well as the rate of cell shortening and rate of cell relengthening compared to WT CMs (**Fig. 4D and 4E**). Peak shortening is calculated from the percent shortening of length data (**Fig. 4D**). The highest and lowest value reached by the transient.

We then investigated Ca^{2+} handling properties of individual CM from 1α-OHase$^{-/-}$ mice (**see Text S1 for detail**). Analysis of Ca^{2+} transients indicated decreased peak systolic Ca^{2+}, measured as Fura-2 ratios in CM from 1α-OHase$^{-/-}$ compared to WT group CM (**Fig. 4F**). The rate of Ca^{2+} transient decay (*tau*, exponential decay of time constant, the speed of relaxation/ calcium uptake) was also significantly reduced in 1α-OHase$^{-/-}$ CMs (**Fig. 4G**) which was calculated by the ionoptix program from the transient, with a reduced time to peak (TTP) and a decrease in relaxation rate (Ca^{2+} efflux) (**Fig. 4H and 4I**). Caffeine causes Ca^{2+} release from the sarcoplasmic reticulum (SR) of mammalian muscle. Thus, to evaluate the SR Ca^{2+} load, we tested caffeine-induced Ca^{2+} release amount from SR in WT and 1α-OHase$^{-/-}$ CMs. We found that CMs from 1α-OHase$^{-/-}$ mice presented a decreased caffeine-induced Ca^{2+} transient compared to WT CMs (**Fig. 4J**). These findings demonstrated profound Ca^{2+} handling abnormalities in 1α-OHase$^{-/-}$ mice CMs, which may contribute to the development of fulminant heart failure after TAC.

The expression level and the activity of sarcoplasmic reticulum Ca^{2+} ATPase (SERCA) is significantly decreased in pressure overload-induced hypertrophy and during heart failure in animals and human, which correlate with decreased myocardial dysfunction [22,23]. To further elucidate the mechanism underlying the defective Ca^{2+} handling, we examined the SERCA2a protein expression level in these mice. We found that 1α-OHase$^{-/-}$ mice showed significant decreased SERCA2a expression after TAC compared to WT mice (**Fig. 5A and 5B**). Phospholamban (PLB) interacts with SERCA and inhibits its Ca^{2+} transport rate, and the relative abundance of SERCA and PLB maintains Ca^{2+} homeostasis and CM contractility. Therefore, SERCA/PLB ratio reflects Ca^{2+} transport capacity of the SR [24]. At baseline, 1α-OHase$^{-/-}$

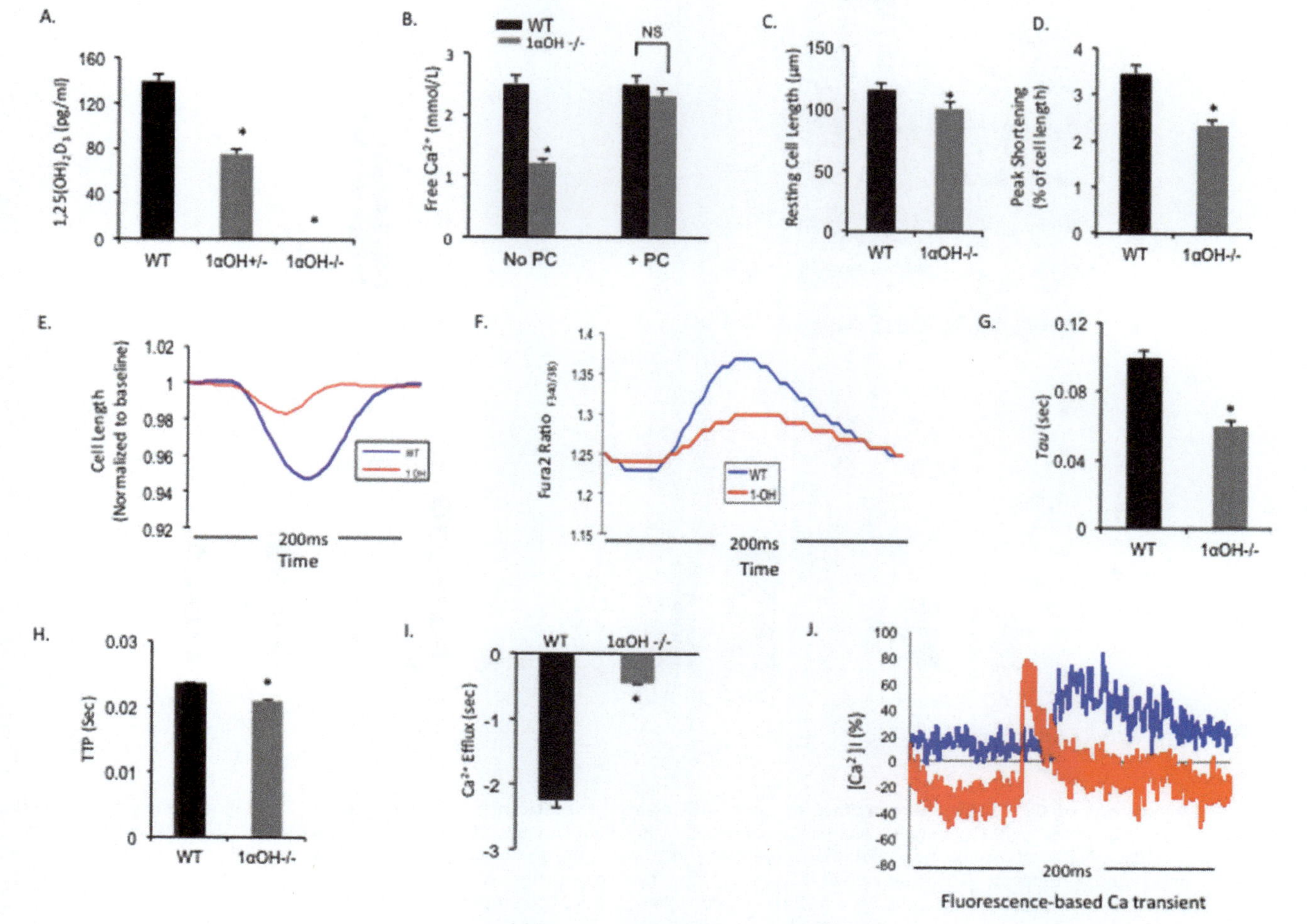

Figure 4. Contractile function and Ca^{2+} transient parameters in isolated CMs from 1αOHase −/− mice. (A and B) Baseline 1, 25$(OH)_2D_3$ (A) and free Ca^{2+} (B) level in WT and 1αOHase −/− mice serums. *, $p<0.05$ compared to WT, N = 6–8 mice. (C) Resting cell length (D) and peak shortening (% of cell length) from isolated CMs obtained from WT and 1αOHase −/− mice. *, $p<0.05$ compared to WT. Ten twitches per CMs were collected for each mouse heart. N = 6–8 mice/group. (E) Continuous measurement of cell contractility from isolated CMs obtained from WT (blue line) and 1αOHase$^{-/-}$ (red line) mice. *, $p<0.05$ compared to WT. Ten twitches per CMs were collected for each mouse heart. N = 6–8 mice/group. (F) Representative Fura 2 ratio (F340/380) from isolated CMs obtained from WT (blue line) and 1αOHase -/- (red line) mice. Data shows that the twitch peak amplitudes are significantly different between WT and 1αOHase -/- CMs, which indicate severely defective Ca^{2+} handling in 1αOHase$^{-/-}$ CMs. (G–I) The rate of Ca^{2+} transient decay (*Tau*) (G), time to peak contraction (TTP) (H), and return velocity to baseline or Ca^{2+} efflux in WT and 1αOHase$^{-/-}$ CMs. *, $p<0.05$ compared to WT. N = 10 CMs/mouse heart. N = 6–8 mice/group. (J) Representative traces of Ca^{2+} transients evoked by 10 mM caffeine recorded in WT (blue line) and 1αOHase$^{-/-}$ (red line) mice CMs.

mouse hearts showed significant increase in PLB, which decreased after TAC (**Fig. 5A and 5B**). SERCA/PLB ratio was also significantly decreased in 1α-OHase$^{-/-}$ mice compared to WT mice (**Fig. 5C**). This may explain the difference in SR Ca^{2+} load and contractile function between WT and 1α-OHase$^{-/-}$ mice CMs, and the depressed levels of SERCA2a may contribute to the severity of heart failure after TAC in 1α-OHase$^{-/-}$ mice.

The Na^{+}- Ca^{2+}-exchanger (NCX) is the dominant myocardial Ca^{2+} efflux mechanism. Ca^{2+} removal from the cytosol occurs by activity of the SR Ca^{2+} pump and by exchange of Ca^{2+} for sodium by the sarcolemmal NCX [25]. The decrease in PLB might lead to a higher activation of the remaining SERCA pumps and increase the activity of NCX [26]. At baseline, there were no significant difference in expression of NCX between the WT and 1α-OHase$^{-/-}$ mice (**Fig. 5A and 5B**). However, we found significant up-regulation of NCX expression in banded WT and 1α-OHase$^{-/-}$ mice with significant 4-folds increase seen in 1α-OHase$^{-/-}$ mice. A relative increase in NCX is expected when SR function is impaired [27]. The function of ryanodine receptor 2 (RyR2) (the cardiac isoform) is to allow Ca^{2+}-induced Ca^{2+} release that brings about contraction, while myocyte relaxation results in RyR2 closure accompanied by the Ca^{2+} re-uptake into SR through the SERCA [28]. After TAC, there was a moderate decrease in RyR2 expression in both WT and 1α-OHase$^{-/-}$ mice (**Fig. 5A and 5B**).

Treatment with PC attenuates cardiac dysfunction after TAC in 1α-OHase -/- mice

The responses of 1α-OHase$^{-/-}$ mice to TAC in our previous experiments may be compounded by their baseline cardiac hypertrophy. Thus, we further determined the specific role of defective vitamin D to pathological conditions by first using "rescue" vitamin D protocol as described previously in 1α-OHase$^{-/-}$ mice, where vitamin D deficiency and its non-cardiac phenotype were both corrected [29]. From 28–30 days of life, 1-α-OHase$^{-/-}$ mice were treated with an initial "rescue" dose of 500 ng/kg of PC, followed by a daily "maintenance" dose of 200 ng/kg from 5 to 8 weeks of age. At 8 weeks, the animals were

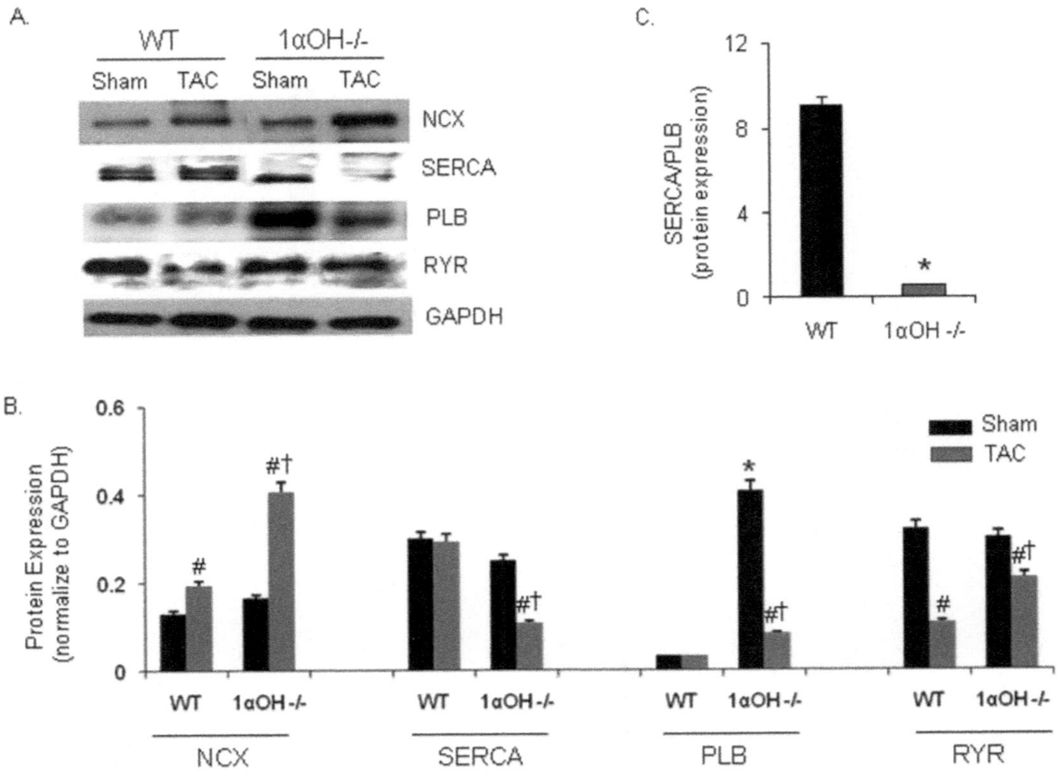

Figure 5. Expressions of Ca^{2+} regulatory protein in mice with altered metabolism of Vitamin D. (A) Representative western blots of various Ca^{2+} handling proteins. (B) Quantitative analysis of various Ca^{2+} handling proteins. NCX = Na^{+}/Ca^{2+} exchanger, SERCA2a = sarcoplasmic reticulum Ca^{2+} ATPase, PLB = phospholamban, and RYR = ryanodine receptor. GAPDH = glyceraldehyde 3-phosphate dehydrogenase. GAPDH was used as internal loading control. *, $p<0.05$ compared to WT. #, $p<0.05$ compared to sham. †, $p<0.05$ compared to WT TAC. N = 8–10. (C) Quantitative analysis of SERCA/PLB protein expression ratio. *, $p<0.05$ compared to WT. #, $p<0.05$ compared to sham, N = 8–10.

divided into the following groups: 1) Vehicle + Sham, 2) Vehicle + TAC, 3) PC + Sham, and 4) PC+TAC. For the vehicle conditions, maintenance doses of PC were changed to vehicle injections, while the PC dose was maintained for PC groups. TAC resulted in a significant increase in HW/BW and LW/BW ratios in mice receiving vehicle for 4 weeks compared to the sham operated mice (**Fig. 6A and 6B**). In mice treated with PC, there was a significant 18% attenuation of TAC-induced HW/BW ratio increase compared to the vehicle treated animals. Histological examination demonstrated that interstitial fibrosis induced by TAC in vehicle-administered 1α-OHase$^{-/-}$ mice were significantly inhibited in PC treated group after TAC (**Fig. 6C**). TAC-induced increases in ANF and β-MHC gene expression, which were both attenuated by PC treatment (**Fig. 6D and 6E**).

We found that decreased fractional shortening after TAC in vehicle treated mice was significantly improved with vitamin D replacement in 1α-OHase$^{-/-}$ mice (**Fig. 6G**). In addition, we observed reduced stroke volume and cardiac output in vehicle treated group after TAC. These parameters also improved after vitamin D replacement (**Fig. 6G and 6H**). Thus, vitamin D replacement resulted in significant attenuation of cardiac dysfunction after TAC in 1α-OHase$^{-/-}$ mice.

Treatment with PC attenuates defective Ca^{2+} handling associated with defective vitamin D signaling

To further assess the effect of vitamin D replacement on CMs contractility in 1α-OHase$^{-/-}$ mice contraction parameters, we performed Ca^{2+} handling analysis of isolated CMs in1α-OHase$^{-/-}$ mice with or without PC treatment. We found that vitamin D replacement attenuated hypocontractility and increased peak shortening in PC treated 1α-OHase$^{-/-}$ mice (**Fig. 6I and 6J**). Rate of relaxation was significantly increased with PC treatment and the rate of Ca^{2+} transient decay (*tau*) was significantly improved (**Fig. 6K and 6L**). Treatment with PC also normalized the PTH level in 1α-OHase$^{-/-}$ mice (**Fig. 7**). These findings suggest that the pathological response in 1α-OHase$^{-/-}$ mice is mainly due to defective vitamin D signaling and associated Ca^{2+} handling, and correcting these abnormalities could rescue these pathological responses.

Discussion

In this study, we demonstrated that vitamin D deficiency is associated with cardiac hypertrophy at baseline results in an exaggerated progression to heart failure after pressure overload in 1α-OHase$^{-/-}$ mice. We also found that there is defective Ca^{2+} handling in 1α-OHase$^{-/-}$ mice, with structural and functional cardiac abnormalities in these mice. These cardiac Ca^{2+} handling abnormalities were completely corrected with vitamin D replacement in 1α-OHase$^{-/-}$ mice. Thus, our studies strongly support the notion that vitamin D deficiency is an under-recognized, non-classic risk factor for developing heart failure that is readily correctable.

Vitamin D is known for its primary role in Ca^{2+} and bone homeostasis [30]. Biological activities of vitamin D are mediated by a hormonally active 1, 25-dihydroxyvitamin D_3 that is converted from 25-hydroxyvitamin D_3 by 1α-OHase. It binds to

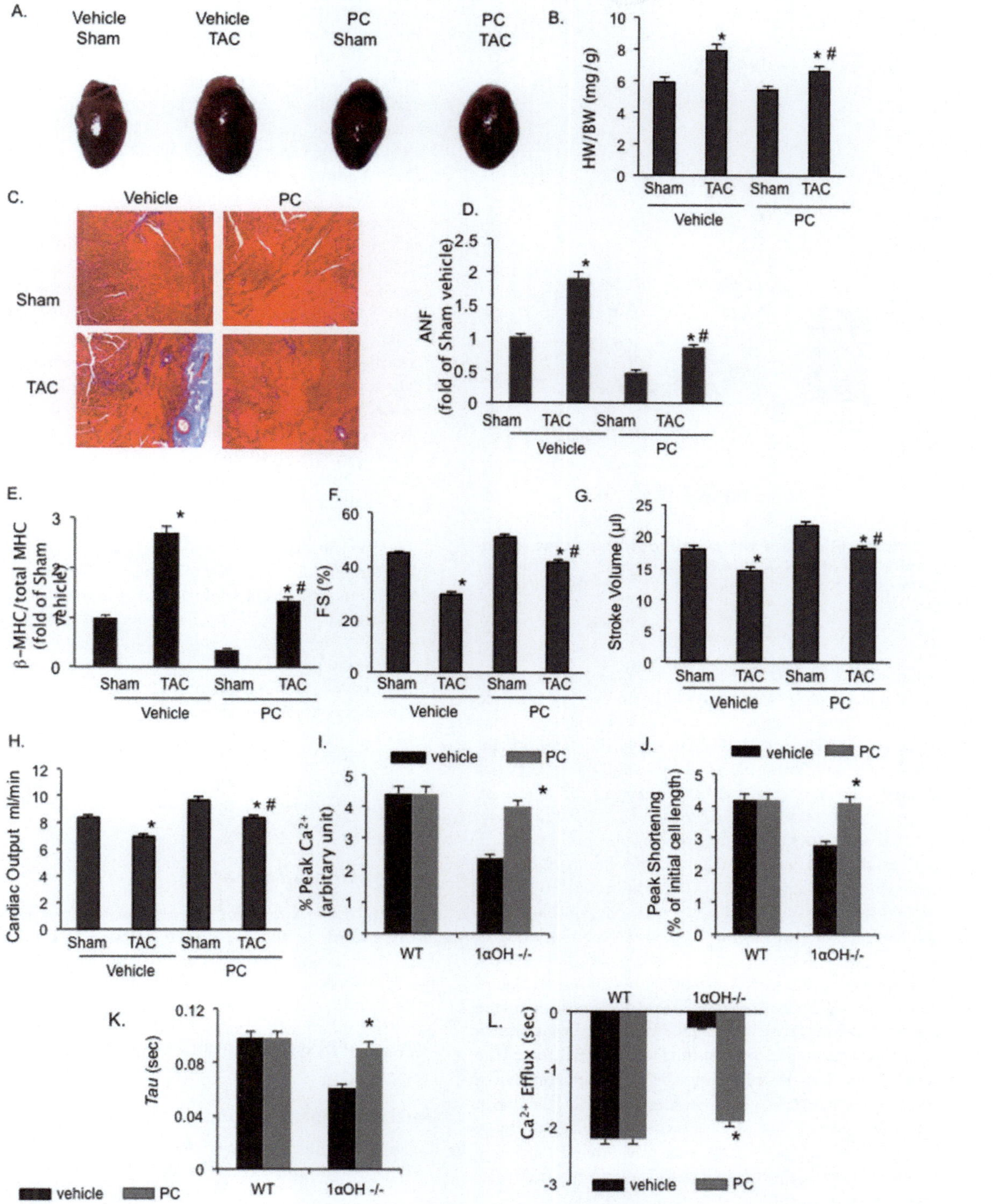

Figure 6. Effect of paricalcitol on cardiac dysfunction parameters. (A) Representative hearts in 1α-OHase$^{-/-}$ mice with or without PC treatment after 4 weeks of sham or TAC. (B) HW/BW ratio in 1α-OHase$^{-/-}$ mice with or without PC treatment after 4 weeks of sham or TAC. *, $p<0.05$ compared to Sham. #, $p<0.05$ compared to vehicle TAC. N = 8–10. (C) Representative Masson-Trichrome heart staining in 1α-OHase$^{-/-}$ mice with or without PC treatment after 4 weeks of sham or TAC. (D and E) Real-time PCR mRNA expression of ANF (D) and of ß-MHC to total MHC ratio (E) after 4 weeks of sham or TAC in 1α-OHase$^{-/-}$ mice with or without PC treatment. *, $p<0.05$ compared to Sham. #, $p<0.05$ compared to vehicle TAC. N = 8–10. (F–H) Fractional shortening (F), stroke volume (G) and cardiac output (H) in 1α-OHase -/- mice with or without PC treatment after 4 weeks of sham or TAC. *, $p<0.05$ compared to Sham. #, $p<0.05$ compared to vehicle TAC. N = 8–10. Effect of paricalcitol on defective calcium handling in 1αOHase −/− mice. (I–L). The % peak Ca^{2+} (I), % peak shortening (J), the rate of Ca^{2+} transient decay (*Tau*) (K), and the return velocity to baseline or Ca^{2+} efflux (L) in 1α-OHase$^{-/-}$ mice with or without PC treatment. *, $p<0.05$ compared to vehicle treated mice group, N = 20 CMs/mouse from 6–8 mice/group.

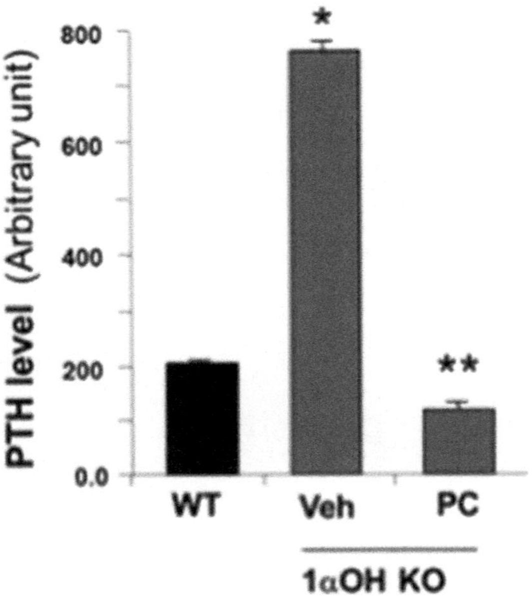

Figure 7. Paricalcitol restore the parathyroid hormone in 1α-OHase$^{-/-}$ mice this model. PTH level in 1α-OHase$^{-/-}$ mice with or without PC treatment. *, $p<0.05$ compared to WT. **, $p<0.05$ compared to vehicle. N = 8–10.

a specific high-affinity vitamin D receptor (VDR), a member of the superfamily of nuclear receptors for steroid hormones [4]. Vitamin D plays an important physiological role in controlling cardiac functions and vitamin D-dependent signaling systems are present in cardiac myocytes and fibroblasts [31]. Vitamin D deficiency has been associated with abnormal cardiac relaxation, proliferation, and increased cardiac renin gene expression [32,33]. Previously, we showed that vitamin D therapy prevents the progression to cardiac hypertrophy [34], and attenuates the development of heart failure in salt sensitive rat model [35]. In addition, 1α-OHase -/- mice developed hypertension, cardiac hypertrophy, and impaired cardiac systolic function, possibly due to the activation of the RAS [8]. Clinically, vitamin D deficiency has been associated with the increased prevalence of myocardial dysfunctions and heart failure [36,37]. Since the critical conversion of the storage form to the active form of vitamin D by 1α-OHase occurs in the kidney, patients with CKD are typically vitamin D deficient. In fact, the prevalence of cardiac hypertrophy and cardiac dysfunction is over 80% in these patients [38,39], and vitamin D therapy has been shown to improve survival and decrease cardiovascular mortality [6,7]. These findings suggest that the role of vitamin D signaling may be significant in the heart, and vitamin D deficiency may offer novel therapeutic target in the treatment of heart failure.

CM contraction is regulated by the interplay between Ca^{2+}, contractile proteins, and the intracellular handling of Ca^{2+}, whereas abnormal Ca^{2+} homeostasis is primarily responsible for depression of CM contractility [22,23]. In several animal and human models of cardiac hypertrophy and heart failure, the whole-cell $[Ca^{2+}]_i$ transient is altered [40,41]. Decreases in SERCA pump expression and activity have been observed in a variety of animal and human models of heart failure and a degree of decrease in SERCA level and its activity, closely correlate with a decreased myocardial function [27]. Thus, these data suggest that alterations in Ca^{2+} handling proteins are important contributors to cardiac dysfunction and heart failure. We found profound Ca^{2+} transient abnormalities, contractile abnormalities and altered expression of various Ca^{2+} handling regulatory proteins in vitamin D deficient CMs, which became exaggerated after TAC. Abnormalities in Ca^{2+} homeostasis, as seen in vitamin D deficiency, may lead to a chronic defect in E–C coupling, which may in turn lead to cardiac dysfunction. Particularly, decreased SERCA and SERCA/PLB expression in 1α-OHase$^{-/-}$ mice supports the hypothesis that alterations in abundance or activity of molecules that regulate systolic and diastolic Ca^{2+} are centrally involved in depressed contractility in hypertrophied and failing hearts.

The key role of cardiac hypertrophy in the pathogenesis of heart disease underscores the need to identify the cellular and molecular mechanisms responsible for both cardiac hypertrophy and its progression to heart failure. A better understanding of disease progression may facilitate the development of novel therapeutic modalities, as well as the development of better guidelines for the prevention of cardiac hypertrophy. Our findings contribute to a better understanding of disease progression that are involved in vitamin D signaling and the development of heart failure. Our finding provides evidences that Ca^{2+} homeostasis and Ca^{2+} handling mediate structural and functional cardiac abnormalities in vitamin D deficient 1α-OHase$^{-/-}$ mice and development of cardiac hypertrophy.

Supporting Information

Table S1 Comparison of cardiomyocytes resting sarcomere length in 0.5 Hz paced cells in WT and 1αOH$^{-/-}$. Sarcomere length of 1α-OHase$^{-/-}$ and WT CMs, raw value in 0.5 Hz paced.

Text S1 Supplemental Information.

Author Contributions

Conceived and designed the experiments: SC RSA PMK. Performed the experiments: SC SB QK JYL SSS. Analyzed the data: SC FdM. Contributed reagents/materials/analysis tools: SC SB QK JYL SSS. Wrote the paper: SC PMK.

References

1. Wang TJ, Pencina MJ, Booth SL, Jacques PF, Ingelsson E, et al. (2008) Vitamin D deficiency and risk of cardiovascular disease. Circulation 117: 503–511.
2. Zittermann A (2006) Vitamin D and disease prevention with special reference to cardiovascular disease. Prog Biophys Mol Biol 92: 39–48.
3. Park CW, Oh YS, Shin YS, Kim CM, Kim YS, et al. (1999) Intravenous calcitriol regresses myocardial hypertrophy in hemodialysis patients with secondary hyperparathyroidism. Am J Kidney Dis 33: 73–81.
4. Demay MB (2006) Mechanism of vitamin D receptor action. Ann N Y Acad Sci 1068: 204–213.
5. McCullough PA, Jurkovitz CT, Pergola PE, McGill JB, Brown WW, et al. (2007) Independent components of chronic kidney disease as a cardiovascular risk state: results from the Kidney Early Evaluation Program (KEEP). Arch Intern Med 167: 1122–1129.
6. Teng M, Wolf M, Lowrie E, Ofsthun N, Lazarus JM, et al. (2003) Survival of patients undergoing hemodialysis with paricalcitol or calcitriol therapy. N Engl J Med 349: 446–456.
7. Teng M, Wolf M, Ofsthun MN, Lazarus JM, Hernan MA, et al. (2005) Activated injectable vitamin D and hemodialysis survival: a historical cohort study. J Am Soc Nephrol 16: 1115–1125.
8. Zhou C, Lu F, Cao K, Xu D, Goltzman D, et al. (2008) Calcium-independent and 1,25(OH)2D3-dependent regulation of the renin-angiotensin system in 1alpha-hydroxylase knockout mice. Kidney Int 74: 170–179.

9. Wehrens XH, Lehnart SE, Reiken SR, Marks AR (2004) Ca2+/calmodulin-dependent protein kinase II phosphorylation regulates the cardiac ryanodine receptor. Circ Res 94: e61–70.
10. Chien KR, Ross J, Jr., Hoshijima M (2003) Calcium and heart failure: the cycle game. Nat Med 9: 508–509.
11. Dardenne O, Prud'homme J, Arabian A, Glorieux FH, St-Arnaud R (2001) Targeted inactivation of the 25-hydroxyvitamin D(3)-1(alpha)-hydroxylase gene (CYP27B1) creates an animal model of pseudovitamin D-deficiency rickets. Endocrinology 142: 3135–3141.
12. McMullen JR, Sherwood MC, Tarnavski O, Zhang L, Dorfman AL, et al. (2004) Inhibition of mTOR signaling with rapamycin regresses established cardiac hypertrophy induced by pressure overload. Circulation 109: 3050–3055.
13. McMullen JR, Shioi T, Zhang L, Tarnavski O, Sherwood MC, et al. (2003) Phosphoinositide 3-kinase(p110alpha) plays a critical role for the induction of physiological, but not pathological, cardiac hypertrophy. Proc Natl Acad Sci U S A 100: 12355–12360.
14. Bae S, Siu PM, Choudhury S, Ke Q, Choi JH, et al. (2010) Delayed activation of caspase-independent apoptosis during heart failure in transgenic mice overexpressing caspase inhibitor CrmA. Am J Physiol Heart Circ Physiol 299: H1374–1381.
15. Choudhury S, Bae S, Ke Q, Lee JY, Kim J, et al. (2011) Mitochondria to nucleus translocation of AIF in mice lacking Hsp70 during ischemia/reperfusion. Basic Res Cardiol 106: 397–407.
16. Rigor DL, Bodyak N, Bae S, Choi JH, Zhang L, et al. (2009) Phosphoinositide 3-kinase Akt signaling pathway interacts with protein kinase Cbeta2 in the regulation of physiologic developmental hypertrophy and heart function. Am J Physiol Heart Circ Physiol 296: H566–572.
17. Shioi T, Kang PM, Douglas PS, Hampe J, Yballe CM, et al. (2000) The conserved phosphoinositide 3-kinase pathway determines heart size in mice. EMBO J 19: 2537–2548.
18. Bassani JW, Bassani RA, Bers DM (1995) Calibration of indo-1 and resting intracellular [Ca]i in intact rabbit cardiac myocytes. Biophys J 68: 1453–1460.
19. Di Rosa M, Malaguarnera M, Nicoletti F, Malaguarnera L (2011) Vitamin D3: a helpful immuno-modulator. Immunology 134: 123–139.
20. Hoenderop JG, Dardenne O, Van Abel M, Van Der Kemp AW, Van Os CH, et al. (2002) Modulation of renal Ca2+ transport protein genes by dietary Ca2+ and 1,25-dihydroxyvitamin D3 in 25-hydroxyvitamin D3-1alpha-hydroxylase knockout mice. FASEB J 16: 1398–1406.
21. Xue Y, Karaplis AC, Hendy GN, Goltzman D, Miao D (2005) Genetic models show that parathyroid hormone and 1,25-dihydroxyvitamin D3 play distinct and synergistic roles in postnatal mineral ion homeostasis and skeletal development. Hum Mol Genet 14: 1515–1528.
22. Del Monte F, Hajjar RJ (2008) Intracellular devastation in heart failure. Heart Fail Rev 13: 151–162.
23. Morgan JP (1991) Abnormal intracellular modulation of calcium as a major cause of cardiac contractile dysfunction. N Engl J Med 325: 625–632.
24. Pieske B, Kretschmann B, Meyer M, Holubarsch C, Weirich J, et al. (1995) Alterations in intracellular calcium handling associated with the inverse force-frequency relation in human dilated cardiomyopathy. Circulation 92: 1169–1178.
25. Bers DM (2000) Calcium fluxes involved in control of cardiac myocyte contraction. Circ Res 87: 275–281.
26. Kubo H, Margulies KB, Piacentino V, 3rd, Gaughan JP, Houser SR (2001) Patients with end-stage congestive heart failure treated with beta-adrenergic receptor antagonists have improved ventricular myocyte calcium regulatory protein abundance. Circulation 104: 1012–1018.
27. Hasenfuss G (1998) Alterations of calcium-regulatory proteins in heart failure. Cardiovasc Res 37: 279–289.
28. Asahi M, Sugita Y, Kurzydlowski K, De Leon S, Tada M, et al. (2003) Sarcolipin regulates sarco(endo)plasmic reticulum Ca2+-ATPase (SERCA) by binding to transmembrane helices alone or in association with phospholamban. Proc Natl Acad Sci U S A 100: 5040–5045.
29. Dardenne O, Prudhomme J, Hacking SA, Glorieux FH, St-Arnaud R (2003) Rescue of the pseudo-vitamin D deficiency rickets phenotype of CYP27B1-deficient mice by treatment with 1,25-dihydroxyvitamin D3: biochemical, histomorphometric, and biomechanical analyses. J Bone Miner Res 18: 637–643.
30. Dusso AS, Brown AJ, Slatopolsky E (2005) Vitamin D. Am J Physiol Renal Physiol 289: F8–28.
31. Chen S, Glenn DJ, Ni W, Grigsby CL, Olsen K, et al. (2008) Expression of the vitamin d receptor is increased in the hypertrophic heart. Hypertension 52: 1106–1112.
32. Lee W, Kang PM (2010) Vitamin D deficiency and cardiovascular disease: Is there a role for vitamin D therapy in heart failure? Curr Opin Investig Drugs 11: 309–314.
33. Xiang W, Kong J, Chen S, Cao L-P, Qiao G, et al. (2005) Cardiac hypertrophy in vitamin D receptor knockout mice: role of the systemic and cardiac renin-angiotensin systems. American Journal of Physiology - Endocrinology And Metabolism 288: E125–E132.
34. Bodyak N, Ayus JC, Achinger S, Shivalingappa V, Ke Q, et al. (2007) Activated vitamin D attenuates left ventricular abnormalities induced by dietary sodium in Dahl salt-sensitive animals. Proc Natl Acad Sci U S A 104: 16810–16815.
35. Bae S, Yalamarti B, Ke Q, Choudhury S, Yu H, et al. (2011) Preventing progression of cardiac hypertrophy and development of heart failure by paricalcitol therapy in rats. Cardiovasc Res 91: 632–639.
36. Gotsman I, Shauer A, Zwas DR, Hellman Y, Keren A, et al. (2012) Vitamin D deficiency is a predictor of reduced survival in patients with heart failure; vitamin D supplementation improves outcome. Eur J Heart Fail 14: 357–366.
37. Holick MF (2007) Vitamin D deficiency. N Engl J Med 357: 266–281.
38. Pilz S, Tomaschitz A, Marz W, Drechsler C, Ritz E, et al. (2011) Vitamin D, cardiovascular disease and mortality. Clin Endocrinol (Oxf) 75: 575–584.
39. Vacek JL, Vanga SR, Good M, Lai SM, Lakkireddy D, et al. (2012) Vitamin D Deficiency and Supplementation and Relation to Cardiovascular Health. Am J Cardiol 109: 359–363.
40. Beuckelmann DJ, Nabauer M, Erdmann E (1992) Intracellular calcium handling in isolated ventricular myocytes from patients with terminal heart failure. Circulation 85: 1046–1055.
41. Perreault CL, Shannon RP, Komamura K, Vatner SF, Morgan JP (1992) Abnormalities in intracellular calcium regulation and contractile function in myocardium from dogs with pacing-induced heart failure. J Clin Invest 89: 932–938.

8

Electrophysiological and Structural Remodeling in Heart Failure Modulate Arrhythmogenesis. 1D Simulation Study

Juan F. Gomez, Karen Cardona, Lucia Romero, Jose M. Ferrero Jr., Beatriz Trenor*

Instituto de Investigación en Ingeniería Biomédica, Universitat Politècnica de València, Valencia, Spain

Abstract

Background: Heart failure is a final common pathway or descriptor for various cardiac pathologies. It is associated with sudden cardiac death, which is frequently caused by ventricular arrhythmias. Electrophysiological remodeling, intercellular uncoupling, fibrosis and autonomic imbalance have been identified as major arrhythmogenic factors in heart failure etiology and progression.

Objective: In this study we investigate *in silico* the role of electrophysiological and structural heart failure remodeling on the modulation of key elements of the arrhythmogenic substrate, i.e., electrophysiological gradients and abnormal impulse propagation.

Methods: Two different mathematical models of the human ventricular action potential were used to formulate models of the failing ventricular myocyte. This provided the basis for simulations of the electrical activity within a transmural ventricular strand. Our main goal was to elucidate the roles of electrophysiological and structural remodeling in setting the stage for malignant life-threatening arrhythmias.

Results: Simulation results illustrate how the presence of M cells and heterogeneous electrophysiological remodeling in the human failing ventricle modulate the dispersion of action potential duration and repolarization time. Specifically, selective heterogeneous remodeling of expression levels for the Na^+/Ca^{2+} exchanger and SERCA pump decrease these heterogeneities. In contrast, fibroblast proliferation and cellular uncoupling both strongly increase repolarization heterogeneities. Conduction velocity and the safety factor for conduction are also reduced by the progressive structural remodeling during heart failure.

Conclusion: An extensive literature now establishes that in human ventricle, as heart failure progresses, gradients for repolarization are changed significantly by protein specific electrophysiological remodeling (either homogeneous or heterogeneous). Our simulations illustrate and provide new insights into this. Furthermore, enhanced fibrosis in failing hearts, as well as reduced intercellular coupling, combine to increase electrophysiological gradients and reduce electrical propagation. In combination these changes set the stage for arrhythmias.

Editor: Alexander V. Panfilov, Gent University, Belgium

Funding: This work was partially supported by (i) the "VI Plan Nacional de Investigación Científica, Desarrollo e Innovación Tecnológica" from the Ministerio de Economía y Competitividad of Spain (grant number TIN2012-37546-C03-01) and the European Commission (European Regional Development Funds – ERDF - FEDER), (ii) the Dirección General de Política Científica de la Generalitat Valenciana (grant number GV/2013/119), and (iii) Programa Prometeo (PROMETEO/2012/030) de la Conselleria d'Educació Formació I Ocupació, Generalitat Valenciana. The funders had no role in study design, data collection and analysis, decision to publish, or preparation of the manuscript.

Competing Interests: The authors have declared that no competing interests exist.

* Email: btrenor@gbio.i3bh.es

Introduction

Heart failure (HF) is a clinical syndrome characterized by the marked and progressive inability of the ventricles to fill and generate adequate cardiac output to meet the demands of cellular metabolism that may have significant variability in its etiology [1]. HF is a final common pathway of a multitude of cardiac pathologies. Congenital cardiac abnormalities, valve disease, hypertension, dilated cardiomyopathy, hypertrophic cardiomyopathy, arrhythmogenic right ventricular cardiomyopathy, and ischemic damage can all result eventually in HF. The primary electrophysiological changes and the mechanisms for arrhythmogenesis associated with HF depend on its etiology [2]. Thus, HF is not characterized by a single set of electrophysiological changes. However, there are a number of consistent findings thought to be important for arrhythmogenesis. These include: ion channel remodeling, enhanced cellular uncoupling, altered calcium homeostasis, extracellular matrix changes, and increased sympathetic nerve activity [2].

Marked ion channel remodeling in failing human hearts has been described in several experimental studies [3–11]. However detailed studies focusing heterogeneous remodeling within the ventricular free wall are lacking [12–16]. This study was undertaken to evaluate how transmural heterogeneous remodeling of selected ion channels in failing hearts modulates electrophysiological dispersion in the ventricular myocardium, which is known to set the stage for malignant arrhythmias [17–19].

Furthermore, structural remodeling and cellular uncoupling [30–34] in failing hearts have long been known to contribute to arrhythmogenesis [20–22]. However, proliferation of fibroblasts and their possible electrical interaction with cardiac myocytes [23–29] has only recently emerged as a plausible pro-arrhythmic factor. These factors are known to alter electrical patterns of propagation and dispersion.

Enhanced dispersion of repolarization in the failing heart, due to a heterogeneous distribution of action potential duration (APD) through the myocardial wall, is thought to be an important contributor to arrhythmia [17–19,30]. However, a recent experimental study by Glukhov et al. [31] reported that transmural APD gradients were decreased in the failing ventricle compared with non-failing hearts.

Computational and theoretical analyses may provide useful insights into the mechanisms responsible for this controversy. Mathematical models of disease-specific AP in human heart are powerful tools for improvement of basic understanding of the ionic mechanism(s) of dysfunction in disease, such as arrhythmias and HF. Furthermore, anatomically detailed multiscale models (from cell to organ dimensions) often can provide complementary approach to clinical and physiological measurements with the common goal of helping to optimize medical devices and pharmacological treatments (see [32,33] for review).

In the present study, the electrophysiological activity of a transmural one dimensional wedge was simulated using well-justified modifications on recent mathematical models of human ventricular AP [34,35] in an attempt to replicate the experimentally reported human HF phenotypes. The influence of electrophysiological and structural remodeling on transmural dispersion of repolarization, Ca^{2+} transients, and electrical conduction properties were the foci of this work. New insights include: the effects of (i) transmural heterogeneous remodeling of SERCA pump and Na^{+}/Ca^{2+}, (ii) the presence of M cells, and (iii) the presence of fibrosis and cellular uncoupling, on repolarization and Ca^{2+} transient gradients.

Methods

Cellular models

Simulations of the electrophysiological activity of endocardial and epicardial human ventricular myocytes were carried out using one of the latest human ventricular AP models, developed by Grandi et al. (GPB model) [34], and characterized by a thorough description of intracellular calcium handling. The O'Hara et al. ventricular AP model (ORd) [35] was also employed to simulate the electrical activity of epicardial, endocardial, and M cells, defined as midmyocardial cells with prolonged APD [36]. Indeed, GPB model does not include a formulation for M cells. ORd model is based on experimental data taken from 140 non-diseased human hearts. It can reproduce the electrophysiological behavior of all three types of human ventricular myocytes, in accordance with experimental observations.

Model of ventricular fibroblast

To simulate the electrical activity of fibroblasts, the formulation of MacCannell et al. [37] was used, which is based on experimental data from adult rat ventricles [38]. Specifically, the active fibroblast model includes a time and voltage-dependent potassium current (I_K), a voltage-dependent inward-rectifying K^+ current (I_{K1}), as well as a Na^+/K^+ pump (I_{NaK}), and a background sodium current ($I_{b,Na}$), with a membrane capacitance of 6.3 pF. The uncoupled resting membrane potential of the active ventricular fibroblast is −49.6 mV.

Homogeneous electrophysiological remodeling in heart failure

To simulate the electrical activity of human ventricular failing myocytes, GPB and ORd models were modified. Quite extensive parameters were changed (based on experimental data from human when it was possible) to describe the hallmark characteristics of failing cardiac tissues and cells, such as AP prolongation and alteration of Ca^{2+} handling [39,40]. A detailed description of these HF models was previously published by our group [41,42]. The entire set of currents and parameter modifications (applied homogeneously in all types of cells) are summarized in Table 1. As mentioned, ORd model includes an electrical description for M cells so that heterogeneous HF remodeling in endocardial, M, and epicardial cells was possible to be defined.

Heterogeneous electrophysiological remodeling in heart failure

Experimental studies describing the functional features and changes in expression levels of ion channels across the ventricular free wall in the failing human heart are scarce [12–16]. Furthermore, extrapolating protein expression levels to channel functional activity is not trivial. Thus, on the basis of the limited literature, we proposed a heterogeneous model of HF based on our previous work [43], where specific parameters were differently altered in epicardial, endocardial, and M cells. Specifically, the activity of the Na^+/Ca^{2+} exchanger (I_{NCX}), which shows a significant upregulation in failing myocytes, was increased 2-fold in epicardial cells and 1.6-fold in M and endocardial cells [15,43], as shown in Table 2. Heterogeneous downregulation of the SERCA pump (I_{SERCA}) has also been described experimentally [16], and was applied in our simulations as follows: a 55% reduction in endocardial cells, a 25% reduction in epicardial cells and a 40% reduction in M cells (see Table 2). These changes which strongly modulate Ca^{2+} transient, were considered as a starting point for heterogeneous remodeling. Transmural heterogeneous remodeling of K^+ currents has also been reported in the human failing ventricular wall, mainly the transient outward K^+ current (I_{to}) [20,44]. Heterogeneous remodeling of I_{to} would surely have an impact on early repolarization; however this is out of the scope of the present work.

Computational methods

To carry out these simulations in strand models of human ventricle we used ELVIRA software [45]. This is based on a pseudo-adaptive finite element method in space and time to solve anisotropic reaction–diffusion equations with highly nonlinear reactive terms. The reaction-diffusion equation (1) governs AP propagation through the multicellular strand. The strand was spatially discretized into linear elements ($\Delta x = 0.01$ cm) delimited by two nodes, one in each of the element ends, where the ionic model is solved. The temporal resolution was fixed to $t = 0.002$ ms to ensure convergence. The scheme accounts for the anisotropy of the media and incorporates an adaptive time step algorithm to integrate the stiff reactive term associated with the ionic currents. The resolution of the monodomain equation (1) is based on the technique of operator splitting.

Table 1. Heart failure ionic remodeling.

Ionic Parameter modified	% in the HF model compared to the normal model		Experimental conditions
	GPB model	ORd model	
I_{NaL}	200%	180%	Isolated cardiomyocytes from LV mid-myocardium of failing dog hearts [88] Whole cell voltage clamp (room temperature) [3]
τ_{hL}	200%	180%	Isolated cardiomyocytes from LV mid-myocardium of failing dog hearts [88] Whole cell voltage clamp (room temperature) [3]
I_{to}	40%	40%	Isolated cardiomyocytes from LV mid-myocardium of failing human hearts. Whole cell voltage clamp (room temperature) [4]
I_{K1}	68%	68%	Review article. Several species [5]
I_{NaK}	90%	70%	Measurements of human myocardial [7] Na,K-ATPase concentration in failing hearts [5]Review article. Several species [6]
I_{Nab}	0	100%	Simulation of human HF [89]
I_{Cab}	153%		Simulation of human HF [89]
I_{NCX}	175%	175%	Simulation of human HF [90]
J_{SERCA}	50%	50%	Isolated cardiomyocytes from LV of failing human hearts. Measurements of Ca^{2+}uptake rates by the SR (37°C) [8]
I_{leak}	300%	130%	Review article [9]
EC_{50SR}	89%		Review article [10]Isolated cardiomyocytes from LV of failing rabbit hearts. Measurements of RyR sensitivity to SR Ca^{2+} [91]
CaMKa		150%	Review article [10]. Transgenic mice [11]
$J_{rel,NP,\infty}$ Ca^{2+} sensitivity		80%	Review article [92]

Changes in original Grandi et al. (GPB) [34] and O'Hara et al. (ORd) [35] models to simulate heart failure (HF) phenotype. The modified parameters are: the late Na^+ current (I_{NaL}), the time constant of inactivation of the I_{NaL} (τ_{hL}), the transient outward K^+ current (I_{to}), the inward rectifier K^+ current (I_{K1}), the Na^+/K^+ pump current (I_{NaK}), the background Ca^{2+} current (I_{Cab}), the Na^+/Ca^{2+} exchanger (I_{NCX}), the sarcoplasmic reticulum (SR) Ca^{2+} pump (J_{SERCA}), the SR Ca^{2+} leak current (I_{leak}), the Ca^{2+} sensitivity of SR Ca^{2+} fluxes (EC_{50SR}), the Ca^{+2}calmodulin-dependent protein kinase II, and the non-phosphorylated Ca^{2+} release, via ryanodine receptors ($J_{rel,NP,\infty}$).

$$\nabla(\tilde{D}\nabla V_m)=\frac{dV_m}{dt}+\frac{I_{ion}}{C_m}+\frac{I_{stm}}{C_m} \quad (1)$$

$$n\cdot(\tilde{D}\nabla V_m)=0 \quad (2)$$

Where V_m is membrane potential in (V), $\tilde{D}=\frac{\tilde{\sigma}}{S_V C_m}$ in (m^2/s) is the diffusion conductivity tensor,$\tilde{\sigma}$ is the conductivity tensor in (S.m), S_V is the surface to volume ratio of the cell in (m^{-1}), C_m in (F) is the membrane capacity, I_{ion} in (A) is the ionic total current, and I_{stm} in (A) is the stimulus current. Equation (1) has boundary conditions (2). Further information can be found in [45].

The ionic model that is solved in each node of the discretized domain changes depending on the described cell (myocyte [34,35] or fibroblast [37]). Temporal equations are computed using a

Table 2. Heart failure heterogeneous transmural ionic remodeling.

Remodeled Current	% in the HF model compared to the normal GPB/ORd models			Experimental conditions
	Epi	M	Endo	
I_{NCX}	200%	160%	160%	Simulation of human HF [89]. The functional activity of the Na^+-Ca^{2+} exchanger was determined by measuring the Na^+-dependent Ca^{2+} uptake into membrane vesicles prepared from human left ventricular samples[93]. Isolated cardiomyocytes from failing canine hearts. Data of transmural NCX mRNA, protein levels, and current [15]. Cellular and transmural 1D simulations of HF using ventricular AP canine model [94].
I_{SERCA}	75%	60%	45%	Isolated cardiomyocytes from LV of failing human hearts. Measurements of Ca^{2+}uptake rates by the SR (37°C) [8]. Endocardial strip preparations from human failing hearts. Measurements of Ca^{2+}uptake in myocardial homogenates (37°C) [95]. LV from human failing hearts. Measurements of Ca^{2+}uptake [96]. Explanted human failing hearts. Data of transmural protein levels of SERCA2a [16].

Changes in original Grandi et al. (GPB) [34] and O'Hara et al. (ORd) [35] models to simulate heart failure (HF) heterogeneous remodeling. The heterogeneously modified parameters are: the Na^+/Ca^{2+} exchanger (I_{NCX}), the sarcoplasmic reticulum (SR) Ca^{2+} pump (J_{SERCA}). Different percentages of these currents with respect to the control value were used in epicardium, endocardium and M-cells (in the case of the ORd model).

semi-implicit numerical method (implicit for the parabolic equation and explicit for ionic models at each node).

Human ventricular transmural strand models

To simulate the electrical activity of a transmural wedge preparation, a heterogeneous one dimensional strand composed of 165 cells was considered as in [35,46,47]. This corresponds to a thickness of 1.65 cm, which is within the range of 1 to 2 cm reported for the width of the human left ventricular wall [48]. The strand was divided into 82 endocardial cells and 83 epicardial cells, each myocyte being driven by GPB formulation [34]. The diffusion tensor ($\tilde{D}$) in normal conditions (NC) for myocyte cells was set to $D_M = D_{xx} = 0.0006$ cm/ms resulting in a conduction velocity (CV) of 50 cm/s as in experimental measurements of transmural conduction [49]. The intercellular uncoupling observed in failing hearts was modeled by a two-fold decrease in diffusion coefficient, i.e. intercellular conductivity was halved ($D_M = 0.0003$ cm/ms), in accordance with experimental measurements in the human failing heart reporting a 50% reduction in connexin43 protein levels [50]. To test other degrees of intercellular uncoupling, mild uncoupling ($D_M = 0.00045$ cm/ms) and severe uncoupling ($D_M = 0.00025$ cm/ms) were also considered. The effect of fibroblasts within the strand was simulated by (i) randomly distributing fibroblasts (diffuse fibrosis) or (ii) considering small localized clusters (patchy fibrosis) [51,52]. Diffuse fibrosis is defined as small deposits of fibrous tissue. Fibroblasts were thus randomly distributed within the strand so that some nodes were assigned to the fibroblast ionic model and the rest of the nodes to the myocyte ionic model. As in [53], a fibrotic content of 10% or 20% corresponds to the percentage of nodes assigned to the fibroblast ionic model. For each fibrotic content 11 random configurations were simulated (see Figures S1 and S2 in File S1). Patchy fibrosis, i.e. larger clusters of fibrous tissue, was simulated with clusters of 25 interconnected fibroblasts, introduced within the ventricular strand. Fibroblasts were electrotonically coupled to surrounding cells (myocytes or other fibrotic cells) by considering a lower conductivity tensor with respect to conductivity tensor between myocytes. The diffusion coefficient in fibroblast elements was decreased three-fold with respect to myocytes, based on experimental data [27]. To test the effects of the heterogeneous electrophysiological remodeling characteristic of HF, multicellular strands containing also M cells were considered. For this purpose, one dimensional simulations were performed using a heterogeneous multicellular strand, which resembles some functional features of a ventricular transmural wedge preparation, as described in O'Hara et al. [35]. This strand was composed by 60 endocardial, 45 M, and 65 epicardial cells governed by ORd formulation. Stimuli were applied at the extreme endocardial end in all configurations with a basic cycle length (BCL) of 1000 ms. Parameters were measured for the last stimulation, after steady state was reached, i.e. after 200 s and 750 s in the cellular strands using GPB and ORd models, respectively.

Parameter definition

APD at 90% of repolarization (APD_{90}) was computed in myocytes of the strand, then APD dispersion was calculated as the difference between the maximum and minimum APD_{90} along the strand. Border effects were avoided by eliminating 15 cells in each end of the strand for the computation of dispersion. Repolarization time (RT) for a cell was measured by adding APD_{90} of this cell to the time needed by the wavefront to reach the cell. Transmural dispersion of repolarization (TDR) was then computed as the difference between the maximum and minimum RT along the multicellular strand. Ca^{2+} transient duration was measured as the time from the upstroke to 80% of recovery ($CaTD_{80}$) as in [54], and the voltage-calcium delay was defined as the delay between the upstrokes of AP and Ca^{2+} transient (AP-Ca delay) [54]. $CaTD_{80}$ and AP-Ca delay dispersions were computed as the difference between the maximum and minimum $CaTD_{80}$ and AP-Ca delay, respectively, along the multicellular strand.

The effective refractory period (ERP) was measured as the minimum time between two consecutive stimuli that resulted in propagation of the AP wave across the strand. Conduction velocity (CV) was measured between the 15th and 150th myocytes (to avoid edge effects), as the distance between cells divided by the difference between the times of maximum depolarization upstroke. The safety factor (SF) for conduction is a quantitative parameter based on the source-sink relationship of electric charge between adjacent cardiac cells. The value of the SF indicates the success or failure in AP propagation. Several definitions of the SF have been published [55–57], and the formulation proposed by Romero and coworkers [58] (SF_m), described in equation (3), was chosen because of its computational advantages. This formulation of the SF was proposed by Shaw and Rudy [56], however, Romero et al. [58] changed the definition of the integration domain, optimizing its calculation and saving computational resources.

$$SF_m = \frac{\int_A I_C dt + \int_A I_{out} dt}{\int_A I_{in} dt} \quad A|t \in [t_{1\%}, t_{V\max}] \tag{3}$$

where I_c stands for the capacitive current, I_{in} is the axial current that enters the cell, I_{out} is the axial current that leaves the cell, $t_{1\%}$ in the instant when membrane potential reaches 1% of its maximum and $t_{V\max}$ is the instant of maximal V_m.

Statistical analysis

SPSS Statistics 17.0 software (IBM SPSS Statistics) was used for student t-test. Values are expressed as mean±SD. $p<0.05$ was considered significant.

Results

Effects of electrophysiological remodeling on transmural repolarization gradients

To assess the influence of HF induced electrophysiological remodeling on repolarization gradients, detailed simulations of the action potential conduction and repolarization in human ventricular transmural wedge preparations were carried out using our modified GPB and ORd AP models. Figure 1 shows the results obtained in a wedge composed by endocardial and epicardial myocytes using GPB model. As depicted in panel A, APD_{90} is longer in the failing endocardial and epicardial myocytes (red line) than in normal conditions (blue line) at a stimulation rate of 1 Hz. Note also that APD dispersion is increased in HF to 24 ms versus 20 ms in control conditions. In addition, as shown in panel B, repolarization time along the strand is delayed in failing myocytes (red line). Transmural dispersion of repolarization was slightly decreased in HF with respect to control conditions.

Similar simulations were conducted using the modified ORd model to assess whether this pattern of results were model-dependent. From Figure 2 (panels A and B) it is clear that for ORd model values of APD and repolarization time are also lengthened in HF compared with NC. As expected, some differences with respect to GPB results were observed. The increase in APD dispersion was more pronounced in HF when ORd model was used. TDR increased in HF whereas the opposite result was

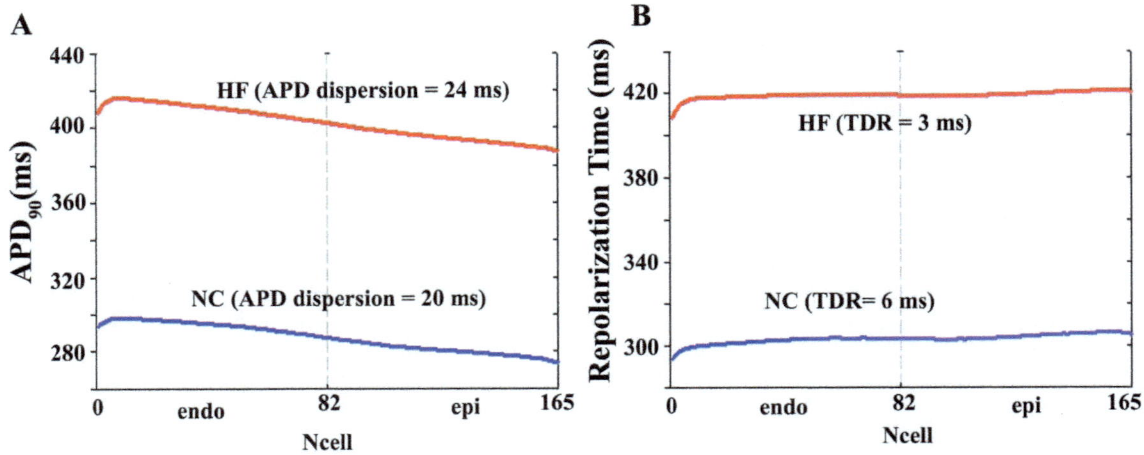

Figure 1. Action potential duration and repolarization time in normal and failing conditions. A. Action potential duration (APD_{90}) measured along a transmural ventricular strand, composed by 82 endocardial and 83 epicardial cells, in normal conditions (NC, blue line) and in heart failure conditions (HF, red line). APD dispersion is indicated in ms for each curve. B. Repolarization time calculated along the ventricular strand in normal (blue line) and failing (red line) conditions. Transmural dispersion of repolarization (TDR) was measured in ms. Simulations were conducted using Grandi et al. (GPB) action potential model [34].

obtained with the GPB model. Significant differences in the formulation of repolarizing currents of ORd and GPB models, as described with detail in [59] are likely responsible for these differences. Especially, the fact that ORd model considers transmural differences in 11 ionic currents, while GPB model distinguishes only between I_{to} in epicardial and endocardial myocytes, might be responsible for the different behaviors of the models in terms of APD transmural gradients and TDR.

To analyze the influence of M cells on repolarization gradients in the failing tissue, a transmural wedge in which M cells were also implemented. In this analysis only ORd model was used, as GPB model does not include any AP formulation for this type of cells. APD dispersion and TDR along a transmural ventricular strand comprising M cells are shown in Figure 2 (panels C and D). The presence of M cells prolongs APD throughout the fiber and increases its dispersion (panel C) in both control and HF. Repolarization time is also increased at each fixed location in the strand and TDR also increased (panel D). However, the relative increase of APD dispersion and TDR in HF with respect to NC, in the presence of M cells is very similar to these changes in their absence. Thus, as expected from their intrinsic properties, M cells increase global repolarization gradients but do not increase the relative changes due to HF electrophysiological remodeling (with respect to control).

Effects of heterogeneous electrophysiological remodeling on transmural repolarization gradients

Several experimental studies [12–16] have reported differences in the remodeling across the transmural ventricular free wall in failing hearts. To analyze how heterogeneous remodeling can affect APD_{90} and corresponding repolarization time gradients, simulations were performed using HF models with spatially heterogeneous remodeling across the ventricular strand, as described in the Methods section. Figure 3 shows the simulation results for GPB model in endocardium and epicardium (blue bars), for ORd model in endocardium and epicardium (red bars), and for ORd model also including M cells (green bars). In the case of GPB model, heterogeneous remodeling of I_{NCX} decreased APD dispersion to 19 ms versus 24 ms corresponding to homogeneous HF remodeling and 20 ms corresponding to normal conditions (panel C Figure 3). Similarly, using ORd model, heterogeneous remodeling of I_{NCX} and/or I_{SERCA} decreased APD dispersion with respect to homogeneous HF remodeling, regardless of the absence (red bars) or presence (green bars) of M cells. TDR (Figure 3 panel D) was also modulated by heterogeneous remodeling and was decreased with respect to homogeneous remodeling when ORd model was used. In general, in the presence of M cells, the values of APD dispersion and TDR are higher, and heterogeneous HF remodeling does not bring these values lower than control values.

Effects of heterogeneous electrophysiological remodeling on transmural dispersion of Ca^{2+} transients

Because the heterogeneous remodeling that is the focus of the paper is limited to I_{NCX} and I_{SERCA}, which strongly affect Ca^{2+} transients, we also analyzed Ca^{2+} homeostasis. Figure 4 depicts Ca^{2+} transients in three different myocytes phenotypes within the transmural strand under normal conditions (blue), and for homogeneous (red) and heterogeneous (pink) HF remodeling. As observed experimentally in HF, the amplitude of Ca^{2+} transients is decreased, and the rise and decay rates are slowed. Figure 5 depicts the values of diastolic Ca^{2+} in panel A, systolic Ca^{2+} in panel B, Ca^{2+} duration ($CaTD_{80}$) in panel C, and the delay between AP and Ca^{2+} upstrokes (AP-Ca delay) in panel D, along the transmural strand. Significant differences in these magnitudes are observed along the ventricular strand in normal conditions (blue lines) and also after HF remodeling (red lines for homogeneous HF and pink lines for heterogeneous HF). The dispersion of $CaTD_{80}$ and AP-Ca delay were calculated for the different AP models (panels E and F in Figure 3). HF increased $CaTD_{80}$ dispersion in both models, which was strongly modulated by heterogeneous remodeling of I_{NCX} and I_{SERCA}. AP-Ca delay dispersion was increased or unaltered in HF using GPB or ORd models, respectively. Again, heterogeneous remodeling modulated AP-Ca delay, especially when GPB model was used.

Heterogeneous remodeling in failing hearts has been considered an important contributor to the HF phenotype and likely a major factor for modulation of transmural repolarization and Ca^{2+} transient gradients, as illustrated in our simulations (see Figure 3). The presence of M-cells also contributes to this modulation, by

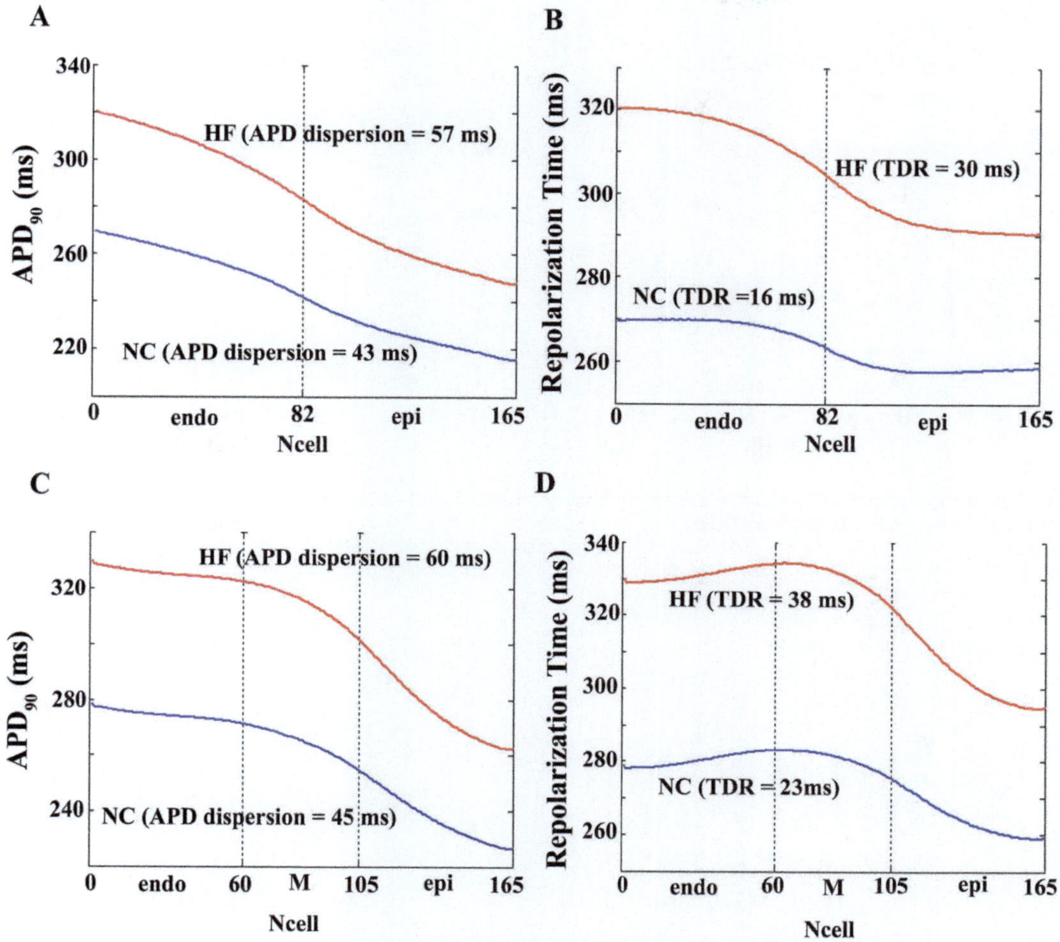

Figure 2. Action potential duration and repolarization time in normal and failing conditions including M cells influence. Panels A and C. Action potential duration (APD_{90}) measured along a transmural ventricular strand, in normal conditions (NC, blue line) and in heart failure conditions (HF, red line). APD dispersion is indicated in ms for each curve. Panels B and D. Repolarization time calculated along the ventricular strand in normal (blue line) and failing (red line) conditions. Transmural dispersion of repolarization (TDR) was measured in ms. The ventricular strands are composed by 82 endocardial and 83 epicardial cells (panels A and B) and by 60 endocardial, 45 M-, and 65 epicardial cells (panels C and D). All simulations were conducted using O'Hara et al. (ORd) action potential model [35].

maintaining higher gradients. However, there is limited electrophysiological data from the human heart, and further experimental studies, similar to [54], are needed to fully determine how heterogeneous remodeling modulates APD gradients, TDR and Ca^{2+} transients changes. Specifically, measurements of AP and Ca^{2+} transients transmural gradients and their relation to protein expression levels or activity of the SERCA pump and I_{NCX} in a transmural wedge of the failing heart would be very valuable.

Effects of structural remodeling on repolarization gradients and impulse conduction

The effect of fibrosis within the strand was evaluated in a transmural ventricular wedge composed by endocardial and epicardial cells. GPB model was used because the effects of electrophysiological remodeling in repolarization gradients were less pronounced than in ORd model and we were interested in evaluating whether structural remodeling could significantly increase these gradients and/or alter action potential conduction. When clusters of fibroblasts were inserted randomly in the strand, marked differences in APD and repolarization time resulted, as shown in Figure 6. When fibrosis was present in the failing strand (10% of fibrotic content), APD dispersion went up to 70 ms, compared to 24 ms with HF electrophysiological remodeling. When intercellular uncoupling was also introduced, the APD dispersion increased even more to 92 ms.

A similar pattern of change could be observed in TDR (see Figure 6 panel B). Transmural dispersion of repolarization was also significantly enhanced when the fibrotic content was 10%, as shown in Figure 6 panel B and even more when intercellular uncoupling was considered. Thus, inserted fibrosis and intercellular uncoupling increased TDR and APD dispersion. Nevertheless, when the fibrotic content was further enhanced to 20%, APD dispersion and TDR were decreased with respect to 10% fibrosis, showing a biphasic behavior with fibrotic content, as shown in Figure 7A and 7B. This tendency was maintained for different uncoupling degrees. The values of APD dispersion and TDR shown correspond to one of the random configurations (configuration 1) for each fibrotic content (10% and 20%). Additional random configurations were simulated and the results are shown in the Supporting Information (see Tables S1 and S2 in File S1 for normal intercellular coupling and Tables S3, S4, S5, and S6 in File S1 for the different degrees of intercellular uncoupling and fibrosis). A statistical analysis was also performed and APD

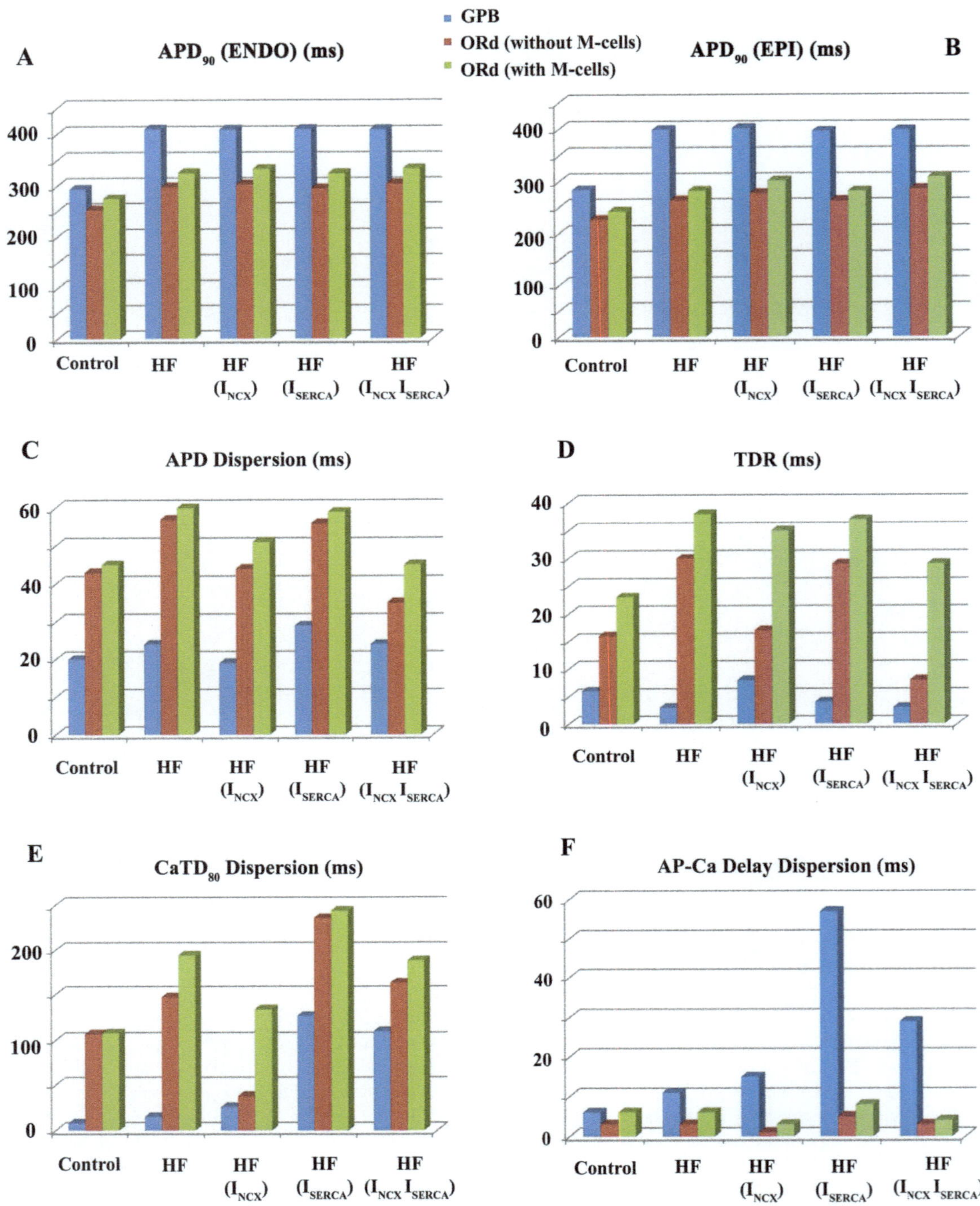

Figure 3. Biomarkers in normal, homogeneous and heterogeneous remodeling failing conditions with GPB, ORd (without M cells), and ORd (with M cells) models. Electrophysiological properties measured in a one dimensional transmural ventricular strand under different pathological conditions. The ventricular strands were composed by 82 endocardial and 83 epicardial cells. All simulations were conducted using Grandi et al. (GPB) action potential model [34] (blue bars), O'Hara et al. [35] model (ORd) without M-cells (red bars) and ORd model with M cells (green bars). The cases considered were: normal conditions (Control), electrical homogeneous heart failure remodeling (HF), electrical heterogeneous heart failure remodeling on I_{NCX} (HF I_{NCX}), electrical heterogeneous heart failure remodeling on I_{SERCA} (HF I_{SERCA}), and electrical heterogeneous heart failure remodeling on I_{NCX} and I_{SERCA} simultaneously (HF $I_{NCX}I_{SERCA}$). The mean action potential duration (APD) along the endocardial (panel A) and epicardial (panel B) strand was measured at 90% repolarization. Dispersion in APD (panel C) was measured along the entire strand as the difference between maximal and minimal APD, avoiding first and last fifteen cells. Transmural dispersion of repolarization (TDR) (panel D) was measured by adding the APD to the time of depolarization of each cell. The calcium transient duration ($CaTD_{80}$) (panel E) was measured from the upstroke to 80% of calcium transient amplitude, dispersion was assessed as in APD. AP-Ca delay (panel F) was measured as the difference between the upstroke in AP and in calcium transient along the entire strand, dispersion was also evaluated as in APD (see Methods section for details).

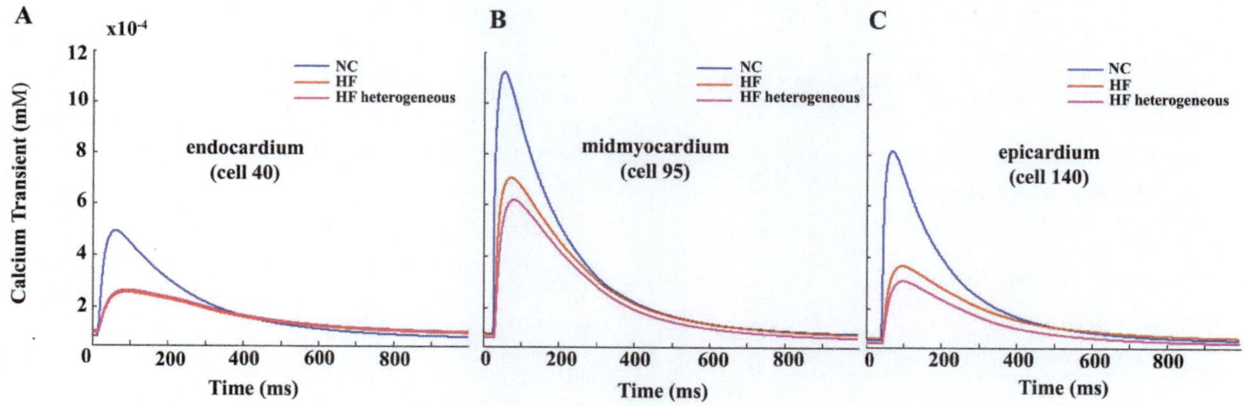

Figure 4. Calcium transient representation under normal and failing conditions. Ca^{2+} transient representation in an endocardial cell (#40) (panel A), in a midmyocardial cell (#95) (panel B), and in an epicardial cell (#140) (panel C) of a heterogeneous ventricular strand for normal conditions (NC blue lines), homogeneous failing conditions (HF red lines), and heterogeneous heart failure (HF) remodeling (magenta lines). Simulations were performed using O'Hara et al. model [35].

dispersion and TDR mean values were lower in the case of 20% of fibrotic content with respect to 10% fibrosis, regardless of the degree of cellular uncoupling (see Tables S1, S2, S3, S4, S5, and S6 in File S1 and Figures S3, S4, S5, S6, S7, S8, S9, and S10 in File S1, however only in the case of APD dispersion this difference was statistically different ($p<0.05$).

The excitability and conduction properties were also analyzed in the presence of HF electrophysiological remodeling, fibrosis and/or intercellular uncoupling. Figure 6 panel C shows the color-coded resting membrane potential (V_{rest}) in each cell of the unidimensional strand in HF without fibrosis, in HF with 10% fibrosis, and in HF with 20% fibrosis after a period of stabilization.

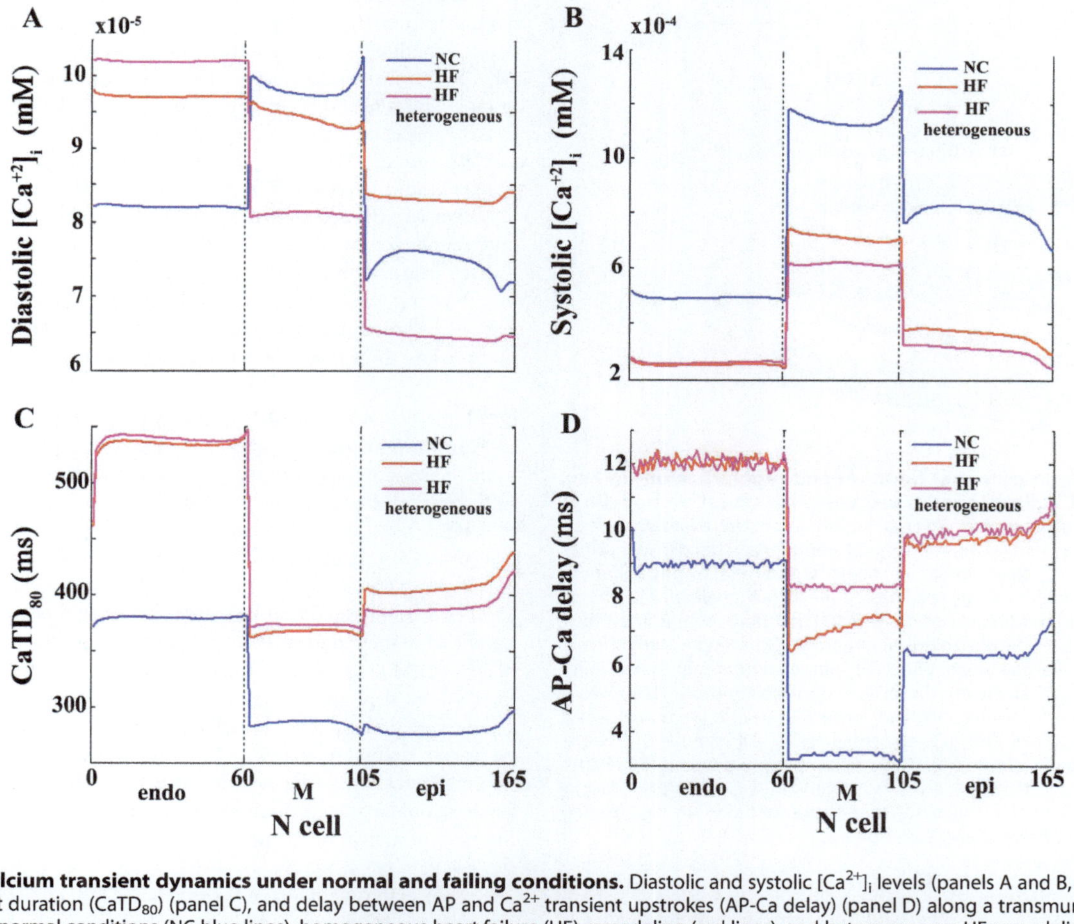

Figure 5. Calcium transient dynamics under normal and failing conditions. Diastolic and systolic $[Ca^{2+}]_i$ levels (panels A and B, respectively), Ca^{2+} transient duration ($CaTD_{80}$) (panel C), and delay between AP and Ca^{2+} transient upstrokes (AP-Ca delay) (panel D) along a transmural ventricular strand under normal conditions (NC blue lines), homogeneous heart failure (HF) remodeling (red lines), and heterogeneous HF remodeling conditions (pink lines). Simulations were performed using O'Hara et al. model [35].

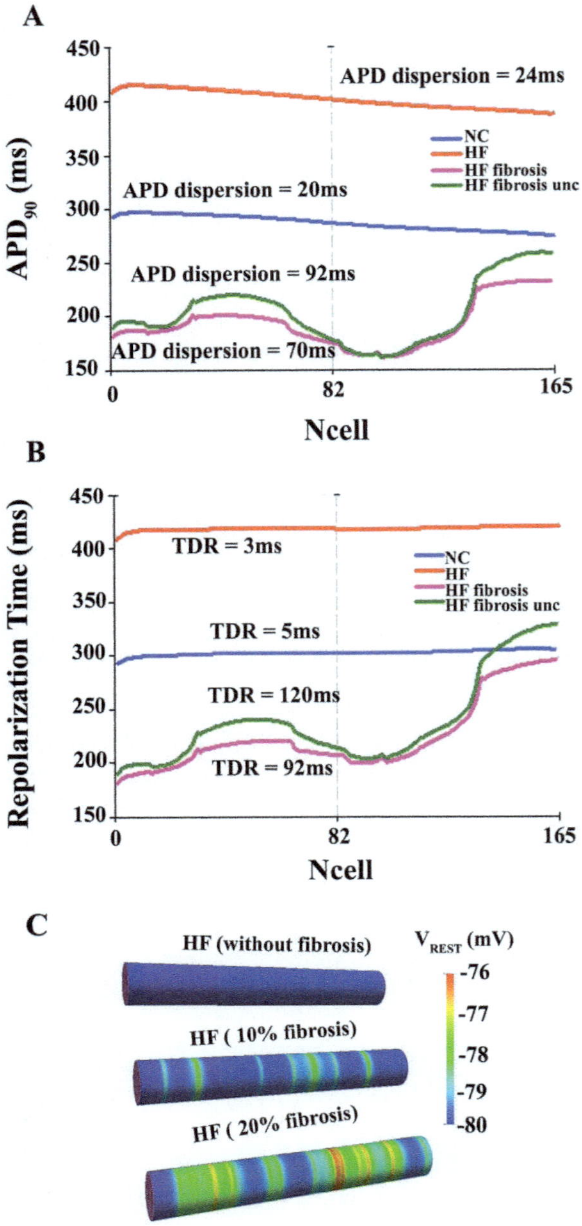

Figure 6. Action potential duration and repolarization time in normal and failing conditions with structural remodeling. Action potential duration (APD_{90}) (panel A) and repolarization time (panel B) measured along transmural ventricular strands, in normal conditions (NC, blue lines), in heart failure electrophysiological remodeling conditions (HF, red lines), in heart failure electrophysiological remodeling conditions with fibrosis 10% (HF fibrosis, pink lines), and in heart failure electrophysiological remodeling conditions with fibrosis 10% and intercellular uncoupling (HF fibrosis unc, green lines). APD dispersion and transmural dispersion of repolarization (TDR) were measured in ms for each curve. The ventricular strands were composed by 82 endocardial and 83 epicardial cells. All simulations were conducted using Grandi et al. (GPB) action potential model [34]. Panel C shows in a color code the resting potential (V_{rest}) along the failing ventricular strand after achieving steady state conditions in the absence of fibrosis, 10% fibrosis, and 20% fibrosis.

As expected, V_{rest} increases with the fibrotic content. Figure 7 panel C shows that HF alone (filled circle with 0% of fibrosis) did not alter significantly CV with respect to control (white circle) but did increase the effective refractory period with respect to control (444 ms vs. 320 ms; results not shown). However, when fibrosis and intercellular uncoupling were considered, separately or concomitantly, the decrease of CV was more pronounced and synergistic. With regard to ERP, uncoupling alone had no significant effect, whereas fibrosis reduced it significantly (results not shown).

The safety in conduction was also evaluated, using the safety factor indicator (see Methods section). As show in Figure 8, the safety factor was very slightly reduced when HF electrophysiological remodeling was considered (red line) with respect to control conditions (blue line). However, when clustered fibrosis was introduced in the HF strand, safety factor was decreased yielding a value approx. 1 in the fibroblasts clusters, indicating that conduction is still possible but less safe. Thus, fibrosis slows CV and the quantity of charge that is able to be transmitted to the next cell is seriously compromised. When the fibrotic cluster was big enough, conduction was blocked.

Discussion

Major findings

This computational work, made possible by using two recent, comprehensive, and complimentary mathematical models of the human ventricular AP, provides important new insights into the role of HF-induced electrophysiological and structural remodeling in the modulation of transmural gradients for late repolarization, intracellular Ca^{2+} transient, and action potential conduction. The principal findings and insights from our work are (i) the demonstration that HF heterogeneous remodeling of I_{NCX} and I_{SERCA} modulates Ca^{2+} transient duration and the dispersion of AP-Ca^{2+} transient upstrokes delay. In addition, (ii) simulated homogeneous electrophysiological remodeling during HF increases APD dispersion (more significantly in ORd model than in GPB model), and (iii) HF structural remodeling enhances repolarization gradients and decreases CV and ERP. (iv) We suggest also that although M cells are known to contribute to the increase of APD and repolarization dispersion, they do not to alter the relative change from normal tissue to failing tissue; and (v) confirmation for the first time of the hypothesis that heterogeneous HF remodeling modulates repolarization gradients and can bring them below the values corresponding to normal conditions.

Electrophysiological gradients in heart failure

Transmural heterogeneities of repolarization play a critical role in the genesis of polymorphic ventricular tachycardia (PVT) in HF [19]. Several experimental studies [19,30,31,54] have addressed the impact of the dispersion of repolarization time in the transmural ventricular wall on the generation of reentrant activity in different animal species. In their study on dog ventricle, Akar et al. [19] demonstrated that spatial gradients of repolarization were significantly increased in HF because of the marked prolongation of APD in M cells and concluded that this was directly responsible for PVT generation. In the human right ventricle Lou et al. [30] also observed an increase in APD gradients in HF and related it to increased arrhythmogenesis. In contrast, Coronel et al. [60] observed that in the pig ventricle it is not only the repolarization gradient but also the restitution characteristics in combination with the time of arrival of the premature wavefront, which determines the occurrence of reentry.

Recent experiments have shown that TDR and APD gradient are reduced as a result of heart failure [31,54]. These studies examined APD prolongation and dispersion of repolarization in coronary artery-perfused left ventricular wedge preparations from

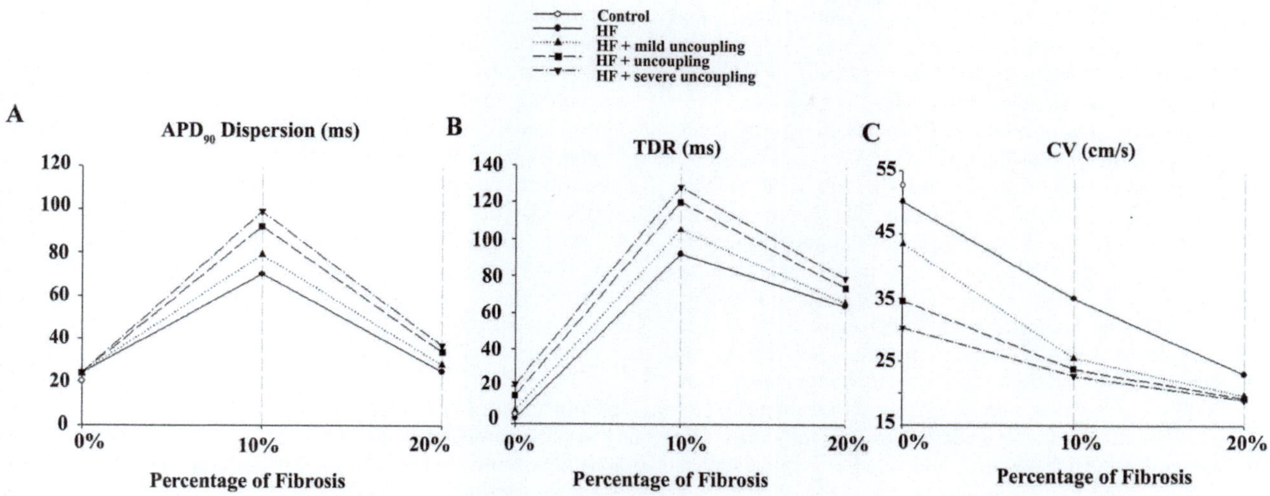

Figure 7. Biomarkers in normal and failing conditions adding structural remodeling with GPB. Electrophysiological properties measured in a one dimensional transmural ventricular strand under different pathological conditions. The ventricular strands were composed by 82 endocardial and 83 epicardial cells. All simulations were conducted using Grandi et al. (GPB) action potential model [34]. The cases considered were: normal conditions (NC) (white circle), electrical heart failure remodeling (HF) (solid line), electrical heart failure remodeling and mild uncoupling (dotted line), normal uncoupling (dashed line) and severe uncoupling (dotted-dashed line). Different degrees of fibrosis were considered: 10% and 20%. Action potential duration (APD) dispersion (panel A), transmural dispersion of repolarization (TDR) (panel B), and conduction velocity (CV) (panel C) along the whole strand were measured (see Methods section for details).

the human heart using optical mapping [31]. In these preparations APs were prolonged in HF in a transmurally heterogeneous manner, with the greatest prolongation occurring in the subepicardial layer, so that APD gradients from subendocardium to subepicardium were significantly decreased in failing compared with non-failing hearts. No significant M cell contribution could be identified in these HF wedges. Their identification of M cells was based on the local APD gradient between the areas of delayed repolarization (M cells) and the neighboring myocardium, taking into account intrinsic cellular properties and extrinsic coupling properties of the tissue. M cell islands were found in non-diseased hearts but this was not the case for the failing ones. Although M cells are present in the canine myocardium [19,61], there is no evidence of the existence of this type of cells under failing conditions in human myocardium [30,31,54]. In the present study we analyzed the role of M cells and heterogeneous ionic remodeling in the modulation of repolarization gradients. Our results revealed increased APD dispersion under HF conditions assuming homogeneous remodeling with respect to control conditions. The presence of M cells increased general repolarization gradients but did not alter the relative change in HF with respect to control observed in the absence of M cells.

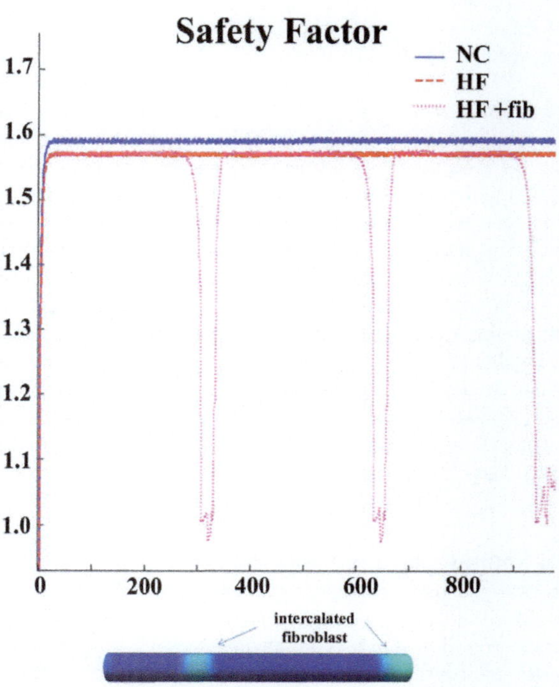

Figure 8. Safety factor for conduction in normal, failing conditions, and with fibrosis inserted. Safety factor (SF) calculated in a fiber of 900 endocardial cells under normal conditions (blue continuous line), when heart failure electrophysiological remodeling is considered (red dashed line), and when clustered fibrosis and concomitant heart failure electrophysiological remodeling are present (pink dotted line).

Assessing the importance of heterogeneous remodeling on the modulation of repolarization gradients was a major highlight in our simulations. Although changes in mRNA and protein expression across the transmural wall have been reported in failing human hearts [12–16,20], much more experimental work is required to demonstrate how heterogeneous functional ionic remodeling can alter APD dispersion. Our theoretical results suggest that transmural heterogeneous remodeling of I_{NCX} and/or I_{SERCA} decreased APD dispersion with respect to homogeneous HF remodeling, regardless of the absence (Figure 3 red bars) or presence (Figure 3 green bars) of M cells. Furthermore, in the absence of M cells, dispersion of repolarization in the heterogeneously remodeled failing tissue, could be brought to lower values than in normal conditions. Thus, this is a plausible explanation for decreased APD dispersion and repolarization gradients in the experimental work of Glukhov et al. [21]. TDR was also modulated by heterogeneous remodeling and was decreased with respect to homogeneous remodeling when ORd model was used.

In the presence of M cells TDR values were higher, and heterogeneous HF remodeling did not bring these values lower than in normal conditions as in [31], where M cells were absent.

The effects of heterogeneous remodeling on Ca^{+2} gradients were also analyzed. It is well known that myocytes in the failing heart exhibit abnormal intracellular Ca^{+2} transients, due in part to the decreased functional expression of the SR Ca^{+2} ATPase (SERCA2a), the enhanced sodium (Na^{+}/Ca^{+2}) exchanger function [62–64], and the aberrant SR Ca^{+2} leak, due to altered ryanodine receptor (RyR) function [65,66]. Transmural differences in regulation of these Ca^{2+}-cycling proteins were found in the failing ventricle [15,16]. Our results accurately reproduce some of these features: the amplitude of Ca^{+2} transients decreases, and the rise and decay rates are slowed down, in accordance with experimental results [8,67]. Furthermore, homogeneous HF remodeling increases $CaTD_{80}$ dispersion, which is strongly modulated by heterogeneous remodeling of I_{NCX} and I_{SERCA}. Experimentally, Lou et al. [54] found that the gradient of $CaTD_{80}$ was lower in failing conditions. Our results can account for this only if heterogeneous remodeling (I_{NCX}) and no M cells were considered in the analysis using ORd model. In our simulations AP-Ca delay dispersion was slightly increased (GPB) or unaltered (ORd), and heterogeneous remodeling lowered it below the values corresponding to the normal heart (ORd). Lou et al. [54] obtained a slightly lower gradient of AP-Ca delay in failing conditions than in normal conditions. Thus, heterogeneous remodeling could be a possible explanation for these results. Furthermore, heterogeneous remodeling of I_{to} [44], which was not considered in the present work, could also have a role in the modulation of Ca^{2+} transient waveform through changes in early repolarization [68].

The role of structural remodeling in heart failure

In HF significant microanatomical remodeling related to arrhythmogenesis has been observed [69,70]. The proliferation of fibroblasts and intercellular uncoupling during HF has been the focus of experimental [12,50,71–75] and simulation [29,76,77] studies. Experimental work has provided some insights into how gap junctions between myocytes are modified in the failing heart. Specifically, the proteins connexin 43 and 45 (Cx43, Cx45), are reduced and reorganized [21,27,50,75,78]. Furthermore, it has been hypothesized that cardiac fibroblasts and myocytes could be coupled to each other through gap junctions and modify electrical signal propagation actively, not only as passive insulators. Several experimental studies in vitro [24–28] corroborate this active interaction between both kinds of cells; however, experimental results in vivo with human cardiac tissue have not been reported. In a variety of species the degree of coupling between myocytes and fibroblasts has been analyzed [23,29,37,52,76,79–81], and a wide range of values were found. In the absence of definitive data, modeling provides a powerful tool to explore repolarization abnormalities under such hypothetical conditions. Our simulation results showed that the presence of fibrosis significantly modified APD dispersion, TDR and other biomarkers (Figure 7). Inserted fibrosis and intercellular uncoupling increased TDR and APD dispersion, and a biphasic behavior was detected depending on the quantity of fibrotic content. This result might be related to the previous simulation studies reporting that intermediate fibrosis increases the vulnerability to reentry in a virtual infarcted rabbit heart [76] and in a virtual guinea pig fibrotic heart [77]. This is also illustrated in our accompanying paper [82] in the setting of simulated human heart failure. Excitability was also altered in the presence of fibroblasts through the elevation of the resting potential as reported before [37,80,83]. Thus, structural remodeling modified the electrical properties of the cardiac tissue generating a substrate for arrhythmogenesis [28,76,77,84], as we illustrated in our accompanying paper [82]. A local decrease in CV when fibrosis was inserted concomitant with intercellular uncoupling was found in our simulations and is in agreement with experimental results [21,24,25,84–86]. In addition, the ERP was enhanced by ionic remodeling present in HF in agreement with experimental results [21] but was decreased as the fibrotic content increased. This effect may favor the vulnerability to reentry [87], as was reported in other simulation studies [76,77]. In this study we also demonstrated for the first time that the safety factor for conduction was reduced in the presence of fibrotic clusters, as stated in Glukhov et al. [21], and propagation block could be elicited.

Limitations of the study

Several limitations need to be considered, when drawing inference from mathematical modeling. Our myocyte model for HF based on changes in the ion channel parameters has the inherited limitations described in [41]. Mainly, data from a large number of experimental studies were taken into account, thus resulting in a high variability not only in the ionic remodeling but also in the stage and etiology of HF and its phenotype. For this reason, a sensitivity analysis was performed in our previous work [42], where the experimental variability in ionic remodeling was taken into account and yielded values of APD_{90} and other HF biomarkers within experimental observations. In addition, our HF model was implemented employing two different human AP models: GPB and ORd. These two models were built and validated on the basis of extensive human data. However, there are important discrepancies in their formulations of K^{+} currents and Ca^{2+} handling, leading to differences in the simulation results regarding repolarization and Ca^{2+} transient behavior. Thus, caution should be exercised when comparing simulation results. With regard to heterogeneous remodeling, only the changes in I_{NCX} and I_{SERCA} were applied heterogeneously within the ventricular wall, on the basis of the limited human data available. Experimental results carried out in human hearts have also reported a transmural heterogeneous remodeling in K^{+} currents [20,44]. Although transmural differences in the remodeling of transient outward K^{+} current would have affect mainly early repolarization, which was out of the scope of the present analysis, they might also have an impact on Ca^{2+} transient waveform and its dispersion within the ventricular wall [68]. Further combinations of heterogeneous remodeling will be considered in our future work. Finally, to simulate the interaction between human ventricular myocytes and fibroblasts we used an ionic fibroblast model [37] based on experimental data from adult rat fibroblasts, as no voltage clamp data or ionic models of human ventricular fibroblasts have been published so far. Possible inter-species differences might affect the results of our simulations.

Clinical implications and conclusions

This study aimed to investigate *in silico* the effects of microanatomical and electrophysiological remodeling on the functional properties (phenotype) of the human failing ventricle. Two of the most recent and detailed human AP models (GPB and ORd) were modified to mimic HF phenotype.

Transmurally heterogeneous HF induced ionic remodeling modulated repolarization and Ca^{2+} transient gradients, which could be driven to values lower than the gradients corresponding to normal tissue. In contrast, homogeneous HF ionic remodeling, intercellular uncoupling, and fibrosis increased these gradients. Structural remodeling also altered conduction properties setting the substrate for arrhythmogenesis. Our findings may have important consequences for the treatment and prevention of human HF-induced arrhythmias and its potential contribution to mortality. Pharmacological modulation of intercellular coupling with rotigaptide, an antiarrhythmic substance increasing gap junctional conductance, may have beneficial effects in patients with heart failure. The concomitant reduction of the amount of fibrosis might be successful in these patients but requires further investigation.

Supporting Information

File S1 Figure S1, Random configurations for 10% fibrosis in the multicellular strand. The multicellular strand is composed by 165 nodes, where the fibroblast model is solved in 10% of the nodes (light color) and the myocyte AP model is solved in the rest of the nodes (blue). See Methods for details. Figure S2, Random configurations for 20% fibrosis in the multicellular strand. The multicellular strand is composed by 165 nodes, where the fibroblast model is solved in 20% of the nodes (light color) and the myocyte AP model is solved in the rest of the nodes (blue). See Methods for details. Figure S3, APD dispersion for normal coupling. Boxplots showing action potential duration (ADP) dispersion for low fibrosis (10%) and high fibrosis (20%), and $D_M = 0.0006$ cm/ms. Figure S4, TDR for normal coupling. Boxplots showing transmural dispersion (TDR) for low fibrosis (10%) and high fibrosis (20%), and $D_M = 0.0006$ cm/ms. Figure S5, APD dispersion for severe uncoupling. Boxplots showing action potential duration (ADP) dispersion for low fibrosis (10%) and high fibrosis (20%), and $D_M = 0.00025$ cm/ms. Figure S6, TDR for severe uncoupling. Boxplots showing transmural dispersion (TDR) for low fibrosis (10%) and high fibrosis (20%), and $D_M = 0.00025$ cm/ms. Figure S7, APD dispersion for intermediate uncoupling. Boxplots showing action potential duration (ADP) dispersion for low fibrosis (10%) and high fibrosis (20%), and $D_M = 0.0003$ cm/ms. Figure S8, TDR for intermediate uncoupling. Boxplots showing transmural dispersion (TDR) for low fibrosis (10%) and high fibrosis (20%), and $D_M = 0.0003$ cm/ms. Figure S9, APD dispersion for mild uncoupling. Boxplots showing action potential duration (ADP) dispersion for low fibrosis (10%) and high fibrosis (20%), and $D_M = 0.00045$ cm/ms. Figure S10, TDR for mild uncoupling. Boxplots showing transmural dispersion (TDR) for low fibrosis (10%) and high fibrosis (20%), and $D_M = 0.00045$ cm/ms. Table S1, APD dispersion and TDR for 10% fibrosis. Action potential duration (APD) dispersion and transmural dispersion (TDR) for the random configurations corresponding to a fibrotic content of 10% and normal intercellular coupling ($D_M = 0.0006$ cm/ms). Table S2, APD dispersion and TDR for 20% fibrosis. Action potential duration (APD) dispersion and transmural dispersion (TDR) for the random configurations corresponding to a fibrotic content of 20% and normal intercellular coupling ($D_M = 0.0006$ cm/ms). Table S3, APD dispersion for 10% fibrosis and intercellular uncoupling. Action potential duration (APD) dispersion for the random configurations corresponding to a fibrotic content of 10% and several degrees of intercellular uncoupling (D_M in cm/ms). Table S4, TDR for 10% fibrosis and intercellular uncoupling. Transmural dispersion of repolarization (TDR) for the random configurations corresponding to a fibrotic content of 10% and several degrees of intercellular uncoupling (D_M in cm/ms). Table S5, APD dispersion for 20% fibrosis and intercellular uncoupling Action potential duration (APD) dispersion for the random configurations corresponding to a fibrotic content of 20% and several degrees of intercellular uncoupling (D_M in cm/ms). Table S6, TDR for 20% fibrosis and intercellular uncoupling. Transmural dispersion of repolarization (TDR) for the random configurations corresponding to a fibrotic content of 20% and several degrees of intercellular uncoupling (D_M in cm/ms).

Author Contributions

Conceived and designed the experiments: BT. Performed the experiments: JFG KC. Analyzed the data: JFG KC BT JMF. Contributed reagents/materials/analysis tools: JFG LR JMF. Wrote the paper: JFG BT.

References

1. Coronel R, de Groot JR, van Lieshout JJ (2001) Defining heart failure. Cardiovasc Res 50: 419–422.
2. Coronel R, Wilders R, Verkerk AO, Wiegerinck RF, Benoist D, et al. (2013) Electrophysiological changes in heart failure and their implications for arrhythmogenesis. Biochim Biophys Acta 1832: 2432–2441.
3. Maltsev VA, Silverman N, Sabbah HN, Undrovinas AI (2007) Chronic heart failure slows late sodium current in human and canine ventricular myocytes: implications for repolarization variability. Eur J Heart Fail 9: 219–227.
4. Beuckelmann DJ, Nabauer M, Erdmann E (1993) Alterations of K+ currents in isolated human ventricular myocytes from patients with terminal heart failure. Circ Res 73: 379–385.
5. Tomaselli GF, Marban E (1999) Electrophysiological remodeling in hypertrophy and heart failure. Cardiovasc Res 42: 270–283.
6. Tomaselli GF, Zipes DP (2004) What causes sudden death in heart failure? Circ Res 95: 754–763.
7. Bundgaard H, Kjeldsen K (1996) Human myocardial Na,K-ATPase concentration in heart failure. Mol Cell Biochem 163–164: 277–283.
8. Piacentino V III, Weber CR, Chen X, Weisser-Thomas J, Margulies KB, et al. (2003) Cellular basis of abnormal calcium transients of failing human ventricular myocytes. Circ Res 92: 651–658.
9. Bers DM, Despa S, Bossuyt J (2006) Regulation of Ca2+ and Na+ in normal and failing cardiac myocytes. Ann N Y Acad Sci 1080: 165–177.
10. Antoons G, Oros A, Bito V, Sipido KR, Vos MA (2007) Cellular basis for triggered ventricular arrhythmias that occur in the setting of compensated hypertrophy and heart failure: considerations for diagnosis and treatment. J Electrocardiol 40: S8–14.
11. Sossalla S, Maurer U, Schotola H, Hartmann N, Didie M, et al. (2011) Diastolic dysfunction and arrhythmias caused by overexpression of CaMKIIdelta(C) can be reversed by inhibition of late Na(+) current. Basic Res Cardiol 106: 263–272.
12. Soltysinska E, Olesen SP, Christ T, Wettwer E, Varro A, et al. (2009) Transmural expression of ion channels and transporters in human nondiseased and end-stage failing hearts. Pflugers Arch 459: 11–23.
13. Walmsley J, Rodriguez JF, Mirams GR, Burrage K, Efimov IR, et al. (2013) mRNA expression levels in failing human hearts predict cellular electrophysiological remodeling: a population-based simulation study. PLoS One 8: e56359.
14. Ambrosi CM, Yamada KA, Nerbonne JM, Efimov IR (2013) Gender differences in electrophysiological gene expression in failing and non-failing human hearts. PLoS One 8: e54635.
15. Xiong W, Tian Y, DiSilvestre D, Tomaselli GF (2005) Transmural heterogeneity of Na+-Ca2+ exchange: evidence for differential expression in normal and failing hearts. Circ Res 97: 207–209.
16. Prestle J, Dieterich S, Preuss M, Bieligk U, Hasenfuss G (1999) Heterogeneous transmural gene expression of calcium-handling proteins and natriuretic peptides in the failing human heart. Cardiovasc Res 43: 323–331.
17. Wit AL, Coromilas J (1993) Role of alterations in refractoriness and conduction in the genesis of reentrant arrhythmias. Implications for antiarrhythmic effects of class III drugs. Am J Cardiol 72: 3F–12F.
18. Akar FG, Yan GX, Antzelevitch C, Rosenbaum DS (2002) Unique topographical distribution of M cells underlies reentrant mechanism of torsade de pointes in the long-QT syndrome. Circulation 105: 1247–1253.
19. Akar FG, Rosenbaum DS (2003) Transmural electrophysiological heterogeneities underlying arrhythmogenesis in heart failure. Circ Res 93: 638–645.
20. Holzem KM, Efimov IR (2012) Arrhythmogenic remodelling of activation and repolarization in the failing human heart. Europace 14 Suppl 5: v50–v57.
21. Glukhov AV, Fedorov VV, Kalish PW, Ravikumar VK, Lou Q, et al. (2012) Conduction remodeling in human end-stage nonischemic left ventricular cardiomyopathy. Circulation 125: 1835–1847.
22. Spach MS, Boineau JP (1997) Microfibrosis produces electrical load variations due to loss of side-to-side cell connections: a major mechanism of structural heart disease arrhythmias. Pacing Clin Electrophysiol 20: 397–413.
23. Kohl P, Camelliti P, Burton FL, Smith GL (2005) Electrical coupling of fibroblasts and myocytes: relevance for cardiac propagation. J Electrocardiol 38: 45–50.

24. Gaudesius G, Miragoli M, Thomas SP, Rohr S (2003) Coupling of cardiac electrical activity over extended distances by fibroblasts of cardiac origin. Circ Res 93: 421–428.
25. Miragoli M, Gaudesius G, Rohr S (2006) Electrotonic modulation of cardiac impulse conduction by myofibroblasts. Circ Res 98: 801–810.
26. Miragoli M, Salvarani N, Rohr S (2007) Myofibroblasts induce ectopic activity in cardiac tissue. Circ Res 101: 755–758.
27. Vasquez C, Moreno AP, Berbari EJ (2004) Modeling fibroblast-mediated conduction in the ventricle. Computers in Cardiology Proceedings 31: 349–352.
28. Zlochiver S, Munoz V, Vikstrom KL, Taffet SM, Berenfeld O, et al. (2008) Electrotonic myofibroblast-to-myocyte coupling increases propensity to reentrant arrhythmias in two-dimensional cardiac monolayers. Biophys J 95: 4469–4480.
29. Jacquemet V, Henriquez CS (2008) Loading effect of fibroblast-myocyte coupling on resting potential, impulse propagation, and repolarization: insights from a microstructure model. Am J Physiol Heart Circ Physiol 294: H2040–H2052.
30. Lou Q, Janks DL, Holzem KM, Lang D, Onal B, et al. (2012) Right ventricular arrhythmogenesis in failing human heart: the role of conduction and repolarization remodeling. Am J Physiol Heart Circ Physiol 303: H1426–H1434.
31. Glukhov AV, Fedorov VV, Lou Q, Ravikumar VK, Kalish PW, et al. (2010) Transmural dispersion of repolarization in failing and nonfailing human ventricle. Circ Res 106: 981–991.
32. Vigmond E, Vadakkumpadan F, Gurev V, Arevalo H, Deo M, et al. (2009) Towards predictive modelling of the electrophysiology of the heart. Exp Physiol 94: 563–577.
33. Clayton RH, Bernus O, Cherry EM, Dierckx H, Fenton FH, et al. (2011) Models of cardiac tissue electrophysiology: progress, challenges and open questions. Prog Biophys Mol Biol 104: 22–48.
34. Grandi E, Pasqualini FS, Bers DM (2010) A novel computational model of the human ventricular action potential and Ca transient. J Mol Cell Cardiol 48: 112–121.
35. O'Hara T, Virag L, Varro A, Rudy Y (2011) Simulation of the undiseased human cardiac ventricular action potential: model formulation and experimental validation. PLoS Comput Biol 7: e1002061.
36. Antzelevitch C (2010) M cells in the human heart. Circ Res 106: 815–817.
37. MacCannell KA, Bazzazi H, Chilton L, Shibukawa Y, Clark RB, et al. (2007) A mathematical model of electrotonic interactions between ventricular myocytes and fibroblasts. Biophys J 92: 4121–4132.
38. Chilton L, Ohya S, Freed D, George E, Drobic V, et al. (2005) K+ currents regulate the resting membrane potential, proliferation, and contractile responses in ventricular fibroblasts and myofibroblasts. Am J Physiol Heart Circ Physiol 288: H2931–H2939.
39. Beuckelmann DJ, Nabauer M, Erdmann E (1992) Intracellular calcium handling in isolated ventricular myocytes from patients with terminal heart failure. Circulation 85: 1046–1055.
40. Janse MJ (2004) Electrophysiological changes in heart failure and their relationship to arrhythmogenesis. Cardiovasc Res 61: 208–217.
41. Trenor B, Cardona K, Gomez JF, Rajamani S, Ferrero JM Jr., et al. (2012) Simulation and mechanistic investigation of the arrhythmogenic role of the late sodium current in human heart failure. PLoS One 7: e32659.
42. Gomez JF, Cardona K, Romero L, Saiz J, Belardinelli L, et al. (2012) Increase in late sodium current and cellular uncoupling exacerbates transmural dispersion of repolarization in heart failure. 39: 233–236.
43. Gomez JF, Cardona K, Romero L, Saiz J, Trenor B (2013) Heterogeneous electrical remodeling of the failing heart modulates the arrhythmogenic substrate. Computing in Cardiology Proceedings 40: 49–52.
44. Ohler A, Amos GJ, Wettwer E, Ravens U (1994) Frequency-dependent effects of E-4031, almokalant, dofetilide and tedisamil on action potential duration: no evidence for "reverse use dependent" block. Naunyn Schmiedebergs Arch Pharmacol 349: 602–610.
45. Heidenreich EA, Ferrero JM, Doblare M, Rodriguez JF (2010) Adaptive macro finite elements for the numerical solution of monodomain equations in cardiac electrophysiology. Ann Biomed Eng 38: 2331–2345.
46. Gima K, Rudy Y (2002) Ionic current basis of electrocardiographic waveforms: a model study. Circ Res 90: 889–896.
47. Moreno JD, Yang PC, Bankston JR, Grandi E, Bers DM, et al. (2013) Ranolazine for Congenital and Acquired Late INa-Linked Arrhythmias: In Silico Pharmacological Screening. Circ Res 113: e50–e61.
48. Remy-Jardin M, Remy J (2014) Integrated Cardiothoracic Imaging with MDCT. Springer.
49. Taggart P, Sutton PM, Opthof T, Coronel R, Trimlett R, et al. (2000) Inhomogeneous transmural conduction during early ischaemia in patients with coronary artery disease. J Mol Cell Cardiol 32: 621–630.
50. Dupont E, Matsushita T, Kaba RA, Vozzi C, Coppen SR, et al. (2001) Altered connexin expression in human congestive heart failure. J Mol Cell Cardiol 33: 359–371.
51. Kawara T, Derksen R, de Groot JR, Coronel R, Tasseron S, et al. (2001) Activation delay after premature stimulation in chronically diseased human myocardium relates to the architecture of interstitial fibrosis. Circulation 104: 3069–3075.
52. Tanaka K, Zlochiver S, Vikstrom KL, Yamazaki M, Moreno J, et al. (2007) Spatial distribution of fibrosis governs fibrillation wave dynamics in the posterior left atrium during heart failure. Circ Res 101: 839–847.
53. Majumder R, Nayak AR, Pandit R (2012) Nonequilibrium arrhythmic states and transitions in a mathematical model for diffuse fibrosis in human cardiac tissue. PLoS One 7: e45040.
54. Lou Q, Fedorov VV, Glukhov AV, Moazami N, Fast VG, et al. (2011) Transmural heterogeneity and remodeling of ventricular excitation-contraction coupling in human heart failure. Circulation 123: 1881–1890.
55. Delgado C, Steinhaus B, Delmar M, Chialvo DR, Jalife J (1990) Directional differences in excitability and margin of safety for propagation in sheep ventricular epicardial muscle. Circ Res 67: 97–110.
56. Shaw RM, Rudy Y (1997) Electrophysiologic effects of acute myocardial ischemia: a theoretical study of altered cell excitability and action potential duration. Cardiovasc Res 35: 256–272.
57. Boyle PM, Vigmond EJ (2010) An intuitive safety factor for cardiac propagation. Biophys J 98: L57–L59.
58. Romero L, Trenor B, Alonso JM, Tobon C, Saiz J, et al. (2009) The relative role of refractoriness and source-sink relationship in reentry generation during simulated acute ischemia. Ann Biomed Eng 37: 1560–1571.
59. Elshrif MM, Cherry EM (2014) A quantitative comparison of the behavior of human ventricular cardiac electrophysiology models in tissue. PLoS One 9: e84401.
60. Coronel R, Wilms-Schopman FJ, Opthof T, Janse MJ (2009) Dispersion of repolarization and arrhythmogenesis. Heart Rhythm 6: 537–543.
61. Undrovinas AI, Belardinelli L, Undrovinas NA, Sabbah HN (2006) Ranolazine improves abnormal repolarization and contraction in left ventricular myocytes of dogs with heart failure by inhibiting late sodium current. J Cardiovasc Electrophysiol 17 Suppl 1: S169–S177.
62. Armoundas AA, Hobai IA, Tomaselli GF, Winslow RL, O'Rourke B (2003) Role of sodium-calcium exchanger in modulating the action potential of ventricular myocytes from normal and failing hearts. Circ Res 93: 46–53.
63. Hobai IA, O'Rourke B (2001) Decreased sarcoplasmic reticulum calcium content is responsible for defective excitation-contraction coupling in canine heart failure. Circulation 103: 1577–1584.
64. O'Rourke B, Kass DA, Tomaselli GF, Kaab S, Tunin R, et al. (1999) Mechanisms of altered excitation-contraction coupling in canine tachycardia-induced heart failure, I: experimental studies. Circ Res 84: 562–570.
65. Marx SO, Gaburjakova J, Gaburjakova M, Henrikson C, Ondrias K, et al. (2001) Coupled gating between cardiac calcium release channels (ryanodine receptors). Circ Res 88: 1151–1158.
66. Yano M, Ono K, Ohkusa T, Suetsugu M, Kohno M, et al. (2000) Altered stoichiometry of FKBP12.6 versus ryanodine receptor as a cause of abnormal Ca(2+) leak through ryanodine receptor in heart failure. Circulation 102: 2131–2136.
67. Pieske B, Maier LS, Bers DM, Hasenfuss G (1999) Ca2+ handling and sarcoplasmic reticulum Ca2+ content in isolated failing and nonfailing human myocardium. Circ Res 85: 38–46.
68. Sah R, Ramirez RJ, Backx PH (2002) Modulation of Ca(2+) release in cardiac myocytes by changes in repolarization rate: role of phase-1 action potential repolarization in excitation-contraction coupling. Circ Res 90: 165–173.
69. Cutler MJ, Rosenbaum DS, Dunlap ME (2007) Structural and electrical remodeling as therapeutic targets in heart failure. J Electrocardiol 40: S1–S7.
70. Gonzalez A, Ravassa S, Beaumont J, Lopez B, Diez J (2011) New targets to treat the structural remodeling of the myocardium. J Am Coll Cardiol 58: 1833–1843.
71. McSpadden LC, Kirkton RD, Bursac N (2009) Electrotonic loading of anisotropic cardiac monolayers by unexcitable cells depends on connexin type and expression level. Am J Physiol Cell Physiol 297: C339–C351.
72. Thompson SA, Copeland CR, Reich DH, Tung L (2011) Mechanical coupling between myofibroblasts and cardiomyocytes slows electric conduction in fibrotic cell monolayers. Circulation 123: 2083–2093.
73. Akar FG, Nass RD, Hahn S, Cingolani E, Shah M, et al. (2007) Dynamic changes in conduction velocity and gap junction properties during development of pacing-induced heart failure. Am J Physiol Heart Circ Physiol 293: H1223–H1230.
74. Fontes MS, van Veen TA, de Bakker JM, van Rijen HV (2011) Functional consequences of abnormal Cx43 expression in the heart. Biochim Biophys Acta
75. Kostin S, Rieger M, Dammer S, Hein S, Richter M, et al. (2003) Gap junction remodeling and altered connexin43 expression in the failing human heart. Mol Cell Biochem 242: 135–144.
76. McDowell KS, Arevalo HJ, Maleckar MM, Trayanova NA (2011) Susceptibility to arrhythmia in the infarcted heart depends on myofibroblast density. Biophys J 101: 1307–1315.
77. Xie Y, Garfinkel A, Camelliti P, Kohl P, Weiss JN, et al. (2009) Effects of fibroblast-myocyte coupling on cardiac conduction and vulnerability to reentry: A computational study. Heart Rhythm 6: 1641–1649.
78. Poelzing S, Rosenbaum DS (2004) Altered connexin43 expression produces arrhythmia substrate in heart failure. Am J Physiol Heart Circ Physiol 287: H1762–H1770.
79. Rook MB, van Ginneken AC, de JB, el Aoumari A, Gros D, et al. (1992) Differences in gap junction channels between cardiac myocytes, fibroblasts, and heterologous pairs. Am J Physiol 263: C959–C977.

80. Jacquemet V, Henriquez CS (2007) Modelling cardiac fibroblasts: interactions with myocytes and their impact on impulse propagation. Europace 9 Suppl 6: vi29–vi37.
81. Sachse FB, Moreno AP, Seemann G, Abildskov JA (2009) A model of electrical conduction in cardiac tissue including fibroblasts. Ann Biomed Eng 37: 874–889.
82. Gomez JF, Cardona K, Martinez L, Rajamani S, Belardinelli L, et al. (2014) Electrophysiological and structural remodeling in heart failure modulate arrhythmogenesis. 2D simulaton study. PLoS One 9 (7) e103273.
83. Nayak AR, Shajahan TK, Panfilov AV, Pandit R (2013) Spiral-wave dynamics in a mathematical model of human ventricular tissue with myocytes and fibroblasts. PLoS One 8: e72950.
84. Wiegerinck RF, van Veen TA, Belterman CN, Schumacher CA, Noorman M, et al. (2008) Transmural dispersion of refractoriness and conduction velocity is associated with heterogeneously reduced connexin43 in a rabbit model of heart failure. Heart Rhythm 5: 1178–1185.
85. Rohr S (2004) Role of gap junctions in the propagation of the cardiac action potential. Cardiovasc Res 62: 309–322.
86. Fast VG, Darrow BJ, Saffitz JE, Kleber AG (1996) Anisotropic activation spread in heart cell monolayers assessed by high-resolution optical mapping. Role of tissue discontinuities. Circ Res 79: 115–127.
87. Qu Z, Karagueuzian HS, Garfinkel A, Weiss JN (2004) Effects of Na(+) channel and cell coupling abnormalities on vulnerability to reentry: a simulation study. Am J Physiol Heart Circ Physiol 286: H1310–H1321.
88. Undrovinas AI, Maltsev VA, Sabbah HN (1999) Repolarization abnormalities in cardiomyocytes of dogs with chronic heart failure: role of sustained inward current. Cell Mol Life Sci 55: 494–505.
89. Priebe L, Beuckelmann DJ (1998) Simulation study of cellular electric properties in heart failure. Circ Res 82: 1206–1223.
90. Winslow RL, Rice J, Jafri S, Marban E, O'Rourke B (1999) Mechanisms of altered excitation-contraction coupling in canine tachycardia-induced heart failure, II: model studies. Circ Res 84: 571–586.
91. Curran J, Brown KH, Santiago DJ, Pogwizd S, Bers DM, et al. (2010) Spontaneous Ca waves in ventricular myocytes from failing hearts depend on Ca(2+)-calmodulin-dependent protein kinase II. J Mol Cell Cardiol 49: 25–32.
92. George CH (2008) Sarcoplasmic reticulum Ca2+ leak in heart failure: mere observation or functional relevance? Cardiovasc Res 77: 302–314.
93. Reinecke H, Studer R, Vetter R, Holtz J, Drexler H (1996) Cardiac Na+/Ca2+ exchange activity in patients with end-stage heart failure. Cardiovasc Res 31: 48–54.
94. Iyer V, Heller V, Armoundas AA (2012) Altered spatial calcium regulation enhances electrical heterogeneity in the failing canine left ventricle: implications for electrical instability. J Appl Physiol 112: 944–955.
95. Hasenfuss G, Reinecke H, Studer R, Meyer M, Pieske B, et al. (1994) Relation between myocardial function and expression of sarcoplasmic reticulum Ca(2+)-ATPase in failing and nonfailing human myocardium. Circ Res 75: 434–442.
96. Schwinger RH, Bohm M, Schmidt U, Karczewski P, Bavendiek U, et al. (1995) Unchanged protein levels of SERCA II and phospholamban but reduced Ca2+ uptake and Ca(2+)-ATPase activity of cardiac sarcoplasmic reticulum from dilated cardiomyopathy patients compared with patients with nonfailing hearts. Circulation 92: 3220–3228.

Quantification of Left Ventricular Torsion and Diastolic Recoil Using Cardiovascular Magnetic Resonance Myocardial Feature Tracking

**Johannes T. Kowallick[1,8]⁹, Pablo Lamata[2,7]⁹, Shazia T. Hussain[3], Shelby Kutty[4], Michael Steinmetz[5,8], Jan M. Sohns[1,8], Martin Fasshauer[1,8], Wieland Staab[1,8], Christina Unterberg-Buchwald[6,8], Boris Bigalke[7,9], Joachim Lotz[1,8], Gerd Hasenfuß[6,8], Andreas Schuster[6,7,8]*

1 Institute for Diagnostic and Interventional Radiology, Georg-August-University Göttingen, Göttingen, Germany, **2** Department of Computer Science, University of Oxford, Oxford, United Kingdom, **3** Papworth Hospital NHS Trust, Papworth Everard, Cambridgeshire, United Kingdom, **4** Children's Hospital and Medical Center, University of Nebraska College of Medicine, Omaha, Nebraska, United States of America, **5** Department of Pediatric Cardiology and Intensive Care Medicine, Georg-August-University Göttingen, Göttingen, Germany, **6** Department of Cardiology and Pneumology, Georg-August-University Göttingen, Göttingen, Germany, **7** Division of Imaging Sciences and Biomedical Engineering, The Rayne Institute, St. Thomas' Hospital, King's College London, London, United Kingdom, **8** DZHK (German Centre for Cardiovascular Research), partner site Göttingen, Göttingen, Germany, **9** Medizinische Klinik III, Kardiologie und Kreislauferkrankungen, Eberhard-Karls-Universität Tübingen, Tübingen, Germany

Abstract

Objectives: Cardiovascular magnetic resonance feature tracking (CMR-FT) offers quantification of myocardial deformation from routine cine images. However, data using CMR-FT to quantify left ventricular (LV) torsion and diastolic recoil are not yet available. We therefore sought to evaluate the feasibility and reproducibility of CMR-FT to quantify LV torsion and peak recoil rate using an optimal anatomical approach.

Methods: Short-axis cine stacks were acquired at rest and during dobutamine stimulation (10 and 20 $\mu g \cdot kg^{-1} \cdot min^{-1}$) in 10 healthy volunteers. Rotational displacement was analysed for all slices. A complete 3D-LV rotational model was developed using linear interpolation between adjacent slices. Torsion was defined as the difference between apical and basal rotation, divided by slice distance. Depending on the distance between the most apical (defined as 0% LV distance) and basal (defined as 100% LV distance) slices, four different models for the calculation of torsion were examined: Model-1 (25–75%), Model-2 (0–100%), Model-3 (25–100%) and Model-4 (0–75%). Analysis included subendocardial, subepicardial and global torsion and recoil rate (mean of subendocardial and subepicardial values).

Results: Quantification of torsion and recoil rate was feasible in all subjects. There was no significant difference between the different models at rest. However, only Model-1 (25–75%) discriminated between rest and stress (Global Torsion: $2.7\pm1.5°cm^{-1}$, $3.6\pm2.0°cm^{-1}$, $5.1\pm2.2°cm^{-1}$, $p<0.01$; Global Recoil Rate: $-30.1\pm11.1°cm^{-1}s^{-1}$, $-46.9\pm15.0°cm^{-1}s^{-1}$, $-68.9\pm32.3°cm^{-1}s^{-1}$, $p<0.01$; for rest, 10 and 20 $\mu g \cdot kg^{-1} \cdot min^{-1}$ of dobutamine, respectively). Reproducibility was sufficient for all parameters as determined by Bland-Altman analysis, intraclass correlation coefficients and coefficient of variation.

Conclusions: CMR-FT based derivation of myocardial torsion and recoil rate is feasible and reproducible at rest and with dobutamine stress. Using an optimal anatomical approach measuring rotation at 25% and 75% apical and basal LV locations allows effective quantification of torsion and recoil dynamics. Application of these new measures of deformation by CMR-FT should next be explored in disease states.

Editor: Zhuoli Zhang, Northwestern University Feinberg School of Medicine, United States of America

Funding: AS was funded by the Research program of the Faculty of Medicine of the Georg-August-University in Göttingen. PL holds a Sir Henry Dale Fellowship jointly funded by the Wellcome Trust and the Royal Society (Grant Number 099973/Z/12/Z). The authors are grateful for the financial support provided by the DZHK (German Centre for Cardiovascular Research). The funders had no role in study design, data collection and analysis, decision to publish, or preparation of the manuscript.

Competing Interests: The authors have declared that no competing interests exist.

* Email: andreas_schuster@gmx.net

⁹ These authors contributed equally to this work.

Introduction

The prevalence of heart failure including systolic and diastolic functional impairments continues to increase representing a major health problem [1,2]. Several diagnostic techniques have been proposed to study systolic and diastolic myocardial performances [3,4,5].

Left ventricular (LV) systolic torsion and diastolic recoil describe the myocardial twisting and untwisting motion resulting from apical counter-clockwise and basal clockwise rotation during systole (when viewed from the apex and normalized for LV length). Torsion and recoil rate have shown to be sensitive markers for systolic and diastolic dysfunction [6,7,8]. The phenomenon can be captured by the simple twist angle (difference in apical and basal rotation) [9,10], the circumferential-longitudinal shear angle [11,12] or torsion (twist per cardiac length) [13,14]. Recent studies showed that torsion might represent an important compensatory mechanism to maintain an adequate systolic function in patients with chronic hypertension as examined in a large community-based population based on cardiovascular magnetic resonance (CMR) myocardial tagging [14,15]. Recoil rate seems particularly appealing to study diastolic function. Its applicability has been demonstrated in isolated diastolic dysfunction [16], in heart failure with preserved ejection fraction [17] and heart disease characterized by both systolic and diastolic dysfunction such as hypertrophic cardiomyopathy (HCM) [18]. CMR myocardial tagging is considered the reference standard for the evaluation of torsion at the current time. However, this technique has not found widespread implementation into clinical routine since practical obstacles, e.g. the need for additional sequence acquisition and time-consuming post-processing limit its clinical applicability. Recent advances in LV deformation quantification based on CMR feature tracking (CMR-FT) allow straightforward quantification of myocardial physiology from routine steady-state free precession (SSFP) images [19,20]. The technique has been used to analyse ventricular strain in health and disease [21,22]. However, the feasibility of CMR-FT for quantitative assessment of LV torsion has never previously been demonstrated.

We therefore aimed to first develop a model that allows uniform selection of apical and basal slices at standardized LV levels and to evaluate its feasibility and reproducibility to quantify LV systolic torsion and diastolic recoil at rest and during dobutamine stress using CMR-FT.

Materials and Methods

Ten healthy volunteers underwent CMR on a 1.5 Tesla scanner (Intera R 12.6.1.3, Philips Medical Systems, Best, The Netherlands). The study protocol was approved by the Institutional Review Board at the University of Nebraska Medical Center and complies with the Declaration of Helsinki. Written informed consent was obtained from all participants.

CMR Imaging

All CMR measurements were performed in the supine position using a 5-channel cardiac surface coil. LV dimensions and function were assessed with an ECG- gated SSFP cine sequence during brief periods of breath-holding in 12 to 14 equidistant short-axis planes (slice thickness 8 mm; gap 1–2 mm) completely covering the LV. The field of view was 360×480 mm and matrix size 196×172. Dobutamine stress imaging was performed as previously described [23]. Complete short-axis stacks were acquired at rest and with 10 and 20 $\mu g \cdot kg^{-1} \cdot min^{-1}$ of dobutamine.

Haemodynamic analysis

End-diastolic (EDV) and end-systolic volume (ESV), stroke volume (SV), ejection fraction and cardiac index (CI), were calculated using MassK-Mode in QMass Version 7.6 (Medis Medical Systems, Leiden, The Netherland). Ventricular volumes were adjusted to body surface area. All parameters were analysed at rest, 10 and 20 $\mu g \cdot kg^{-1} \cdot min^{-1}$ of dobutamine stress. Furthermore, heart rate and mean blood pressure were measured at rest and with both levels of dobutamine stimulation.

Cardiac magnetic resonance myocardial feature tracking

Myocardial feature tracking was performed using dedicated software (TomTec Imaging Systems, 2D CPA MR, Cardiac Performance Analysis, Version 1.1.2.36, Unterschleissheim, Germany). All short-axis slices were included in the analysis between the most apical slice showing LV cavity at end-systole and the most basal slice including a complete circumference of myocardium at end-systole. LV endocardial and epicardial borders were manually traced in all slices using a point-and-click approach with the initial contour set at end-diastole. Endocardial and epicardial border surfaces were manually delineated and the automated tracking algorithm was applied. The software automatically tracks 48 subendocardial and subepicardial tissue voxels throughout the cardiac cycle. Tracking performance was visually reviewed to ensure accurate tracking of the ventricular myocardium. In case of insufficient border tracking manual adjustments were made to the initial contour and the algorithm was reapplied. Tracking was repeated for three times in each short-axis view and results were based on the average of the three repeated measures.

Definition of torsion and recoil rate

Torsion and peak recoil rate were calculated using MATLAB software (The Math Works, MA, USA). Averaged LV rotation profiles were calculated from the angular displacement of all 48 tissue voxels in all slices. LV rotation was averaged across the three repeated measurements. The rotation of points that would typically be located in between adjacent slices was linearly interpolated resulting in a complete 3D LV model of angular displacement (**Figure 1**). When viewed from the apex, LV torsion was calculated as the difference in counter-clockwise apical rotation (ϕ_{apex}) and clockwise rotation at the base (ϕ_{base}) divided by the inter-slice distance (D) [13,14]:

$$LV\ Torsion = \frac{\phi_{apex} - \phi_{base}}{D}$$

The distance (D) was calculated as the sum of the slice thickness (8 mm) and gap (1–2 mm) of imaging planes that were located in between the basal and apical slices where rotation was measured [14] (**Figure 2 and 3**). Depending on these measurement positions of rotation obtained at different LV locations and the distance between the most apical (defined as 0% of LV distance) and the most basal slice (defined as 100% of LV distance) the following four methods to calculate torsion were examined: Model 1 (difference in rotation between 25% and 75%), model 2 (difference in rotation between 0% and 100%), model 3 (difference in rotation between 25% and 100%) and model 4 (difference in rotation between 0% to 75%) (**Figure 3**). The analysis included subepicardial and subendocardial torsion as well as LV global torsion (averaged subendocardial and subepicardial torsion). Furthermore, subendocardial, subepicardial and global peak recoil

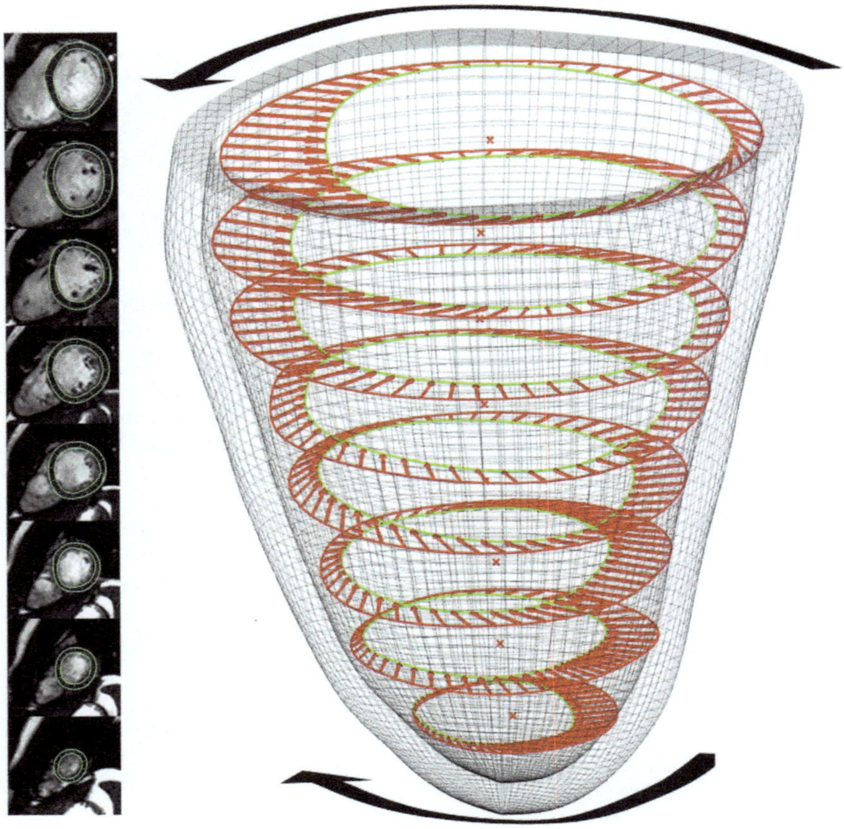

Figure 1. 3 D model of LV rotational displacement. Rotation between time points (angular difference between red and green contours) is computed in each slice, and it is then linearly interpolated between slices. The 3D ventricular model is automatically fitted to the contours [48] and is used here only for illustration purposes, and not for the definition of the location of the most apical and basal points.

rates were calculated from the maximum slope ($-d\theta/dt$) of the diastolic limb of the torsion-time curve (**Figure 2**).

Statistical Analysis

Statistical analysis was performed using Microsoft Excel and IBM SPSS Statistics version 22 for Macintosh. Data are expressed as mean (± standard deviation). Differences of torsion and peak recoil rate calculated between models 1–4 were assessed by the Friedman test. Pairwise comparisons between variables at rest and with increasing levels of dobutamine were evaluated using the Wilcoxon test. All statistical tests with p values <0.05 were considered statistically significant.

Two independent observers analysed all cases to assess inter-observer variability (JTK & AS). Intra-observer variability was derived from the repeated analysis by the first observer (JTK) after four weeks. The intra- and inter-observer variability were assessed by intraclass correlation coefficients (ICC) using a model of absolute agreement. Agreement was considered excellent when ICC>0.74, good when ICC = 0.60–0.74, fair when ICC = 0.40–0.59, and poor when ICC<0.4 [24]. Furthermore, Bland Altman analysis [25] and coefficients of variation (CoV) were calculated. The CoV was defined as the standard deviation of the differences divided by the mean [26].

Results

The image quality was sufficient to perform CMR-FT in all subjects and for all slices at rest and during dobutamine stress. CMR-FT post-processing took 10 to 12 minutes for a LV short-axis stack on average including adjustments if necessary. Participant demographics are summarised in **table 1**.

Haemodynamic response to dobutamine

There were no side effects to dobutamine exposure. There was a significant increase of cardiac output, mean blood pressure and ejection fraction between rest and both levels of dobutamine as well as between 10 and 20 $\mu g \cdot kg^{-1} \cdot min^{-1}$ of dobutamine. Stroke volume increased significantly between rest and both levels of dobutamine, whilst no further increase was observed between 10 and 20 $\mu g \cdot kg^{-1} \cdot min^{-1}$ of dobutamine (**table 2**).

Torsion and recoil rate at rest

Inter-slice distances used for torsion calculation were 2.9±0.4 cm (model 1), 5.8±0.7 cm (model 2) and 4.4±0.5 cm (model 3 and 4). There was no significant difference of endocardial, epicardial or global torsion and endocardial and global recoil rate between the models 1–4 at rest. Results are displayed in **table 3**. There was a significant difference ($p = 0.02$) of epicardial recoil rate between model 2 (0–100%) and model 4 (0–75%).

Torsion and recoil rate during dobutamine stress

Table 4 summarises torsion and recoil rate parameters at rest and during dobutamine stress as calculated by the different models. The mean inter-slice distance during dobutamine exposure was slightly lower compared with rest due to increased

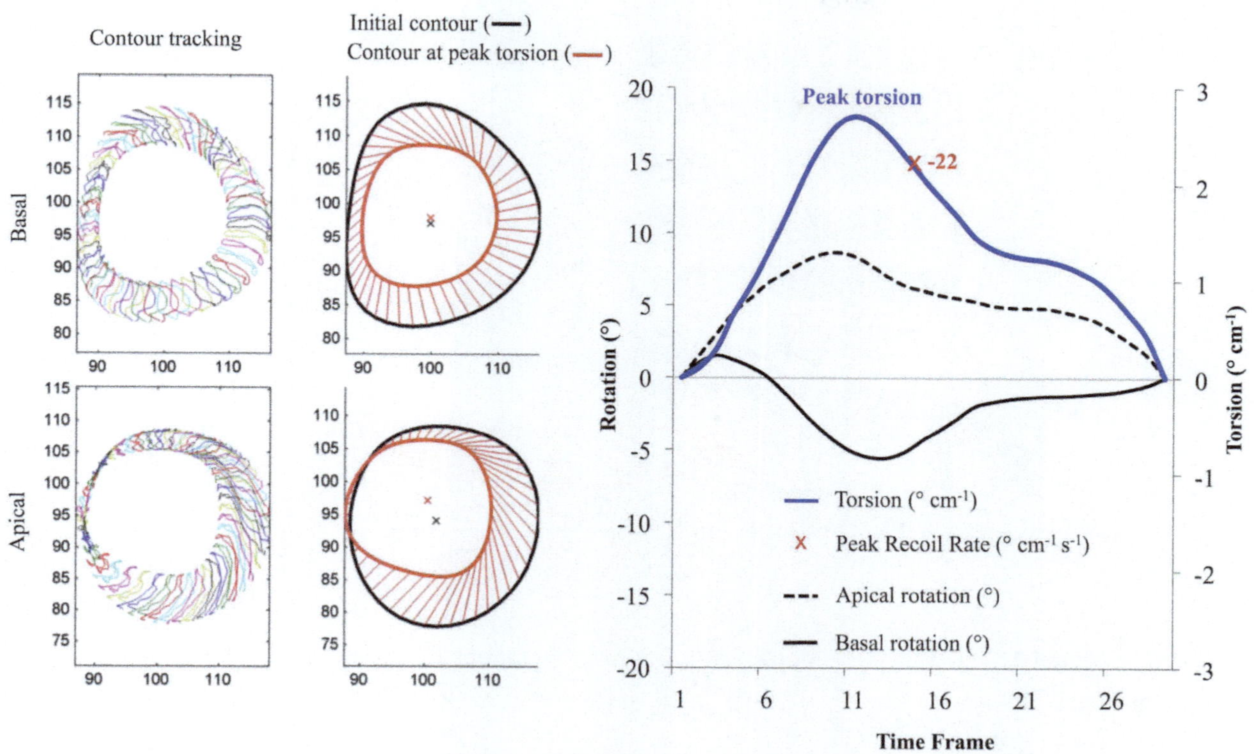

Figure 2. Evaluation of rotation. Rotational displacement (degrees) of 48 voxels was tracked throughout the cardiac cycle (**left**). Left ventricular torsion (° cm^{-1}) was calculated as the difference in counter-clockwise (positive) apical rotation and clockwise (negative) rotation at the base, divided by the inter-slice distance (**right**).

longitudinal shortening with stress. The inter-slices distances were 2.8±0.3 cm (model 1), 5.6±0.6 cm (model 2) and 4.2±0.4 cm (model 3 and 4) for measurements during 10 and 20 μg·kg^{-1}·min^{-1} of dobutamine.

Model 1 (25–75%) was the only approach that revealed significantly increased torsion and recoil rate (subendocardial, subepicardial and global) between rest and both levels of dobutamine as well as between 10 and 20 μg·kg^{-1}·min^{-1} of dobutamine except there was no significant difference of subepicardial torsion ($p = 0.33$) and global torsion ($p = 0.06$) between rest and 10 μg·kg^{-1}·min^{-1} of dobutamine (**Figure 4**). The increase of torsion during dobutamine stress was more pronounced on the subendocardial as compared to the subepicarial level. All other models showed only partly significant results or trends towards increased torsion and recoil rates as outlined in **table 4**.

Reproducibility

Bland Altman analysis, ICC and CoV are displayed in **table 5**. There was no difference in reproducibility between rest and dobutamine stimulation. ICC for model 1 (25–75%) and model 3 (25–100%) consistently showed values above 0.85. The model 2 (0–100%) and 4 (0–75%) showed slightly higher inter-observer variability for subendocardial torsion with ICC of 0.78 and 0.79, respectively.

Discussion

Myocardial twisting and untwisting represent fundamental mechanisms of LV systolic and diastolic function. It has been suggested that even up to 40% of stroke volume is produced from systolic twisting forces [27]. The subsequent fast untwisting during early diastole is a major indicator of the restoring forces that contribute to rapid diastolic filling [28,29]. In a clinical context, a simple, quick and robust quantification of LV twisting and untwisting motion is therefore desirable. The present study applied CMR-FT to assess both systolic torsion and diastolic recoil directly from routine SSFP cine images to capture these phenomena and demonstrates several important findings. CMR-FT based quantification of myocardial twisting motion as assessed with torsion and diastolic recoil is feasible and reproducible. Furthermore, we were able to show that CMR-FT allows discrimination of both systolic torsion and diastolic recoil at rest and dobutamine stress when using standardized analyses based on rotation measurements at 25% and 75% LV distance.

Feasibility of CMR-FT derived torsion

The presented approach used a complete LV rotational model to define exact apical and basal slice positions by assessing rotational profiles of all short-axis slices of a short-axis stack with subsequent linear interpolation of inter-slice rotation between adjacent slices. This approach appears suitable since several studies revealed strict linear progression of rotation from base to apex [10,12,14]. Previous reports have shown that the amount of LV rotation is highly dependent on the site of measurements at apical and basal levels. This needs to be taken into account when calculating the simple twist angle [10]. We therefore applied torsion (twist normalized to inter-slice distance) to quantify the myocardial twisting motion since this technique is supposed to be less influenced by the variation in rotation as compared to the simple twist definition (difference in apical and basal rotation) [30]. The results of our study indicate, that in fact CMR-FT

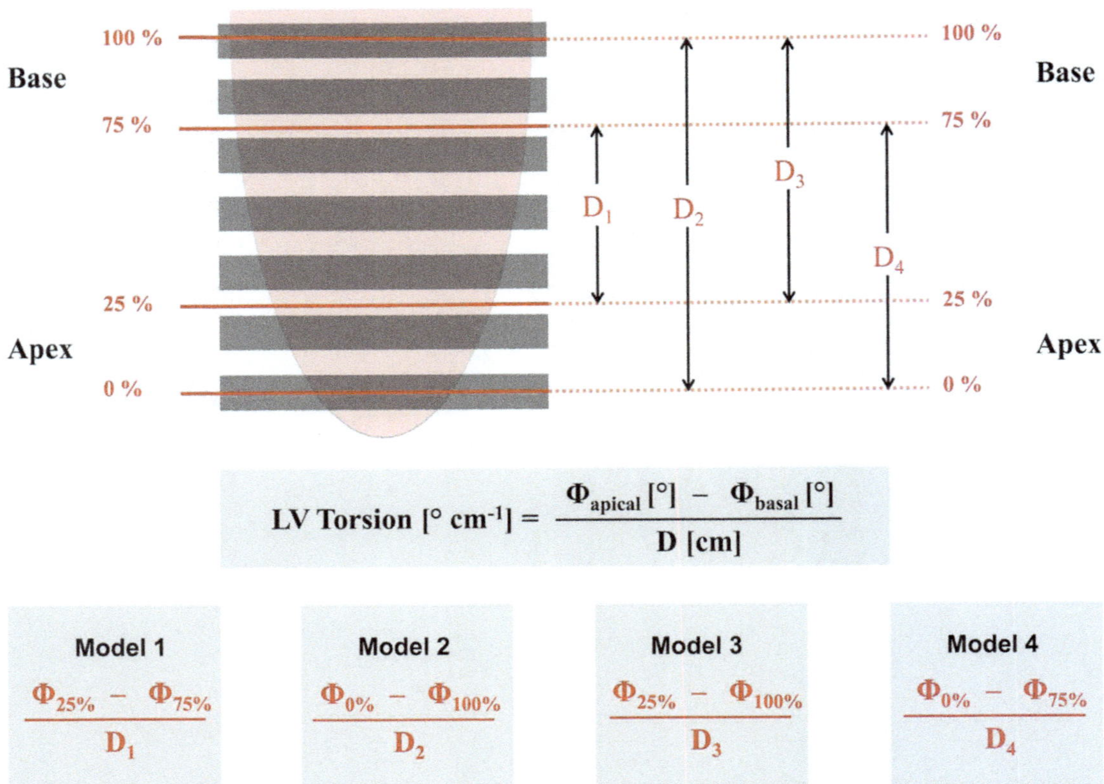

Figure 3. Definitions to calculate torsion. CMR feature tracking was performed in all slices of a short-axis stack. Four models (1–4) to calculate torsion were evaluated. Left ventricular (LV) torsion was calculated as the difference in counter-clockwise apical rotation (ϕ_{apex}) and clockwise rotation at the base (ϕ_{base}), divided by the inter-slice distance (D). The rotation of points at 0% ($\phi_{0\%}$) and 100% ($\phi_{100\%}$) distance correspond to the most apical and most basal levels. The rotation of points at 25% ($\phi_{25\%}$) and 75% ($\phi_{75\%}$) distance correspond to points that are typically located in between slices (linearly interpolated from adjacent slices). This approach allows generating constant distances (D_1-D_4) between corresponding apical and basal slices independently of varying cardiac anatomy.

quantification of torsion at rest is not that dependant on measurement positions since we have not detected any significant differences between the four examined models that used rotation from different standardized LV levels serving for the calculation of torsion. However, differences in recoil rate were more pronounced. Hence, quantification of recoil rate might be more dependent on the exact slice position as compared to quantification of torsion. This is particularly important when quantification of diastolic function is required which underpins the need for a method allowing a uniform slice selection at standardized LV levels. It is important to note that our methodology allows accurate, specific assessments of LV torsion and diastolic recoil at different levels throughout the myocardial wall which could be particularly valuable in the assessment of myocardial diseases that predominantly affect the endocardial layer such as subendocardial myocardial infarction, cardiac amyloid or endomyocardial fibrosis.

Table 1. Subject characteristics.

Demographics	Healthy volunteers
Study population	N = 10
Gender (f/m)	5/5
Age (y)	40.6 (23–51)
LV-EDV (ml/m^2)	51.0 (7.5)
LV-ESV (ml/m^2)	21.7 (5.1)
LV-CI (l/min/m^2)	2.0 (0.4)
LV-EF (%)	57.9 (5.6)

Continuous variable are expressed as mean (standard deviation), age is expressed as median (range).
f: female, m: male, EDV: end-diastolic volume, ESV: end-systolic volume, CI: cardiac index, EF: ejection fraction.

Table 2. Volumetric and hemodynamic response to 10 and 20 μg $kg^{-1}min^{-1}$ of dobutamine.

Parameter	Level of dobutamine (μg kg^{-1} min^{-1})			P value		
	Rest	10	20	Rest vs. 10	Rest vs. 20	10 vs. 20
LV-CI (l/min/m²)	2.0 (0.4)	3.3 (0.8)	4.2 (0.6)	**<0.01**	**<0.01**	**<0.01**
LV-EDV (ml/m²)	51.0 (7.5)	52.7 (9.1)	43.8 (15.4)	0.33	**<0.05**	**<0.01**
LV-ESV (ml/m²)	21.7 (5.1)	14.4 (5.9)	11.4 (4.6)	**<0.01**	**<0.01**	**<0.01**
LV-SV (ml/m²)	29.4 (4.1)	38.3 (7.4)	37.3 (6.5)	**<0.01**	**<0.01**	0.24
LV-EF (%)	57.9 (5.6)	72.9 (9.5)	77.0 (5.7)	**<0.01**	**<0.01**	**<0.05**
Mean BP (mmHg)	91.5 (10.2)	98.6 (10.4)	102.9 (10.7)	**<0.01**	**<0.05**	**<0.05**
Heart Rate	69.3 (10.3)	85.2 (16.6)	112.8 (11.9)	**<0.01**	**<0.01**	**<0.01**

Bold p values indicate a significance level <0.05.
BP: blood pressure, other abbreviations as in table 1.

Reproducibility of CMR-FT derived torsion

CMR-FT represents a relatively novel approach to quantify myocardial deformation. Previous CMR-FT studies primarily focused on ventricular strain measurements. The reported amount of reproducibility and repeatability varies between studies with most studies reporting reasonable reproducibility of global strain levels [19,31,32,33]. Therefore, intra- and inter-observer variability for torsion and recoil rate needs to be taken into special consideration. In order to maximise reproducibility all measurements were repeated three times and corresponding averaged rotational profiles were included in the calculation of torsion. As a result, all torsion and recoil rate parameters were highly reproducible on an intra-observer and inter-observer level. We found slightly lower reproducibility of model 2 (0–100%) and model 4 (0–75%) as compared to model 1 (25–75%) or model 3 (25–100%). Both, model 2 and model 4, involve rotational measurements taken from the most apical slice included in the calculation of torsion. As described in previous reports, reproducibility for CMR-FT derived strain parameters was lower at apical myocardial levels than at mid-ventricular or basal levels [34]. Our study shows that this holds true for apical and basal rotation assessment with CMR-FT and emphasises to rather include apical rotation from a slice position at 25% LV distance instead of using the most apical slice of a short-axis stack.

Torsion as a function of dobutamine exposure

Previous studies investigated the effect of inotropic stimulation with dobutamine on LV torsion in a canine model and found increased torsion paralleled by accelerated recoil rate [35,36]. The findings were confirmed in a human model using echocardiographic speckle tracking [37]. The authors found that subepicardial torsion remained unchanged during low dose dobutamine infusion and increased with higher doses of dobutamine. In contrast, subendocardial torsion already increased during low dose dobutamine infusion [37]. In the present study, we showed that model 1 (25–75%) using the shortest distance between apical and basal slices, consistently revealed significant increases of subendocardial and global torsion as well as accelerated recoil rate (subendocardial, subepicardial and global) with increasing levels of dobutamine. Conversely, subepicardial torsion only increased with the application of an intermediate dose of dobutamine, which is in accordance with the published findings by Akagawa et al. [37]. The other models using either the most apical or basal slice did not reliably differentiate torsion and recoil rate between rest and pharmacological stress and only showed non-significant trends towards increased torsion and recoil rates. This is most likely explained by through-plane motion causing loss of tracked features from the imaging plane. This might be particularly pronounced in the very apical and basal LV slices since longitudinal shortening is increased during dobutamine stress and may explain the need to

Table 3. Torsion and recoil rate.

	Model 1 (25–75%)	Model 2 (0–100%)	Model 3 (25–100%)	Model 4 (0–75%)	P value
Torsion Endo (°/cm)	3.0 (1.9)	3.6 (1.6)	3.6 (1.7)	3.4 (2.0)	0.72
Torsion Epi (°/cm)	2.3 (1.3)	2.7 (0.9)	2.6 (1.4)	2.6 (0.8)	0.37
Global Torsion (°/cm)	2.7 (1.5)	3.2 (1.2)	3.1 (1.5)	3.0 (1.3)	0.56
Recoil Rate Endo (°/cm/s)	−34.2 (10.3)	−46.2 (18.3)	−42.2 (9.7)	−45.5 (24.7)	0.56
Recoil Rate Epi (°/cm/s)	−26.1 (14.6)	−26.4 (9.3)	−24.8 (12.5)	−31.4 (10.6)*	**0.048**
Global Recoil Rate (°/cm/s)	−30.1 (11.1)	−36.3 (12.7)	−33.5 (9.1)	−38.5 (16.4)	0.29

Baseline values for torsion and recoil rate in comparison between the four models.
Variables are given as mean (SD)
***p = 0.022 vs. Model 2**
Bold p values indicate a significance level <0.05.
Endo: subendocardial, Epi: subepicardial, Global: average of subendocardial and subepicardial, rest: measurement at rest, 10: level of 10 μg kg^{-1} min^{-1} of dobutamine, 20: level of 20 μg kg^{-1} min^{-1} of dobutamine.

Table 4. Comparison of torsion and recoil rate between rest and stimulation with dobutamine.

		Level of dobutamine ($\mu g\ kg^{-1} min^{-1}$)			P value		
		rest	10	20	Rest vs. 10	Rest vs. 20	10 vs. 20
Model 1 (25–75%)	**Torsion Endo (°/cm)**	3.0 (1.9)	4.6 (2.5)	6.0 (2.4)	**0.02**	**<0.01**	**0.02**
	Torsion Epi (°/cm)	2.3 (1.3)	2.7 (1.5)	4.1 (2.2)	0.33	**0.01**	**0.03**
	Global Torsion (°/cm)	2.7 (1.5)	3.6 (2.0)	5.1 (2.2)	0.06	**<0.01**	**0.01**
	Recoil Rate Endo (°/cm/s)	−34.2 (10.3)	−53.6 (14.8)	−79.1 (35.1)	**0.01**	**<0.01**	**0.04**
	Recoil Rate Epi (°/cm/s)	−26.1 (14.6)	−40.3 (19.2)	−58.6 (32.3)	**0.02**	**<0.01**	**0.04**
	Global Recoil Rate (°/cm/s)	−30.1 (11.1)	−46.9 (15.0)	−68.9 (32.3)	**<0.01**	**<0.01**	**0.03**
Model 2 (0–100%)	**Torsion Endo (°/cm)**	3.6 (1.6)	5.2 (2.5)	5.8 (2.5)	0.14	0.09	0.51
	Torsion Epi (°/cm)	2.7 (0.9)	3.8 (2.0)	3.9 (1.8)	0.29	0.06	0.45
	Global Torsion (°/cm)	3.2 (1.2)	4.5 (2.2)	4.8 (1.9)	0.17	0.07	0.51
	Recoil Rate Endo (°/cm/s)	−46.2 (18.3)	−72.7 (37.9)	−82.6 (32.9)	0.17	0.047	0.33
	Recoil Rate Epi (°/cm/s)	−26.4 (9.3)	−49.0 (34.0)	−55.5 (28.0)	0.047	**<0.01**	0.39
	Global Recoil Rate (°/cm/s)	−36.3 (12.7)	−60.8 (34.7)	−69.1 (28.3)	0.11	**0.02**	0.39
Model 3 (25–100%)	**Torsion Endo (°/cm)**	3.6 (1.7)	4.8 (2.6)	6.1 (3.0)	0.07	**<0.01**	0.09
	Torsion Epi (°/cm)	2.6 (1.4)	2.9 (1.4)	3.9 (2.1)	0.51	**0.02**	**0.03**
	Global Torsion (°/cm)	3.1 (1.5)	3.8 (2.0)	5.0 (2.4)	0.07	**<0.01**	**0.02**
	Recoil Rate Endo (°/cm/s)	−42.2 (9.7)	−62.9 (29.7)	−69.5 (25.0)	**0.02**	**0.02**	0.45
	Recoil Rate Epi (°/cm/s)	−24.8 (12.5)	−37.8 (18.5)	−48.3 (25.3)	**0.02**	**0.01**	0.07
	Global Recoil Rate (°/cm/s)	−33.5 (9.1)	−50.4 (23.6)	−58.9 (24.6)	**0.01**	**0.01**	0.33
Model 4 (0–75%)	**Torsion Endo (°/cm)**	3.4 (2.0)	5.4 (2.5)	5.5 (3.0)	0.17	0.11	0.96
	Torsion Epi (°/cm)	2.6 (0.8)	4.0 (2.3)	4.1 (1.7)	0.24	**0.02**	0.20
	Global Torsion (°/cm)	3.0 (1.3)	4.7 (2.3)	4.8 (1.8)	0.14	**0.047**	0.88
	Recoil Rate Endo (°/cm/s)	−45.5 (24.7)	−69.8 (39.4)	−99.5 (45.6)	0.24	**0.01**	0.11
	Recoil Rate Epi (°/cm/s)	−31.4 (10.6)	−55.0 (34.7)	−70.4 (38.4)	0.06	**<0.01**	0.14
	Global Recoil Rate (°/cm/s)	−38.5 (16.4)	−62.4 (36.4)	−84.9 (38.9)	0.09	**0.01**	0.11

Bold p values indicate a significance level <0.05. Abbreviations as in table 3.

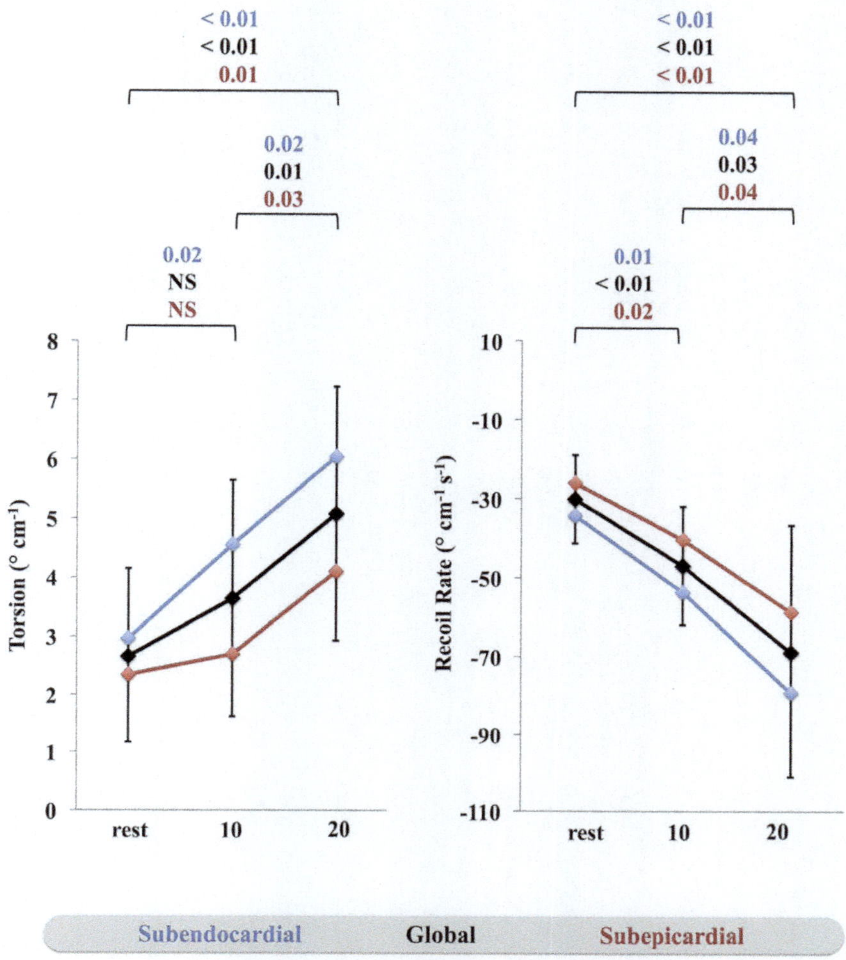

Figure 4. Torsion and recoil rate during dobutamine stress. Torsion and recoil rate (blue: subendocardial; red: subepicardial, black: global) as derived using model 1 (25–75%) in comparison between rest and increasing levels of dobutamine. A p-value <0.05 was considered statistically significant.

measure torsion from positions a bit farer away from the apex and the base.

CMR-FT in the context of existing methods to calculate torsion

Previously described CMR based modalities for the study of myocardial twisting and untwisting motion include myocardial tagging [10,38], tissue phase mapping [39] and displacement encoding with stimulated echoes (DENSE) [40]. Although accelerated techniques have been reported for myocardial tagging [41,42], all mentioned approaches commonly require additional sequence acquisitions and are usually associated with time-consuming post-processing both limiting their clinical applicability. In contrast, CMR-FT allows direct quantification of myocardial motion from standard SSFP images, which are widely available since they are generally part of every clinical CMR volumetric examination. From a clinical perspective, evaluation of myocardial torsion using CMR-FT has the potential to be integrated into a given clinical CMR protocol. Speckle-tracking echocardiography is another technique that has proved feasible for the quantification of myocardial rotation [8,10,43]. Speckle tracking echocardiography is widely available and benefits from high temporal resolution but suffers from limited image quality especially occasionally poor acoustic windows [23]. In general echocardiography does not allow a reliable and uniform selection of apical and basal slices in individual subjects, which has proved to be crucial for a robust quantification of myocardial twisting motion as expressed by our data and in previous reports [10]. Furthermore it is challenging to quantify torsion (twist per length) with speckle-tracking echocardiography, since the assessment of the inter-slice distance between apical and basal slices is generally not possible. Speckle-tracking echocardiography is therefore limited to the simple twist definition, which is even more dependent on the exact slice locations and difficult to reproduce in longitudinal studies [30]. Notwithstanding these considerations, several echocardiography speckle tracking based studies have shown the feasibility of twisting and untwisting motion quantification in various heart diseases. These involve conditions with a predominant diastolic involvement such as heart failure with preserved ejection fraction [17], diseases with predominant systolic involvement such as ischemic cardiomyopathy [44] and also diseases that equally affect systole and diastole such as hypertrophic cardiomyopathy [45] or cardiac amyloidosis [46]. Whether or not such assessments could also be derived from CMR-FT torsion and diastolic recoil measurements need to be investigated with future research studies.

Table 5. Reproducibility for all four models to calculate torsion and diastolic recoil rate.

		Model 1 (25–75%)			Model 2 (0–100%)			Model 3 (25–100%)			Model 4 (0–75%)		
		Mean Difference (SD)	**ICC (95%CI)**	**CoV (%)**	**Mean Difference (SD)**	**ICC (95%CI)**	**CoV (%)**	**Mean Difference (SD)**	**ICC (95%CI)**	**CoV (%)**	**Mean Difference (SD)**	**ICC (95%CI)**	**CoV (%)**
Intra-observer	**Torsion Endo (°/cm)**	0.02 (1.36)	0.92 (0.83–0.96)	30.14	−0.06 (0.79)	0.97 (0.94–0.99)	16.09	−0.16 (0.83)	0.97 (0.95–0.99)	16.91	0.00 (1.04)	0.96 (0.91–0.98)	21.80
	Torsion Epi (°/cm)	−0.02 (0.91)	0.94 (0.87–0.97)	29.81	0.05 (0.42)	0.99 (0.97–0.99)	12.23	0.03 (0.51)	0.98 (0.95–0.99)	16.50	−0.02 (0.61)	0.97 (0.94–0.99)	16.99
	Global Torsion (°/cm)	0.00 (1.05)	0.93 (0.86–0.97)	27.65	−0.01 (0.50)	0.98 (0.96–0.99)	12.07	−0.06 (0.49)	0.99 (0.97–0.99)	12.14	−0.01 (0.66)	0.97 (0.94–0.99)	15.81
	Recoil Rate Endo (°/cm/s)	6.48 (15.24)	0.92 (0.82–0.96)	25.88	0.98 (23.49)	0.91 (0.81–0.96)	34.73	−2.82 (10.88)	0.95 (0.90–0.98)	19.17	−0.56 (31.59)	0.88 (0.75–0.95)	44.29
	Recoil Rate Epi (°/cm/s)	−0.44 (9.74)	0.96 (0.92–0.98)	23.50	−0.81 (11.72)	0.95 (0.90–0.98)	27.11	−1.64 (7.51)	0.96 (0.92–0.98)	20.79	−3.80 (16.43)	0.93 (0.85–0.97)	32.63
	Global Recoil Rate (°/cm/s)	3.02 (9.68)	0.96 (0.92–0.98)	19.30	0.09 (15.77)	0.94 (0.87–0.97)	28.44	−2.23 (7.89)	0.96 (0.92–0.98)	16.97	−2.18 (21.34)	0.91 (0.82–0.96)	35.08
Inter-observer	**Torsion Endo (°/cm)**	0.07 (1.58)	0.89 (0.77–0.95)	35.30	0.94 (1.33)	0.85 (0.54–0.94)	30.35	0.52 (1.18)	0.94 (0.85–0.97)	25.84	0.62 (1.89)	0.80 (0.59–0.91)	42.31
	Torsion Epi (°/cm)	−0.15 (0.74)	0.96 (0.92–0.98)	23.55	0.35 (0.78)	0.94 (0.85–0.97)	23.73	0.21 (0.50)	0.98 (0.94–0.99)	16.54	0.14 (1.03)	0.93 (0.85–0.97)	29.61
	Global Torsion (°/cm)	−0.04 (1.07)	0.93 (0.86–0.97)	28.04	0.64 (0.97)	0.89 (0.68–0.96)	25.33	0.37 (0.70)	0.96 (0.91–0.99)	18.44	0.38 (1.35)	0.86 (0.71–0.93)	33.78
	Recoil Rate Endo (°/cm/s)	8.09 (17.07)	0.90 (0.76–0.95)	28.60	−9.31 (17.17)	0.91 (0.77–0.96)	27.47	−0.70 (8.61)	0.97 (0.94–0.99)	14.89	−7.01 (25.30)	0.89 (0.76–0.95)	37.15
	Recoil Rate Epi (°/cm/s)	−0.05 (9.42)	0.96 (0.93–0.98)	22.63	−5.35 (12.64)	0.93 (0.85–0.97)	30.85	−2.35 (7.02)	0.97 (0.93–0.98)	19.61	−6.42 (16.56)	0.92 (0.82–0.96)	33.77
	Global Recoil Rate (°/cm/s)	4.02 (10.76)	0.95 (0.90–0.98)	21.24	−7.33 (10.86)	0.95 (0.82–0.98)	21.00	−1.52 (6.02)	0.98 (0.96–0.99)	12.86	−6.71 (17.38)	0.92 (0.83–0.96)	29.67

ICC: Intraclass-correlation coefficient; CoV: coefficient of variation; SD: standard deviation; CI: confidence interval. Other abbreviations as in table 3.

Regarding longitudinal assessments, previous studies applied myocardial tagging to investigate the inter-study reproducibility for quantitative analysis of torsion and recoil rate and found good reproducibility for torsion whilst peak recoil rate was only poorly reproducible [38]. In fact, the study of recoil rate may require a more strict definition of measurement positions at apical and basal levels. This may be challenging using myocardial tagging, since this is usually performed at 3 LV levels only (apical, mid-ventricular and basal) and therefore subject to manual planning of slice positions. In contrast, we have now introduced a CMR-FT based technique that allows a uniform and exact definition of apical and basal slice positions independent of different heart sizes. Future work will need to address whether this approach positively impacts on inter-study reproducibility of torsion and of recoil rate in particular.

Limitations

The sample size of this feasibility study was relatively small. Notwithstanding this fact the results demonstrate feasibility and good reproducibility for torsion and diastolic recoil quantification with CMR-FT from routine cine images. Ideally we would have compared our results to myocardial tagging representing the reference standard for such acquisitions. However, given the necessity to obtain a whole SSFP short-axis stack at rest and with different levels of dobutamine we felt that the acquisition of an equal number of tagged images would have resulted in scanning times difficult to tolerate during dobutamine stimulation.

A general limitation of CMR based quantification of myocardial twisting motion is the current lack of standardized methods. Future studies will need to compare CMR-FT derived torsion and recoil rate with parameters from myocardial tagging using equal computation (twist per length) [38] or alternative computational methods e.g. the circumferential-longitudinal shear angle [11,12] which has not been addressed in the present study. However, there is evidence to suggest that twisting mechanics as assessed by torsion (twist per length) and shear angle deliver somewhat similar results [15]. The individual merits of both methods remain to be addressed in future investigations. A further limitation of both, conventional myocardial tagging and CMR-FT is the two-dimensional acquisition technique. We developed a pseudo three-dimensional mesh of myocardial torsion based on linear interpolation. However, this method does not compensate for through plane motion. Previous studies compared 2D and 3D derived torsion measured by myocardial tagging [47] and found that through plane motion did not significantly impact on 2D torsion since both methods showed reasonable agreement. The authors concluded to rather use the faster and easier 2D method for calculation of LV torsion. If this also holds true for 2D derived torsion from CMR-FT remains to be addressed in future investigations.

The clinical applicability of CMR-FT derived torsion and diastolic recoil assessment will depend on the speed of the analysis. At the present time the result files originating from CMR-FT are analysed using an in-house module for MATLAB. Future software developments will need to incorporate both post-processing steps in a single application to further minimize post-processing time.

Finally the current work aimed to determine the feasibility and reproducibility to quantify torsion and recoil rate from CMR-FT in a collective of healthy volunteers at rest and during dobutamine stress. Future research needs to prospectively validate this novel technique in pathologies such as coronary artery disease, heart failure or valvular disease.

Conclusions

CMR-FT allows derivation of myocardial torsion directly from standard SSFP cine images. Torsion and recoil rate calculated from apical and basal slices with 25–75% distance consistently discriminated between rest and increasing levels of dobutamine. Reproducibility was good to excellent for all torsion and recoil rate parameters, but was especially high when using an apical level at 25% LV distance instead of the most apical slice. When using CMR-FT to quantify myocardial torsion, it is therefore suggested to select apical and basal slices at standardized 25% and 75% levels. The analysis of myocardial torsion and recoil motion based on CMR-FT may have potential clinical and research applications when exact quantification of systolic and diastolic function is required. Future validation studies in larger cohorts should follow to establish the clinical utility and the prognostic implications of this technique.

Author Contributions

Conceived and designed the experiments: JTK PL AS. Performed the experiments: JTK PL STH SK BB AS. Analyzed the data: JTK PL AS. Contributed reagents/materials/analysis tools: MS JMS MF WS CUB JL GH. Wrote the paper: JTK PL AS.

References

1. Murray CJ, Lopez AD (1997) Alternative projections of mortality and disability by cause 1990–2020: Global Burden of Disease Study. Lancet 349: 1498–1504.
2. Owan TE, Hodge DO, Herges RM, Jacobsen SJ, Roger VL, et al. (2006) Trends in prevalence and outcome of heart failure with preserved ejection fraction. The New England journal of medicine 355: 251–259.
3. Karamitsos TD, Francis JM, Myerson S, Selvanayagam JB, Neubauer S (2009) The role of cardiovascular magnetic resonance imaging in heart failure. Journal of the American College of Cardiology 54: 1407–1424.
4. Kowallick JT, Edelmann F, Lotz J, Lamata P, Schuster A (2014) Imaging Diastolic Dysfunction with Cardiovascular Magnetic Resonance. Journal of Cardiology and Therapy 1: 58–64.
5. Pennell DJ (2010) Cardiovascular magnetic resonance. Circulation 121: 692–705.
6. Delhaas T, Kotte J, van der Toorn A, Snoep G, Prinzen FW, et al. (2004) Increase in left ventricular torsion-to-shortening ratio in children with valvular aortic stenosis. Magnetic resonance in medicine: official journal of the Society of Magnetic Resonance in Medicine/Society of Magnetic Resonance in Medicine 51: 135–139.
7. Dong SJ, Hees PS, Siu CO, Weiss JL, Shapiro EP (2001) MRI assessment of LV relaxation by untwisting rate: a new isovolumic phase measure of tau. American journal of physiology Heart and circulatory physiology 281: H2002–2009.
8. Opdahl A, Remme EW, Helle-Valle T, Edvardsen T, Smiseth OA (2012) Myocardial relaxation, restoring forces, and early-diastolic load are independent determinants of left ventricular untwisting rate. Circulation 126: 1441–1451.
9. Swoboda PP, Larghat A, Zaman A, Fairbairn TA, Motwani M, et al. (2014) Reproducibility of myocardial strain and left ventricular twist measured using complementary spatial modulation of magnetization. Journal of magnetic resonance imaging: JMRI 39: 887–894.
10. Goffinet C, Chenot F, Robert A, Pouleur AC, le Polain de Waroux JB, et al. (2009) Assessment of subendocardial vs. subepicardial left ventricular rotation and twist using two-dimensional speckle tracking echocardiography: comparison with tagged cardiac magnetic resonance. European heart journal 30: 608–617.
11. Russel IK, Gotte MJ, Kuijer JP, Marcus JT (2008) Regional assessment of left ventricular torsion by CMR tagging. Journal of cardiovascular magnetic resonance: official journal of the Society for Cardiovascular Magnetic Resonance 10: 26.
12. Buchalter MB, Weiss JL, Rogers WJ, Zerhouni EA, Weisfeldt ML, et al. (1990) Noninvasive quantification of left ventricular rotational deformation in normal humans using magnetic resonance imaging myocardial tagging. Circulation 81: 1236–1244.
13. Sorger JM, Wyman BT, Faris OP, Hunter WC, McVeigh ER (2003) Torsion of the left ventricle during pacing with MRI tagging. Journal of cardiovascular magnetic resonance: official journal of the Society for Cardiovascular Magnetic Resonance 5: 521–530.
14. Yoneyama K, Gjesdal O, Choi EY, Wu CO, Hundley WG, et al. (2012) Age, sex, and hypertension-related remodeling influences left ventricular torsion assessed by tagged cardiac magnetic resonance in asymptomatic individuals: the multi-ethnic study of atherosclerosis. Circulation 126: 2481–2490.

15. Donekal S, Venkatesh BA, Liu YC, Liu CY, Yoneyama K, et al. (2014) Interstitial Fibrosis, Left Ventricular Remodeling, and Myocardial Mechanical Behavior in a Population-Based Multiethnic Cohort: The Multi-Ethnic Study of Atherosclerosis (MESA) Study. Circulation Cardiovascular imaging 7: 292–302.
16. Park SJ, Miyazaki C, Bruce CJ, Ommen S, Miller FA, et al. (2008) Left ventricular torsion by two-dimensional speckle tracking echocardiography in patients with diastolic dysfunction and normal ejection fraction. Journal of the American Society of Echocardiography: official publication of the American Society of Echocardiography 21: 1129–1137.
17. Wang J, Khoury DS, Yue Y, Torre-Amione G, Nagueh SF (2008) Preserved left ventricular twist and circumferential deformation, but depressed longitudinal and radial deformation in patients with diastolic heart failure. European heart journal 29: 1283–1289.
18. Abozguia K, Nallur-Shivu G, Phan TT, Ahmed I, Kalra R, et al. (2010) Left ventricular strain and untwist in hypertrophic cardiomyopathy: relation to exercise capacity. American heart journal 159: 825–832.
19. Hor KN, Gottliebson WM, Carson C, Wash E, Cnota J, et al. (2010) Comparison of magnetic resonance feature tracking for strain calculation with harmonic phase imaging analysis. JACC Cardiovascular imaging 3: 144–151.
20. Kowallick JT, Kutty S, Edelmann F, Chiribiri A, Villa A, et al. (2014) Quantification of left atrial strain and strain rate using Cardiovascular Magnetic Resonance myocardial feature tracking: a feasibility study. Journal of cardiovascular magnetic resonance: official journal of the Society for Cardiovascular Magnetic Resonance 16: 60.
21. Morton G, Schuster A, Jogiya R, Kutty S, Beerbaum P, et al. (2012) Inter-study reproducibility of cardiovascular magnetic resonance myocardial feature tracking. Journal of cardiovascular magnetic resonance: official journal of the Society for Cardiovascular Magnetic Resonance 14: 43.
22. Schuster A, Paul M, Bettencourt N, Morton G, Chiribiri A, et al. (2013) Cardiovascular magnetic resonance myocardial feature tracking for quantitative viability assessment in ischemic cardiomyopathy. International journal of cardiology 166: 413–420.
23. Nagel E, Lehmkuhl HB, Bocksch W, Klein C, Vogel U, et al. (1999) Noninvasive diagnosis of ischemia-induced wall motion abnormalities with the use of high-dose dobutamine stress MRI: comparison with dobutamine stress echocardiography. Circulation 99: 763–770.
24. Oppo K, Leen E, Angerson WJ, Cooke TG, McArdle CS (1998) Doppler perfusion index: an interobserver and intraobserver reproducibility study. Radiology 208: 453–457.
25. Bland JM, Altman DG (1986) Statistical methods for assessing agreement between two methods of clinical measurement. Lancet 1: 307–310.
26. Grothues F, Smith GC, Moon JC, Bellenger NG, Collins P, et al. (2002) Comparison of interstudy reproducibility of cardiovascular magnetic resonance with two-dimensional echocardiography in normal subjects and in patients with heart failure or left ventricular hypertrophy. The American journal of cardiology 90: 29–34.
27. Esch BT, Warburton DE (2009) Left ventricular torsion and recoil: implications for exercise performance and cardiovascular disease. Journal of applied physiology 106: 362–369.
28. Burns AT, La Gerche A, Prior DL, Macisaac AI (2009) Left ventricular untwisting is an important determinant of early diastolic function. JACC Cardiovascular imaging 2: 709–716.
29. Moon MR, Ingels NB, Jr., Daughters GT, 2nd, Stinson EB, Hansen DE, et al. (1994) Alterations in left ventricular twist mechanics with inotropic stimulation and volume loading in human subjects. Circulation 89: 142–150.
30. Young AA, Cowan BR (2012) Evaluation of left ventricular torsion by cardiovascular magnetic resonance. Journal of cardiovascular magnetic resonance: official journal of the Society for Cardiovascular Magnetic Resonance 14: 49.
31. Schuster A, Kutty S, Padiyath A, Parish V, Gribben P, et al. (2011) Cardiovascular magnetic resonance myocardial feature tracking detects quantitative wall motion during dobutamine stress. Journal of cardiovascular magnetic resonance: official journal of the Society for Cardiovascular Magnetic Resonance 13: 58.
32. Schuster A, Morton G, Hussain ST, Jogiya R, Kutty S, et al. (2013) The intra-observer reproducibility of cardiovascular magnetic resonance myocardial feature tracking strain assessment is independent of field strength. European journal of radiology 82: 296–301.
33. Singh A, Steadman CD, Khan JN, Horsfield MA, Bekele S, et al. (2014) Intertechnique agreement and interstudy reproducibility of strain and diastolic strain rate at 1.5 and 3 tesla: A comparison of feature-tracking and tagging in patients with aortic stenosis. Journal of magnetic resonance imaging: JMRI.
34. Wu L, Germans T, Guclu A, Heymans MW, Allaart CP, et al. (2014) Feature tracking compared with tissue tagging measurements of segmental strain by cardiovascular magnetic resonance. Journal of cardiovascular magnetic resonance: official journal of the Society for Cardiovascular Magnetic Resonance 16: 10.
35. Buchalter MB, Rademakers FE, Weiss JL, Rogers WJ, Weisfeldt ML, et al. (1994) Rotational deformation of the canine left ventricle measured by magnetic resonance tagging: effects of catecholamines, ischaemia, and pacing. Cardiovascular research 28: 629–635.
36. Rademakers FE, Buchalter MB, Rogers WJ, Zerhouni EA, Weisfeldt ML, et al. (1992) Dissociation between left ventricular untwisting and filling. Accentuation by catecholamines. Circulation 85: 1572–1581.
37. Akagawa E, Murata K, Tanaka N, Yamada H, Miura T, et al. (2007) Augmentation of left ventricular apical endocardial rotation with inotropic stimulation contributes to increased left ventricular torsion and radial strain in normal subjects: quantitative assessment utilizing a novel automated tissue tracking technique. Circulation journal: official journal of the Japanese Circulation Society 71: 661–668.
38. Donekal S, Ambale-Venkatesh B, Berkowitz S, Wu CO, Choi EY, et al. (2013) Inter-study reproducibility of cardiovascular magnetic resonance tagging. Journal of cardiovascular magnetic resonance: official journal of the Society for Cardiovascular Magnetic Resonance 15: 37.
39. Codreanu I, Robson MD, Golding SJ, Jung BA, Clarke K, et al. (2010) Longitudinally and circumferentially directed movements of the left ventricle studied by cardiovascular magnetic resonance phase contrast velocity mapping. Journal of cardiovascular magnetic resonance: official journal of the Society for Cardiovascular Magnetic Resonance 12: 48.
40. Haggerty CM, Kramer SP, Binkley CM, Powell DK, Mattingly AC, et al. (2013) Reproducibility of cine displacement encoding with stimulated echoes (DENSE) cardiovascular magnetic resonance for measuring left ventricular strains, torsion, and synchrony in mice. Journal of cardiovascular magnetic resonance: official journal of the Society for Cardiovascular Magnetic Resonance 15: 71.
41. Reyhan M, Ennis DB (2013) Quantitative assessment of systolic and diastolic left ventricular twist using Fourier Analysis of Stimulated echoes (FAST) and CSPAMM. Journal of magnetic resonance imaging: JMRI 37: 678–683.
42. Reyhan M, Natsuaki Y, Ennis DB (2012) Fourier analysis of STimulated echoes (FAST) for the quantitative analysis of left ventricular twist. Journal of magnetic resonance imaging: JMRI 35: 587–593.
43. Notomi Y, Lysyansky P, Setser RM, Shiota T, Popovic ZB, et al. (2005) Measurement of ventricular torsion by two-dimensional ultrasound speckle tracking imaging. Journal of the American College of Cardiology 45: 2034–2041.
44. Bansal M, Leano RL, Marwick TH (2008) Clinical assessment of left ventricular systolic torsion: effects of myocardial infarction and ischemia. Journal of the American Society of Echocardiography: official publication of the American Society of Echocardiography 21: 887–894.
45. Notomi Y, Martin-Miklovic MG, Oryszak SJ, Shiota T, Deserranno D, et al. (2006) Enhanced ventricular untwisting during exercise: a mechanistic manifestation of elastic recoil described by Doppler tissue imaging. Circulation 113: 2524–2533.
46. Karabay CY, Kocabay G (2011) Left ventricular torsion by two-dimensional speckle tracking echocardiography in patient with a-type amyloid heart disease. Journal of the American Society of Echocardiography: official publication of the American Society of Echocardiography 24: 818 e815–819.
47. Russel IK, Tecelao SR, Kuijer JP, Heethaar RM, Marcus JT (2009) Comparison of 2D and 3D calculation of left ventricular torsion as circumferential-longitudinal shear angle using cardiovascular magnetic resonance tagging. Journal of cardiovascular magnetic resonance: official journal of the Society for Cardiovascular Magnetic Resonance 11: 8.
48. Lamata P, Sinclair M, Kerfoot E, Lee A, Crozier A, et al. (2014) An automatic service for the personalization of ventricular cardiac meshes. Journal of the Royal Society, Interface/the Royal Society 11: 20131023.

10

A Randomized Pilot Trial of Remote Ischemic Preconditioning in Heart Failure with Reduced Ejection Fraction

Michael A. McDonald[1]*, Juarez R. Braga[1], Jing Li[2], Cedric Manlhiot[2], Heather J. Ross[1], Andrew N. Redington[2]

1 Division of Cardiology, Peter Munk Cardiac Centre, University of Toronto, Toronto, Canada, **2** Division of Cardiology, Hospital for Sick Children, University of Toronto, Toronto, Canada

Abstract

Background: Remote ischemic preconditioning (RIPC) induced by transient limb ischemia confers multi-organ protection and improves exercise performance in the setting of tissue hypoxia. We aimed to evaluate the effect of RIPC on exercise capacity in heart failure patients.

Methods: We performed a randomized crossover trial of RIPC (4×5-minutes limb ischemia) compared to sham control in heart failure patients undergoing exercise testing. Patients were randomly allocated to either RIPC or sham prior to exercise, then crossed over and completed the alternate intervention with repeat testing. The primary outcome was peak VO2, RIPC versus sham. A mechanistic substudy was performed using dialysate from study patient blood samples obtained after sham and RIPC. This dialysate was used to test for a protective effect of RIPC in a mouse heart Langendorff model of infarction. Mouse heart infarct size with RIPC or sham dialysate exposure was also compared with historical control data.

Results: Twenty patients completed the study. RIPC was not associated with improvements in peak VO2 (15.6+/−4.2 vs 15.3+/−4.6 mL/kg/min; $p = 0.53$, sham and RIPC, respectively). In our Langendorff sub-study, infarct size was similar between RIPC and sham dialysate groups from our study patients, but was smaller than expected compared to healthy controls (29.0%, 27.9% [sham, RIPC] vs 51.2% [controls]. We observed less preconditioning among the subgroup of patients with increased exercise performance following RIPC ($p < 0.04$).

Conclusion: In this pilot study of RIPC in heart failure patients, RIPC was not associated with improvements in exercise capacity overall. However, the degree of effect of RIPC may be inversely related to the degree of baseline preconditioning. These data provide the basis for a larger randomized trial to test the potential benefits of RIPC in patients with heart failure.

Trial Registration: ClinicalTrials.gov NCT01128790

Editor: Yoshihiro Fukumoto, Kurume University School of Medicine, Japan

Funding: The authors have no funding or support to report.

Competing Interests: Andrew Redington is co-holder of a patent and shareholder in a company developing an automated remote preconditioning device. There was no commercial funding or other involvement for this project and an automated device was not used in this study.

* Email: Michael.mcdonald@uhn.on.ca

Introduction

Exercise impairment in patients with chronic heart failure (HF) is associated with significant morbidity and mortality [1–4]. Objective measures of exercise capacity continue to be important predictors of clinical outcomes, and are widely used to risk stratify HF patients for advanced therapies, including cardiac transplantation [3–5]. The effects of chronic left ventricular dysfunction and HF on exercise capacity are multifactorial, and relate to diminished cardiac output and to alterations in peripheral and respiratory skeletal muscle structure and function [6–9]. Notably, improvements in skeletal muscle function and exercise capacity are associated with improvements in left ventricular function [10], reduced hospitalization [11], and better transplant-free survival [12]. It follows that interventions to improve exercise capacity may translate into significant clinical benefits in the HF population.

Remote ischemic preconditioning (RIPC) is a well-described protective mechanism in which a transient, sub-lethal reduction in blood flow to tissues in one area of the body renders other remote tissues more resistant to subsequent episodes of prolonged ischemia [13]. Although the precise mechanisms are not fully defined, the remote ischemic preconditioning stimulus appears to trigger release of circulating factors [14–16] that result in downstream effects on mitochondrial function within the target organ(s) [13]. Early clinical application of RIPC in cardiac patients has been encouraging; transient limb ischemia, typically involving 2–4 cycles of 5–10 minutes each, has been shown to limit myocardial injury in the setting of elective cardiac or vascular surgery, as well as percutaneous coronary intervention for angina or acute myocardial infarction [17–21].

To date, the impact of RIPC in HF patients has not been explored. However, 'local' ischemic preconditioning of the legs improved maximal power output and maximal oxygen consumption during subsequent bicycle ergometry in healthy volunteers [22]. Recent work from members of our group has demonstrated that RIPC can improve maximal performance in highly trained swimmers, suggesting a salutary effect on peripheral skeletal, respiratory and cardiac muscle function under conditions of exercise induced hypoxic ischemia [23]. We therefore sought to determine whether RIPC would be associated with improvements in exercise capacity in patients with HF due to left ventricular systolic dysfunction.

Methods

The protocol for this trial and supporting CONSORT checklist are available as supporting information; see Checklist S1 and Protocol S1.

Ethics Statement

All patients provided written informed consent, and the study protocol was approved by the Research Ethics Board of the University Health Network, and registered prior to initiation (Identifier: NCT01128790, registered December 2009 at ClinicalTrials.gov). The CONSORT 2010 Statement for clinical trials was followed for the reporting of our study results herein. There are currently no ongoing clinical trials of RIPC intervention from our group at this time.

Patient Population

We performed a randomized, controlled, crossover pilot trial of patients recruited from the Heart Function Clinic at the Toronto General Hospital, a University of Toronto affiliated teaching hospital. The Heart Function Clinic is a large volume multidisciplinary clinic that manages of a broad spectrum of HF patients, including those with advanced HF referred for consideration of transplantation or mechanical circulatory support.

Ambulatory clinic patients scheduled for routine cardiopulmonary stress testing were approached for study inclusion if they met all of the following criteria: ≥18 years of age, left ventricular ejection fraction (LVEF) <40%, history of New York Heart Association (NYHA) class II–IV symptoms, HF for at least 12 weeks, and clinical stability. Patients were initially excluded for any of the following reasons: ischemic cardiomyopathy, cardiovascular related hospitalization within the preceding four weeks, diabetes, peripheral neuropathy, inability to exercise or other contraindications to stress testing, inability or unwillingness to participate in serial exercise testing. Patients were enrolled and followed from September 2009 to February 2011. Following study initiation, there were comparatively few patients from our clinic population with non-ischemic cardiomyopathy who met all other inclusion criteria, and we therefore modified our protocol to include patients with stable underlying coronary disease that were otherwise eligible. All other exclusion criteria were maintained throughout the study.

Study Protocol

Patients were approached for participation and consent was obtained prior to their scheduled cardiopulmonary exercise test. Immediately prior to testing, patients were randomized by one of the investigators (MM or JB) in a 1:1 ratio by computer generated allocation sequence, to the order in which they received either RIPC intervention or sham intervention. Patients then crossed over to receive the alternate intervention at a dedicated follow-up visit for repeat exercise testing. Where possible, patients were scheduled for a second exercise study within four weeks to minimize the potential impact of disease progression or any interim therapeutic intervention on exercise capacity. Throughout the duration of the trial, patients were unaware of the expected effects of the sham or RIPC treatment and investigators (other than those performing the intervention) remained blinded to treatment assignment.

The RIPC stimulus consisted of four cycles of 5 minutes of upper limb ischemia followed by 5 minutes of reperfusion. A blood pressure cuff was placed over the upper arm, and limb ischemia was achieved by inflating the cuff 20 mmHg above the systolic pressure. The sham intervention consisted of four cycles of 5 minutes of blood pressure cuff inflation to only 10 mmHg, interspersed with 5 minutes of cuff deflation to simulate reperfusion. After completing four cycles of either intervention, 30 mL of blood was drawn, placed on ice and transferred to the investigators' laboratory as part of the pre-specified mechanistic sub-study. Immediately thereafter, patients completed a cardiopulmonary exercise test with respiratory gas analysis according to a routine stationary bicycle ramp protocol (10 Watt per minute incremental workload). Testing was symptom limited after achieving a diagnostic workload, defined as a respiratory exchange ratio >1.05. A dedicated exercise physiologist who was unaware of the treatment assignment supervised all tests, and a blinded investigator (HR) reported the results.

The primary outcome measure was peak oxygen consumption (VO2) measured in milliliters of oxygen consumed per kilogram of body mass per minute (mL/kg/min) during peak exercise following sham intervention compared to peak VO2 following RIPC intervention. Secondary outcomes included a comparison of exercise duration, workload achieved, ventilatory anaerobic threshold, absolute peak VO2, and the slope of the minute ventilation (VE) to carbon dioxide production (VCO2) ratio. As this pilot study was exploratory in nature and undertaken for feasibility, no sample size calculations were performed. We estimated that 20 patients with paired exercise data would represent an adequate sample to inform future trial design and generate appropriate study hypotheses.

Sub-study Protocol

We conducted a pre-specified sub-study to assess whether HF patients elaborate circulating protective factor(s) in response to a RIPC stimulus. The animal protocols used for this study were approved by the Animal care and Use Committee of the Hospital for Sick Children in Toronto and conformed with the Guide for the Care and Use of Laboratory Animals published by the National Institutes of Health (publication # 85-23, revised 1996). The 30 mL of blood drawn immediately following the RIPC or sham intervention was collected in heparinized tubes and placed on ice. It was subsequently centrifuged at 3000 rpm for 20 minutes at room temperature and the plasma fraction was dialyzed against a 20 fold volume of Krebs-Henseleit solution across a 12–14 kDa dialysis membrane. The dialysate was then prepared for use in a mouse heart Langendorff model as previously described [23]. Briefly, the dialysate was made isotonic and adjusted to pH 7.4 with sodium bicarbonate and glucose. Prior to perfusion of the mouse hearts, D-glucose, NaHCO3 and EDTA were added to a final concentration of 15 mM, 25 mM and 0.5 mM in the dialysate, respectively. Mice were anesthetized with pentobarbital in standard fashion and the hearts were excised, cannulated at the aorta, and perfused with modified Krebs-Ringer buffer at 37°C. A water-filled latex balloon was inserted into the left ventricle, connected to a pressure transducer and maintained at 7–10 mmHg to allow beat to beat measurement of left ventricular pressures (PowerLab data acquisition system AD Instruments; Colorado Springs, CO, USA). Dialysate derived from each patient for both sham and RIPC conditions was used to perfuse 2–4 mouse hearts, and data from each preparation was averaged.

Following a 20 minute stabilization period, the hearts were perfused with the study patient dialysate solution and then subjected to 30 minutes of no-flow ischemia followed by 60 minutes of reperfusion. After completing the protocol, the hearts were frozen at −80°C. Each heart was then sectioned into 1 mm thick slices and stained with 1.25% 2,3,5-triphynyltetrazolium chloride to distinguish areas of infarcted tissue (white colour) from non-infarcted tissue (red colour). The slices were formalin fixed and scanned into Photoshop. Using this method, it was possible to trace the area of infarcted tissue and express this as a proportion of the total area of LV myocardium at risk. The primary endpoint of this Langendorff sub-study was infarct area in hearts perfused with sham dialysate versus infarct area in hearts perfused with RIPC dialysate. Secondary endpoints included LV developed pressure, LV end-diastolic pressure, maximum rate of systolic pressure rise (dP/dt max) and fall (dP/dt min). Infarct size observed after sham or RIPC dialysate exposure in heart failure patients described above was also compared with infarct size observed using an identical sham and RIPC procedure to prepare dialysate from 4 healthy subjects serving as historical controls (4 males, age range 25–50 years).

Statistical Analysis

Continuous data are reported as means with standard deviation, and categorical data are reported as frequencies. Normality of the distribution of continuous variables was tested using the Shapiro-Wilks test. Differences in exercise outcomes between sham control and RIPC intervention were assessed using paired t-tests. Logistic regression model was used to identify factors associated with response to RIPC, with relative difference between RIPC and Sham used as a dependent variable and each categorical variable or each tertile of continuous variables as independent predictors. A p-value of <0.05 was considered significant for all comparisons. All analyses were performed using SPSS for Windows v 11.0 (SPSS Inc., Chicago, IL).

Results

Main Study

Figure 1 outlines the patient flow through the study. In total, 22 patients consented to participate from September 2009 to January 2011, and all 22 were randomized and subsequently completed the assigned first intervention prior to undergoing the initial cardiopulmonary exercise stress test. Two patients, both allocated to the initial sham control group, withdrew from the study and declined to undergo follow-up exercise testing. Therefore, the final study population included in the analysis consisted of 20 patients who completed the protocol with both sham and RIPC interventions.

The baseline characteristics of the study patients are shown in Table 1. As outlined, the majority were males with non-ischemic cardiomyopathy. All patients were treated with beta blockers and ACE inhibitors, 70% required loop diuretics, and a large proportion of patients had received a defibrillator and/or cardiac resynchronization therapy. Although all patients had previously been characterized as NYHA class II, III, or IV, most were minimally symptomatic at the time of enrollment.

The majority of patients in this study (16/20) completed sequential cardiopulmonary exercise tests within 30 days as planned. Two patients were unable to return for scheduled follow-up testing for logistical reasons and completed the protocol within 90 days, and an additional two patients completed follow-up by 180 days. There were no adverse effects observed for any of our study patients. The results for the primary outcome, peak VO2 for RIPC compared to sham intervention, are shown in Figure 2 and Table 2. Overall, RIPC prior to cardiopulmonary exercise testing was not associated with improvements in peak VO2 in this population (15.6+/−4.2 mL/kg/min vs 15.3+/−4.6 mL/kg/min; $p = 0.53$, for sham and RIPC, respectively). With respect to the secondary outcomes, there was no observed benefit of RIPC on exercise duration, workload achieved, anaerobic threshold, or VE/CO2 slope (Table 2). Excluding patients that did not complete the protocol within 30 days had no impact on our results. Moreover, post-hoc exploratory analysis did not identify any baseline clinical characteristics, (including age, gender, duration of heart failure, functional class, BNP level) associated with an improved peak VO2 following RIPC intervention. Finally, the sequence of testing did not appear to have an effect on our results, as there were no significant differences in peak VO2 from the initial exercise study compared to the follow-up study, irrespective of the treatment allocation.

Langendorff Sub Study

In the Langendorff study, there was no significant difference in infarct area between mouse hearts perfused with sham dialysate and those perfused with RIPC dialysate (29.0+/−7.9% versus 27.9+/−6.8%; $p = 0.62$). Additionally, the secondary endpoint hemodynamic measurements were not significantly different at any stage following perfusion with either sham or RIPC derived dialysate.

Using this Langendorff model, we undertook a further exploratory comparison of infarct size following perfusion with dialysate derived from our heart failure study population versus infarct size following perfusion with dialysate derived from plasma from healthy controls undergoing sham/RIPC intervention. The infarct size observed in hearts perfused with dialysate from our heart failure patients was nearly 45% less than the infarct size observed in hearts perfused with healthy control dialysate following sham intervention. Moreover, the infarct area seen in our study approximates the infarct area seen with exposure to dialysate from healthy control subjects following RIPC intervention (Figure 3).

In order to determine whether the apparent lack of effect of RIPC in our study population could be explained by a high degree of baseline preconditioning, we assessed infarct size in the Langendorff model according to clinical response to RIPC treatment. In this post hoc analysis, mouse infarct size was significantly smaller among the subgroup of patients who had no improvement in exercise capacity following RIPC intervention, suggesting that the overall absence of a clinical response to RIPC in our study population may relate to a higher degree of preconditioning at baseline for the majority of patients (Figure 4).

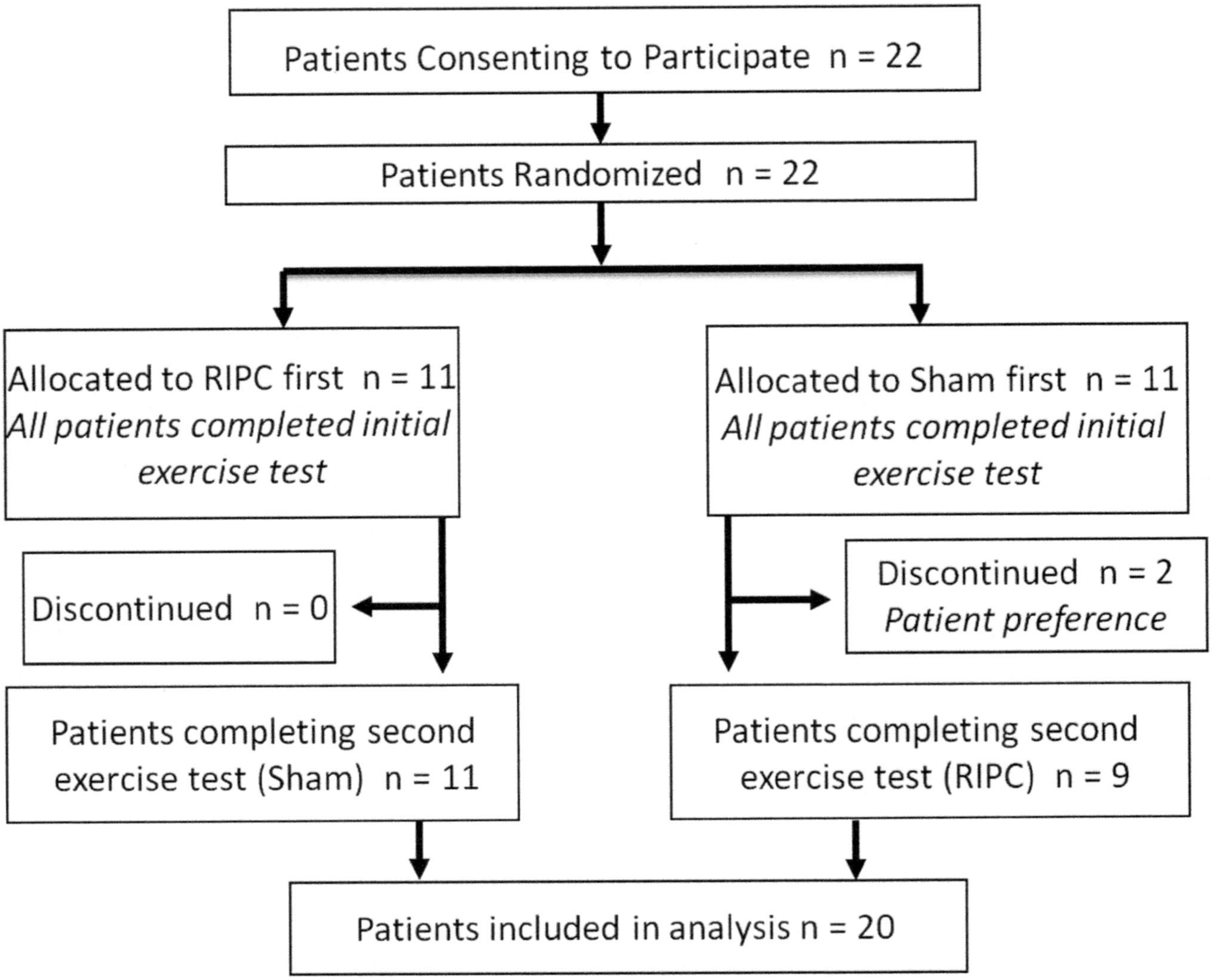

Figure 1. Patient flow through the study. 22 patients consented to participate in the study. Two patients declined repeat testing and were excluded from the analysis; 20 patients complete the study protocol with paired testing.

Discussion

In this randomized crossover pilot study, RIPC was not associated with improvements in objective measures of exercise capacity in ambulatory HF patients with left ventricular dysfunction. Specifically, there was no overall benefit with respect to any of the prognostically important exercise variables, including peak VO2, exercise duration, workload achieved or VE/VCO2 slope during cardiopulmonary stress testing. A principle finding from our Langendorff sub-study was that RIPC in this study population does not appear to confer additional protection against ischemia reperfusion injury through release of circulating preconditioning factor(s). This observation is in contrast with the effects of RIPC in a healthy control population [23]; moreover our results suggest that patients with chronic HF may already be relatively preconditioned.

To our knowledge, this is the first clinical trial to evaluate the effect of RIPC in a heart failure population. There is a growing body of evidence that suggests RIPC induced by transient limb ischemia, similar to the protocol used in our study, is associated with a significant reduction in end organ injury due to a variety of ischemic stressors. One of the earliest clinical studies of RIPC was a randomized controlled trial of 37 pediatric patients undergoing cardiopulmonary bypass for corrective cardiac surgery [17]. In this study, four 5-minute cycles of limb ischemia and reperfusion resulted in less troponin elevation, lower inotrope requirements, and better lung function in the early post-operative setting. RIPC with lower limb ischemia was also shown to attenuate myocardial and renal injury in a randomized controlled trial of 82 patients undergoing elective abdominal aortic aneurysm repair [19]. These early trials have supported the observation that RIPC confers multisystem protection in an ischemic environment.

Maximal exercise performance is limited by 'relative' ischemia of skeletal muscle and is associated with tissue hypoxia and lactic acid accumulation, and thus can be considered a form of ischemic stress. Recently, the potential benefits of ischemic preconditioning have extended into the domain of exercise performance in healthy individuals. de Groot and colleagues showed that ischemic preconditioning of each leg prior to bicycle exercise testing improved both maximal workload and maximal oxygen consumption [22] in healthy volunteers. Members of our group have shown that RIPC induced by transient upper limb ischemia immediately

Table 1. Baseline characteristics of the study population.

Age (years)	56.3+/−11.8
Male	18 (90)
Duration of heart failure (months)	71.3+/−63.4
Etiology:	
Ischemic	4 (20)
Non-ischemic	16 (80)
LVEF (%)	29.3+/−6.8
NYHA functional class:	
I	5 (25)
II	10 (50)
III	5 (25)
IV	-
HTN*	3 (15)
Smoking history:	
Never	11 (55)
Prior	8 (40)
Current	1 (5)
Atrial fibrillation	6 (30)
Medications:	
ACE inhibitor/ARB†	20 (100)
Beta blocker	20 (100)
Spironolactone	10 (50)
Digoxin	7 (35)
Loop diuretic	14 (70)
Nitrate	2 (10)
AICD‡	12 (60)
CRT'	5 (25)
Systolic blood pressure (mmHg)	105.7+/−12.8
Diastolic blood pressure (mmHg)	69+/−9.9
Heart rate (beats/min)	64.8+/−7.8
Height (cm)	178.6+/−8.6
Weight (kg)	94.7+/−22.5
Hemoglobin (g/L)	145.4+/−14.8
Serum creatinine (μmol/L)	94+/−22.5
Serum sodium (mmol/L)	138.5+/−2.7
BNP# (pg/mL)	Range 10.0–1616.0

(N = 20).
Values are expressed as means +/− standard deviation, or numbers and percentages.
*HTN: hypertension.
†ARB: angiotensin receptor blocker.
‡AICD: automated implantable cardioverter-defibrillator.
'CRT: cardiac resynchronization therapy.
#BNP: B-type natriuretic peptide.

prior to exercise was associated with significant improvements in competitive swim times in elite athletes [23]. Furthermore, dialyzed serum taken from the swimmers following RIPC (but not serum taken before) was shown to carry a circulating "protective factor" that significantly reduced infarct size in a mouse Langendorff model of ischemia-reperfusion [23], confirming the importance of humoral-mediated pathways discussed earlier [14–16]. Prior to performing our study, we hypothesized that RIPC may have a favorable impact on exercise capacity of HF patients who are subject to musculoskeletal and cardiac ischemia as they reach an anaerobic state at peak exercise. These patients have poor exercise tolerance secondary to reduced cardiac output, abnormalities in myocyte fibre composition, and reduced mitochondrial density [7–9]. Any intervention to improve exercise performance in a HF population with various physiologic limitations could potentially translate into important clinical benefits.

Why then was there no overall impact of RIPC on exercise capacity in this study, despite using a conventional preconditioning protocol? The answer to this question may be multifactorial, but

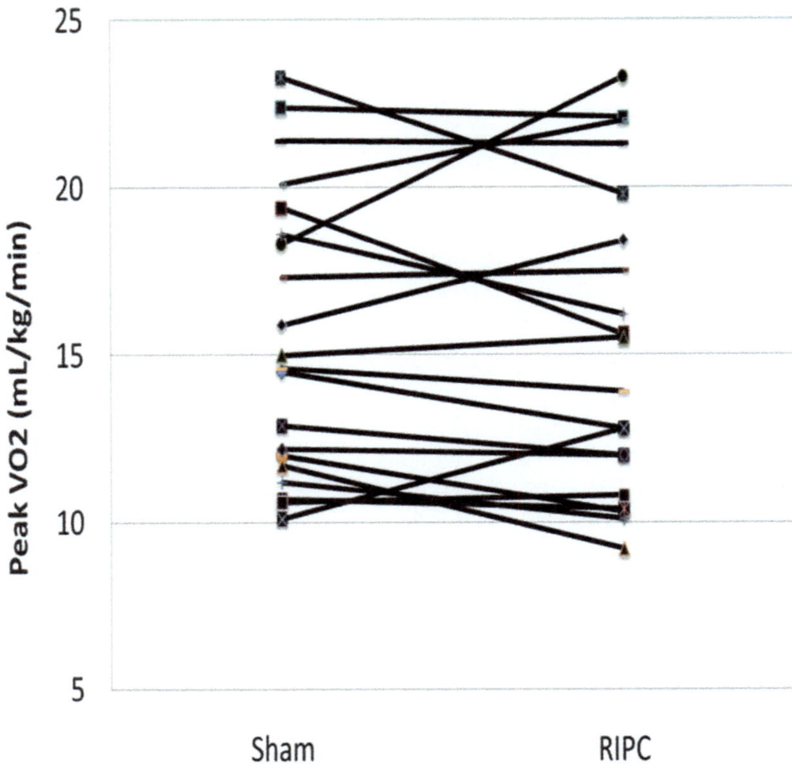

Figure 2. Individual exercise test results for sham versus RIPC intervention. Peak VO2 is shown for all study subjects undergoing exercise stress testing immediately following sham and RIPC interventions.

our Langendorff study provides important new evidence to suggest that these patients may already be in a 'preconditioned state'. Indeed, our results show that plasma obtained after sham intervention already contained dialyzable circulating cardioprotective factors characteristic of those liberated by remote preconditioning stimuli [14–16]. Consequently, overall the level of cardioprotection observed in control dialysate from the heart failure patients was similar to that seen after RIPC in normal volunteers, and was unaffected by additional RIPC. The reason for this is less clear however. There is emerging evidence that vigorous exercise in healthy subjects itself is a stimulus for release of cardioprotective factors [24]. We speculate that daily activities in HF patients may act as a similar stimulus to the release of cardioprotective factors as a result of skeletal muscle ischemia. It is also possible that the heart may act as a paracrine organ for the release of cardioprotective factors. For example, Dickson and colleagues have shown that coronary effluent from hearts subjected to brief periods of ischemia is cardioprotective in an untreated acceptor heart [25].

Irrespective of where the circulating factors originate, our data do suggest that there may be a subgroup of heart failure patients that might respond to RIPC. Although the numbers were small, when we compared those that had significantly improved exercise performance with RIPC, versus those that did not, there was also a

Table 2. Exercise performance of Sham control versus RIPC intervention.

	Sham	RIPC	P value
Peak VO2 (ml/kg/min)	15.6+/−4.2	15.3+/−4.6	0.53
Secondary Endpoints:			
Exercise duration (minutes)	10.3+/−3.0	11.0+/−3.0	0.13
Workload (watts)	108.5+/−29.8	103.0+/−32.6	0.07
AT* (ml/kg/min)	9.6+/−2.6	9.6+/−3.0	0.98
Peak VO2† (L/min)	1.45+/−0.36	1.42+/−0.42	0.39
VE/VECO2‡ slope	28.7+/−4.3	29.9+/−5.4	0.06

(N = 20).
Values expressed as means +/− standard deviation.
*AT: anaerobic threshold.
†VO2: oxygen uptake.
‡VE/VCO2: minute ventilation - carbon dioxide production ratio.

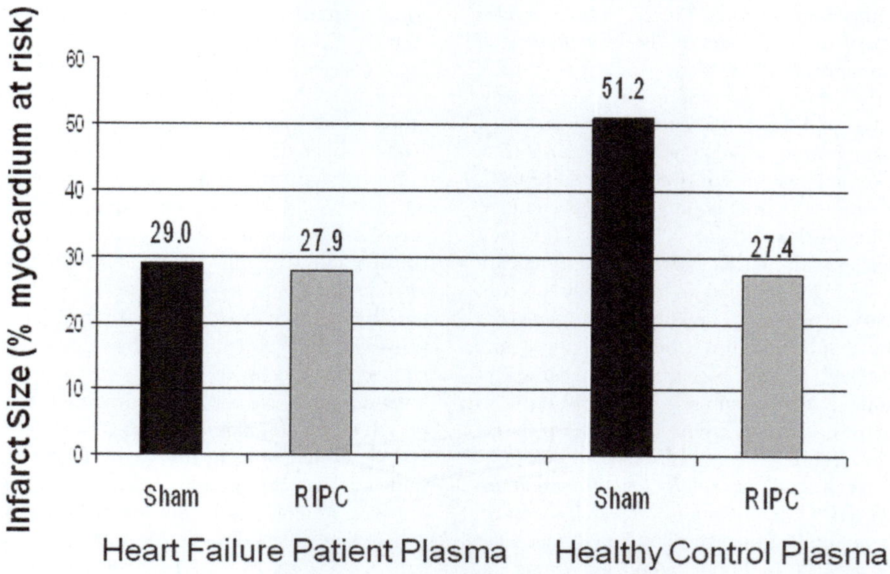

Figure 3. Langendorff mouse heart infarct size after perfusion with dialysate from heart failure patients versus healthy controls. Heart failure patient dialysate, irrespective of RIPC or sham treatment, reduced infarct to the same extent as the dialysate from RIPC-treated healthy controls, as compared to sham treated healthy controls.

significant difference in the level of cardioprotection afforded by their plasma dialysate in the mouse Langendorff studies. Plasma from patients that showed improvement in exercise capacity had lower baseline protection against ischemia, suggesting that their degree of baseline preconditioning was lower, and hence their capacity to respond to RIPC was higher.

It is also important to note, that while we were able to demonstrate the presence of circulating cardioprotective factors in vitro, we cannot confirm that they are the same as those induced by RIPC, nor can we confirm that they have any effect in-vivo in our HF patients. In pre-clinical studies, older age and underlying cardiac dysfunction have been shown to result in abnormal mitochondrial permeability transition pore and kATP channel

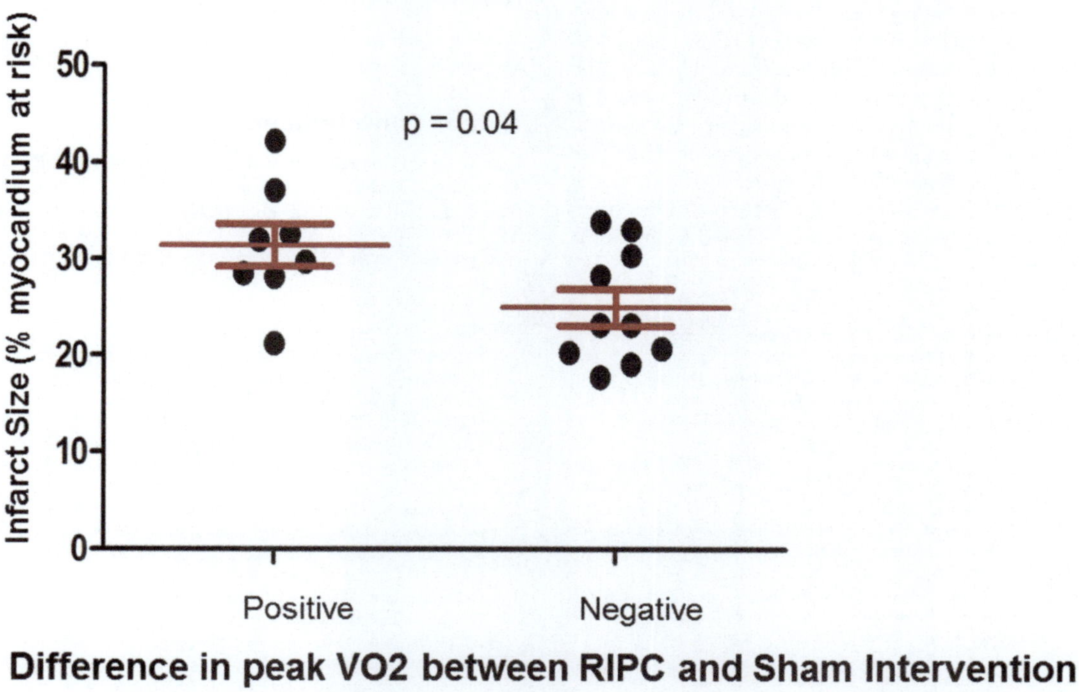

Figure 4. Infarct size stratified by the effect of RIPC on exercise performance. In the Langendorff model, mean infarct size was significantly smaller after perfusion with dialysate from the subgroup of patients who had no improvement in exercise performance following RIPC treatment. Data are presented as mean +/− SD % of infarcted myocardium.

function that may blunt the effects of RIPC [26,27]. There are also well documented ultrastructural changes in peripheral skeletal muscle associated with impairments in oxidative capacity [7–9,28], and the implications for ischemic preconditioning remain unclear. Failing myocardium also undergoes ultrastructural adaptation characterized by fetal gene reprogramming, with a decreased rate of aerobic metabolism and relative resistance to ischemia [29,30]. Coupled with the observation that mitochondrial kATP channels are endogenously activated in heart failure [27], all of this data suggest that in the clinical domain, RIPC may not yield significant additional protection from ischemic stress in a relatively 'preconditioned' HF state. While our pilot data show that there appears to be a subgroup of patients that benefit most from RIPC (those with low baseline preconditioning), in the absence of a clinical test of 'pre-existing preconditioning' the widespread adoption of RIPC as a clinical tool will require demonstration of effect in large, unselected, cohort studies. In this regard, it is likely that our study was underpowered to detect a small, but still meaningful difference in peak VO2 between RIPC intervention and sham control exercise tests. Based on the results from our pilot data, future trials would need an approximately 4–5 fold our sample size to have at least 80% power to detect a clinically important difference of 1–2 mL/kg/min in peak VO2. Smaller degrees of improvement would not likely translate into better transplant free survival [12].

Our study has a number of important limitations that may warrant caution in the interpretation of our results. Our post-hoc subgroup analysis of 'responders' versus 'non-responders' to RIPC, is not only somewhat artificial in terms of examining responses in a binary fashion, but also does not allow meaningful analysis of factors associated with those response, beyond the reported differences in cardioprotective activity of their plasma. A number of comorbidities and medications have been associated with either blunted or enhanced responses to ischemia-reperfusion injury and preconditioning [31,32]. As we did not exclude patients with comorbidities such as hypertension, dyslipidemia or left ventricular hypertrophy, and we did not perform a medication washout prior to testing, it is possible that our results may have been confounded. The impact of residual medications such as ACE inhibitors and statins in the Langendorff perfusate is indeterminate, and it is conceivable that these therapies may have modified the preconditioning response in the mouse heart. Although our model has previously been used to demonstrate the presence of a humoral mediator of RIPC [23], it is also possible that some of the larger sized key mediators of preconditioning were filtered from plasma while preparing the dialysate. For example, Giricz and colleagues recently demonstrated that extracellular vesicles (exosomes and microvesicles) may be necessary to confer protection in a rat heart Langendorff model of ischemic preconditioning [33]. Furthermore, we did not measure lactic acid levels to confirm a state of relative hypoxia with anaerobic metabolism at peak exercise. However, our cardiopulmonary exercise protocol with respiratory gas analysis did allow for an estimation of anaerobic threshold as a surrogate for lactic acidosis. Finally, patients in our trial had considerable variability in their inter-test intervals. Although we attempted to repeat paired exercise tests within 4 weeks from enrollment, we were unable to achieve this for all patients, providing the opportunity for bias due to changes in treatment or clinical status between tests.

In summary, we conducted the first randomized controlled trial of RIPC in ambulatory patients with HF and left ventricular systolic dysfunction. In this study, RIPC was not associated with improvements in objective measures of exercise capacity. The apparent absence of an effect of RIPC may relate to a high degree of baseline preconditioning in our patient population, and those with lesser degrees may be benefit with RIPC. However large, adequately powered clinical trials and further mechanistic translational studies are needed before the effects of RIPC in HF can be established definitively.

Supporting Information

Checklist S1 CONSORT Checklist relevant to the main study protocol.

Protocol S1 Study rationale and summary of the study and sub-study protocols.

Acknowledgments

We wish to thank Michael Walker for his expertise in exercise physiology and cardiopulmonary stress testing

Author Contributions

Conceived and designed the experiments: MM HR AR. Performed the experiments: MM JB JL. Analyzed the data: MM JB JL CM. Contributed reagents/materials/analysis tools: JL HR AR. Wrote the paper: MM CM AR.

References

1. McElroy PA, Janicki JS, Weber KT (1988) Cardiopulmonary exercise testing in congestive heart failure. Am J Cardiol 62: 35A–40A.
2. Mancini DM, Eisen H, Kussmaul W, Mull R, Edmunds LH Jr, et al (1991) Value of peak exercise oxygen consumption for optimal timing of cardiac transplantation in ambulatory patients with heart failure. Circulation 83: 778–86.
3. Pardaens K, Van Cleemput J, Vanhaecke J, Fagard RH (2000) Peak oxygen uptake better predicts outcome than submaximal respiratory data in heart transplant candidates. Circulation 101: 1152–57.
4. O'Neill JO, Young JB, Pothier CE, Lauer MS (2005) Peak oxygen consumption as a predictor of death in patients with heart failure receiving beta-blockers. Circulation 111: 2313–18.
5. Aaronson KD, Schwartz JS, Chen TM, Wong KL, Goin JE, et al (1997) Development and prospective validation of a clinical index to predict survival in ambulatory patients referred for cardiac transplant evaluation. Circulation 95: 2660–67.
6. Wilson JR, Martin JL, Ferraro N (1984) Impaired skeletal muscle nutritive flow during exercise in patients with congestive heart failure: role of cardiac pump dysfunction as determined by the effect of dobutamine. Am J Cardiol 53: 1308–15.
7. Mancini DM, Coyle E, Coggan A, Beltz J, Ferraro N, et al (1989) Contribution of intrinsic skeletal muscle changes to 31P NMR skeletal muscle metabolic abnormalities in patients with chronic heart failure. Circulation 80: 1338–46.
8. Duscha BD, Kraus WE, Keteyian SJ, Sullivan MJ, Green HJ, et al (1999) Capillary density of skeletal muscle: a contributing mechanism for exercise intolerance in class II–III chronic heart failure independent of other peripheral alterations. J Am Coll Cardiol 33: 1956–63.
9. Hambrecht R, Fiehn E, Yu J, Niebauer J, Weigl C, et al (1997) Effects of endurance training on mitochondrial ultrastructure and fibre type distribution in skeletal muscle of patients with stable chronic heart failure. J Am Coll Cardio 29: 1067–73.
10. Haykowsky MJ, Liang Y, Pechter D, Jones LW, McAlister FA, et al (2007) A meta-analysis of the effect of exercise training on left ventricular remodeling in heart failure patients. The benefit depends on the type of training performed. J Am Coll Cardiol 49: 2329–36.
11. O'Connor CM, Whellan DJ, Lee KL, Keteyian SJ, Cooper LS, et al (2009) Efficacy and safety of exercise training in patients with chronic heart failure: HF-ACTION randomized controlled trial. JAMA 301: 1439–50.
12. Stevenson LW, Steimle AE, Fonarow G, Kermani M, Kermani D, et al (1995) Improvement in exercise capacity of candidates awaiting heart transplantation. J Am Coll Cardiol 25: 163–70.
13. Kharbanda RK, Nielsen TT, Redington AN (2009) Translation of remote ischaemic preconditioning into clinical practice. Lancet 374: 1557–65.
14. Shimizu M, Tropak M, Diaz RJ, Suto F, Surendra H, et al (2009) Transient limb ischaemia remotely preconditions through a humoral mechanism acting

directly on the myocardium ; evidence suggesting cross-species protection. Clin Sci (Lond) 117: 191–200.
15. Steensrud T, Li J, Dai X, Manlhiot C, Kharbanda RK, et al (2010) Pretreatment with the nitric oxide donor SNAP or nerve transection blocks humoral preconditioning by remote limb ischemia or intra-arterial adenosine. Am J Physiol 299: H1598–603.
16. Redington KL, Disenhouse T, Strantzas SC Gladstone R, Wei C, et al (2012) Remote cardioprotection by direct peripheral nerve stimulation and topical capsaicin is mediated by circulating humoral factors. Basic Res Cardiol 107: 1–10.
17. Cheung MM, Kharbanda RK, Konstantinov IE, Shimitzu IE, Shimizu M, et al (2006) Randomized controlled trial of the effects of remote ischemic preconditioning on children undergoing cardiac surgery: first clinical application in humans. J Am Coll Cardiol 47: 2277–82.
18. Venugopal V, Hausenloy DJ, Ludman A, Di Salvo C, Kolvekar S, et al (2009) Remote ischaemic preconditioning reduces myocardial injury in patients undergoing cardiac surgery with cold-blood cardioplegia: a randomised controlled trial. Heart 95: 1567–71.
19. Ali ZA, Callaghan CJ, Lim E, Ali AA, Nouraei SA, et al (2007) Remote ischemic preconditioning reduces myocardial and renal injury after elective abdominal aortic aneurysm repair: a randomized controlled trial. Circulation 116(11 Suppl): I98–105.
20. Hoole SP, Heck PM, Sharples L, Khan SN, Duehmke R, et al (2009) Cardiac remote ischemic preconditioning in coronary stenting (CRISP Stent) study: a prospective randomized control trial. Circulation 119: 820–7.
21. Botker HE, Kharbanda R Schmidt MR, Bottcher M, Kaltoft AK, et al (2010) Remote ischaemic conditioning before hospital admission, as a complement to angioplasty, and effect on myocardial salvage in pateints with acute myocardial infarction: a randomized trial. Lancet 375: 727–34.
22. de Groot PC, Thijssen DH, Sanchez M, Ellenkamp R, Hopman MT (2010) Ischemic preconditioning improves maximal performance in humans. Eur J Appl Physio 108: 141–6.
23. Jean-St-Michel E, Manlhiot C, Li J, Tropak M, Michelsen MM, et al (2011) Remote preconditioning improves maximal performance in highly-trained athletes. Med Sci Sports Exerc 43: 1280–6.
24. Michelsen MM, Stottrup NB, Schmidt MR, Lofgren B, Jensen RV, et al (2012) Exercise induced cardioprotection is medicated by a bloodborne, transferable factor. Basic Res Cardiol 107: 1–9.
25. Dickson EW, Lorbar M, Porcaro WA, Lee WJ, Blehar DJ, et al (1999) Rabbit heart can be "preconditioned" via transfer of coronary effluent. Am J Physiol 277:H2451–7.
26. Zhu J, Rebecchi MJ, Tan M, Glass PS, Brink PR, et al (2010) Age-associated differences in activation of Akt/GSK-3beta signaling pathways and inhibition of mitochondrial permeability transition pore opening in the rat heart. J Gerontol A Biol Sci Med Sci 65: 611–9.
27. Maack C, Dabew ER, Hohl M, Schafers HJ, Hohm M (2009) Endogenous activation of mitochondrial katp channels protects human failing myocardium from hydroxyl radical-induced stunning. Circ Res 105: 811–7.
28. Hambrecht R, Niebauer J, Fiehn E, Kalberer B, Offner B, et al (1995) Physical training in patients with stable chronic heart failure: effects on cardiorespiratory fitness and ultrastructural abnormalities of leg muscles. J Am Coll Cardiol 25: 1239–49.
29. Rajabi M, Kassiotis C, Razeghi P, Taegtmeyer H (2007) Return to the fetal gene program protects the stressed heart: a strong hypothesis. Heart Fail Rev 12: 331–43.
30. Ostadal B, Ostadalova I, Kolar F, Charvatova Z, Netuka I (2009) Ontogenetic development of cardiac tolerance to oxygen deprivation – possible mechanisms. Physiol Res 58 Suppl 2: S1–12.
31. Hausenloy DJ, Botker HE, Condorelli G, Ferdinandy P, Garcia-Dorado D, et al (2013) Translating cardioprotection for patient benefit: position paper from the Working Group of Cellular Biology of the Heart of the European Society of Cardiology. Cardiovasc Res 98: 7–27.
32. Ferdinandy P, Schultz R, Baxter GF (2007) Interaction of cardiovascular risk factors with myocardial ischemia/reperfusion injury, preconditioning, and postconditioning. Pharmcol Rev 59: 418–58.
33. Giricz A, Varga ZV, Baranyai T, Sipos P, Paloczi K, et al (2014) Cardioprotection by remote ischemic preconditioning of the rat heart is mediated by extracellular vesicles. J Mol Cell Cardiol 68: 75–78.

11

Response of Various Conduit Arteries in Tachycardia- and Volume Overload-Induced Heart Failure

Xiao Lu[1], Zhen-Du Zhang[1], Xiaomei Guo[1], Jenny Susana Choy[1], Junrong Yang[1], Mark Svendsen[1], Ghassan Kassab[1,2,3]*

1 Department of Biomedical Engineering, Indiana University Purdue University Indianapolis, Indianapolis, Indiana, United States of America, **2** Department of Surgery, Indiana University Purdue University Indianapolis, Indianapolis, Indiana, United States of America, **3** Cellular and Integrative Physiology, Indiana University Purdue University Indianapolis, Indianapolis, Indiana, United States of America

Abstract

Although hemodynamics changes occur in heart failure (HF) and generally influence vascular function, it is not clear whether various HF models will affect the conduit vessels differentially or whether local hemodynamic forces or systemic factors are more important determinants of vascular response in HF. Here, we studied the hemodynamic changes in tachycardia or volume-overload HF swine model (created by either high rate pacing or distal abdominal aortic-vena cava fistula, respectively) on carotid, femoral, and renal arteries function and molecular expression. The ejection fraction was reduced by 50% or 30% in tachycardia or volume-overload model in four weeks, respectively. The LV end diastolic volume was increased from 65±22 to 115±78 ml in tachycardia and 67±19 to 148±68 ml in volume-overload model. Flow reversal was observed in diastolic phase in carotid artery of both models and femoral artery in volume-overload model. The endothelial function was also significantly impaired in carotid and renal arteries of tachycardia and volume-overload animals. The endothelial dysfunction was observed in femoral artery of volume-overload animals but not tachycardia animals. The adrenergic receptor-dependent contractility decreased in carotid and femoral arteries of tachycardia animals. The protein expressions of NADPH oxidase subunits increased in the three arteries and both animal models while expression of MnSOD decreased in carotid artery of tachycardia and volume-overload model. In conclusion, different HF models lead to variable arterial hemodynamic changes but similar vascular and molecular expression changes that reflect the role of both local hemodynamics as well as systemic changes in HF.

Editor: Xun Ai, Loyola University Chicago, United States of America

Funding: This research was supported by the National Institute of Health-National Heart, Lung, and Blood Institute Grant R01 HL084529-01. The funders had no role in study design, data collection and analysis, decision to publish, or preparation of the manuscript.

Competing Interests: The authors have declared that no competing interests exist.

* Email: gkassab@iupui.edu

Introduction

Heart failure (HF) is one of the leading causes of cardiovascular morbidity and mortality in Western countries. HF is accompanied by alteration of hemodynamic conditions, which is due to the triggers of complex reflex changes in the sympathetic, endocrine, and rennin systems [1–3]. HF is also associated with subcellular abnormalities that are associated with cardiac hypertrophy and vascular dysfunctions.

A critical effect of HF is reduced blood flow in the cardiovascular system resulting from mild to severe reduction in cardiac output (CO). The reduction of CO in HF is usually accompanied by low ejection fraction (EF) and consequently reduced wall shear stress (WSS). In these patients, the heart usually beats faster to compensate for compromised EF. This often leads to transient retrograde flow and negative WSS in arteries during each cardiac cycle. The alteration of WSS may cause endothelial cell dysfunctions [4] which likely contributes to vascular pathophysiology of HF including increased total peripheral resistance which in turn affects the heart through increase in afterload. Endothelial dysfunction can be due to increased reactive oxygen species (ROS) generation and reduced nitric oxide (NO) bioavailability. The specific mechanisms responsible for the interplay between hemodynamic (low and reverse flows) and vascular dysfunction in HF remain relatively unknown. Although increased oxidative stress with reduced nitric oxide (NO) bioavailability has been proposed as a potential mechanism in HF [5], it is unclear which factors are primary in the initiation and progression of vascular dysfunction in HF. It is also not clear whether the etiology of HF affects the conduit arteries differentially.

The objective of present study is to understand whether the specific etiology of HF affects the conduit vessels with varying distance from the heart differentially despite a similar end stage of heart function. An additional objective was to determine whether local or systemic factors are more important determinants of vascular function in animal models of tachycardia and volume overload-induced HF. Accordingly, we studied cardiac function of tachycardia and volume-overload animals and associated hemodynamic parameters in carotid, femoral, and renal arteries. The vascular function and proteins expression of eNOS and NADPH oxidase of various arteries were determined to assess the various biomarkers of blood vessels in the two different HF models.

Materials and Methods

Domestic swine (55 to 65 kg) were provided by Michigan State University and housed at Indiana University School of Medicine Facilities (Laboratory Animal Resource Center). The pigs had ad libitum access to water and food. A room temperature of 20–22°C and humidity of 30% to 70% were maintained. The animals were carefully checked for preexisting diseases and acclimated for at least 3 days before undergoing the surgical procedure. All animal experiments were performed in accordance with national and local ethical guidelines, including the Principles of Laboratory Animal Care, the Guide for the Care and Use of Laboratory Animals and the National Society for Medical Research, and an approved Indiana University School of Medicine IACUC protocol (Permit Number:3051) regarding the use of animals in research.

Tachycardia Model

Six animals were used in a pacing-induced tachycardia model. The pigs were fasted overnight and surgical anesthesia was induced with TKX (Telazol 10 mg/kg, Ketamine 5 mg/kg, Xylazine 5 mg/kg) and maintained with isoflurane 1–2%. Ventilation was provided with a respirator to maintain physiological P_{CO2} and P_{O2} at approximately 35 and 100 mmHg, respectively. Electrocardiographic (ECG) leads were attached to the animal limbs and cardiac electrical signals were monitored on a Physio-Control Lifepak 9P defibrillator. Body temperature was maintained at 37°C to 38°C and pH at 7.4±0.1. The anesthesia was monitored and recorded once per every 10 minutes during the procedure. The adequacy of anesthesia was confirmed by stability of respiration and heart rate, absence of palpebral reflex and jaw tone, and no limb withdrawal reflex.

A thoracotomy was performed along the fourth intercostal space and the chest cavity was opened to fully expose the heart. Two platinum pacemaker electrodes (Medtronic, Minneapolis, MN) were placed on the surface in the lateral LV free wall at 0.5 cm apart and secured by suture. The pace maker was placed in a percutaneous pocket near the neck for easy access. The function of the pace maker was tested and the pacing threshold was determined. Pacing was started one or two weeks after the animals were completely recovered from surgery. The initial pacing rate was set at 210 beats/min for one week followed by 190 beats/min for underwent additional three weeks as described earlier [6]. Five animals served as sham which received open-chest surgery without implantation of a pace-maker.

Volume-overload Model

Seven animals were anesthetized similar to those described above. An incision was made in the mid abdomen and the aorta and vena cava were exposed near the common iliac artery. The adventitia of the aorta and vena cave was removed over an area twice as long and twice as wide as the arteriotomy. Both aorta and adjacent vena cava were partially occluded with tissue clamps. An incision (1 cm long) was made on vena cava wall on the occluded side to open the cava cavity. From the inside of the vena cava cavity, another small incision was made on vena cava wall and through the adjacent, occluded aorta wall. A 2.5 mm aortic punch (Medtronic, Minneapolis, MN) was then used to create the aortic-vena cava (A-V) fistula at diameter of 6 mm. The free edges of the fistula of cava and aorta was sutured together (7/0 suture), to maintain the incision open (A-V fistula). The first incision made on vena cava was closed with 7/0 suture. The animal was then heparinized (100 U/kg) and the clamp released. The patency of the fistula was ensured after 20 minutes of observations and the abdomen was subsequently closed layer by layer. The animals were given Plavix (75 mg/day) and Asprin (81 mg/day) with food daily to prevent clotting and maintain an open fistula. Five animals served as sham that underwent the open-abdominal surgery and the dissection of abdominal aorta and vena cava without the A-V fistula.

Echocardiography and blood flow measurement

Echocardiography (Philips Ultrasound, Bothell, WA) was performed weekly to evaluate the heart function. Animals were maintained under light anesthesia with 1–2% Isoflurane and 100% oxygen by mask. The animals were then placed on sling for echocardiography. For tachycardia HF animals, the pace maker was turned off for 30 min to attain stable conditions during imaging. After the echocardiographic measurements, the pace maker was turned back on.

In the terminal study, the animals were placed under general anesthesia after the echocardiography procedure described above. The pace maker was turned off and blood sample was collected. One of each carotid, femoral, and renal arteries was carefully exposed. A perivascular ultrasonic flow probe (Transonic Systems Inc. Ithaca, NY) was placed around the middle portion of each vessel segment. The incisions were approximated and the vessels were allowed to recover for at least 30 min. The blood flow of these vessels was then recorded for an additional 30 min. After flow measurements, the vessels were excised for analysis of proteins expression and vascular function.

In vitro isovolumic myography

The functions of endothelial and smooth muscle cells in vessels from control or paced animals were tested using an isovolumic myograph [7]. In these experiments, the vessel contraction was maintained under isovolumic conditions during the test, and the changes of lumen pressure represented the degree of contraction or dilation of the vessels. The details of method for the isovolumic myograph and testing protocol have been described previously [7]. Briefly, the vessel segments were quickly removed from animals before termination and placed in 4°C saline. The surrounding connective tissues were carefully removed under a microscope and all branches of the vessel were ligated. The vessel was then transferred into the myograph bath chamber filled with physiological salt solution (PSS: in mmol/L: 142 NaCl, 4.7 KCl, 2.7 Sodium HEPES, 3 HEPES acid, 1.17 $MgSO_4$, 2.79 $CaCl_2$, 5.5 Glucose) and cannulated at two ends to tubes containing PSS. The vessel was stretched to its in vivo length and equilibrated for 40 min with intravascular pressure set at 10 mmHg while the chamber temperature was gradually increased to 37°C. The intravascular pressure was increased to 80% of physiological pressure during the testing. Phenylephrine (PE) and acetylcholine (ACh) dose-response contraction and dilation experiments were performed on each vessel, respectively. The overall contractility of the vessel segment was tested with 60 mM KCl introduced into the chamber. The endothelium-independent vasorelaxation in response to sodium nitroprusside was performed to verify whether vascular smooth muscle (VSM) developed resistance to nitric oxide.

Western blotting analysis

Stored artery segments were homogenized in lysis buffer containing 50 mM glycerophosphate, 100 μM sodium orthovanadate, 2 mM magnesium chloride, 1 mM EGTA, 0.5% Triton X-100, 1 mM DL-dithiothreitol, 20 μM pepstatin, 20 μM leupeptin, 0.1 U/ml aprotinin, and 1 mM phenylmethylsulfonyl fluoride and then incubated on ice for 1 hr. The sample was centrifuged at 1,000 *g* for 15 min at 1°C, and the supernatant was

Table 1. Ratio of heart weight to body weight and plasma angiotensin II in sham, tachycardia (Tachy) and volume-overload (VOL) HF animals.

	Sham	Tachy	VOL	P value
Heart/body (g/kg)	2.7±0.02	4.2±0.62	4.1±0.5	<0.05
RV/LV (g/g)	0.32±0.03	0.5±0.06	0.5±0.16	<0.05
LV/BW (g/kg)	2.0±0.03	2.8±0.35	2.7±0.17	<0.05
RV/BW (g/kg)	0.65±0.05	1.4±0.3	1.4±0.43	<0.05
Ang II (ng/ml)	0.09±0.08	0.343±0.219	0.263±0.176	<0.05

P value is the comparison of tachycardia and volume-overload groups with sham. RV: right ventricle. LV: left ventricle. BW: body weight Ang II: angiotensin II.

collected. The total protein was measured by a BCA kit (Bio-Rad). To examine each protein expression, equal amounts of protein (50 µg) from each sample were loaded on each lane and electrophoresed in 4–20% Tris-Glycine gel (Invitrogen) and then transferred onto a polyvinylidene difluoride membrane (Millipore). After being incubated for 2 hrs in 6% dried milk in TBS-Tween buffer, the membrane was incubated overnight at 4°C with specific primary antibody in blocking buffer (anti-p47^{phox} and anti-gp91^{phox}, Santa Cruz Biotech at 1:200 dilution, MnSOD 1:1000 dilution, Enzo; eNOS 1:300 dilution, BD). The membrane was then rinsed and incubated with horseradish peroxidase-conjugated secondary antibody (Santa Cruz Biotechnology) for 2 hrs at 1:5,000 dilutions in blocking buffer. All samples from each group were also probed with anti-GAPDH antibody (1:5000, Abcam) to correct for sample loading.

ELISA analysis

Blood samples were centrifuged and plasma was collected and stored in -80°C until ELISA analysis. The 96-well plates precoated with angiotensin II specific antibody were used to measure Angiotensin II in plasma (Abcam's Angiotensin II Human *in vitro* ELISA kit). Standards or test samples were added to the wells of the plates and subsequently an angiotensin II specific biotinylated detection antibody was added and then followed by washing with wash buffer. Streptavidin-Peroxidase Complex was added and unbound conjugates were washed away with buffer. TMB was then used to visualize Streptavidin-Peroxidase enzymatic reaction.

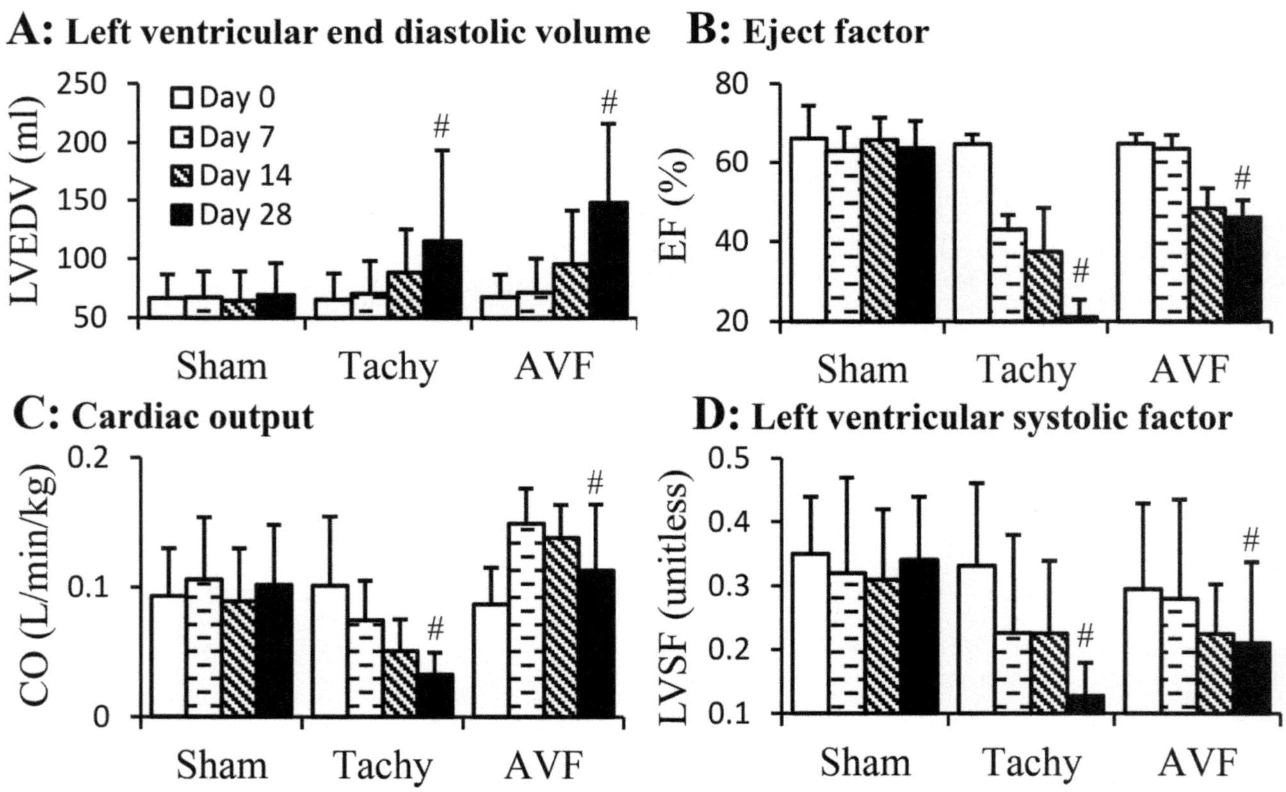

Figure 1. Cardiac parameters of tachycardia and volume-overload models over the four weeks duration. A: left ventricular end diastolic volume (LVEDV); B: ejection fraction (EF); C: cardiac output (CO); D: left ventricular systolic factor (LVSF). Sham, sham group; Tachy, tachycardia group; VOL, volume-overload group. #: $p<0.05$, One-way ANOVA analysis with post-hoc (Bonferroni) tests to verify the variation of cardiac parameters in time course.

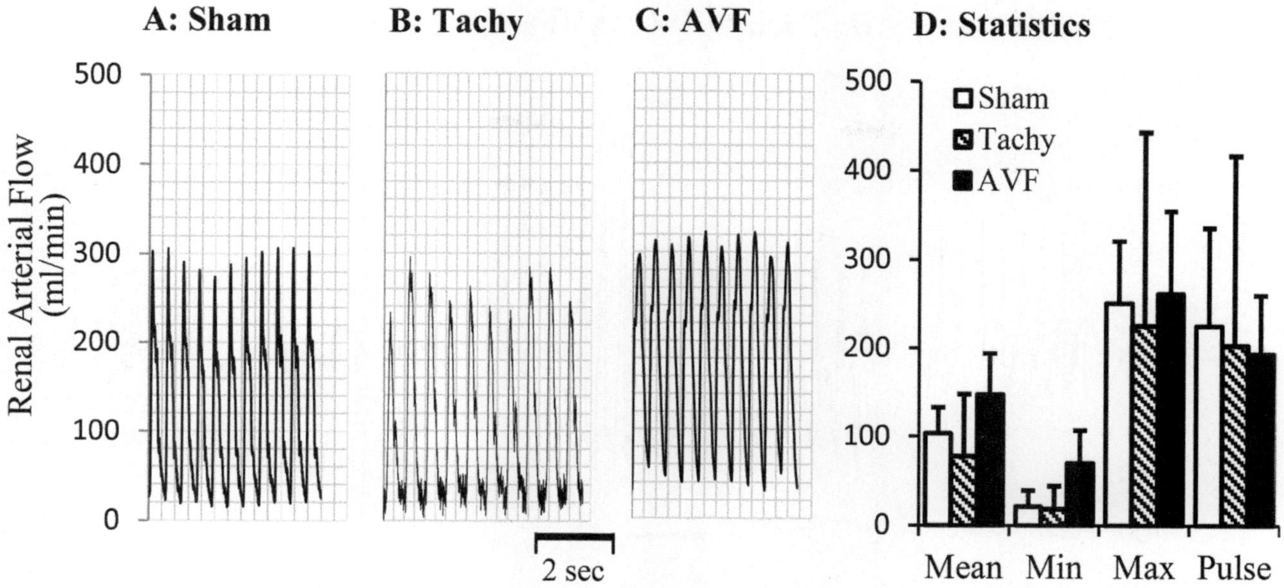

Figure 2. Blood flow in renal arteries at day 28. A representative tracing of blood flow inform A: sham animal; B: tachycardia animal; C: volume-overload animal. D: Statistical data (mean±SD) of blood flow at day 28. Pulse flow is defined maximal flow to minus minimal flow. Sham, sham group; Tachy, tachycardia group; VOL, volume-overload group. *: $p<0.05$, Student's t-test in comparison with sham.

TMB was catalyzed by Streptavidin-Peroxidase to produce a blue color product that changed into yellow after adding acidic stop solution. The density of yellow coloration was directly proportional to the amount of angiotensin II captured in plate.

Data Analysis

All data were expressed as mean±standard deviation (SD). Students' t-test was used to detect differences between pairwise groups. Variance analysis (One-way ANOVA) with post-hoc (Bonferroni) tests was used in time course and Two-way ANOVA with post-hoc (Tukey's) test was used in dose-dependent comparisons. $P<0.05$ was considered statistically significant.

Results

In the tachycardia and volume-overload induced HF, the ratios of heart weight to body weight were increased significantly in the 4 week duration in comparison with sham animals (Table 1). This increase occurred in both left and right ventricles but predominately in right ventricle (Table 1). In tachycardia induced HF model, all animals tolerated the rapid pacing and 50% of the animals had abdominal ascites (500–3000 ml) by the end of 4

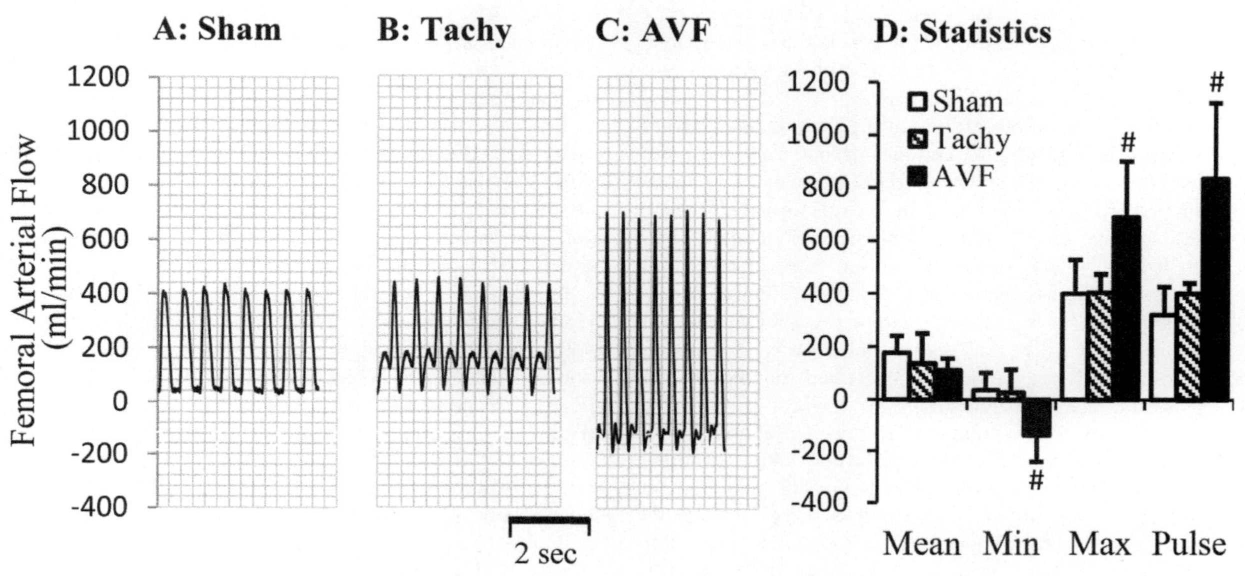

Figure 3. Blood flow in femoral artery at day 28. A representative tracing of blood flow inform A: sham animal; B: tachycardia animal; C: volume-overload animal. D: Statistical data (mean±SD) of blood flow at day 28. Pulse flow is defined maximal flow to minus minimal flow. Sham, sham group; Tachy, tachycardia group; VOL, volume-overload group. *: $p<0.05$, Student's t-test in comparison with sham.

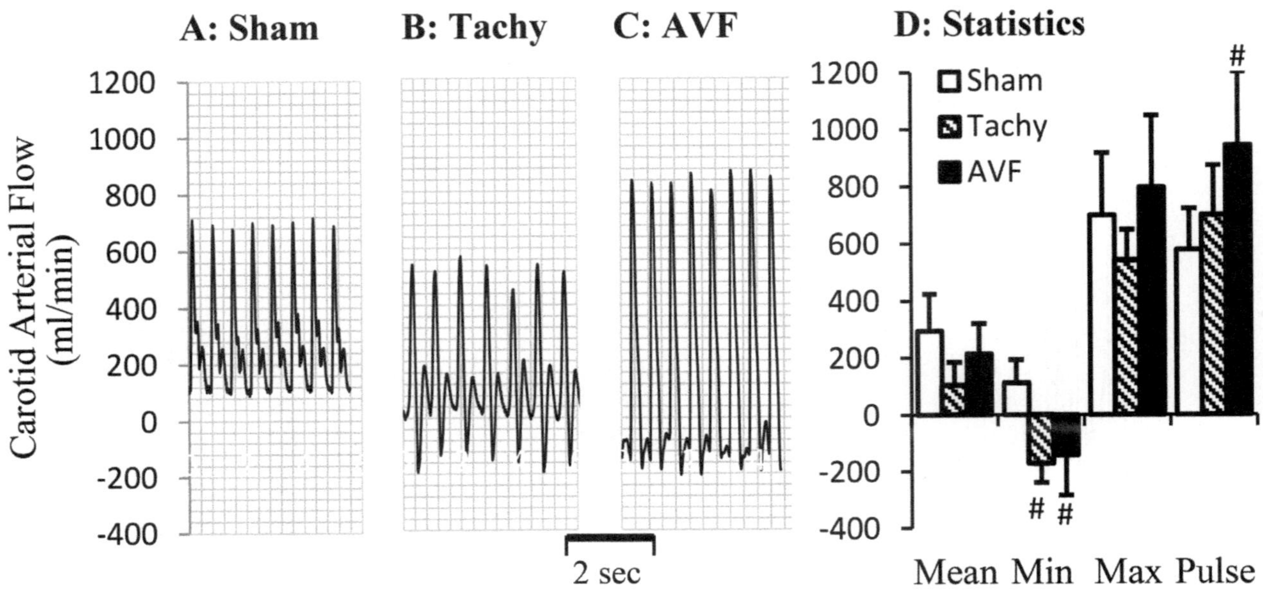

Figure 4. Blood flow measured in carotid artery at day 28. A representative tracing of blood flow from A: sham animal; B: tachycardia animal; C: volume-overload animal. D: Statistical data (mean±SD) of blood flow at day 28. Pulse flow is defined maximal flow to minus minimal flow. Sham, sham group; Tachy, tachycardia group; VOL, volume-overload group. *: $p<0.05$, Student's t-test in comparison with sham.

weeks. In volume-overload induced HF model, the animals developed edema, respiratory distress, and ascites (700–3,700 mml) in 4 weeks. We also found that the level of Angiotensin II in plasma increased in both tachycardia and volume-overload groups in comparison with sham (Table 1).

The parameters of cardiac function from echocardiography are represented in Figure 1. The left ventricular end diastolic volume (LVEDV) significantly increased ($p<0.05$) in both tachycardia and volume-overload HF (Figure 1A). The ejection fraction (EF) decreased significantly ($p<0.05$) in both tachycardia and volume-overload induced HF (Figure 1B). The cardiac output (CO) decreased monotonically in tachycardia animals but increased in the first postoperative week and decreased in following weeks of volume-overload animals (Figure 1C). The left ventricular systolic factor (LVSF) also decreased ($p<0.05$) in both tachycardia and volume overload induced HF (Figure 1D).

The blood flows in various arteries at the time of acute studies are represented in Figures 2–4. The mean blood flow and pulse flow (maximal minus minimal flow) in renal artery did not change statistically in both tachycardia (pace maker was turned off during blood flow measurements) and volume-overload animals (Figure 2). In femoral artery, there was no significant flow reversal during diastolic phase in sham and tachycardia animals (Figures 3A, B and D). In A-V fistula volume-overload animals, a significant flow reversal during diastolic phase was observed in femoral artery and the pulse flow increased significantly in tachycardia and volume-overload groups (Figures 3C and D). The significant flow reversal was observed during diastolic phase in carotid artery four weeks after tachycardia and volume-overload but not in sham animals (Figures 4A, B and C). The pulse flows in carotid artery in volume-overload animals were significantly increased in comparison with shams (Figure 4D). The mean flow in carotid artery decreased in tachycardia group in comparison with sham.

The phenylephrine-induced vascular contraction is represented in Figure 5. Phenylephrine activates adrenergic receptor to induce vascular smooth muscle contraction which was blunted in femoral and carotid arteries but not in renal artery of tachycardia animals (Figure 5A–C). The adrenergic receptor dependent contraction did not change in volume-overload (Figure 5A–C). KCl–induced receptor-independent contraction was attenuated in femoral and carotid arteries in volume-overload animals but not in renal artery (Figure 5D). Although the receptor-independent vasoconstriction did not change statistically in the carotid and femoral arteries in tachycardia animals, a decreased tendency was observed (Figure 5D). Based on the contractility analysis, the adrenergic activation of carotid and femoral arteries appears blunted in tachycardia but not in volume-overload animals.

The endothelium-dependent vasodilation in response to acetylcholine (ACh) is represented in Figure 6. The significant attenuation of endothelium-dependent vasodilation was observed in renal and carotid arteries in tachycardia and volume-overload animals (Figure 6A, C). The endothelium-dependent vasodilation of femoral artery was attenuated in volume-overload but not in tachycardia (Figures 6B). The endothelium-independent vasodilation in response to sodium nitroprusside was significantly attenuated in renal and carotid arteries in both tachycardia and volume-overload animals and did not change in femoral artery experimental groups (Figure 6D).

Expressions of several proteins were determined by Western blot in artery segments collected from sham, tachycardia, and volume-overload animals (Figure 7). The expression of eNOS was down-regulated in renal and carotid arteries of tachycardia model (Figure 7A and C) and all three arteries of volume-overload model (Figure 7). The expression of $p47^{phox}$ was up-regulated in all three arteries of tachycardia model (Figure 7) and femoral and carotid arteries of volume-overload model. The expression of $p22^{phox}$ was up-regulated in renal and femoral arteries of tachycardia model and renal and carotid arteries of volume-overload model (Figure 7). The expression of $gp91^{phox}$ was up-regulated in renal and carotid arteries of tachycardia model and femoral artery of volume-overload model (Figure 7). The MnSOD expression was down-regulated in renal and carotid arteries of tachycardia model and carotid artery of volume-overload model (Figure 7).

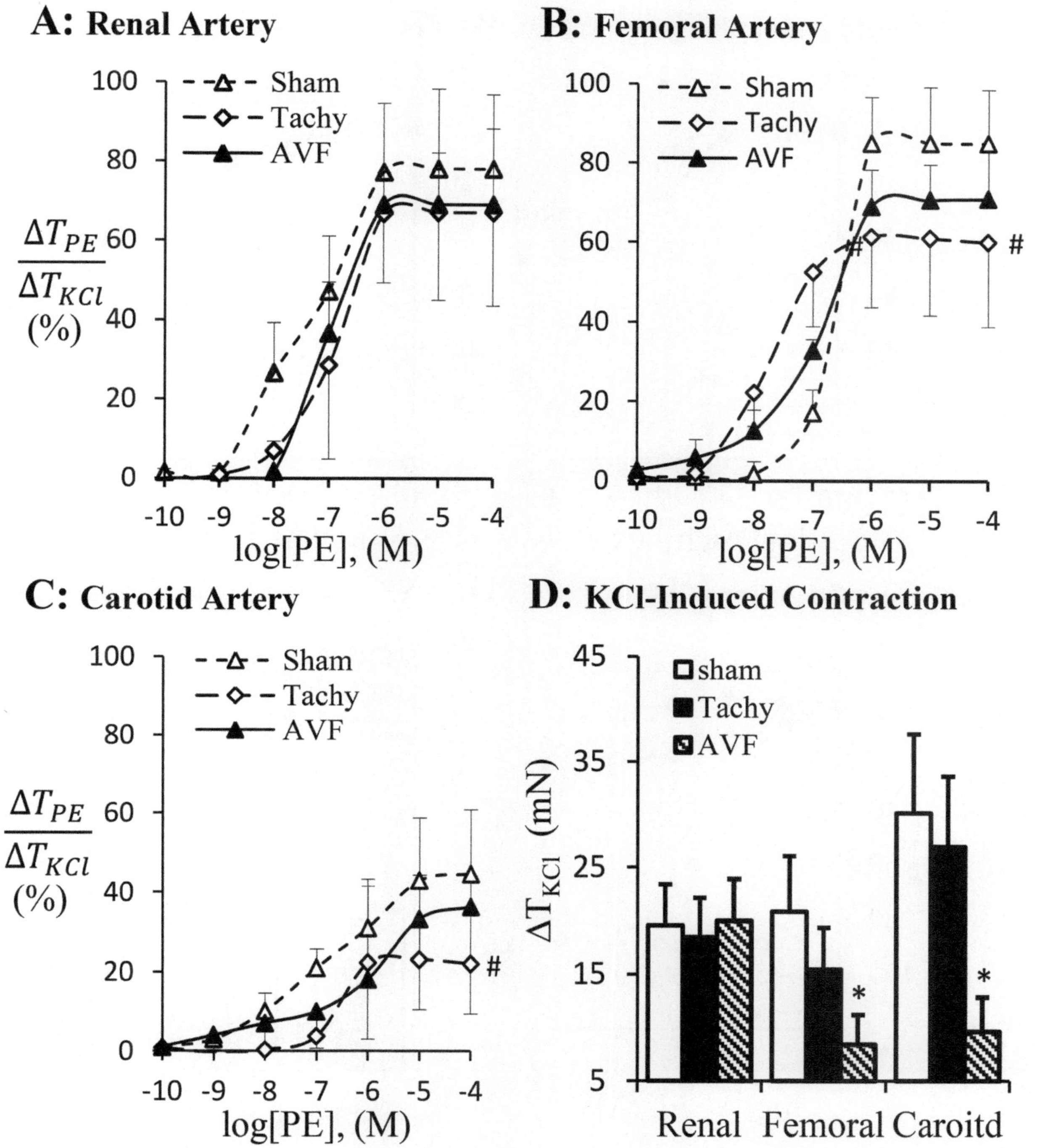

Figure 5. Adrenergic agonist PE-induced arterial contraction was normalized by KCl-induced contraction. A: renal artery contraction; B: femoral artery contraction; C: carotid artery contraction. D: potassium chloride (KCl) induced contraction. Sham, sham group; Tachy, tachycardia group; VOL, volume-overload group. #: $p<0.05$, Two-way ANOVA analysis with post-hoc (Tukey's) test to detect the difference of the dose-dependent groups. *: $p<0.05$ Students' t-test in comparison with sham.

The cardiac function and hemodynamic changes and their effects on vascular functions and molecular expression are summarized in Table 2. The cardiac function at four weeks was consistently compromised in tachycardia and volume-overload HF models. The hemodynamic changes were not consistent in the various vessels in the two animal models while the vascular function and molecular expression changes were fairly consistent with the femoral artery being least affected.

Discussion

In tachycardia and volume-overload HF models, carotid, femoral and renal arteries were exposed to either systemic (Ang. II, plasma oxidative stress, etc.) or systemic plus hemodynamic (flow reversal) factors. We observed that systemic factor alone compromised endothelial function of renal artery and systemic factor plus flow reversal compromised endothelial function of

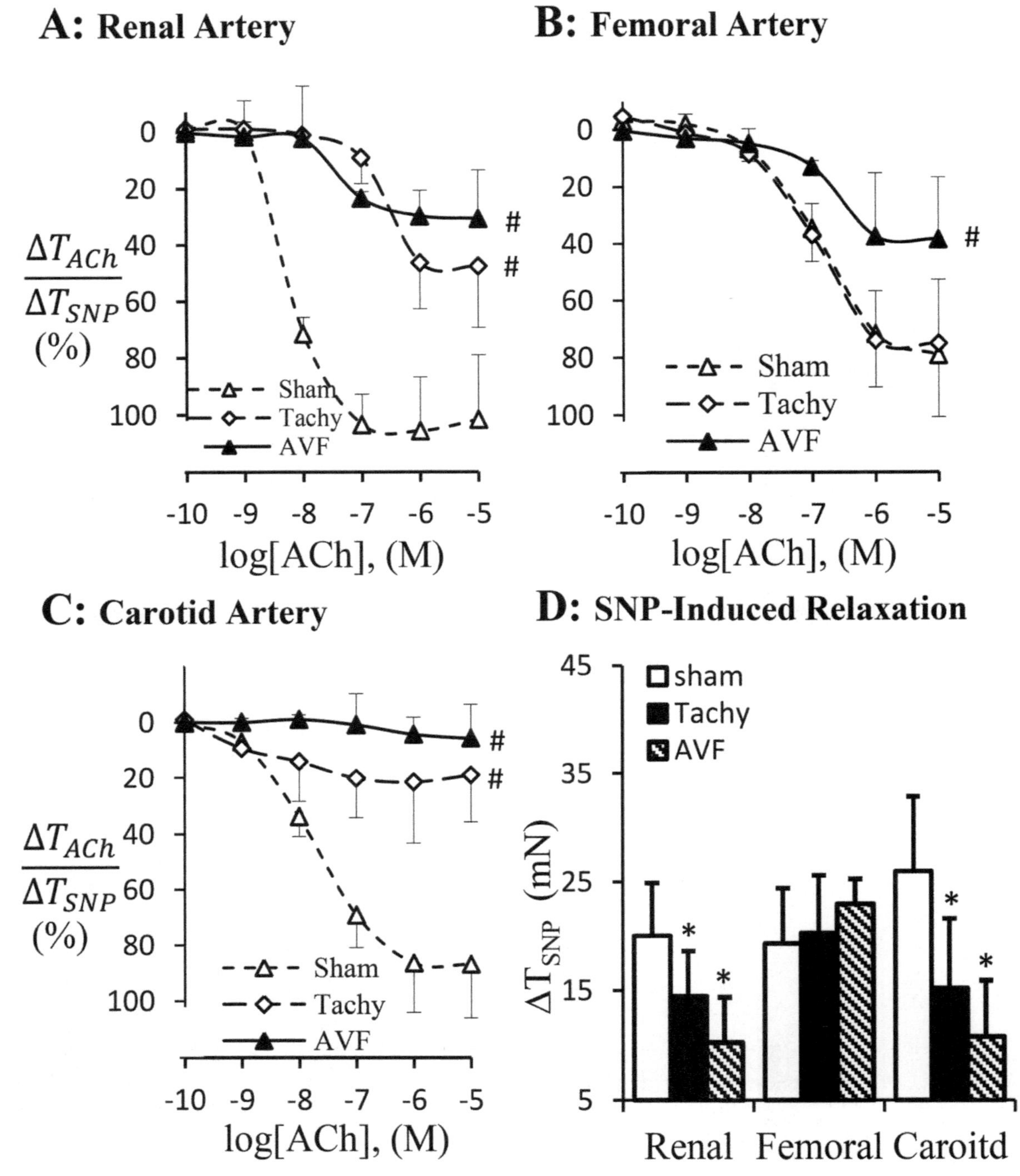

Figure 6. Endothelium-dependent vascular relaxation. Acetylcholine-induced vasodilation was normalized with sodium prusside (SNP, NO donor) induced vasodilation in renal (A), femoral artery (B) and carotid artery (C). D: SNP induced vasodilation. Sham, sham group; Tachy, tachycardia group; VOL, volume-overload group. #: $p<0.05$, Two-way ANOVA analysis with post-hoc (Tukey's) test to detect the difference of the dose-dependent groups. *: $p<0.05$ Students' t-test in comparison with sham.

carotid and femoral arteries. The oxidative stress was increased in all three arteries of tachycardia and volume-overload HF models while adrenergic dependent contraction was decreased in femoral and carotid arteries but remained unchanged in renal arteries of both HF models. The observation underscores different response of various blood vessels to systemic effects. These findings suggest that hemodynamics (flow reversal) is an important regulator of endothelial function and receptor-dependent vasoconstriction in addition to the systemic effects in tachycardia and volume-overload HF models.

Tachycardia or volume-overload HF model induced by either pace maker or A-V fistula have been well established in large and small animals [8,9]. In tachycardia model, the pacing rates vary and the time required to develop HF is different depending on the animal species. We followed a previously used rapid pacing to induce HF in swine with higher rates initially (230 bpm) followed by lower pacing rate at 190 bpm [6]. The tachycardia animals in

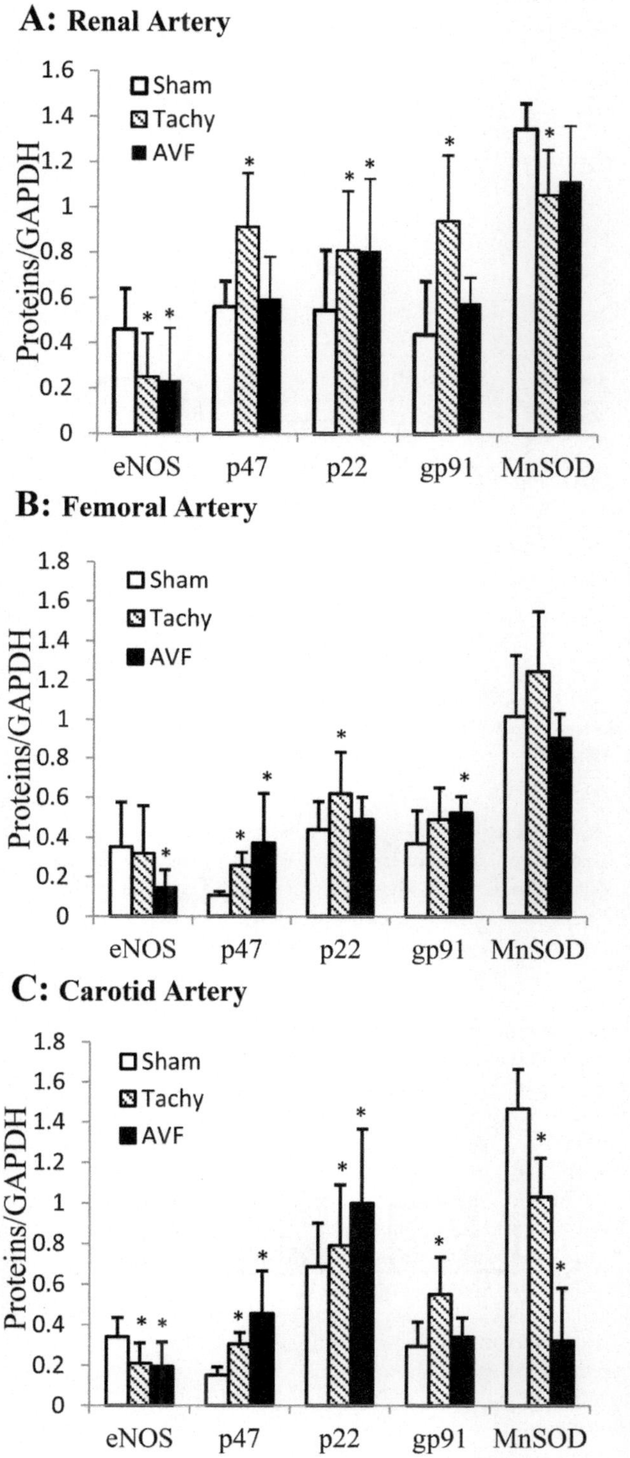

Figure 7. Expression of eNOS, $p47^{phox}$, $p22^{phox}$, $gp91^{phox}$, and MnSOD in various arteries measured by western blotting. A: renal artery; B: femoral artery; C: carotid artery. Equal amount of protein of each sample were used. The results were expressed as ratio of densities of target protein and GAPDH. Sham, sham group; Tachy, tachycardia group; VOL, volume-overload group. *: $p<0.05$ Students' t-test in comparison with sham.

our experiments showed typical changes such as reduced ventricular function [10–12]. As seen in Figure 1, the EF and LVEF were significantly reduced. The hypertrophy of the heart was also observed as shown in Figure 1. The increase of heart weight (Table 1) is predominantly in right ventricle as reported by other groups [12,13]. These findings confirmed that the animals in our present study developed typical changes in tachycardia HF model. For volume-overload model, the EF decreased from 65% to 45%. As shown in Figure 1, the LVEDV was also doubled suggesting a sever LV dilation as shown previously by other groups [12,14]. In our experiments, the volume-overload animals developed significant complications including edema, ascites and respiratory distress. Animals would not survive longer to observe further decrease of EF without medical interventions. Therefore, the EF of HF animal with volume-overload in our study was higher than those reported in humans that are under medical treatment. However, the LV dysfunction was similar to those reported previously [15].

In previous studies, the cardiac and vascular functions in HF have been intensively studied. The increased peripheral artery resistance has been attributed to neurohumoral pathways including the rennin-angiotensin and sympathetic nervous system [1,3]. Our present study suggests that regional blood flow change may also contribute to regulation of vascular function. We have shown previously that acute tachycardia by pacing induced transient hemodynamic changes in medium sized peripheral arteries, including decreased systemic pressure and near-wall retrograde flow or full flow reversal [16]. In tachycardia animals, the flow reversal was found in the carotid artery during diastolic phase but not in the femoral artery. In volume-overload animals, the reversed flow was observed in both femoral and carotid arteries (Figure 3–4). Reverse flow was not observed in renal artery of either HF model. The reason that blood flow reversal is observed in some vessels but not others is because flow pulsatility and transient reversal dependent not only on cardiac hemodynamics (inlet into the vessel) but also the impedance of microcirculation. Although cardiac functions and hemodynamics were affected similarly in the various vessels, the regulation of impedance in various microcirculations is likely very different; e.g., renal microcirculation tone is regulated by various hormones (Ang. II, norepinephrine, etc.) and hence prevents flow reversal. The response of renal artery to various agonists is also different from other peripheral arteries [17–18]. Therefore, Ang. II and oxidative stress in this study result in different vascular dysfunction of renal artery from carotid and femoral arteries. The receptor-independent vasoconstriction which reflects the contractility of vascular smooth muscle was also compromised in the carotid artery of tachycardia and volume-overload animals and femoral artery of only volume-overload animals (Figure 5D). The adrenergic receptor dependent contraction in carotid and femoral arteries, however, was attenuated in tachycardia animals but did not change in volume-overload (Figure 5B and C). The decrease in adrenergic receptor dependent contraction in tachycardia model may indicate blunted adrenergic activation. This implies that adrenergic activation may be more relevant to HF models (tachycardia or volume-overload) and overshadows the hemodynamic contribution (reversal flow and pulse flow). Although the contractility differences (e.g., receptor dependent and independent vasoconstriction) were largely noted for all vessels, the renal arteries in both models were not affected (Table 2). Endothelial dysfunction, however, was observed in the renal artery of tachycardia and volume-overload animals despite the lack of flow reversal, which suggests factors other than local hemodynamics factors. Hence, the endothelial function was compromised in the renal artery but the vascular smooth muscle cell function remained preserved at this duration of the model. Although the impaired endothelial function of renal artery may be one of the

Table 2. Summary of heart and vascular function, hemodynamic, and biochemical changes at 4 weeks of tachycardia and volume-overload.

	Tachycardia			Tachycardia		
LV/BW	↑			↑		
ANG II	↑			↑		
LVEDV	↑			↑		
EF	↓			↓		
CO	↓			↓		
LVSF	↓			↓		
	Renal	**Femoral**	**Carotid**	**Renal**	**Femoral**	**Carotid**
Reversal flow	No	No	Yes	No	Yes	Yes
Pulse flow	—	⇡	⇡	—	↑	↑
EC-dependent vasodilation	↓	—	↓	↓	↓	↓
eNOS expression	↓	—	↓	↓	↓	↓
NADPH oxidase expression	↑	↑	↑	↑	↑	↑
MnSOD expression	↓	—	↓	⇣	—	↓
EC-independent vasodilation	↓	—	↓	↓	—	↓
Receptor-independent vasoconstriction	—	⇣	⇣	—	↓	↓
Adrenergic activation	—	↓	↓	—	⇣	⇣

Notes: The functional and biochemical variations are denoted using ↑ (increase), ↓ (decrease), No (not found), Yes (found), — (no change), ⇡ (increased but not statistically, p values were between 0.051 to 0.063), and ⇣ (decreased but not statistically, p values were between 0.052 to 0.061).

complications of heart failure [19], the cause and effect relations remain unclear.

The primary source of superoxide in endothelial cells stems from NADPH oxidase. NADPH oxidase which has been extensively studied in phagocyte consists of both membrane components ($p22^{phox}$, $gp91^{phox}$ and Rac1) or catalytic core proteins and cytosolic components ($p47^{phox}$ phagocyte oxidase, $p67^{phox}$ phagocyte oxidase, Rac, and Rho GDI) or regulatory subunits [20]. The endothelial NADPH oxidase (Nox) shares many similarities with those of phagocytes. All the classical NADPH oxidase subunits are expressed in endothelial cells [21]. The level of superoxide in tissue depends on the balance between production and removal. SODs are enzymes that catalyze the dismutase of superoxide and serve as important antioxidant [22]. In the present study, we found that the expression of NADPH oxidase subunits increased in all arteries of tachycardia and volume-overload animals, which approximately correlates somewhat with endothelial dysfunction (Figure 7). The decrease in MnSOD in carotid artery and renal artery of tachycardia animals also correlates with endothelial dysfunction (Figure 7). Several lines of evidence support the hypothesis that superoxide likely mediated vascular dysfunctions in our study. First, Ang II has been shown to increase in HF and induce superoxide production in endothelial cells [23]. In combination with increase Nox subunit ($p47^{phox}$) and decreased antioxidant (SOD), Ang II may play an important role in superoxide production of the three arteries. Second, altered hemodynamics may play a major role. We have previously shown evidence that NADPH oxidase has a directional response to shear stress [24]. In the present study, the retrograded flow was observed in carotid artery from tachycardia and volume-overload animals and femoral artery in volume-overload animals.

In summary, the present study investigated the systemic factors (physio-pathological parameters such as circulating Ang. II and oxidative stress), hemodynamic changes and vascular dysfunctions in renal, carotid and femoral arteries in two HF animal models induced by chronic tachycardia and volume-overload. In these models, systemic factors changed significantly and local reverse blood flow was found in carotid and femoral arteries but not in renal artery. The endothelial dysfunction coincided with arteries having flow reversal (femoral and carotid in volume overload and carotid artery of tachycardia model) but was also found in vessels without flow reversal (renal arteries of both tachycardia and volume overload models). This suggests an important role for systemic factors in renal endothelial dysfunction in comparison with carotid and femoral arteries in which systemic factors plus flow reversal result in endothelial dysfunction. Adrenergic dependent vascular smooth muscle activation was compromised in both femoral and carotid arteries of both HF models but not in renal arteries. The molecular expressions were largely similar in all vessels of both HF models. Although tachycardia and volume-overload HF model showed similar impaired of LV dysfunction at four weeks, there was variability in arterial hemodynamics and the functional and molecular expression reflected both the local hemodynamic as well as systemic changes in HF.

Author Contributions

Conceived and designed the experiments: XL GK. Wrote the paper: XL ZDZ GK. Animal Surgery: XL ZDZ XG JSC MS. Ultrasonic image and physiological analysis: ZDZ XL JSC MS. Functional and molecular analysis: XL JY ZDZ.

References

1. Zucker IH, Wang W, Brandle M, Schultz HD, Patel KP (1995) Neural regulation of sympathetic nerve activity in. heart failure. Progress in cardiovascular diseases 37(6): 397–414.
2. Remme WJ (1994) Therapeutic strategies and neurohormonal control in heart failure. European heart journal 15 Suppl D: 129–38.
3. Schrier RW, Abraham WT (1999) Hormones and hemodynamics in heart failure. The New England journal of medicine 341(8): 577–85.
4. Chiu JJ, Chien S (2011) Effects of disturbed flow on vascular endothelium: pathophysiological basis and clinical perspectives. Physiological reviews 91(1): 327–87.
5. Tsutsui H, Kinugawa S, Matsushima S (2011) Oxidative stress and heart failure. Am J Physiol Heart Circ Physiol 301(6): H2181–90.
6. Kostelec M, Covell J, Buckberg GD, Sadeghi A, Hoffman JI, et al. (2006) Myocardial protection in the failing heart: I. Effect of cardioplegia and the beating state under simulated left ventricular restoration. J Thorac Cardiovasc Surg 132(4): 875–83.
7. Lu X, Kassab GS (2007) Vasoactivity of blood vessels using a novel isovolumic myograph. Ann Biomed Eng 35(3): 356–66.
8. Power JM, Tonkin AM (1999) Large animal models of heart failure. Aust N Z J Med 29(3): 395–402.
9. Patten RD, Hall-Porter MR (2009) Small animal models of heart failure: development of novel therapies, past and present. Circ Heart Fail 2(2): 138–44.
10. Paslawska U, Gajek J, Kiczak L, Noszczyk-Nowak A, Skrzypczak P, et al. (2010) Development of porcine model of chronic tachycardia-induced cardiomyopathy. Int J Cardiol.
11. Chow E, Woodard JC, Farrar DJ (1990) Rapid ventricular pacing in pigs: an experimental model of congestive heart failure. Am J Physiol 258(5 Pt 2): H1603–5.
12. Wilson JR, Douglas P, Hickey WF, Lanoce V, Ferraro N, et al. (1987) Experimental congestive heart failure produced by rapid ventricular pacing in the dog: cardiac effects. Circulation 75(4): 857–67.
13. Kawai H, Mohan A, Hagen J, Dong E, Armstrong J, et al. (2000) Alterations in cardiac adrenergic terminal function and beta-adrenoceptor density in pacing-induced heart failure. Am J Physiol Heart Circ Physiol 278(5): H1708–16.
14. Zhang Y, Popovic ZB, Bibevski S, Fakhry I, Sica DA, et al. (2009) Chronic vagus nerve stimulation improves autonomic control and attenuates systemic inflammation and heart failure progression in a canine high-rate pacing model. Circ Heart Fail 2(6): 692–9.
15. Taylor RR, Covell JW, Ross J Jr (1968) Left ventricular function in experimental aorto-caval fistula with circulatory congestion and fluid retention. J Clin Invest 47(6): 1333–42.
16. Zheng H, Huo Y, Svendsen M, Kassab GS (2010) Effect of blood pressure on vascular hemodynamics in acute tachycardia. J Appl Physiol 109(6): 1619–27.
17. Zeigler DW, Johnson JA, Koivunen DG, Siripaisarnpipat S, Fowler WL Jr, et al. (1986) Angiotensin receptors and pressor hyperresponsiveness in renal prehypertensive rabbits. Am J Physiol 251(1 Pt 2): H196–204.
18. Henrion D, Laher I, Laporte R, Bevan JA (1992) Further evidence from an elastic artery that angiotensin II amplifies noradrenaline-induced contraction through activation of protein kinase C. Eur J Pharmacol 224(1): 13–20.
19. Elkayam U, Cohen G, Gogia H, Mehra A, Johnson JV, et al. (1996) Renal vasodilatory effect of endothelial stimulation in patients with chronic congestive heart failure. J Am Coll Cardiol 28(1): 176–82.
20. Babior BM (1999) NADPH oxidase: an update. Blood 93(5): 1464–76.
21. Gorlach A, Brandes RP, Nguyen K, Amidi M, Dehghani F, et al. (2000) A gp91phox containing NADPH oxidase selectively expressed in endothelial cells is a major source of oxygen radical generation in the arterial wall. Circ Res 87(1): 26–32.
22. Afonso V, Champy R, Mitrovic D, Collin P, Lomri A (2007) Reactive oxygen species and superoxide dismutases: role in joint diseases. Joint, bone, spine: revue du rhumatisme 74(4): 324–9.
23. Zhang H, Schmeisser A, Garlichs CD, Plotze K, Damme U, et al. (1999) Angiotensin II-induced superoxide anion generation in human vascular endothelial cells: role of membrane-bound NADH-/NADPH-oxidases. Cardiovasc Res 44(1): 215–22.
24. Godbole AS, Lu X, Guo X, Kassab GS (2009) NADPH oxidase has a directional response to shear stress. Am J Physiol Heart Circ Physiol 296(1): H152–8.

Data-Driven Decisions for Reducing Readmissions for Heart Failure: General Methodology and Case Study

Mohsen Bayati[1], Mark Braverman[2], Michael Gillam[3], Karen M. Mack[3], George Ruiz[3], Mark S. Smith[3], Eric Horvitz[4]*

1 Stanford University, Stanford, California, United States of America, **2** Princeton University, Princeton, New Jersey, United States of America, **3** MedStar Health and Washington Hospital Center, Washington, D. C., United States of America, **4** Microsoft Research and University of Washington School of Medicine, Redmond, Washington, United States of America

Abstract

Background: Several studies have focused on stratifying patients according to their level of readmission risk, fueled in part by incentive programs in the U.S. that link readmission rates to the annual payment update by Medicare. Patient-specific predictions about readmission have not seen widespread use because of their limited accuracy and questions about the efficacy of using measures of risk to guide clinical decisions. We construct a predictive model for readmissions for congestive heart failure (CHF) and study how its predictions can be used to perform patient-specific interventions. We assess the cost-effectiveness of a methodology that combines prediction and decision making to allocate interventions. The results highlight the importance of combining predictions with decision analysis.

Methods: We construct a statistical classifier from a retrospective database of 793 hospital visits for heart failure that predicts the likelihood that patients will be rehospitalized within 30 days of discharge. We introduce a decision analysis that uses the predictions to guide decisions about post-discharge interventions. We perform a cost-effectiveness analysis of 379 additional hospital visits that were not included in either the formulation of the classifiers or the decision analysis. We report the performance of the methodology and show the overall expected value of employing a real-time decision system.

Findings: For the cohort studied, readmissions are associated with a mean cost of \$13,679 with a standard error of \$1,214. Given a post-discharge plan that costs \$1,300 and that reduces 30-day rehospitalizations by 35%, use of the proposed methods would provide an 18.2% reduction in rehospitalizations and save 3.8% of costs.

Conclusions: Classifiers learned automatically from patient data can be joined with decision analysis to guide the allocation of post-discharge support to CHF patients. Such analyses are especially valuable in the common situation where it is not economically feasible to provide programs to all patients.

Editor: Harry Zhang, Old Dominion University, United States of America

Funding: The research was supported as a project at Microsoft Research (http://research.microsoft.com/en-us/), a basic science research unit of Microsoft. Microsoft Research is an open research laboratory (with no publication controls) exploring curiosity-driven research with multiple concentrations in basic and applied computer science. MBa was also a postdoctoral researcher in Microsoft Research during 2007–2009 and received research support from Microsoft Research during 2010–12. MBa also received support by National Science Foundation award number 1216011. MBr was a postdoctoral researcher in Microsoft Research during 2008–2010 and received research support from Microsoft Research during 2010–11. MBr was also supported by a Natural Science and Engineering Research Council of Canada through its Discovery Grant program. MBr was supported by Microsoft Research (http://research.microsoft.com/en-us/) and also by the Natural Science and Engineering Research Council of Canada through its Discovery Grant program, by the Alfred P. Sloan Fellowship and by the National Science Foundation. The funders had no role in study design, data collection and analysis, decision to publish, or preparation of the manuscript.

Competing Interests: The authors declare that no competing interests exist. The authors know of no conflicts with the independent scholarship of the collaborations of researchers at Microsoft Research, Stanford, Princeton, and MedStar Health on this study.

* Email: horvitz@microsoft.com

Introduction

The increasing availability of large quantities of clinical data being captured by electronic health record systems frames opportunities for generating predictive models from that data to enhance healthcare. We first describe the construction of a predictive model that forecasts the likelihood that heart failure patients will be rehospitalized within 30 days of their discharge. Then, we show how the predictive model can be coupled with an automated decision analysis, which uses patient-specific predictions about readmissions within a cost-benefit model, to provide guidance on the patient-specific allocation of readmission reduction programs. We discuss how such a coupling creates a valuable *data to prediction to action* pipeline that can be implemented within a decision-support system to guide interventions. We describe methods for employing a cohort of test patients, held out from the development of the predictive models, to characterize the overall value of using a real-time decision system given uncertainty in costs and efficacies. This approach provides a foundation for understanding the relationship between interventions that promise to reduce readmission rates at some cost and predictive models that provide forecasts about individual patients' readmission risk.

High rates of rehospitalization within 30 days of discharge reported at multiple health centers have motivated studies of the use of predictive models to identify patients at the highest risk for readmission and the feasibility of using these inferred likelihoods to guide clinical decision making. In a 2007 report to the U.S. Congress, the Medicare Payment Advisory Commission (MedPAC) indicated that as much as $12B is spent annually by Medicare on potentially preventable readmissions within 30 days of patient discharge [1]. Beyond monetary costs, readmission within a short time horizon may be an indicator of poor quality of care with implications for the quality and length of patient lives. Incentives that would encourage hospitals to reduce the rates of unnecessary readmissions have been proposed and are being implemented [2].

Numerous programs for reducing readmissions have been implemented and tested over the past twenty years [3–11]. These programs have sought reductions in readmissions via investments in post-discharge care coordination, patient education and self-management support, scheduled outpatient visits, and telemedicine. A recent survey of readmission reduction programs can be found in [12].

Post-discharge intervention studies described in the literature often report some reduction in readmission rates associated with the intervention being studied. Reported reductions in rates of readmission vary from a few percentage points to 50% or more. Reported per-patient intervention costs vary from a low of $180 [13–14] to $1,200 [15]. Results span savings of thousands of dollars per patient to reported net losses. [16].

Even when an intensive post-discharge program is found effective in preventing readmissions, it may be prohibitively expensive to provide such an intervention to an entire patient cohort. However, net savings may be achieved when the same interventions are applied in a selective manner to patients identified as being at high risk for readmission.

Some readmission reduction programs have been implemented as patient-specific, with enrollment of patients into the prevention program determined by risk scores [17–20]. Detailed surveys of such scores are provided in [21–22]. A notable example is LACE [17]. LACE and related scores are designed to be simple enough to be calculated manually at time of discharge.

We give an end-to-end demonstration of the methodology of per-patient cost-benefit analysis based on a risk score that is automatically inferred from EHR data. We perform a sensitivity analysis of the overall effectiveness of readmission reduction programs over reported ranges of efficacies and costs of interventions and probe the expected value of embedding a real-time system providing these automated inferences in the clinical workflow. Finally, we compare the utility of our score for the end-to-end process to that of LACE and show that even relatively modest improvements in prediction quality can make a substantial difference in the utility of an intervention.

The advances introduced include: (1) a means for harnessing data available in the local EHR to build the best possible predictive model based on the locally available data; (2) the ability to embed computational guidance on risk rather than relying on heuristic policies or manual calculations of risk scores; (3) the ability to use local financial data to perform a calibrated cost-benefit analysis that recommends an intervention based on the optimal expected payoff; and (4) the ability to perform offline analyses to probe the value of embedding real-time guidance on interventions in a clinical setting via exploring implications of different combinations of costs and benefits of the interventions. The results highlight the importance of combining predictions with decision analysis.

Materials and Methods

We performed the studies on de-identified patient data drawn from the EHR system for a large tertiary urban hospital serving the Metropolitan Washington DC area. Approval for data access and analysis was granted by hospital's institutional review board.

The patient cohort consists of all Medicare patients who were admitted as inpatients to the hospital during July 1, 2007–June 30, 2010 and were discharged alive with heart failure as their primary diagnosis (ICD9 codes 402.01, 402.11, 402.91, 404.01, 404.03, 404.11, 404.13, 404.91, 404.93, and 428.x).

For each visit we defined a target binary variable to describe the patient's 30-day bounce-back status (bb_{30}). We defined all-cause rehospitalizations occurring within 30 days as $bb_{30}=1$ and no rehospitalization as $bb_{30}=0$. The correct value of bb_{30} was obtained using data files provided by the U.S. Centers for Medicare & Medicaid Services (CMS) to the hospital in April 2011. Our goal was to estimate the probability of $bb_{30}=1$ for patients where the value of bb_{30} is unknown.

We divided the cohort into a derivation cohort, consisting of all visits that started between July 1, 2007–June 30, 2009, and a validation set of all visits that started between August 1, 2009–June 30, 2010. In order to build a predictive model, the following information was extracted from the EHR database for each patient:

- *Patient information*: age, gender, marital status, family support.
- *Visit information*: date, time, duration, type (inpatient, emergency, or outpatient), source (emergency, transfer, etc.).
- *Medical information*: history of diagnoses, lab results, medications, medical history, chief complaint, attending and admitting doctors.

For the analysis of costs, we gathered cost information for these visits from the hospital's administrative database. To be consistent with CMS definitions, we excluded the following visits that did not meet criteria for calculation of hospital readmission rates according to CMS 30-day mortality and readmission patient-level data files sent to the hospital.

- Patient was not enrolled in fee for service (FFS) Parts A and B (the standard U.S. Federal-funded health coverage for those over 65) during the 12 consecutive months prior to the index admission or in the 30 days after discharge.
- Patient died during the index hospitalizations.
- Patent left against medical advice (AMA).
- Patient was transferred to another acute care facility.

- Additional admission within 30 days of discharge from an index admission (an admission cannot be considered both an index admission and a readmission).

Our eligible cohort was reduced to 1,172 hospital visits including 793 visits in the derivation cohort and 379 visits in the validation group. Further refinement of the cohort to account for readmissions of patients to other medical facilities is presented in accompanied Text S1.

Model-building and variable selection

We encoded the information about each visit as a vector of binary variables of size 3,388. The variables were extracted automatically from the patient visit data. We used logistic regression to compute probabilities of rehospitalization for cases in the validation set. Since our model contains a large set of variables relative to the cohort size, we use the LASSO technique to select the most predictive variables and avoid overfitting [23–24]. Overfitting is a challenge in statistics and machine learning that can specialize the predictive model to the training cases and provide predictors that do not ideally generalize to future, previously unseen cases. The optimal parameters of LASSO were selected based on a cross-validation analysis. The details of this analysis are described in the accompanied Text S1.

We also implemented LACE [17] in our cohort and compared its predictive accuracy with the statistical classifier using area under receiver-operator characteristic (ROC) curve and reclassification analysis. Details of this implementation and calibration of both LACE and the classifier is provided in the accompanied Text S1.

From Predictions to Decisions

We coupled the predictive classifier for readmission with a decision model to perform patient-specific decision analyses for guiding post-discharge interventions. The decision model takes into account the predicted probability of readmission, cost and efficacy of applying the intervention, and average cost of readmission and allocates the interventions. We made the following simplifying assumptions:

- The cost of applying an intervention is on a per-patient basis and is the same for all patients. Most prior studies make this assumption. Interventions include assuring an outpatient visit within a specified time frame, rendering additional patient education, performing follow-up phone calls, and providing a fixed number of home visits.
- The expected cost $C_{readmit}$ of readmission is *a priori* the same for all patients. $C_{readmit}$ may include not just the monetary cost of a readmission, but also a penalty for the reduced quality of care associated with presentations warranting avoidable hospital readmissions. $C_{readmit}$ may be set by the hospital using a variety of considerations or just be calculated from past financial data. We obtained $C_{readmit}$ using the latter option by calculating the empirical average readmission costs for patients in the derivation cohort.
- The efficacy of the intervention is *a priori* the same $P_{success}$ for the entire cohort of patients. For example, an intervention that reduces the readmission rate by 25% reduces the readmission risk of each patient to whom it is applied by 25%.

Without the intervention, the expected cost of readmission for a patient whose probability of being readmitted within 30 days is p is

$$C_0(p) = p \times C_{readmit},$$

which is the full cost of a readmission, weighted by the likelihood of the readmission. The intervention adds $C_{intervene}$ to the cost of treatment but promises to reduce the readmission probability to $p(1-P_{success})$, thus bringing the total expected cost to

$$C_1(p) = C_{intervene} + p(1-P_{success})C_{readmit}.$$

The expected cost of the outcomes associated with the cases of intervention and nonintervention as functions of p are plotted in **Figure 1**. The expected utility of the intervention is the difference of these expected values, $U(p) = C_0(p) - C_1(p)$. For low values of p, the intervention is not warranted, as $C_0(p) < C_1(p)$ and $U(p) < 0$. For high values of p, $U(p)$ becomes positive and the intervention becomes beneficial. Note that the expected utilities associated with the intervention and default post-discharge programs cross at a threshold probability, which we denote by p^*. At this probability of readmission, the expected utility for the intervention and default programs are equal. We seek to maximize the overall benefit of the program for all patients by taking patient-specific actions that maximize the net expected benefit for each patient. The ideal policy for maximizing utility is to apply the intervention to patients for whom $U(p) > 0$, or equivalently

$$p \geq p^* = \frac{C_{intervene}}{P_{success} \times C_{readmit}}$$

The predictive model provides patient-specific estimates of the readmission probability p based on the available data, and we use the model to predict for each patient whether $p \geq p^*$.

Finally, to explore the importance of the accuracy of the classifier in this analysis, we repeated the study using the LACE score instead of the output of the learned classifier and compared the results of the two analyses.

Software packages

All statistical analysis including construction of the classifier, cross-validation analysis, model calibration, and decision optimization was performed using R and Matlab.

Results

Model validation

The optimal classifier achieved an overall area under the curve (AUC) of 0.66 on the validation cohort. This is 10% improvement over the predictive model presented in [20], which obtained an AUC equal to 0.60, and an 11% improvement over LACE [17], which had an AUC of 0.59 in the validation cohort. The cross-validation AUC for the classifier and LACE for the derivation cohort is 0.69±0.0198 ($p_{value} < 0.05$) and 0.59±0.0093 ($p_{value} < 0.05$), respectively. The difference is statistically significant ($p_{value} < 0.001$). The fractions of readmissions to outside hospitals in the derivation and validation cohorts are 35.2% and 47.9%, respectively. This significant increase in outside readmissions highlights a major challenge of predicting readmissions in our data as the patient population and patterns of engagements with the hospital has significantly changed. If we remove from the

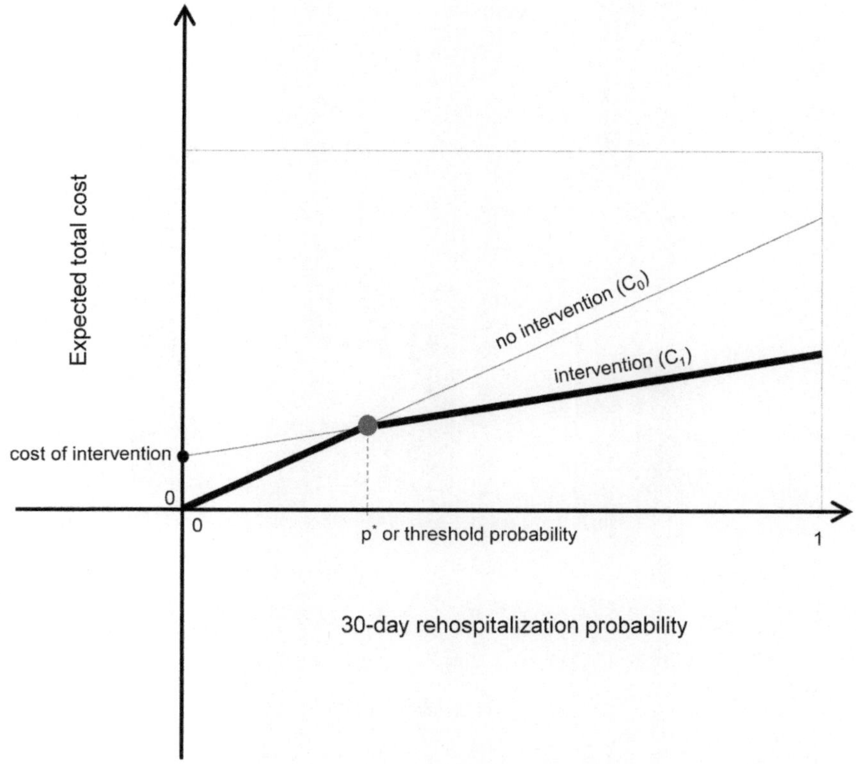

Figure 1. Plots of utility of outcomes for the intervention and no-intervention cases, showing relationship of potential expected utilities of outcomes achieved with a postdischarge program that reduces the rate of readmission versus the default of making no special intervention. Darker lines highlight ideal policy for any predicted likelihood of rehospitalization.

validation cohort all patients who were readmitted to outside hospitals, the AUC of the classifier on the validation cohort is 0.71.

The observed and predicted probabilities of rehospitalization provided by the predictive model for both derivation and validation cohorts are shown in **Figure 2**. The reclassification of patients from the three risk groups obtained by LACE to the three risk groups obtained by the learned classifier is shown in **Table 1**.

Predictive variables

The optimal model automatically selects a subset of 253 variables from 3,388 available variables to avoid overfitting to the derivation data. **Tables 2** and **3** show lists of the variables identified as most influential in predicting rehospitalization within 30 days. The variables are separated into lists of findings that provide the most evidential support for (**Table 2**) and against (**Table 3**) a patient being rehospitalized and are clustered within each list into diagnosed diseases, medications, lab results, and patterns of engagement with the healthcare system. Observations on engagement include such statistics as time since the last hospitalization and the number of hospitalizations in the last year.

Exploring the value of a real-time decision system

The patient-specific decision analyses applied to each of the CHF patients in the validation cohort using the utility model described in the Materials and Methods section identifies patients in the validation cohort who would have received the post-discharge intervention according to a policy of minimizing expected care costs. We compared the efficacy of using such patient-specific decision analyses to the use of a simpler *uniform policy*, where interventions are allocated homogeneously to either all or none of the patients, based on an analysis of which of the two possible uniform policies (*apply to all* versus *apply to none*) has the highest net expected value.

Table 4 compares the percentage of total readmission costs ($1,291,300) that would be saved, as predicted by the model, through using a patient-specific decision analysis as opposed to offering interventions to all patients in a uniform manner for efficacies (reduction in readmission rate) assumed to be 25%, 35% and for costs of intervention set to $800, $1,300, and $1,800. **Table 4** also shows the percentage of total expected readmissions prevented with the patient-specific analysis versus the best uniform policy. **Table 4** also displays the cost savings achieved by the patient-specific decision analysis when LACE is used in place of the statistical classifier. Using the poorer-performing LACE score for identifying patients at risk for readmissions translates into lower savings and narrower bands of usefulness across regimes defined by the costs and efficacies of programs.

We note that information in **Table 4**, representing details about the value and appropriateness of using patient-specific versus uniform policies depends on the costs, efficacies, and the predictive power of the classifier derived from data. Improvements in the accuracy of classifiers lead to greater selectivity in the application of programs and greater overall benefits to patients and hospitals. For example, by using the patient-specific decision analysis in the application of an intervention that costs $1,300 and that is 35% effective, 3.8% of rehospitalization costs can be saved and 18.2% of readmissions can be prevented. However, applying the intervention to all patients does not save dollars. Rather, providing the program to all patients adds 3.2% to the total costs.

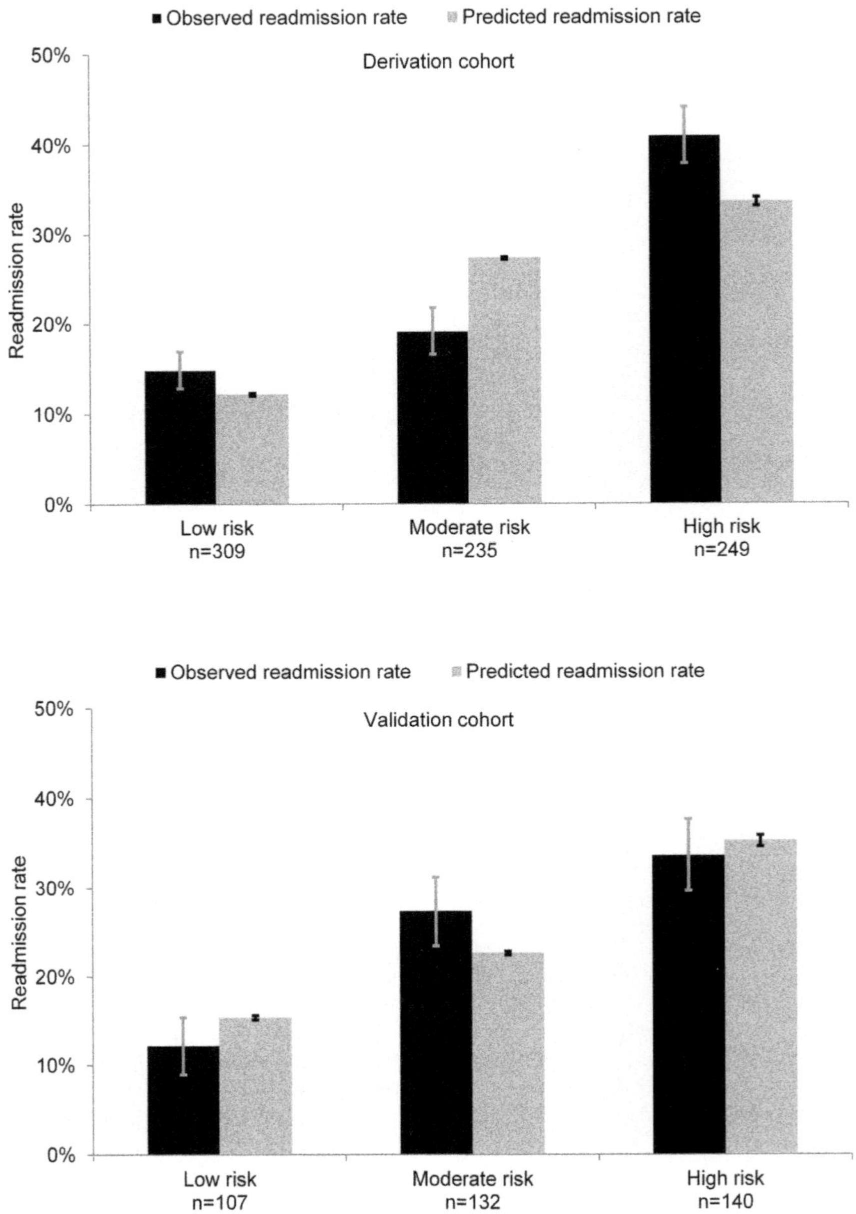

Figure 2. Study of calibration of likelihoods generated by predictive model. Figures show number of patients in each of three risk groups of derivation cohort (top) and validation cohort (bottom) with observed and predicted readmission rates within a margin of error with $p_{value}<0.05$.

Table 1. Reclassification of patients from the three risk groups obtained by LACE to revised risk groups obtained by the classifier.

Reclassification matrix

		Classifier			
		Low risk	**Moderate risk**	**High risk**	**Total reclassified (%)**
LACE	**Low risk (%)**	35.8	36.2	28.0	**64.2**
	Moderate risk (%)	16.8	33.6	49.6	**66.4**
	High risk (%)	0.0	23.5	76.5	**23.5**

Table 2. Top variables selected by machine learning procedure that increase risk of readmission within 30 days.

Top supportive evidence

Variable class	Variable description	Log Odds Ratio	Log Odds Ratio Standard Error[1]
Lab Results	Lymphocyte % is low	0.0128	0.0027
Patterns of Engagement	Patient was admitted in past 6 months	0.0112	0.0031
Lab Results	BUN is high	0.0038	0.0012
Lab Results	Glucose level random is elevated	0.003	0.0012
Lab Results	Monocyte absolute is low	0.0028	0.0012
Other Diagnoses	History of nondependent abuse of drugs (ICD9 305.x)	0.0018	0.001
Other Diagnoses	History of chronic airway obstruction, not elsewhere classified (ICD9 496.x)	0.0017	0.0008
Other Diagnoses	History of gastrointestinal hemorrhage (ICD9 578.x)	0.0014	0.0007
Lab Results	AST is elevated	0.0013	0.0006
Other Diagnoses	History of cardiomyopathy (ICD9 425.x)	0.001	0.0006
Lab Results	Magnesium is low	0.001	0.0006
Lab Results	INR is elevated	0.0009	0.0004
Patterns of Engagement	Patient has been in isolated room in hospital	0.0009	0.0006
Lab Results	BNP is high	0.0007	0.0005

These are variables that receive positive log-odds ratio with the largest magnitude.
1. Obtained from sample standard error for cross-validation odds ratios

Intervention decisions obtained using LACE in lieu of the learned classifier would achieve only 0.5% savings and prevented only 2.6% of readmissions.

Given the ranges of costs and efficacies of post-discharge programs reported in the literature, the efficacy of a specific new program may not be known at the time that a new program is formulated. To build insights about the value of employing a real-time decision system in light of such uncertainty, we introduce an automated analysis of the *net expected value of a decision system* in a clinical environment. For each of a large number of different pairs of assumed efficacy and cost of intervention, we apply the data to prediction to action pipeline for all patients in the validation cohort, using the hospital-specific classifier that we have generated from local data. This sensitivity analysis provides the overall reduction in readmissions or savings for each pair of independently varied cost and efficacy. We performed this analysis and combined the multiple studies into a contour map visualization of the expected savings across the spectrum of cost and efficacy of the intervention. The contour map in **Figure 3**(a) represents the expected reductions in costs achieved with the use of a real-time decision system that performs guidance on patient-specific enrollment versus performing no special intervention for different combinations of cost and efficacies of programs. **Figure 3**(b) considers the boost in savings achieved by using the

Table 3. Top variables selected by machine learning procedure that decrease risk of readmission within 30 days.

Top disconfirming evidence

Variable class	Variable description	Log Odds Ratio	Log Odds Ratio Standard Error[1]
Patterns of Engagement	Number of emergency room visits during past 6 months <2	−0.0607	0.0035
Lab results	Hematocrit % is normal	−0.0442	0.0043
Lab results	BNP is normal	−0.044	0.0049
Lab results	Alkaline phosphatase is normal	−0.0428	0.0033
Lab results	Chloride is normal	−0.0428	0.0042
Cardiac medications	Patient is not on digoxin therapy	−0.0396	0.0039
Lab results	MCHC % is low	−0.0387	0.0039
Changes in lab results	TSH variation during current visit is low	−0.0343	0.003
Changes in lab results	CO2 variation during current visit is low	−0.0318	0.0039
Changes in lab results	RDW variation during current visit is low	−0.0308	0.0038
Changes in lab results	MCV variation during current visit is low	−0.0306	0.0036

These are variables that receive negative log-odds ratio with largest magnitude.
1. Obtained from sample standard error for cross-validation odds ratios

Table 4. Comparison of savings achieved and readmissions prevented for post-discharge programs with different costs and efficacies.

Comparison of savings		Savings or losses				Readmissions prevented		
Cost of intervention	Efficacy	Patient-specific analysis and classifier	Patient-specific analysis and LACE	Intervention applied to all patients	Best uniform policy	Patient-specific analysis and classifier	Patient-specific analysis and LACE	Best uniform policy
$300	25%	16.2%	15.9%	16.2%	16.2%	25.0%	24.5%	25.0%
	35%	26.2%	26.2%	26.2%	26.2%	35.0%	35.0%	35.0%
$800	25%	5.4%	1.3%	1.5%	1.5%	17.4%	2.9%	25.0%
	35%	13.2%	9.1%	11.5%	11.5%	31.4%	22.2%	35.0%
$1,300	25%	0.7%	0.0%	−13.2%	0.0%	5.2%	0.0%	0.0%
	35%	3.8%	0.5%	−3.2%	0.0%	18.2%	2.6%	0.0%
$1,800	25%	0.3%	0.0%	−27.8%	0.0%	0.8%	0.0%	0.0%
	35%	0.8%	0.0%	−17.8%	0.0%	7.3%	0.0%	0.0%

Three policies are compared: patient specific analysis using the classifier, patient-specific analysis using LACE, best uniform policy. For comparison of savings an additional column demonstrates the policy that applies intervention to every patient may lead to loss (or savings).

patient-specific decision guidance over the best uniform policy. The best uniform policy refers to the intervention being performed for all patients or none of the patients, depending on which outcome is better. The contour map demonstrates that the use of a real-time decision-analytic system for guidance would not yield net savings when the intervention is inexpensive and efficient, as it is best in that situation to apply the intervention to the entire population. Likewise, decision-analytic guidance would not be useful when the intervention is very expensive and inefficient, as such a program would not be cost-effective for any patients. However, for interventions with more intermediate costs and efficacies, relative savings of nearly 10% can be realized for the population we have studied, given predictions available from the classifier. **Figure 3**(c) considers the same boost in cost savings achieved by the patient-specific decision analysis over the use of the LACE score. The use of the poorer-performing LACE score for identifying patients at risk for readmissions translates to significantly lower savings and narrower regimes of applicability across regimes defined by the costs and efficacies of programs.

Discussion and Conclusions

Implications for readmission reduction

As demonstrated by the results displayed in **Table 4** and **Figure 3**, selective patient enrollment based on automatic risk stratification, could be applied effectively to take advantage of interventional programs that are too expensive to be applied to the entire population of heart failure patients.

The value of performing patient-specific decision analyses will generally increase with increases in classification accuracy, which can be achieved with larger training sets as well as more complete medical information about individual patients. A readmission prediction study [25] conducted in a Veterans Health Administration (VA) Hospital considered a heart failure patient cohort of $n = 198{,}460$, including data from a cross-hospital EHR containing the long-term medical histories of patients. Using this more extensive data, a statistical classifier was created with an AUC of 0.82. We found that 47% of the readmission patients in our cohort were readmitted to outside medical facilities within 30 days of their initial hospitalization for heart failure. We found that we had sparse EHR data on this substantial proportion of patients and that this may have detracted from the predictive power of our model. The results of the VA study highlight the value of implementing a shared patient database among the different hospitals that patients visit over time.

Analysis and insights enabled by the electronic capture of clinical data

We see the construction and use of predictive models that are custom tailored to populations as having the ability to deliver predictions of higher accuracy than those produced by simpler clinical rules designed for application across all hospitals. We envision that the *data to prediction to action* pipeline will become more widely used as EHR systems become more prevalent. We now outline several benefits of using local patient data to construct classifiers to predict outcomes, as compared to relying on simpler rules such as LACE.

Automated risk calculation

The classifier for predictions is constructed entirely from data available within the EHR. In real-time clinical use, findings on specific patients can be drawn automatically from the EHR, requiring no additional time from the practitioners. The computed risk scores can in turn be used to recommend enrollment into

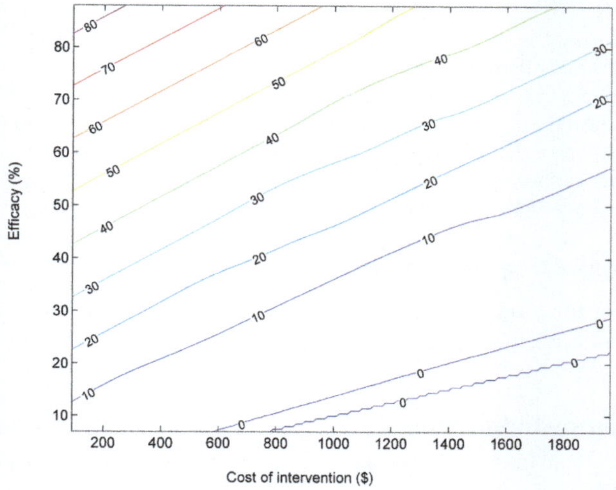

(a)

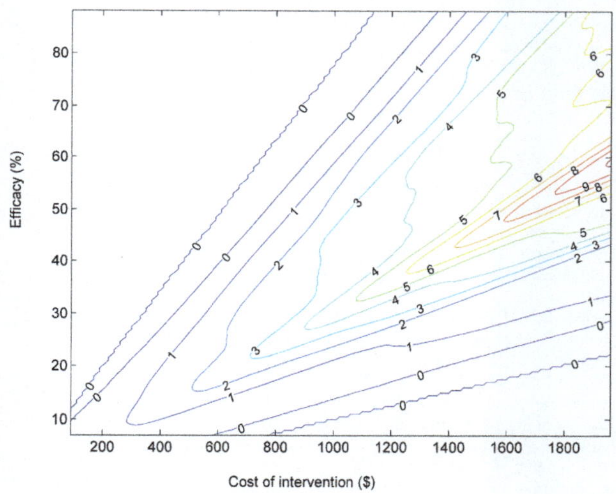

(b)

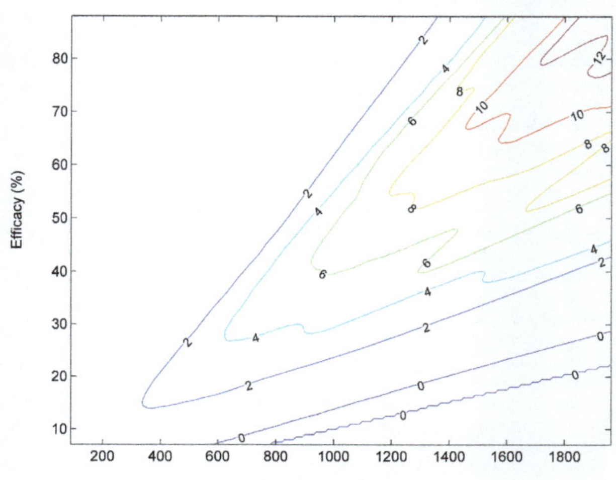

(c)

Figure 3. Contour maps capturing cost savings for ranges of program costs and efficacies: (a) savings with decision analysis over no intervention; (b) savings achieved with automated decision analysis over that of applying best uniform policy; (c) savings achieved with automated decision analysis over the use of LACE score, highlighting value of using more accurate predictive model. The labels on contour maps show percentage savings.

prevention programs as part of the workflow. Currently, such enrollment is performed typically using a pencil-and-paper form, or an application specifically designed for this purpose, and observations about patients and their health are manually entered or checked, making it difficult to consider multiple influencing factors. The risk estimation methods we describe do not place additional demands on practitioners and enable large numbers of patients to be screened for multiple intervention and prevention programs. Such automation also enables valuable data on the efficacy of interventions to be collected and harnessed. Moreover, when data on outcomes associated with interventions is accrued in the EHR, we can extend the methodology described in this paper to estimate both the readmission risk and the likelihood of the intervention succeeding at the level of an individual patient or patient subpopulation, further amplifying the effect of the intervention program.

Emphasis on local data

The predictive model is constructed entirely using local data. If our aim is to make the best possible predictions, taking local populations, data collection, and practice patterns into account will almost always be important in achieving the highest predictive performance. This raises the question of how a model trained within one hospital would perform when validated at a different hospital. As readmission patterns and prevalence vary by hospital and by region [26], a risk-stratification model that is not constructed locally will not be able to take into account the location-specific trends, details of care activities, and patient population. Unlike a generic risk rule, a locally trained classifier will be able to adjust as changes in the hospital's patterns of care occur over time.

Clinical face validity of observations

In reviewing the most predictive variables found by the classifier, we found that low lymphocyte percentage (top variable in **Table 2**) has previously been linked to poor outcomes in early postdischarge period of hospitalized HF patients [27] and low hematocrit (second top variable in **Table 3**) has been related to lower risk of heart failure [28]. However, a benefit of the data-driven approach is that we make use of all available data in constructing a predictive model. This means that we do not restrict the analysis solely to variables that have been found valid in previous studies. This characteristic is important because a learning algorithm may derive significant predictive power from variables that have poor face validity and appear arbitrary. This predictive power can stem from correlations among seemingly irrelevant variables available in the EHR and other, more interpretable variables that are not captured in the patient record. Variables identified as discriminatory may serve as proxies for other variables that would be more understandable, but are not available in the system. For example, in one of our studies on predicting general readmissions to the hospital, we discovered that "cocaine test: negative" raises the likelihood that the patient will be readmitted. A subsequent inquiry revealed that clinicians would be unlikely to administer a cocaine screening unless they had reason to suspect that a patient may be a drug abuser. Thus, the observation that the test was administered at all is linked to a higher-level assessment by the physician that the patient belongs to a vulnerable population—an assessment that is not recorded directly in the health database. Classifiers derived from all of the data available in the EHR will generally perform as well or better than models restricted only to those variables that have widely recognized clinical significance or that mesh with intuition as understandable or obvious indicators of risk with respect to a specific target ailment. We note that great care must be taken in interpreting the clinical relevance of variables flagged by such models as discriminating. Such observations are not necessarily involved in a *causal* manner nor suggest new paths to intervention. Observations identified as useful by the learning procedure may reflect local care patterns and not necessarily correspond to a generalizable risk factor. At the same time, variables identified as discriminating for a given predictive task may unearth new clinical insights and frame directions for study and intervention.

On limitations of local predictive tools

A potential drawback of the analytical pipeline that we have presented versus traditional risk-stratification scores is that its implementation would require some amount of computing resources. As the approach is data driven and relies only on data within the EHR, it can be implemented by the hospital, by the EHR vendor, or by an independent third party, further lowering the cost of implementing such a predictive system.

Another limitation of this study is the fact that it is based on retrospective data. A more rigorous validation would entail performing a randomized controlled experiment. However, the results provide a first step to demonstrate the applicability of risk stratification for guiding allocation of post-discharge interventions in a cost-effective manner.

Supporting Information

Text S1 Supplemental Details to Materials and Methods.

Acknowledgments

We thank Paul Koch, Dobroslav Kolev, and Hank Rappaport for assistance with data access and interpretation.

Author Contributions

Conceived and designed the experiments: M. Bayati M. Braverman MG KMM GR MSS EH. Performed the experiments: M. Bayati M. Braverman EH. Analyzed the data: M. Bayati M. Braverman KMM EH. Contributed reagents/materials/analysis tools: M. Bayati M. Braverman MG KMM MSS EH. Wrote the paper: M. Bayati M. Braverman KMM MSS EH.

References

1. Medicare Payment Advisory Commission (2013) Promoting greater efficiency in Medicare, report to Congress. Medicare Payment Advisory Commission. Available at: http://www.medpac.gov/documents/jun07_entirereport.pdf.
2. Center for Medicare and Medicaid Services (2009) Proposed changes to the hospital inpatient prospective payment system for acute care hospitals. Federal Register. May 22;74(98): 24166. Available at: http://edocket.access.gpo.gov/2009/pdf/E9-10458.pdf.
3. Gonseth J, Guallar-Castillon P, Banegas JR, Rodriguez-Artalejo F (2004) The effectiveness of disease management programmes in reducing hospital re-admission in older patients with heart failure: a systematic review and meta-analysis of published reports. Eur Heart J. 25: 1570–1595.
4. Gwadry-Sridhar F, Flintoft V, Lee DS, Lee H, Guyatt GH (2004) A systematic review and meta-analysis of studies comparing readmission rates and mortality rates in patients with heart failure. Arch Intern Med.164: 2315–2320.
5. Jovicic A, Holroyd-Leduc JM, Straus SE (2006) Effects of self-management intervention on health outcomes of patients with heart failure: A systematic review of randomized controlled trials. BMC Cardiovasc Disord. 6: 43.
6. Koelling T (2005) Multifaceted outpatient support can improve outcomes for people with heart failure: commentary. Evid Based Cardiovasc Med.; 9: 138–141.
7. Krumholz HM, Amatruda J, Smith GL, Mattera JA, Roumanis SA, et al. (2002) Randomized trial of an education and support intervention to prevent readmission of patients with heart failure. J Am Coll Cardiol.39: 83–89.
8. McAlister FA, Lawson FM, Teo KK, Armstrong PW (2001) A systematic review of randomized trials of disease management programs in heart failure. Am J Med. 110: 378–384.
9. Phillips CO, Wright SM, Kern DE, Singa RM, Shepperd S, et al. (2004) Comprehensive discharge planning with postdischarge support for older patients with congestive heart failure: a meta-analysis. JAMA. 291: 1358–1367.
10. Rich M, Beckham V, Wittenberg C, Leven CL, Freedland K., et al. (1995) A multidisciplinary intervention to prevent the readmission of elderly patients with congestive heart failure. N. Engl J Med. 333: 1190–1195.
11. Hernandez AF, Greiner MA, Fonarow GC, Hammill BG, Heidenreich PA, et al. (2010) Relationship between early physician follow-up and 30-day readmission among Medicare beneficiaries hospitalized for heart failure. JAMA. 303: 1716–1722.
12. Boutwell A, Griffin F, Hwu S (2009) Effective interventions to reduce rehospitalizations: a compendium of 15 promising interventions. Cambridge, MA: Institute for Healthcare Improvement;. Available at http://ah.cms-plus.com/files/STAAR_A_Compendium_of_Promising_Interventions.pdf.
13. Anderson C, Deepak B, Amoateng-Adjepong Y, Zarich S (2005) Benefits of comprehensive inpatient education and discharge planning combined with outpatient support in elderly patients with congestive heart failure. Congestive Heart Failure. 11: 315–321.
14. Coleman EA, Parry C, Chalmers S, Min SJ (2006) The care transitions intervention: Results of a randomized controlled trial. JAMA. 166: 1822–1828.
15. Kasper EK, Gerstenblith G, Hefter G, Van Anden E, Brinker JA, et al. (2002) A randomized trial of the efficacy of multidisciplinary care in heart failure outpatients at high risk of hospital readmission. J Am Coll of Cardiol. 39: 471–480.
16. Peikes D, Chen A, Schore J, Brown R (2002) Effects of care coordination on hospitalization, quality of care, and health care expenditures among Medicare beneficiaries: 15 randomized trials. JAMA. 301: 603–618.
17. Van Walraven C, Dhalla IA, Bell Ch, Etchells E, Stiell IG (2010) Derivaiton and validation of an index to predict early death or unplanned readmission after discharge from hospital to the community. CMAJ. 6: 51–557.
18. Amarasingham R, Moore BJ, Tabak YP, Drazner MH, Clark CA, et al. (2010) An automated model to identify heart failure patients at risk for 30-day readmission or death using electronic medical record data. Med Care. 48(11):981–8.
19. Wang L, Porter B, Maynard C, Bryson C, Sun H, et al. (2012) Predicting Risk of Hospitalization or Death Among Patients With Heart Failure in the Veterans Health Administration. Am J Cardiol. 110(9):1342–9.
20. Keenan PS, Normand ST, Lin Z, Drye EE, Bhat KR, et al. (2008) An administrative claims measure suitable for profiling hospital performance on the basis of 30-day all-cause readmission rates among patients with heart failure. Circulation.1: 29–37.
21. Kansagara D, Englander H, Salanitro A, Kagen D, Theobald C, et al. (2011) Risk prediction models for hospital readmission: a systematic review. JAMA. 306(15):1688–1698.
22. Giamouzis G, Kalogeropoulos A, Georgiopoulou V, Smith LS, Dunbar S, et al. (2011) Hospitalization epidemic in patients with heart failure: risk factors, risk prediction, knowledge gaps, and future directions. J Card Fail. 17(1):54–75.
23. Chen S, Donoho D (1994) Basis pursuit, Signals, Systems and Computers, (1):41–44.
24. Tibshirani R (1996) Regression shrinkage and selection via the lasso. J Royal Statistics Society Series B. 58: 267–288.
25. Wang L, Porter B, Maynard C, Bryson C, Sun H, et al. (2012) Predicting risk of hospitalization or death among patients with heart failure in the veterans health administration, Am J Cardiol. 110(9):1342–9.
26. Jencks SF, Williams MV, Coleman EA (2009) Rehospitalizations among patients in the Medicare fee-for-service program. New Engl J Med. 360: 1418–1428
27. Vaduganathan M, Ambrosy A, Greene S, Mentz R, Subacius H, et al. (2012) Predictive value of low relative lymphocyte count in patients hospitalized for heart failure with reduced ejection fraction: insights from the EVEREST trial, Circ Heart Fail. 5(6):750–8.
28. Coglianese E, Qureshi M, Vasan R,Wang Th, Moore L (2012) Usefulness of the Blood Hematocrit Level to Predict Development of Heart Failure in a Community, Am J Cardiol. 109(2): 241–245.

Development of Contrast-Induced Acute Kidney Injury after Elective Contrast Media Exposure in Patients with Type 2 Diabetes Mellitus: Effect of Albuminuria

Jun-qing Yang[1]◔, Peng Ran[1]◔, Ji-yan Chen[1]*, Yi-ting He[2], Li-wen Li[1], Ning Tan[1], Guang Li[1], Shuo Sun[1], Yong Liu[1], Jia-xin Zhan[1], Jian-yi Zheng[1], Ying-ling Zhou[1]*

1 Department of Cardiology, Guangdong Cardiovascular Institute, Guangdong General Hospital, Guangdong Academy of Medical Sciences, Guangzhou, Guangdong, China, **2** Department of Cardiology, Shunde first hospital, Foshan, Guangdong, China

Abstract

Background: The influence of albuminuria and urinary pH on the development of contrast-induced acute kidney disease (CI-AKI) in patients with type 2 diabetes mellitus (T2DM) after elective coronary angiography (CAG) or percutaneous coronary intervention (PCI) is unknown.

Methods: CI-AKI was defined as an increase in serum creatinine $>$26.4 μmol/L or $\geq$50% of baseline value within 48 hours after contrast media exposure. Demographics, traditional risk factors, clinical outcomes and CI-AKI incidence were compared between groups. Univariate analysis and multivariate logistic regression were performed to assess risk factors of CI-AKI.

Results: We observed 597 patients with T2DM after CAG or PCI. Patients were divided into 3 groups based on early morning urinary albumin: negative group (urine dipstick negative, n = 483), trace group (urine dipstick trace, n = 60), and positive group (urine dipstick $\geq$1+, n = 54). CI-AKI occurred in 33 (5.5%) patients, including 19 (3.9%) in the negativealbuminuria group, 4 (6.7%) in the trace group, and 10 (18.5%) in the positive group ($p < 0.001$), respectively. After adjusting for potential confounding risk factors, positive albuminuria (OR = 3.8, 95% CI: 1.5 to 9.2, p = 0.004) and urinary pH$<$6 (OR = 2.4, 95% CI: 1.1 to 5.1, p = 0.020) remained significantly associated with CI-AKI.

Conclusion: Preprocedural albuminuria and urinary pH $<$6 are independent risk factors of CI-AKI in patients with T2DM undergoing elective cardiac catheterization, and may be used to identify patients at high risk of post-procedural CI-AKI.

Editor: Emmanuel A. Burdmann, University of Sao Paulo Medical School, Brazil

Funding: The work was supported by Science and Technology Planning Project of Guangdong Province (grant NO.: 2008A030201002), Guangdong Cardiovascular Institute; and Guangdong Provincial Cardiovascular Clinical Medicine Research Fund (grant NO.: 2009X41), Guangzhou, China. The funders had no role in study design, data collection and analysis, decision to publish, or preparation of the manuscript.

Competing Interests: The authors have declared that no competing interests exist.

* Email: gdphospital@163.com (JYC); gdghospital@163.com (YLZ)

◔ These authors contributed equally to this work.

Introduction

Contrast-induced acute kidney injury (CI-AKI) is a leading cause of nosocomial acute renal failure [1,2]. It is associated with poor outcomes, including dialysis and in-hospital [3] and 1–2 year mortality [4,5]. Furthermore, it prolongs hospitalization and increases medical costs [6].

Albuminuria is common in patients with type 2 diabetes (T2DM). Previous studies have demonstrated that increased albuminuria and reduced estimated glomerular filtration rate (eGFR) are independent risk factors for acute kidney injury [7], and cardiovascular and renal events [8] in T2DM patients. However, the impact of albuminuria on the prevalence of CI-AKI in T2DM patients is unclear, and few studies have investigated the relationship between urinary albumin levels and CI-AKI. In addition, the pathogenesis of CI-AKI may include free radicals production, which is promoted by the acidic environment in the urinary tubule [9]. Urinary pH may be associated with CI-AKI.

Therefore, we investigated influence of urinary albumin levels and urinary pH on the incidence of CI-AKI in T2DM patients who underwent elective CAG or PCI.

Methods

Study protocol

We conducted an observational study in consecutive patients with T2MD and who underwent elective CAG or PCI at the Guangdong Cardiovascular Institute of Guangdong General Hospital, Guangdong Academy of Medical Sciences, between August 2009 and August 2012. The study protocol was approved by the Guangdong General Hospital ethics committee, and all patients provided a written informed consent.

T2DM patients undergoing CAG or PCI were enrolled. Exclusion criteria were: 1) age <18years; 2) eGFR<15 ml/min/1.73 m^2; 3) dialysis; 4) nephrotic syndrome; 5) nephropyelitis; 6) emergency CAG or PCI; 7) cardiac shock; 8) severe aortic valve disease; 9) multiple myeloma; 10) severe hepatic insufficiency; 11) acute stroke; 12) diabetic ketoacidosis; 13) iodic contrast administration during the preceding 7 days; 14) coronary revascularization surgery; 15) nonsteroidal anti-inflammatory drugs (NSAIDs) use within 48 hours before the procedure; 16) severe sepsis; 17) pregnancy; 18) allergy to contrast medium.

Routine urinalysis of early morning urine samples which involved urinary albumin and pH was performed upon hospital admission and before the procedure. Serum creatinine was measured as part of routine clinical care upon admission, and daily for 2 days after the procedure. Urinary albumin and pH were tested using an Urisys-2400 automatic analyzer (Roche Diagnostics, Basel, Switzerland), a Miditrom Junior analyzer (Roche Diagnostics, Basel, Switzerland), or a COBAS U411 analyzer (Roche Diagnostics, Basel, Switzerland). eGFR was estimated using the abbreviated Modification of Diet in Renal Disease (MDRD) formula [10].

CAG or PCI was performed using standard techniques [11]. The dose and types of contrast medium were left to the discretion of the interventional cardiologist. The use of aspirin, clopidogrel, β-blockers, angiotensin-converting enzyme inhibitors (ACEIs)/ angiotensin receptor blockers (ARBs), calcium channel blockers (CCBs), diuretics, intra-aortic balloon pump (IABP) or vascular active drugs was also left to the discretion of the interventional and/or clinical cardiologist. Patients received perioperative hydration for 8–36 hours with normal saline at a rate of 1 ml/ kg/hour. The hydration rate was reduced by half in patients with a left ventricular ejection fraction (LVEF) <35% or NYHA class III–IV at admission.

T2DM was defined as fasting plasma glucose ≥126 mg/dl (7.0 mmol/L); or 2-h plasma glucose ≥200 mg/dl (11.1 mmol/L) during an oral glucose tolerance test; or in a patient with classic symptoms of hyperglycemia or hyperglycemic crisis, a random plasma glucose ≥200 mg/dl (11.1 mmol/L) [12], a previous diagnosis or received treatment was also accepted. Anemia was defined as baseline hematocrit <39% for men and <36% for women. Hypotension was defined as systolic blood pressure (SBP) <80 mmHg for at least 1 hour requiring inotropic support with medications or intra-aortic balloon pump (IABP) within 24 hours periprocedurally. Congestive heart failure was defined as New York Heart Association functional classification III/IV and/or history of pulmonary edema [13].

Endpoints

Primary endpoints. The primary endpoint was the occurrence of CI-AKI, was defined as an increase in serum creatinine > 26.4 μmol/L or ≥50% of baseline value within 48 hours after contrast media exposure [14].

Secondary endpoints. Secondary endpoints were absolute change in serum creatinine within 48 hours, in-hospital death and dialysis. The cause of death was ascertained from discharge documents and discussion with attending physician.

Follow-up

Follow-up was performed at an outpatient clinic visit or via telephone interviews. Cardiac death was defined as any death with a demonstrable cardiac cause or any death that was not clearly attributable to a non-cardiac cause [15]. All-cause death, cardiac death, and dialysis were adjudicated by two experienced cardiologists who were blinded to angiographic and biochemical data.

Statistical analysis

SPSS 19.0 was used for statistical analysis. Patients were divided into three groups according to early morning urinary albumin assessment by routine urinalysis: negative group (urine dipstick negative), trace group (urine dipstick trace), and positive group (urine dipstick ≥1+). Data are presented as mean ± standard deviation (SD) for normally distributed data, or medians and interquartile ranges (IQR) for unevenly distributed data. Categorical data are expressed as numbers (%). Demographics, traditional risk factors, clinical outcomes and CI-AKI incidence were compared between groups. Chi-square tests or Fisher exact tests were used for categorical data, as appropriate. Normally distributed variables were compared by one-way ANOVA (with Bonferroni correction for comparisons between groups if the ANOVA p-value was <0.05), or by the Kruskal-Wallis test for unevenly distributed data.Risk factors were initially screened for univariate association with CI-AKI at a p value <0.20, and identified variables were then assessed in a forward stepwise manner using a p-value criterion of <0.05. The final model included the important baseline characteristics. Multivariate logistic regression analysis was performed to identify independent risk factors for CI-AKI. Cumulative event curves were constructed using the Kaplan-Meier survival method, and cumulative event rates were compared using the log-rank test. All p-values were two-tailed, and a p-value <0.05 was considered statistically significant.

Results

A total of 597 patients with T2DM after elective CAG or PCI were included; 173 (29.0%) were female, and the overall patient age was 65.1±10.1 years. Baseline patient eGFR and serum creatinine were were 77.8 ml/min/1.73 m^2 (IQR 61.6–96.7 ml/ min/1.73 m^2) and 84.0 μmol/L (IQR 70.5–106.0 μmol/L), respectively. Overall, 33 patients (5.5%) developed CI-AKI

Baseline characteristics

Table 1 shows the baseline characteristics of the study population. There were significant differences among negative, trace and positive groups including: serum creatinine { 82.0(IQR 68.0–101.0)μmol/L vs. 94.4(IQR 75.3–113.5)μmol/L vs. 117.6(IQR 95.3–190.0)μmol/L, p<0.001}, urea nitrogen {4.8(IQR 3.8–6.2) mmol/L vs. 5.4(IQR 4.4–7.0)mmol/L vs.7.4(IQR 5.0–9.8) mmol/L, p<0.001}, eGFR { 80.2 (IQR 64.0–98.9)ml/min/1.73 m^2 vs.72.3(IQR 50.6–97.3)ml/min/1.73 m^2 vs.54.5(IQR 31.1–74.8) ml/min/1.73 m^2, p<0.001}, the proportion of preoperative congestive heart failure (13.0% vs.16.7% vs. 25.9%, p = 0.011), anemia (36.5% vs.40.0% vs. 66.7%,p<0.001), hypertension (67.9% vs.75.0% vs. 88.9%, p = 0.001), hypoalbuminemia (36.2±4.6 g/L vs. 33.7±4.3 g/L vs. 31.3±4.9 g/L, p<0.001), SBP(133.2±20.0 mmHg vs. 137.6±20.1 mmHg vs. 141.8±27.1 mmHg, p = 0.002), HbA1c (7.6±1.5% vs. 8.5±2.2% vs. 7.8±1.6, p = 0.014), and use of diuretics (13.9% vs.18.3% vs. 38.9%, p<0.001). There was no difference in age, LVEF, periprocedural hypotension, periprocedural IABP, urinary pH, history of myocardial infarction, or hyperlipidemia.

Procedural characteristics

Table 2 lists the procedural characteristics of the patients. Compared with the negative and trace groups, the patients in the positive urine albumin group were hydrated with higher volumes

Table 1. Baseline Characteristics.

characteristics	Urinary Albumin				p			
	All (N = 597)	Negative (N = 483)	Trace (N = 60)	Positive (N = 54)	All	Negative vs. Trace	Trace vs. Positive	Positive vs. Negative
Female, n(%)	173(29.0%)	151(31.3%)	9(15.0%)	13(24.1%)	0.046	-	-	-
Age, years	65.1±10.1	65.0±10.1	64.7±10.0	66.5±9.5	0.541	-	-	-
eGFR,	77.8	80.2	72.3	54.5	<0.001*	-	-	-
ml/min/1.73 m^2	(61.6-96.7)	(64.0-98.9)	(50.6-97.3)	(31.1-74.8)				
SBP, mmHg	134.4±21.0	133.2±20.0	137.6±20.6	141.8±27.1	0.002	0.378#	0.838#	0.012#
DBP, mmHg	77.1±11.9	77.1±11.9	76.6±10.8	78.0±13.5	0.737	-	-	-
HR, bpm	74.7±11.7	74.6±11.3	75.1±11.4	75.7±14.1	0.461	-	-	-
LVEF, %	59.2±12.8	59.7±12.7	57.2±13.4	57.4±12.5	0.120	-	-	-
Hypotension, n(%)	14(2.3%)	12(2.5%)	1(1.7%)	1(1.9%)	0.682	-	-	-
IABP, n(%)	10(1.7%)	7(1.4%)	1(1.7%)	2(3.7%)	0.260	-	-	-
Congestive heart failure, n(%)	87(14.6%)	63(13.0%)	10 (16.7%)	14(25.9%)	0.011	-	-	-
Medical history								
Smoking, n(%)	20(34.3%)	162(33.5%)	28(46.7%)	15(27.8%)	0.965	-	-	-
Hypertension, n(%)	421(70.5%)	328(67. 9%)	45(75.0%)	48(88.9%)	0.001	-	-	-
Dyslipidemia, n(%)	82(13.7%)	69(14.3%)	6(10.0%)	7(13.0%)	0.555	-	-	-
Anemia, n(%)	235(39.6%)	175(36.5%)	24(40.0%)	36(66.7%)	<0.001	-	-	-
MI history, n(%)	87(14.6%)	66(13.7%)	8(13.3%)	13(24.1%)	0.075	-	-	-
CABG history, n(%)	7(1.2%)	6(1.2%)	1(1.7%)	0(0.0%)	0.552	-	-	-
Laboratory measurements								
SCr, μmol/L	84.0 (70.5-106.0)	82.0 (68.0–101.0)	94.4 (75.3–113.5)	117.6 (93.5–190.0)	<0.001*	-	-	-
BUN, mmol/L	5(4.0–6.4)	4.8(3.8–6.2)	5.4(4.4–7.0)	7.4(5.0–9.8)	<0.001*	-	-	-
TC, mmol/L	4.3±1.1	4.2±1.1	4.2±1.0	4.5±1.1	0.211	-	-	-
LDL-C, mmol/L	2.4(1.9–3.0)	2.4(1.9–3.0)	2.3(1.8–3.2)	2.5(2.0–3.1)	0.871*	-	-	-
TG, mmol/L	1.4(1.0–1.9)	1.4(1.0–1.9)	1.5(1.0–1.8)	1.5(1.2–2.6)	0.158*	–	-	-
HbA1c, %	7.7±1.6	7.6±1.5	8.5±2.2	7.8±1.6	0.014	<0.001#	0.029#	1.000#
Urinary PH<6,n(%)	179(30.0%)	140(29.0%)	20(33.3%)	19(35.2%)	0.271	-	-	-
PH<5.5	155	27	13	15				
PH = 5.5	24	13	7	4				
Hematocrit (%)	38.0±4.8	38.0±4.6	39.0±4.4	35.0±6.2	<0.001	1.000#	0.002#	<0.001#
Hemoglobin, g/L	129.2±16.5	130.22±15.4	132.0±16.2	116.8±20.6	<0.001	1.000#	<0.001#	<0.001#
Albumin, g/L	35.5±4.8	36.2±4.6	33.7±4.3	31.3±4.9	<0.001	0.049#	0.097#	<0.001#
Medicine usage								
ACEI/ARB, n (%)	531(88.9%)	434(89.9%)	49(81.7%)	48(88.9%)	0.351	-	-	-

Table 1. Cont.

characteristics	Urinary Albumin				p			
	All (N = 597)	Negative (N = 483)	Trace (N = 60)	Positive (N = 54)	All	Negative vs. Trace	Trace vs. Positive	Positive vs. Negative
β-blocker, n (%)	515(86.3%)	421(87.2%)	52(86.7%)	42(77.8%)	0.087	-	-	-
CCB, n (%)	156(26.2%)	116(24.1%)	18(30.0%)	22(40.7%)	0.007	-	-	-
Diuretics, n (%)	99(16.6%)	67(13.9%)	11(18.3%)	21(38.9%)	<0.001	-	-	-
Statin, n (%)	584(97.8%)	473(97.9%)	60(100.0%)	51(94.4%)	0.289	-	-	-
Insulin, n (%)	175 (29.3%)	125 (25.9%)	26 (43.3%)	24(44.4%)	<0.001	-	-	-
α-glycosidase inhibitors, n (%)	341(57.1%)	284(58.8%)	33(55.0%)	24(44.4%)	0.046	-	-	-
Sulfonylureas, n(%)	169(28.3%)	147(30.4%)	17(28.3%)	5(9.3%)	0.003	-	-	-
Repaglinide/Nateglinide, n(%)	80 (13.4%)	67 (13.9%)	8 (13.3%)	5 (9.3%)	0.381	-	-	-
Thiazolidinediones, n(%)	13(2.2%)	11(2.3%)	2 (3.3%)	0 (0%)	0.453	-	-	-

1. Data are expressed as number (%), or mean±SD for normally distributed data, or median (IQR) for unevenly distributed data.
2.* P was tested by Kruskal-Wallis test.
3. # P was tested by Bonferroni correction.
4. Chi-square test or Fisher exact test was used for the frequency of distribution. Means were compared by One-way ANOVA for normally distributed data.
5. SBP: Systolic blood pressure. DBP: diastolic blood pressure. BUN: blood urea nitrogen. LVEF: left ventricular ejection fraction; ACEI/ARB: angiotensin-converting enzyme inhibitor/angiotensin receptor blocker. CABG: coronary artery bypass grafting. CCB: Calcium channel blocker. MI: myocardial infarction. HbA1C: glycosylated hemoglobin A1c. LDL-C: low density lipoprotein-cholesterol. TG: Triglycerides.

Table 2. Procedural Characteristics.

Characteristics	Urinary Albumin				*p*
	All (N = 597)	**Negative (N = 483)**	**Trace (N = 60)**	**Positive (N = 54)**	
Number of lesions (n)	2.1±1.1	2.0±1.1	2.0±1.0	2.3±1.1	0.322
Number of stents (n)	1.6±1.4	1.5±1.4	1.6±1.4	1.6±1.2	0.945
Left main lesion (%)	64(10.7%)	54(11.2%)	5(8.3%)	5(9.3%)	0.520
Left main treated (%)	30(5.0%)	28(5.8%)	1(1.7%)	1(1.9%)	0.100
Total stent length (mm)	38.4±36.6	38.1±37.2	40.3±36.4	38.7±32.4	0.912
Contrast Type					0.263
Iopamidol	328(55.1%)	265(55.0%)	33(55.0%)	30(56.6%)	
Iopromide	238(40.0%)	199(41.3%)	23(38.3%)	16(30.2%)	
Iodixanol	25(4.2%)	16(3.3%)	3 (5.6%)	6 (11.3%)	
Contrast volume, ml	130 (80–170)	130 (80–165)	130 (100–150)	135 (77.5–172.5)	0.901*
Intravenous hydration volume, ml	500 (500–1000)	500 (500–1000)	500 (500–1000)	1000(500–1500)	0.002*

1. Data are expressed as number (%), or mean±SD for normally distributed data, or median (IQR) for unevenly distributed data.
2. *P was tested by Kruskal-Wallis test.
3. PCI: percutaneous coronary intervention.

of fluid (500 ml (IQR 500–1000 ml) and 500 ml (IQR 500–1000 ml) vs. 1000 ml (IQR 500–1500 ml); p = 0.002), presumably because patients with albuminuria presented with reduced baseline renal function and underwent longer hydration. There were no differences in the other procedural characteristics.

CI-AKI incidence and in-hospital outcomes

CI-AKI incidence and in-hospital clinical outcomes are displayed in Table 3. The CI-AKI incidence in positive urine albumin group was higher than the negative and trace groups (negative vs. trace vs. positive: 3.9% vs.6.7% vs. 18.5%, p<0.001). A difference was observed in dialysis frequency (0.2% vs. 1.7% vs. 1.9%, p = 0.005). No difference was observed regarding in-hospital death.

Multivariate analysis

Results of multivariate logistic regression analysis have been displayed in Table 4. After adjusting for potential confounding risk factors (Hosmer-Lemeshow Chi-square: 5.2, p = 0.520), and using the negative group as reference, the odds ratio (OR) of CI-AKI was 3.8 (95% CI: 1.5–9.2, p = 0.004) for the positive urine albumin group, but 1.4 (95%CI: 0.4–4.5, p = 0.562) for the trace urine albumin group. The OR of CI-AKI was 2.4 (95% CI: 1.1–5.1, p = 0.020) for urinary pH <6, and 2.5 (95% CI: 1.1–5.7, p = 0.023) for eGFR <60 ml/min/1.73 m^2. However, age >65 years and congestive heart failure were not associated with CI-AKI in this study.

Follow-up

Median follow-up was 23 months (IQR: 16 to 30 months). Clinical outcomes were available for 572 patients (95.8%). Forty-two (7.5%) patients died. Cardiac death occurred in 11 patients in the positive urine albumin group due to refractory heart failure (n = 6), acute myocardial infarction (n = 1), cardiac arrest (n = 1), or other cardiovascular causes (n = 3). In the trace urine albumin group, 4 cardiac deaths were caused by refractory heart failure (n = 1), acute myocardial infarction (n = 1), cardiac arrest (n = 1), or other cardiovascular causes (n = 1). In the negative urine albumin group, 16 cardiac deaths were attributed to refractory heart failure (n = 6), acute myocardial infarction (n = 6), sudden death (n = 2), or other cardiovascular causes (n = 2).

Table 3. CI-AKI incidence and Clinical outcomes in-hospital.

Outcomes	Urinary Albumin				*p*
	All (N = 597)	**Negative (N = 483)**	**Trace (N = 60)**	**Positive (N = 54)**	
CI-AKI					
SCr increase≥26.4μmol/L or ≥50%, n(%)	33(5.5%)	19(3.9%)	4(6.7%)	10(18.5%)	<0.001
SCr increase≥26.4μmol/L, n(%)	31(5.2%)	18(3.7%)	3(5.0%)	10(18.5%)	<0.001
SCr increase≥50%, n(%)	10(1.7%)	6(1.2%)	2(3.3%)	2 (3.7%)	0.101
Absolute change in SCr, μmol/L	1.3(−5.8–10.0)	0.9(−5.5–9.0)	2.3(−6.0–10.0)	10.1(−7.8–20.1)	0.016*
Death, n(%)	3 (0.5%)	1(0.2%)	2(3.3%)	0(0%)	0.280
Dialysis, n(%)	2(0.5%)	0(0%)	1(1.7%)	1(1.9%)	0.005

CI-AKI: contrast-induced acute kidney injury; SCr: serum creatinine;
* P was tested by Kruskal-Wallis test.

Table 4. Univariate and multivariate analyses of predictors for CI-AKI.

Risk factors	Univariate analysis			Multivariate analysis		
	OR	95%CI	*p*	OR	95%CI	*p*
Urinary Albumin			<0.001			0.015
Negative	-	-	-	-	-	-
Trace (vs. Negative)	1.7	0.6–5.3	0.327	1.4	0.4–4.5	0.562
Positive (vs. Negative)	5.6	2.4–12.7	<0.001	3.8	1.5–9.2	0.004
Urinary PH<6.0	3.0	1.5–6.1	0.002	2.4	1.1–5.1	0.020
eGFR<60 ml/min/1.73 m^2	5.0	2.4–10.3	<0.001	2.5	1.1–5.7	0.023
Age>65 years	2.6	1.2–5.8	0.016	1.8	0.8–4.1	0.191
Congestive heart failure*	3.7	1.8–7.9	0.001	2.1	0.9–4.8	0.074

*Congestive heart failure was defined as New York Heart Association functional classification III/IV and/or history of pulmonary edema.
Hosmer-Lemeshow Chi-square: 5.2, $p = 0.520$.

The cumulative rate of all-cause death (33.4% vs. 7.3%, log rank P<0.001) (Fig.1), cardiac death (30.7% vs. 5.2%, log rank P<0.001) (Fig.2) and dialysis (10.9% vs. 0.7%, log rank P< 0.001)(Fig.3) were higher in patients with CI-AKI compared with those without.

Discussion

The present study suggests that pre-procedural urinary albumin levels, urinary pH <6 and eGFR <60 ml/min/1.73 m^2 were independent predictors for CI-AKI in patients with T2DM undergoing elective cardiac catheterization (CAG or PCI).

The mechanism of CI-AKI/contrast-induced nephropathy (CIN) is not clear. However, it probably involves the direct toxic

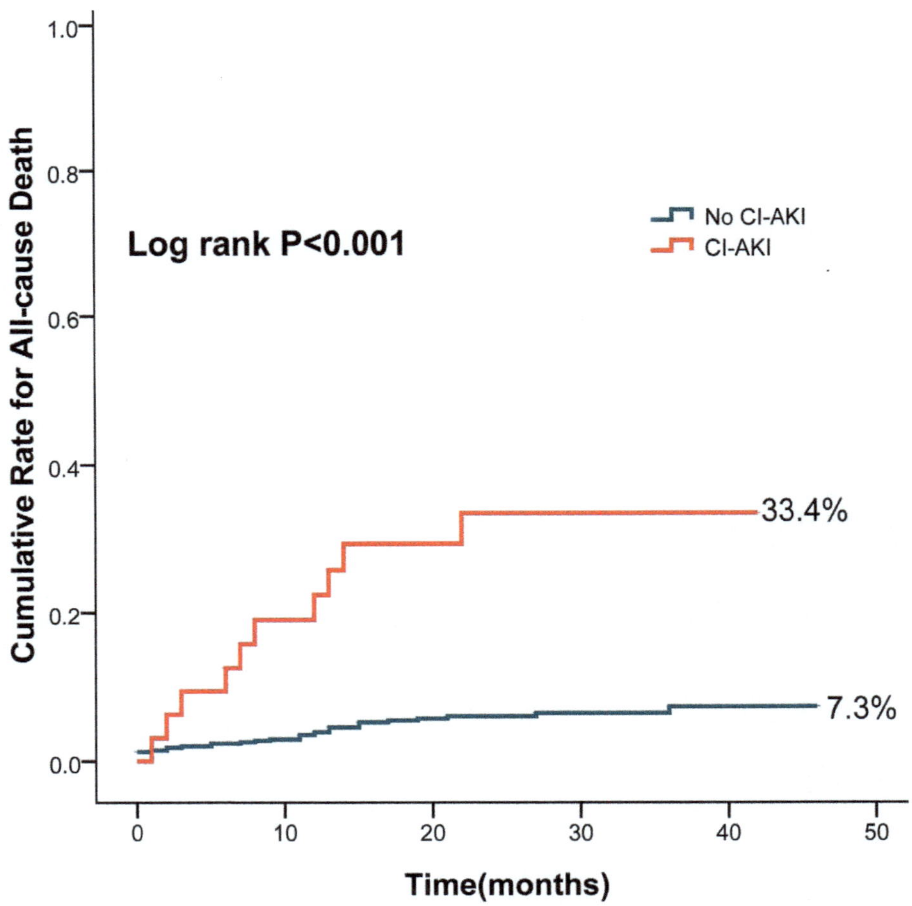

Figure 1. Cumulative rates for all-cause death in patients with CI-AKI and without CI-AKI.

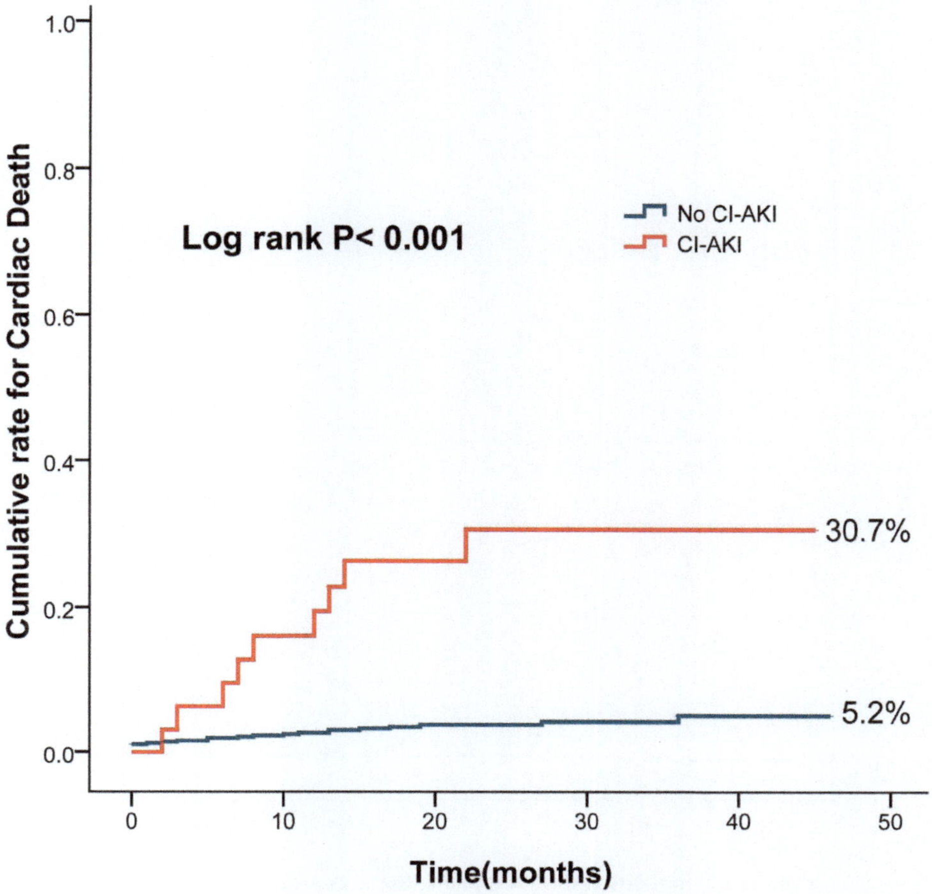

Figure 2. Cumulative rates for cardiac death in patients with CI-AKI and without CI-AKI.

effect of contrast agents and decreased renal medullary blood flow resulting in medullary ischemia that may lead to enhanced ROS formation and oxidative stress.

Many studies have indicated that preexisting renal disease [13,16,17] and T2DM [13,16–20] are risk factors for CI-AKI/CIN. In the Mehran's study, preexisting renal disease including eGFR <60 ml/min/1.73 m^2 or serum creatinine >1.5 mg/dl, is an independent predictor of CIN [13]. European Society of Urogenital Radiology (ESUR) contrast media safety Committee [14] considers that serum creatinine is not an ideal marker for renal function, and support eGFR to identify impaired renal function. In present study, eGFR <60 ml/min/1.73 m^2 was an independent risk factors for CI-AKI (OR = 2.5, 95% CI: 1.1–5.7, P = 0.023). The possible reason is that preexisting renal disease is associated with a decreased vasodilatory response and slower clearance of contrast media compared to normal subjects. Besides, in the Mehran's study [13], T2DM is an independent predictor of CIN. The possible mechanisms are: impaired endothelial function, caused by persistent hyperglycemia [21], leading to impaired renal vasomotor function and renal ischemia; and increased ROS generationas well as preexisting renal failure or metabolic syndrome [17].

Albuminuria may be an additional risk factor for T2DM patients. Albumin is almost totally restricted by the glomerular barrier, filtered albumin is reabsorbed by the proximal tubular cells [22], degraded there, and brings about inflammatory and fibrogenic mediators resulting in inflammation and fibrosis, followed by loss of renal function [22,23]. Albuminuria may contribute to the pathogenesis of CI-AKI/CIN by its toxic effects on the tubular system [24]. Albuminuria could activate Fas-mediated and peroxisome proliferator-activated receptor-γ-dependent apoptosis, and induce proinflammatory molecules, leading to apoptosis and damage of the renal tubular system [25–32]. In addition, albumin overload in proximal tubules could induce ROS formation, which activates NF-κB and consequently evokes NF-κB-dependent inflammatory reactions [33]. Moreover, in animal models of massive proteinuria, excessive oxidative stress induced by oxidized fatty acid was noted in regions with renal tubular damage [34]. Albuminuria and contrast media may share similar effects on kidneys [24], and may coordinate with each other in the pathogenesis of CI-AKI/CIN.

James et al. [7] demonstrated that the incidence of AKI is about 4 times higher in patients with heavy albuminuria (relative risk: 4.4 vs. no albuminuria, 95% CI: 3.7–5.2). Furthermore, long-term outcomes such as dialysis, death and composite renal outcomes are worse in patients with heavy albuminuria. In other studies [8,35–38], similar conclusions were reached, i.e. that albuminuria was an independent risk factor for AKI, renal and cardiovascular events, and all-cause mortality. In addition, albuminuria and eGFR were independently associated with AKI [39]. Chronic kidney disease (CKD) is defined as either kidney damage (proteinuria, hematuria or anatomical abnormality) or eGFR<60 ml/min/1.73 m^2 present on at least 2 occasions for ≥3 months [40]. The diagnosis of proteinuria supports the diagnosis of CKD in T2DM patients, independently of eGFR values [41]. Albuminuria may represent another type of CKD. Albuminuria may be an independent

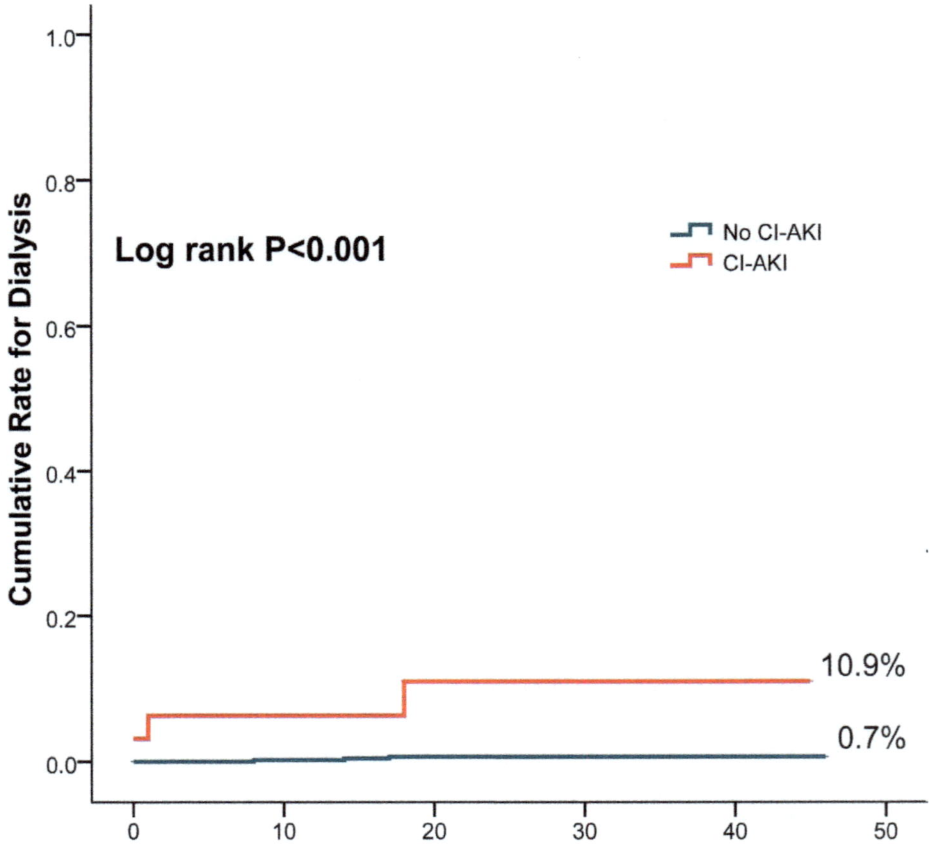

Figure 3. Cumulative rates for dialysis in patients with CI-AKI and without CI-AKI.

predictor for CI-AKI. A recent study [24] concluded that proteinuria may be a new risk factor for CIN in CKD patients; however, the sample size was small. Our data supported the hypothesis that urinary albumin levels were associated with CI-AKI incidence, and that albuminuria was an independent risk factor for CI-AKI in patients with T2DM.

ROS formation plays an important role in the development of CI-AKI/CIN [42] and may be promoted by an acidic urinary environment, but is inhibited by higher pH [22,39], and alkalinizing renal tubular fluid with bicarbonate may reduce injury. As with others, this is the most important mechanism why sodium bicarbonate provided more protection than sodium chloride in animal models for acute ischemic renal failure [43], clinical trials [9,44,45] and meta analyses [46–48] for CIN. Besides, sodium bicarbonate appears capable to scavenge ROS, and increasing urine flow. Additional, sodium bicarbonate avoids the large amounts of chloride which is in isotonic saline that may cause constriction of the renal vasculature. Therefore, guidelines by ESUR contrast media safety Committee considers that sodium bicarbonate seems to provide equal or superior protection to isotonic saline [14]. Actually, urinary pH is used in the diagnosis of renal tubular acidosis (RTA), despite its low specificity. Urinary pH could partly indicate renal tubular fluid pH, and a low urinary pH (<5.5) could be found in various forms of RTA (mostly in types 2 and 4 RTA) [49,50]. In the present study, among patients with urinary pH <6 most (n = 155, 86.59%) were of <5.5, and some may be with RTA. In a recent study[51], CIN incidence was significantly lower in patients with urinary pH >6 (32.8% vs. 2.2% in those with urinary pH >6, P<0.0001). The study by Merten et al. [9] showed that lower post-procedure urinary pH (5.6±0.6 vs.6.5±0.8, P = 0.002) and lower CIN incidence in the group hydrated by sodium bicarbonate compared with sodium chloride. Despite a small sample size (n = 119) and a weak statistical power [52], patients with urinary pH <6 may be a population that could benefit from bicarbonate hydration to prevent CI-AKI/CIN. Another study [53] concluded that daily oral sodium bicarbonate could slow eGFR decline and reduce urinary albumin based on a 5-year follow-up.

Albuminuria and urinary pH <6 are valuable for identifying patients at high risk of CI-AKI. What adds to the value of these parameters is that they are included in the routine test for every patient, and easy to obtain from preoperative urinalysis. Using these existing data, we may assess every patient more accurately and give him/her more precise risk stratification, importantly, with no additional cost and little effort.

Limitations

Our study has several limitations. First, this study was observational, of moderate-scale, and from a single center. Some patients were excluded such as patients with a nephrotic syndrome. The results should be confirmed in a large-scale multicenter clinical trial, including patients excluded from the current analysis. Second, treatment-related details in coronary artery disease were not available. Available information was restricted to cardiovascular drugs used. Finally, the data of some useful biochemical parameters such as cystatin C and urinary albumin/creatinine ratio were lacking in the present study.

Conclusions

Preprocedural albuminuria and urinary pH <6 were independent factors for CI-AKI in T2DM patients undergoing elective cardiac catheterization. Urinary albumin levels and urinary pH may be potential biochemical parameters for screening high-risk patients.

Acknowledgments

We would like to express our deep appreciation to Gary S. Mintz, Cardiovascular Research Foundation, New York, USA, for his insight and editorial assistance.

Author Contributions

Conceived and designed the experiments: JYC YLZ. Performed the experiments: JQY PR. Analyzed the data: JQY PR YTH. Wrote the paper: JQY PR. Contributed to revising manuscript critically for important intellectual content: LWL NT GL YL SS. Contributed to acquisition of data: JXZ JYZ.

References

1. Parfrey P. (2005) The clinical epidemiology of contrast-induced nephropathy. Cardiovasc Intervent Radiol 28 Suppl 2:S3–S11.
2. Mccullough P A, Stacul F, Becker C R, Adam A, Lameire N, et al. (2006) Contrast-Induced Nephropathy (CIN) Consensus Working Panel: executive summary. Rev Cardiovasc Med 7:177–197.
3. Mccullough P A, Wolyn R, Rocher L L, Levin R N, O'Neill WW. (1997) Acute renal failure after coronary intervention: incidence, risk factors, and relationship to mortality. Am J Med 103:368–375.
4. Tublin M E, Murphy M E, Tessler F N. (1998) Current concepts in contrast media-induced nephropathy. AJR Am J Roentgenol 171:933–939.
5. Gupta R, Gurm H S, Bhatt D L, Chew DP, Ellis SG. (2005) Renal failure after percutaneous coronary intervention is associated with high mortality. Catheter Cardiovasc Interv 64:442–448.
6. Weisbord S D, Chen H, Stone R A, Kip K E, Fine M J et al. (2006) Associations of increases in serum creatinine with mortality and length of hospital stay after coronary angiography. J Am Soc Nephrol 17:2871–2877.
7. James M T, Hemmelgarn B R, Wiebe N, Pannu N, Manns BJ et al. (2010) Glomerular filtration rate, proteinuria, and the incidence and consequences of acute kidney injury: a cohort study. Lancet 376:2096–2103.
8. Ninomiya T, Perkovic V, de Galan B E, Zoungas S, Pillai A et al. (2009) Albuminuria and kidney function independently predict cardiovascular and renal outcomes in diabetes. J Am Soc Nephrol, 20:1813–1821.
9. Merten G J, Burgess W P, Gray L V, Holleman J H, Roush T S et al. (2004) Prevention of contrast-induced nephropathy with sodium bicarbonate: a randomized controlled trial. JAMA 291:2328–2334.
10. National Kidney Foundation. (2002) K/DOQI clinical practice guidelines for chronic kidney disease: evaluation, classification, and stratification. Am J Kidney Dis 39:S1–S266.
11. Levine G N, Bates E R, Blankenship J C, Bailey SR, Bittl JA et al. (2011) 2011 ACCF/AHA/SCAI Guideline for Percutaneous Coronary Intervention: executive summary: a report of the American College of Cardiology Foundation/American Heart Association Task Force on Practice Guidelines and the Society for Cardiovascular Angiography and Interventions.Circulation 124:2574–2609.
12. Gavi S, Hensley J. (2009) Diagnosis and management of type 2 diabetes in adults: a review of the ICSI guideline. Geriatrics 64:12–17, 29.
13. Mehran R, Aymong E D, Nikolsky E, Lasic Z, Iakovou I et al. (2004) A simple risk score for prediction of contrast-induced nephropathy after percutaneous coronary intervention: development and initial validation. J Am Coll Cardiol 44:1393–1399.
14. Stacul F, van der Molen A J, Reimer P, Webb J A, Thomsen H S et al. (2011) Contrast induced nephropathy: updated ESUR Contrast Media Safety Committee guidelines. EurRadiol, 21:2527–2541.
15. Yang Z K, Zhang R Y, Hu J, Zhang Q, Ding FH et al. (2013) Impact of successful staged revascularization of a chronic total occlusion in the non-infarct-related artery on long-term outcome in patients with acute ST-segment elevation myocardial infarction. Int J Cardiol 165:76–79.
16. Rihal C S, Textor S C, Grill D E, Berger P B, Ting H H et al. (2002) Incidence and prognostic importance of acute renal failure after percutaneous coronary intervention. Circulation 105:2259–2264.
17. Toprak O, Cirit M, Yesil M, Bayata S, Tanrisev M et al. (2007) Impact of diabetic and pre-diabetic state on development of contrast-induced nephropathy in patients with chronic kidney disease. Nephrol Dial Transplant 22:819–826.
18. Dangas G, Iakovou I, Nikolsky E, Aymong E D, Mintz G S et al. (2005) Contrast-induced nephropathy after percutaneous coronary interventions in relation to chronic kidney disease and hemodynamic variables. Am J Cardiol 95:13–19.
19. Klima T, Christ A, Marana I, Kalbermatter S, Uthoff H et al. (2012) Sodium chloride vs. sodium bicarbonate for the prevention of contrast medium-induced nephropathy: a randomized controlled trial. Eur Heart J 33:2071–2079.
20. Lindsay J, Canos D A, Apple S, Pinnow E, Aggrey G K et al. (2004) Causes of acute renal dysfunction after percutaneous coronary intervention and comparison of late mortality rates with postprocedure rise of creatine kinase-MB versus rise of serum creatinine. Am J Cardiol 94(6):786–789.
21. Kamdar A, Weidmann P, Makoff D L, Massry SG. (1977) Acute renal failure following intravenous use of radiographic contrast dyes in patients with diabetes mellitus. Diabetes 26:643–649.
22. Gorriz J L, Martinez-Castelao A. (2012) Proteinuria: detection and role in native renal disease progression. Transplant Rev (Orlando) 26:3–13.
23. Birn H, Christensen E I. (2006) Renal albumin absorption in physiology and pathology. Kidney Int 69:440–449.
24. Piskinpasa S, Altun B, Akoglu H, Yildirim T, Agbaht K et al. (2013) An uninvestigated risk factor for contrast-induced nephropathy in chronic kidney disease: proteinuria. Ren Fail 35:62–65.
25. Wang Y, Rangan G K, Tay Y C, Wang Y, Harris D C. (1999) Induction of monocyte chemoattractant protein-1 by albumin is mediated by nuclear factor kappaB in proximal tubule cells. J Am Soc Nephrol,10:1204–1213.
26. Erkan E, De Leon M, Devarajan P. (2001) Albumin overload induces apoptosis in LLC-PK(1) cells. Am J Physiol Renal Physiol 280:F1107–F1114.
27. Arici M, Chana R, Lewington A, Brown J, Brunskill N J. (2003) Stimulation of proximal tubular cell apoptosis by albumin-bound fatty acids mediated by peroxisome proliferator activated receptor-gamma. J Am Soc Nephrol 14:17–27.
28. Tang S, Leung J C, Abe K, Chan KW, Chan LY et al. (2003) Albumin stimulates interleukin-8 expression in proximal tubular epithelial cells in vitro and in vivo. J Clin Invest 111:515–527.
29. Zoja C, Morigi M, Figliuzzi M, Bruzzi I, Oldroyd S et al. (1995) Proximal tubular cell synthesis and secretion of endothelin-1 on challenge with albumin and other proteins. Am J Kidney Dis 26:934–941.
30. Cameron J S. (1990) Proteinuria and progression in human glomerular diseases. Am J Nephrol Suppl 1:81–87.
31. Abbate M, Benigni A, Bertani T, Remuzzi G.(1999) Nephrotoxicity of increased glomerular protein traffic. Nephrol Dial Transplant 14:304–312.
32. Ohse T, Inagi R, Tanaka T, Ota T, Miyata T et al. (2006) Albumin induces endoplasmic reticulum stress and apoptosis in renal proximal tubular cells. Kidney Int 70:1447–1455.
33. Morigi M, Macconi D, Zoja C, Donadelli R, Buelli S et al. (2002) Protein overload-induced NF-kappaB activation in proximal tubular cells requires H(2)O(2) through a PKC-dependent pathway. J Am Soc Nephrol 13:1179–1189.
34. Kanaguchi Y, Suzuki Y, Osaki K, Sugaya T, Horikoshi S et al. (2011) Protective effects of L-type fatty acid-binding protein (L-FABP) in proximal tubular cells against glomerular injury in anti-GBM antibody-mediated glomerulonephritis. Nephrol Dial Transplant 26:3465–3473.
35. Grams M E, Astor B C, Bash L D, Matsushita K, Wang Y et al. (2010) Albuminuria and estimated glomerular filtration rate independently associate with acute kidney injury. J Am Soc Nephrol 21:1757–1764.
36. Huang T M, Wu V C, Young G H, Lin YF, Shiao CC et al. (2011) Preoperative proteinuria predicts adverse renal outcomes after coronary artery bypass grafting. J Am Soc Nephrol 22:156–163.
37. Hemmelgarn B R, Manns B J, Lloyd A, James MT, Klarenbach S et al. (2010) Relation between kidney function, proteinuria, and adverse outcomes. JAMA 303:423–429.
38. Hillege H L, Fidler V, Diercks G F, van Gilst WH, de Zeeuw D et al. (2002) Urinary albumin excretion predicts cardiovascular and noncardiovascular mortality in general population. Circulation 106:1777–1782.
39. Hingorani S R, Seidel K, Lindner A, Aneja T, Schoch G et al. (2008) Albuminuria in hematopoietic cell transplantation patients: prevalence, clinical associations, and impact on survival. Biol Blood Marrow Transplant 14:1365–1372.
40. The National Collaborating Centre for Chronic Conditions (UK). (2008) Chronic Kidney Disease: National clinical guideline for early identification andmanagement in adults in primary and secondary care.Royal College of Physicians (UK); Sep.
41. Wijns W, Kolh P, Danchin N, Di Mario C, Falk V et al. (2010) Guidelines on myocardial revascularization. Eur Heart J 31:2501–2555.
42. Heyman S N, Rosen S, Khamaisi M, Idée JM, Rosenberger C et al. (2010) Reactive oxygen species and the pathogenesis of radiocontrast-induced nephropathy. Invest Radiol 45:188–195.

43. Atkins J L.(1986) Effect of sodium bicarbonate preloading on ischemic renal failure. Nephron 44:70–74.
44. Briguori C, Airoldi F, D'Andrea D, Bonizzoni E, Morici N et al. (2007) Renal Insufficiency Following Contrast Media Administration Trial (REMEDIAL): a randomized comparison of 3 preventive strategies. Circulation 115:1211–1217.
45. Recio-Mayoral A, Chaparro M, Prado B, Cózar R, Méndez I et al. (2007) The reno-protective effect of hydration with sodium bicarbonate plus N-acetylcysteine in patients undergoing emergency percutaneous coronary intervention: the RENO Study. J Am Coll Cardiol 49:1283–1288.
46. Meier P, Ko D T, Tamura A, Tamhane U, Gurm HS. (2009) Sodium bicarbonate-based hydration prevents contrast-induced nephropathy: a meta-analysis. BMC Med 7:23.
47. Navaneethan S D, Singh S, Appasamy S, Wing RE, Sehgal AR. (2009) Sodium bicarbonate therapy for prevention of contrast-induced nephropathy: a systematic review and meta-analysis. Am J Kidney Dis 53:617–627.
48. Hogan S E, L'Allier P, Chetcuti S, Grossman PM, Nallamothu BK et al. (2008) Current role of sodium bicarbonate-based preprocedural hydration for the prevention of contrast-induced acute kidney injury: a meta-analysis. Am Heart J 156:414–421.
49. Brown A S. (2010) Renal tubular acidosis. DimensCrit Care Nurs 29:112–119.
50. Smulders Y M, Frissen P H, Slaats E H, Silberbusch J. (1996) Renal tubular acidosis. Pathophysiology and diagnosis. Arch Intern Med 156:1629–1636.
51. Markota D, Markota I, Starcevic B, Tomic M, Prskalo Z et al. (2013) Prevention of contrast-induced nephropathy with Na/K citrate. Eur Heart J 34:2362–2367.
52. Pflueger A, Abramowitz D, Calvin A D. (2009) Role of oxidative stress in contrast-induced acute kidney injury in diabetes mellitus. Med Sci Monit 15:A125–A136.
53. de Brito-Ashurst I, Varagunam M, Raftery M J, Yaqoob MM. (2009)Bicar-Bicarbonate supplementation slows progression of CKD and improves nutritional status. J Am Soc Nephrol 20:2075–2084.

14

Longitudinal Hemodynamic Measurements in Swine Heart Failure Using a Fully Implantable Telemetry System

Jenny S. Choy[1], Zhen-Du Zhang[1], Koullis Pitsillides[2], Margo Sosa[3], Ghassan S. Kassab[1,4,5]*

1 Department of Biomedical Engineering, Indiana University Purdue University Indianapolis, Indianapolis, Indiana, United States of America, **2** Transonic EndoGear Inc., Davis, California, United States of America, **3** Transonic Systems Inc., Ithaca, New York, United States of America, **4** Department of Surgery, Indiana University, Indianapolis, Indiana, United States of America, **5** Department of Cellular and Integrative Physiology, Indiana University, Indianapolis, Indiana, United States of America

Abstract

Chronic monitoring of heart rate, blood pressure, and flow in conscious free-roaming large animals can offer considerable opportunity to understand the progression of cardiovascular diseases and can test new diagnostics and therapeutics. The objective of this study was to demonstrate the feasibility of chronic, simultaneous measurement of several hemodynamic parameters (left ventricular pressure, systemic pressure, blood flow velocity, and heart rate) using a totally implantable multichannel telemetry system in swine heart failure models. Two solid-state blood pressure sensors were inserted in the left ventricle and the descending aorta for pressure measurements. Two Doppler probes were placed around the left anterior descending (LAD) and the brachiocephalic arteries for blood flow velocity measurements. Electrocardiographic (ECG) electrodes were attached to the surface of the left ventricle to monitor heart rate. The telemeter body was implanted in the right side of the abdomen under the skin for approximately 4 to 6 weeks. The animals were subjected to various heart failure models, including volume overload (A-V fistula, n = 3), pressure overload (aortic banding, n = 2) and dilated cardiomyopathy (pacing-induced tachycardia, n = 3). Longitudinal changes in hemodynamics were monitored during the progression of the disease. In the pacing-induced tachycardia animals, the systemic blood pressure progressively decreased within the first 2 weeks and returned to baseline levels thereafter. In the aortic banding animals, the pressure progressively increased during the development of the disease. The pressure in the A-V fistula animals only showed a small increase during the first week and remained stable thereafter. The results demonstrated the ability of this telemetry system of long-term, simultaneous monitoring of blood flow, pressure and heart rate in heart failure models, which may offer significant utility for understanding cardiovascular disease progression and treatment.

Editor: Partha Mukhopadhyay, National Institutes of Health, United States of America

Funding: The authors have no support or funding to report.

Competing Interests: The authors have the following interests. M Sosa is employed by Transonic Systems Inc. and K Pitsillides by Endosomatic Systems Inc. There are no patents, products in development, or marketed products to declare.

* Email: gkassab@iupui.edu

Introduction

Blood pressure, blood flow and heart rate are often altered under different cardiovascular conditions, such as heart failure. The monitoring of these parameters is therefore seminal in the study of cardiovascular physiology, pathogenesis, pharmacology and treatment modalities. Although many methods have been used to perform these measurements, the animals are typically under anesthesia where the normal physiological regulation may be affected [23]. It is desirable to obtain these vitals in conscious animals, which is often achieved by restraining the animals and taking the measurements through indwelling exteriorized catheters and blood pressure cuffs. The restrain of the animals, however, introduces significant stress, and the measurements may be confounded by multiple factors such as increased plasma catecholamine and cortisol [18,21]. In addition, the presence of the indwelling catheters in chronic animal models increases the risk of thrombosis and infection.

Radio-telemetry is an alternative method that addresses some of these shortcomings. It provides continuous recordings without stress from any exogenous factors. This technology has been developed and tested in both small and large animals [2,16,24,25]. Most systems, however, only include channels for blood pressure and/or ECG measurements [9,16,26] or have limited battery power that only last for short periods of time [12,22].

We previously developed an implantable radio-telemetry system with multichannel and long life battery that was tested in normal animals [3]. In the present study, we have developed and tested a telemetry system (EndoGear1) that provides continuous recording of pressure, flow and ECG signals throughout the experimental period in the swine model during the progression of heart failure. The telemetry device has been made smaller and we further reduced the power consumption.

Materials and Methods

Telemetry implant and base station

The telemetry unit, the receiver, and the signal processing stations (Figure 1A) were provided by Transonic EndoGear Inc. The telemetry device consisted of two blood pressure channels, two Doppler-based flow channels, one temperature channel, and one ECG channel. The pressure transducers consisted of two 3Fr Millar pressure sensors, specially designed for the telemetry system, with a very low drift ($\pm$3 mmHg) over a year. The pressure sensors were calibrated before they were implanted in the animals, and recalibrated immediately after they were removed at the end of the study. Prior to the calibration, the sensors were soaked overnight in distilled water. The device was then equilibrated for 2 hrs. in a water bath at 38°C. The ECG component had a two-lead configuration and the electrodes were stainless steel for long-term stability. A temperature sensor embedded in the implant case was used to measure the animals' body temperature.

The implant was powered by a lithium battery (Table 1, Figure 1A), which lasted six to eight weeks depending on the monitoring mode. An automated timed acquisition mode was implemented to allow recording of the signal at different intervals to further extend the battery's life. The battery was attached to the implant through an implantable connector and it was surgically placed in the subcutaneous tissue for easy accessibility if replacement was necessary.

A remotely positioned radio frequency transceiver link was attached to the base station decoder/controller unit through a cable. This allowed the base station decoder/controller unit to be placed in a remote location away from the animals' housing, which minimized the effects of human presence. The transceiver was placed near the animals' cage, which allowed the swine free movement within the pen. The signals were automatically registered and saved in a computer using a data acquisition system (Biopac Systems, Inc., Goleta, CA). An illustration of the telemetry implant in an animal and the data acquisition system are shown in Figure 1B. The telemetry system was described in detail in our previous publication [3]. Table 1 describes the specifications of the telemetry system used in the present study. The system is available through Transonic EndoGear Inc.

Animal preparation

Eight Yorkshire swine (40–55 Kg body weight) of either sex were used in this study. The animals were divided into 3 groups according to the heart failure model: volume overload (arteriovenous, A-V fistula, n = 3), pressure overload (aortic banding, n = 2), and dilated cardiomyopathy (pacing-induced tachycardia, n = 3). The animals were fasted overnight and surgical anesthesia was induced with TKX (Telazol 10 mg/kg, Ketamine 5 mg/kg, Xylazine 5 mg/kg) and maintained with 1–2% Isoflurane-balance O_2. Electrocardiographic (ECG) leads were attached to the swine limbs. Body temperature was maintained at 37.5$\pm$0.5°C and pH at 7.4$\pm$0.1. Heart rate, respiratory rate, SpO_2 and $ETCO_2$ were monitored during the duration of the procedure. All animal experiments were performed in accordance with national and local ethical guidelines, including the Principles of Laboratory Animal Care, the Guide for the Care and Use of Laboratory Animals and the National Association for Biomedical Research [6,14], and an approved Indiana University Purdue University Indianapolis IACUC protocol regarding the use of animals in research.

Telemetry implant

The chest was opened through a median sternotomy under sterile conditions. A subcutaneous pouch was created on the right lumbar area of the abdomen to hold the implant unit and the battery. The flow probes, pressure sensors and ECG leads were tunneled subcutaneously towards the chest and into the chest cavity. The left anterior descending (LAD) artery was dissected free from the surrounding tissue and a 2.5 mm diameter Doppler flow transducer was secured around the artery. The proximal portion of the brachiocephalic artery close to the aortic arch was also dissected free from the surrounding tissue and a 4.5 mm diameter Doppler flow transducer was placed around the artery. The angle of the ultrasonic crystal (0.5 mm in diameter) embedded in the transducer was pre-fixed relative to the blood vessel wall and the space between the crystal and the vessel was filled with ultrasound gel. A Millar pressure sensor was inserted into the left ventricle (LV) through an 18 gauge needle puncture in the free wall close to the apex. Similarly, another pressure sensor was inserted into the aortic arch and advanced towards the descending aorta to measure systemic pressure. The two ECG leads were sutured to the surface of the heart, one close to the base and the other close to the apex. The pressure sensors and ECG electrodes were secured with silk suture on the heart's surface and the connecting cables were secured to the chest wall. All signals were monitored for approximately 15 minutes to attain stability before the chest was closed.

Heart failure models

Volume overload (A-V fistula). After adequate anesthesia, a mid-incision was made on the abdomen. The intestines and bladder were gently moved to one side inside the abdomen to expose the distal aorta and inferior vena cava. Heparin (~100 IU/kg) was administered to achieve an activated clotting time of >200 seconds prior to creation of the fistula. Both aorta and cava were carefully dissected and partially occluded with an atraumatic tissue clamp. A lateral incision (approximately 0.6 mm) was made on both the aorta and the cava and the free edges were sutured together to create the fistula. The clamp was released and the patency of the fistula confirmed.

Pressure overload (Aortic banding). The chest was opened through a mid sternotomy and the heart was cradled using the pericardial sac. The ascending aorta (above the aortic valve) was carefully dissected and a sterile constrictor (made of a cable tie recovered with tygon tubing) was placed around it. A Mikro-tip pressure sensor (Millar Instruments) was inserted into the aorta by needle puncture, and the constrictor was cinched until the aortic pressure doubled the baseline. The pressure was recorded for approximately 15 minutes to ensure stability.

Dilated cardiomyopathy (pacing-induced tachycardia). After opening the chest, two pacemaker leads were secured on the surface of the LV with non-absorbable sutures. The main lead was tunneled through the right fifth intercostal space from the chest cavity to the exterior. The lead was secured to the body of the pacemaker, and the pacemaker was then placed under the skin. The pace pulse was set at 190–230 bpm using a programmer.

All three heart failure models were established one week after the telemetry implant. The animals were followed for 4 to 6 weeks during the progression of the disease.

Statistical analysis

All data were expressed as mean $\pm$ SD. Comparisons of results between two groups were performed by a paired t-test. Multiple

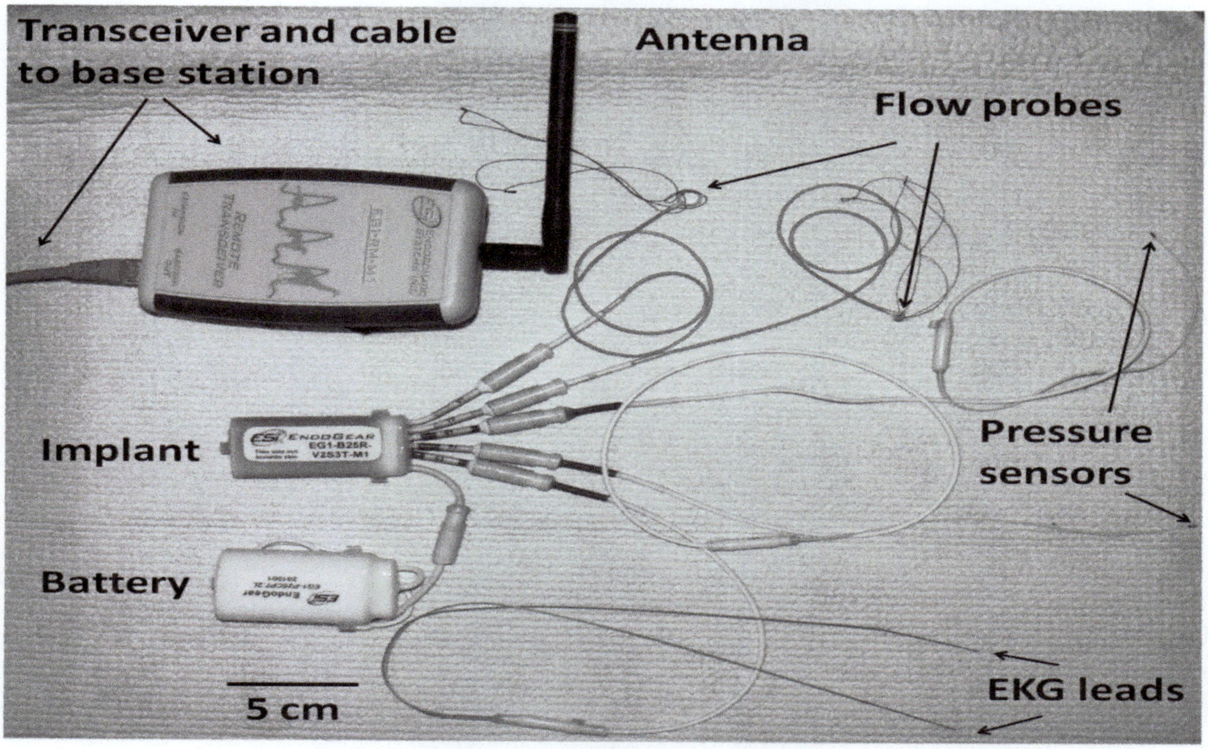

(A)

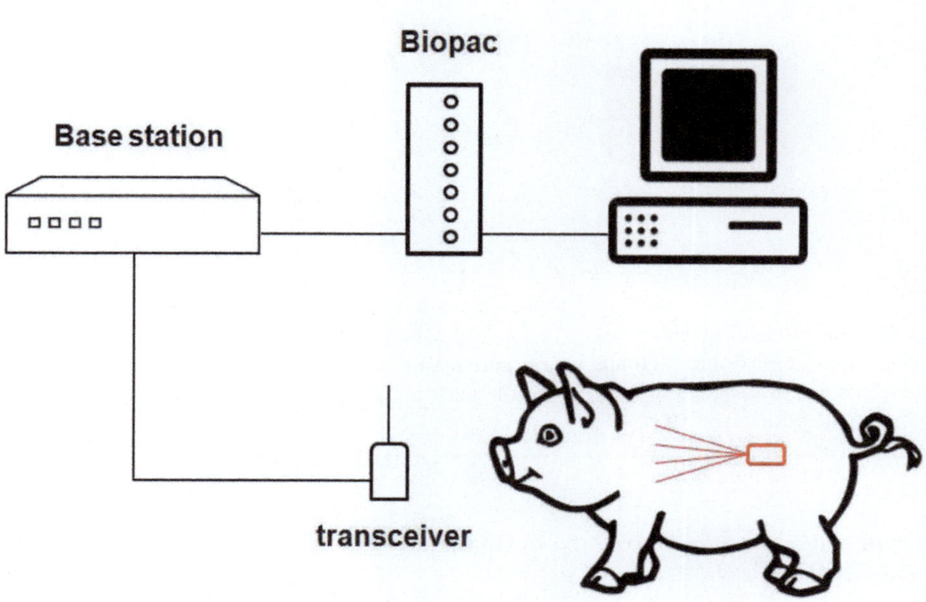

(B)

Figure 1. Components of the telemetry system (A) including the transceiver, the telemeter body, the battery, the Doppler flow probes, and the pressure and ECG sensors. The telemetry system uses detachable connectors for easy replacement of the battery and sensors if necessary. Illustration of the animal monitoring using the telemetry system and a schematic representation of the three heart failure models (B).

Table 1. A summary of the specifications for the EndoGear1 system.

SYSTEM SIGNALS	
Flow Velocity Channels	Configurable; up to 3
Biometric Sensor Channels	Configurable; up to 3
Temperature Channel	Sensor embedded in Implant; 1
Reference Barometric Pressure	Included in Base Station; 1
Signal Sampling Rate (all channels)	Normal: 120 Samples/sec; Reduced: 60 Samples/sec
DOPPLER FLOWMETER	
Ultrasound Frequency	20 MHz
Pulse Repetition Frequency	64 kHz maximum
Range Gate Adjustment Limits	0.7–8 mm in 0.7 mm increments
Doppler Frequency Shift Measured	±20 kHz
Blood Velocity Range	±120 cm/sec
Perivascular Cuff Probes	1.5–8 mm vessel diameter
Piezoelectric Doppler Transducer	0.7 mm diameter
BLOOD PRESSURE	
Range	−50 to 300 mmHg
Intravascular Pressure Sensor	3 French (1 mm diameter) typical
ECG	
Input Impedance	≥10 MΩ
Signal Band	0.5–50 Hz
TEMPERATURE	
Temperature Range	15–50°C
Resolution	0.0625°C
IMPLANT	
Case Volume (without connectors)	25 cc; 2.5″L ×1.25″ W ×0.5″ D
Power Consumption (maximum configuration)	On: 11 mAmp; Sleep: 1.8 mAmp
Battery Power Module	Lithium-thionyl chloride; size A- 3.6 V, AA-2.4 (disposable, non-rechargeable)
BASE STATION	
Dimensions	10.75″ L ×10″ W ×3.2″D
Weight	4 lbs.
Electrical Power	9 Vdc
Analog Output Signal Range	0–5 volts; all channels
Storage Temperature	−10 to 60°C; ≤90% humidity
Operational Temperature	0–40°C
RF TRANSCEIVER	
Operational RF Band (specific)	303, 315, 418, 433, 868, 916 MHz
Range (environmental dependent)	Monopole: 3–6 meters; 1 meter challenged
Planar	1–3 meters; 20–50 cm minimum

group comparisons were performed with analysis of variance (ANOVA). $P<0.05$ was considered statistically significant.

Results

Data acquisition at baseline

After the telemetry device was implanted, the measurements were recorded continuously during the first 24 hrs. to verify the stability of the device. The data were sampled at 100 Hz from the base station decoder/controller analog output using Acqknowledge software version 4 (Biopac Systems, Inc., Goleta, CA). Flow, pressure, and ECG signals were recorded at baseline (before any heart failure model was initiated), as shown in Figure 2A. The ECG signal was amplified and bandpass-filtered between 0.5 and 50 Hz. After the first day of implant, the measurements were continuously recorded for 20 min. every 2 hrs. in the awake, free-ranging animal. As shown in Figure 2, the directions of the maximum and minimum flow wave forms from the LAD and the brachiocephalic arteries were opposite as expected, while the pressure wave forms from the aorta and the LV were in the same direction. In one animal, we changed the telemetry's battery to test the effect of this procedure on the recordings. The wave forms for both flow and pressure before and after battery replacement showed no alteration (tracings not shown).

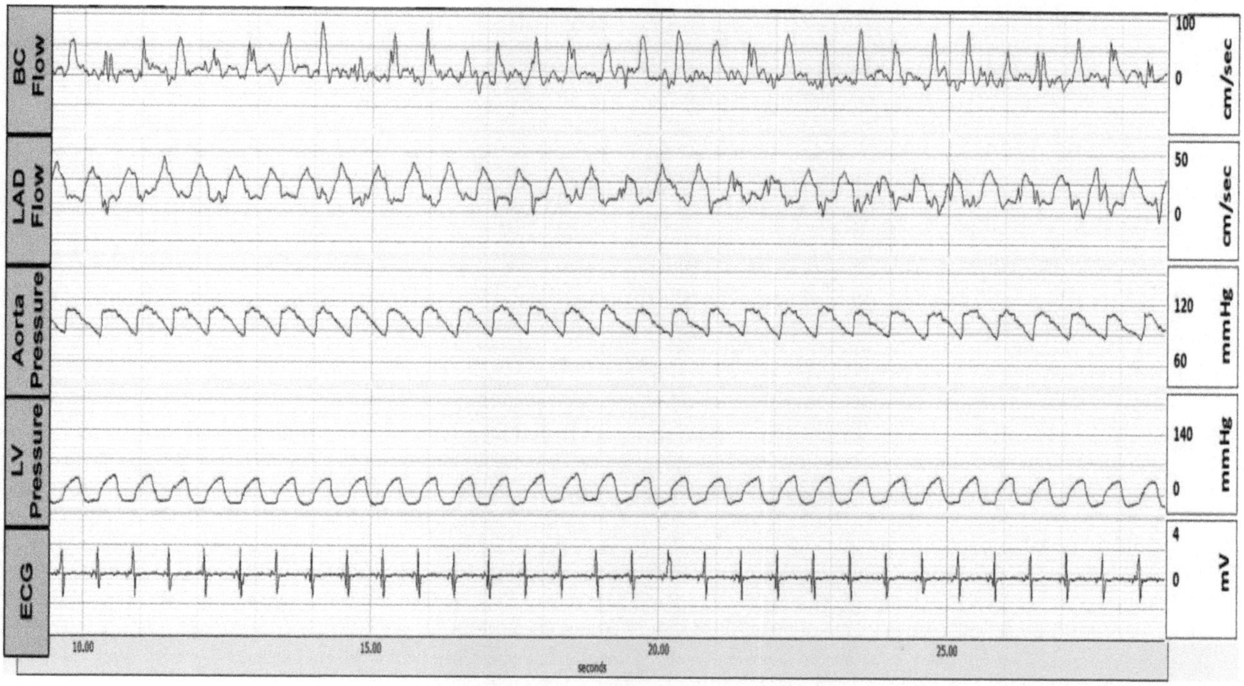

(A)

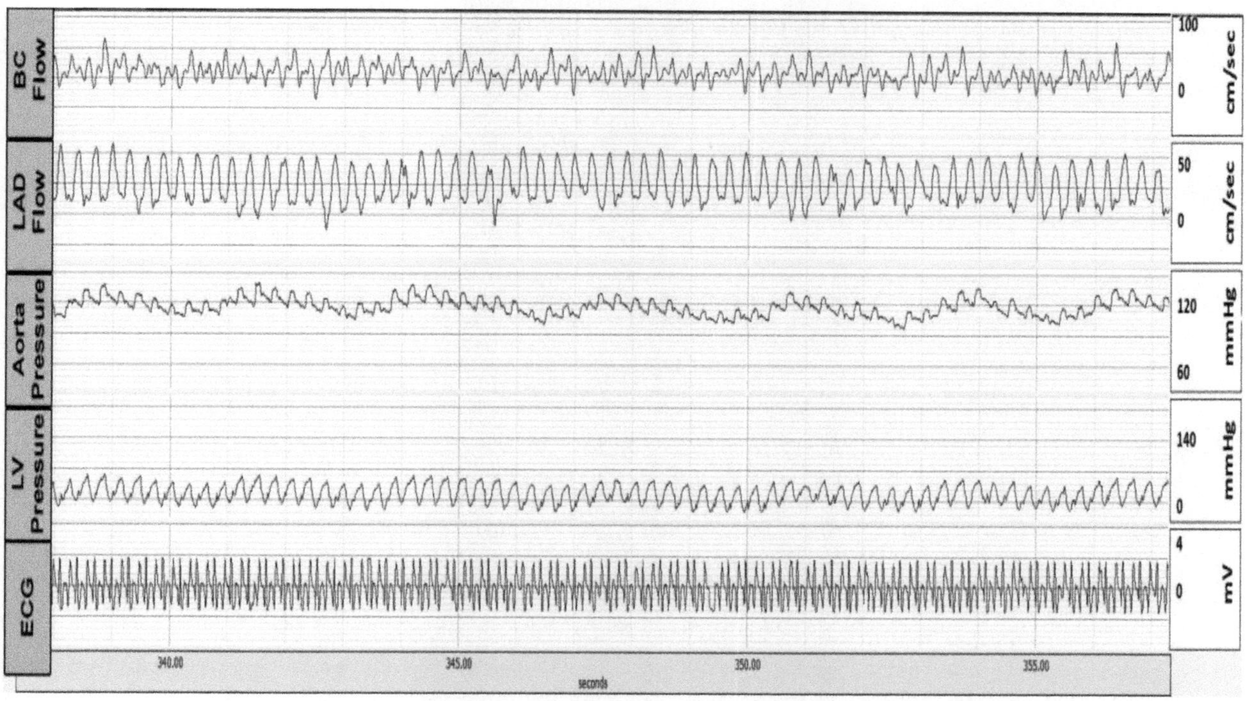

(B)

Figure 2. Baseline tracings of a representative pacing-induced tachycardia animal before the pacemaker was activated (A). Representative tracings when the animal was paced at 190 bpm (B).

Data acquisition during heart failure

All parameters were recorded under resting conditions for 20 minutes every 2 hrs. Once the animals developed end-stage heart failure, the parameters were recorded continuously. Figure 2 and Figure 3 show representative hemodynamic tracings in the awake, untethered swine before the development of heart failure as obtained directly from the telemetry system. Figure 4 shows different pressure changes in the aortic banding, A-V fistula, and pacing-induced tachycardia animals during the development of heart failure. In the aortic banding animals, the left ventricular end-systolic pressure (LVESP, 71±12.4 mmHg at baseline) immediately increased after the stenosis was created and continued to rise progressively during the first (176.1±18.2 mmHg, $p<0.001$) and second (200.3±15.4 mmHg) weeks. Interestingly, during the third week of aortic banding, the LVESP decreased (164.2±7.2 mmHg) significantly ($p<0.001$), and then progressively increased (180.3±26.5 mmHg) again until the end of the study duration (Figure 4A). The left ventricular end-diastolic pressure (LVEDP, 9±5.4 mmHg at baseline) did not change significantly (7.2±3.6 mmHg, $p=0.33$) during the first week post-stenosis but showed a significant increase (11.7±2.3 mmHg, $p<0.05$) during the second week. Thereafter, the LVEDP progressively decreased (8.4±6.6 mmHg) to approximately the baseline values (7.1±12.9 mmHg) by the end of the study (Figure 4B). The mean aortic pressure (MAP, 93±18.6 mmHg at baseline) immediately increased after the stenosis and continued to rise progressively during the first (144.6±24.9 mmHg, $p<0.05$) and second (180±21.9 mmHg) weeks. Similar to the pattern observed for the LVESP, the mean aortic pressure significantly decreased (156.3±14.5 mmHg, $p=0.05$) during the third week, and then progressively increased (187.9±38.9 mmHg) again until the end of the study (Figure 4C).

In the A-V fistula animals, the LVESP (140±12.8 mmHg at baseline) fluctuated during the development of heart failure (125.9±36.4 mmHg at week 1, 146.3±25.7 mmHg at week 2, and 102±38.2 mmHg at week 3), increasing significantly (207.25±17 mmHg, $p<0.001$) by the end of the study (Figure 4A). The LVEDP (21±9.5 mmHg at baseline), progressively decreased to negative values until the third week (0±20 mmHg at week 1, −16.6±16.4 mmHg at week 2, and −6.5±24.7 mmHg at week 3), and then significantly increased (89.5±6.6 mmHg, $p<0.001$) by the end of the study (Figure 4B). The MAP (107±8.3 mmHg at baseline) progressively increased (112±14 mmHg at week 1, 125.3±9.1 mmHg at week 2, and 127.5±2.1 mmHg at week 3, $p<0.05$) during the development of heart failure (Figure 4C).

In the high-rate pacing animals, the LVESP (106±48.8 mmHg at baseline) immediately dropped (70±14.2 mmHg) after initiation of pacing, and monotonically decreased thereafter until the end of the study (49±4.5 mmHg), although the values between baseline and end-stage heart failure were not significantly different ($p=0.18$, Figure 4A). The LVEDP (15±8.5 mmHg at baseline) fluctuated during the development of heart failure (27±6.9 mmHg at week 1, 13±25.3 mmHg at week 2, 24±4.5 mmHg at week 3, and 13±9.5 mmHg at week 4) ending at 32±3.8 mmHg by the end of the study (Figure 4B). The MAP (100±9.9 mmHg at baseline) progressively decreased during the first two weeks of pacing (98±29.1 mmHg at week 1 and 64±2.4 mmHg at week 2), showing a progressive increased (77±10.5 mmHg at week 3, 126±3.2 mmHg at week 4, and 145±4.5 mmHg at week 5, $p<0.05$) until the end of the study (Figure 4C).

Figure 5 shows flow velocity measurements in the LAD and brachiocephalic arteries in the A-V fistula (Figures 5A and 5B, respectively) and aortic banding (Figures 5C and 5D, respectively) animals. In the A-V fistula animals, the LAD max flow velocity (32±9 cm/s at baseline) increased (50.2±9.2 cm/s) during the first week of disease, and thereafter progressively decreased (43.3±2.1 cm/s at week 2, 31.5±0.7 cm/s at week 3, and 7.7±2.5 mmHg at week 4, $p<0.05$) throughout the remainder of the study duration (Figure 5A). The LAD min flow velocity (−4±7.9 cm/s at baseline) also increased (6±3.5 cm/s) during the first week, and thereafter decreased monotonically (3.6±2.9 cm/s at week 2, −1.3±2.5 mmHg at week 3, and −21.7±1.5 cm/s at week 4, $p<0.05$) with the development of heart failure (Figure 5A). The brachiocephalic max flow velocity (87±2.2 cm/s at baseline) progressively decreased (81.3±9.1 cm/s at week 1, 66.8±6.7 cm/s at week 2, 63.5±0.7 cm/s at week 3, and 57.7±9.5 cm/s at week 4, $p<0.05$) during the development of the disease (Figure 5B). The brachiocephalic min flow velocity (−52±1.3 cm/s at baseline) progressively increased during the development of heart failure (−51±6.9 cm/s at week 1, −44.3±5.3 cm/s at week 2, −41.5±4.9 cm/s at week 3, and −31.7±5.8 cm/s at week 4, $p<0.05$). Interestingly, the difference between max and min flow velocity (pulse velocity) decreased with the progression of the disease (Figure 5B).

In the aortic banding animals (Figures 5C and 5D), the LAD max flow velocity (22±6.8 cm/s at baseline) progressively increased after banding (60.3±8.2 cm/s at week 1) but decreased by the end of the study (53.6±8.2 cm/s, $p<0.001$, Figure 5C). The LAD min flow velocity (−10±8.6 cm/s at baseline) progressively decreased during the development of the disease (−20.2±12.8 cm/s at the end) although the values were not significantly different ($p=0.24$, Figure 5C). The progressive increase in negative flow (flow reversal) has been observed in patients with LV hypertrophy in conditions such as aortic stenosis. The brachiocephalic max flow velocity (64±5.3 cm/s at baseline) progressively decreased in the aortic banding animals over the duration of the study (39.4±13 cm/s, $p<0.05$, Figure 5D). The brachiocephalic min flow (−12±2.1 cm/s at baseline) progressively decreased (−33.6±4.7 cm/s, $p<0.001$) during the development of the disease (Figure 5D).

Transient changes were detected by telemetry in the heart failure animals. Figure 6 shows a transient decrease in both aortic and LV pressure (negative pressure) detected by telemetry in one representative animal with high-rate pacing. Figure 6 also shows the corresponding increase in the LAD flow velocity.

Discussion

Longitudinal measurements of hemodynamic vitals in large animal models of cardiovascular chronic disease have numerous utilities. Telemetry has been extensively used in different animal models to understand the progression of cardiovascular diseases. Swine models are commonly used to study the mechanisms of heart failure and to develop new diagnostics and therapies. We have previously demonstrated that a biotelemetry system can reliably monitor blood flow and pressure in freely roaming normal animals [3,8]. In the swine model, the present study demonstrated that continuous recording of pressure, flow, and electrical activity of the heart using an implantable telemetric system effectively revealed hemodynamic changes during the progression of heart failure. The data were recorded while the animals were freely ranging in the cage, and the telemetry receiver provided good quality signals to the software allowing reliable data analysis. The surgical procedure to implant the telemetry device unlikely affected the cardiovascular physiology and disease progression, and when properly implanted, the telemetric system and the connecting cables did not impede proper visualization of the heart during echocardiography.

The development of implantable biotelemetry systems has been pursued for several decades [3,7,10,11,25]. One of the major challenges, however, has been the high power requirements for multiple channels to measure both blood flow and pressure simultaneously [12,22], which can limit the applicability of the telemetry in many studies that require animal monitoring for extended periods of time. The telemetry system used in the present

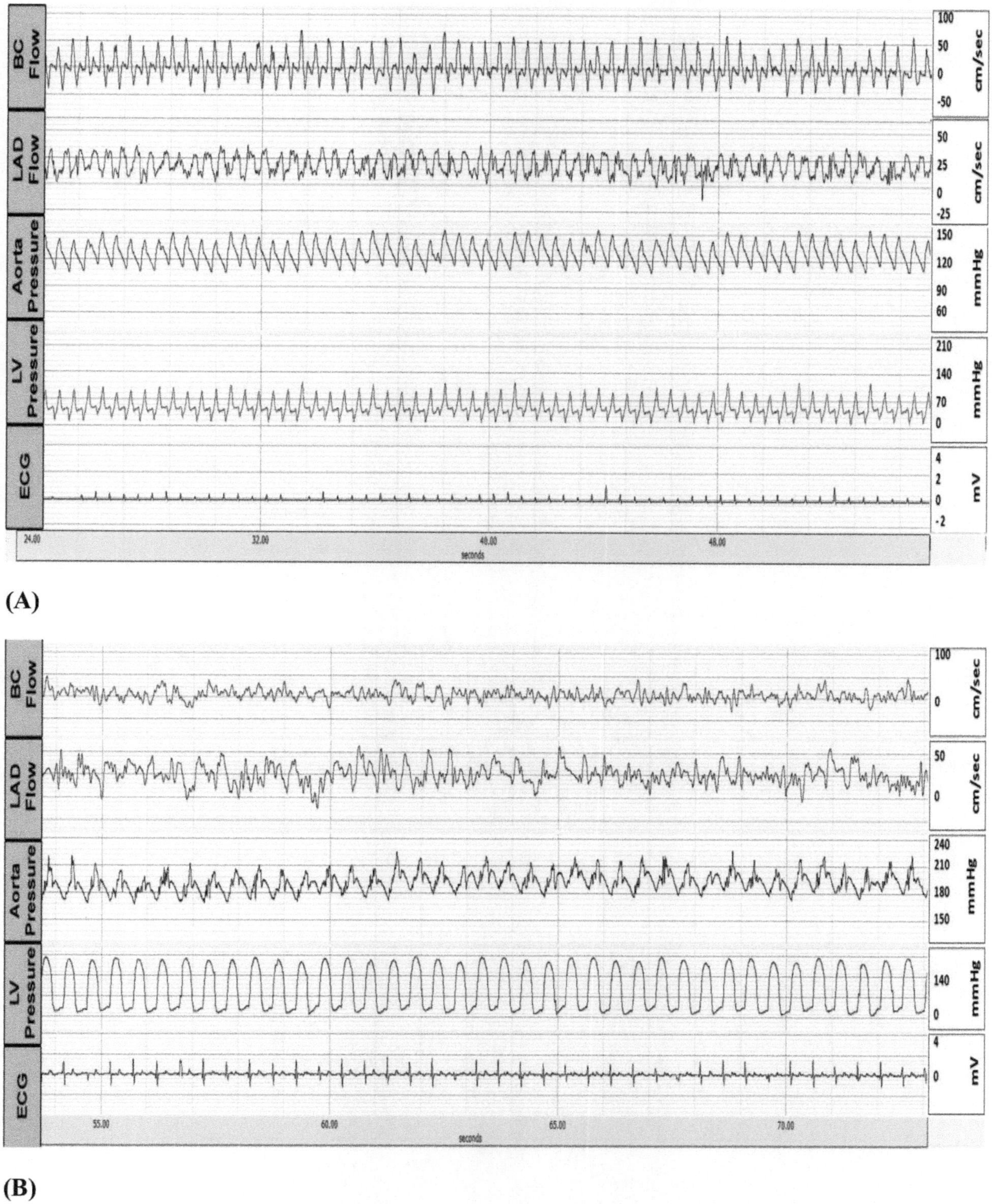

Figure 3. Representative tracings of telemetric recordings in an animal with volume overload - A-V fistula (A). Representative tracings of telemetric recordings in an animal with pressure overload - aortic banding (B).

study not only provides multichannel simultaneous recordings for flow, pressure, and ECG but also a longer battery life (up to 6 weeks) that can be replaced to allow longer recording time without affecting data collection.

There are no bandwidth bottlenecks with the telemetry system because all the physiological signals including the Doppler flow velocity measurements are processed to derive their final low bandwidth state. This in turn is more suitable for a telemetry

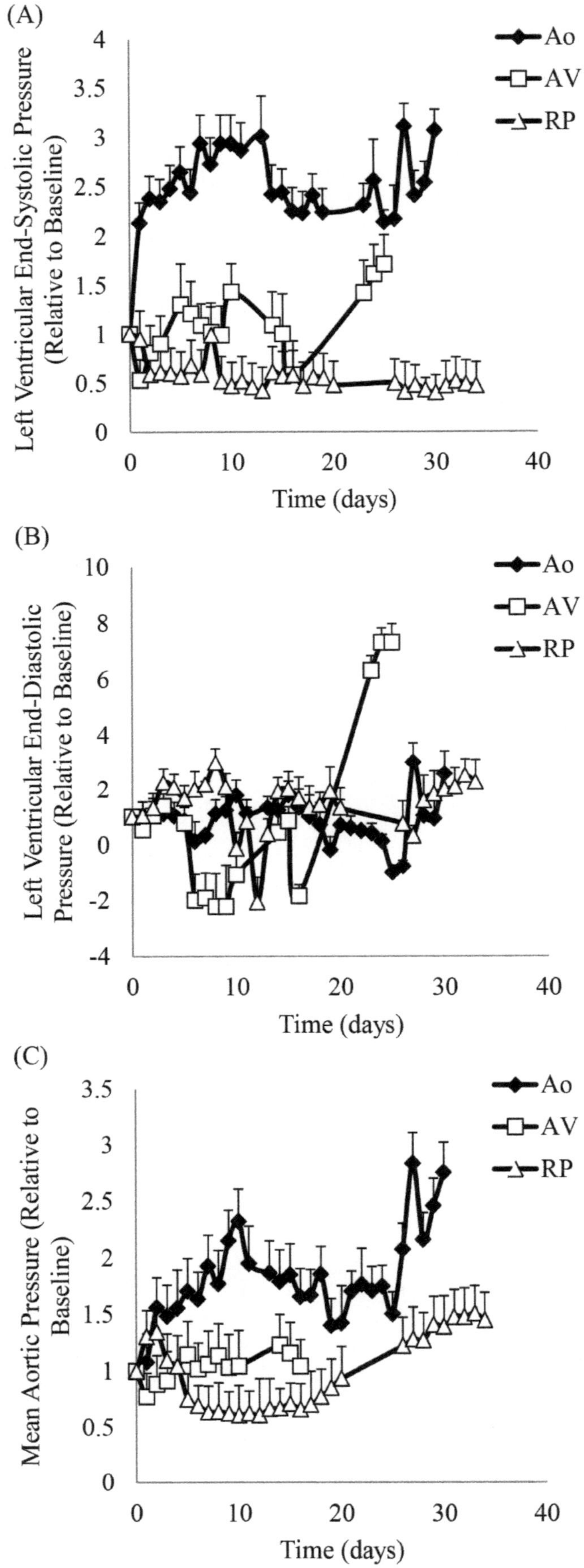
(A)
Left Ventricular End-Systolic Pressure (Relative to Baseline)
Time (days)
Ao
AV
RP
(B)
Left Ventricular End-Diastolic Pressure (Relative to Baseline)
Time (days)
Ao
AV
RP
(C)
Mean Aortic Pressure (Relative to Baseline)
Time (days)
Ao
AV
RP

Figure 4. Measurements of A) left ventricular end-systolic pressure (LVESP), B) left ventricular end-diastolic pressure (LVEDP), and C) mean aortic pressure in animals with volume overload, pressure overload and dilated cardiomyopathy. All measurements are relative to baseline.

system since low bandwidth also translates to lower power in the radio frequency transmitter and therefore extends battery life.

There are several differences (including size, hardware and software design) between the telemetry system presented here (Table 1) and the one previously developed by our group [3]. The present telemetry is approximately 3 times smaller than its predecessor and uses a new connector system. The hardware design uses 25% higher Doppler excitation voltage to accommo-

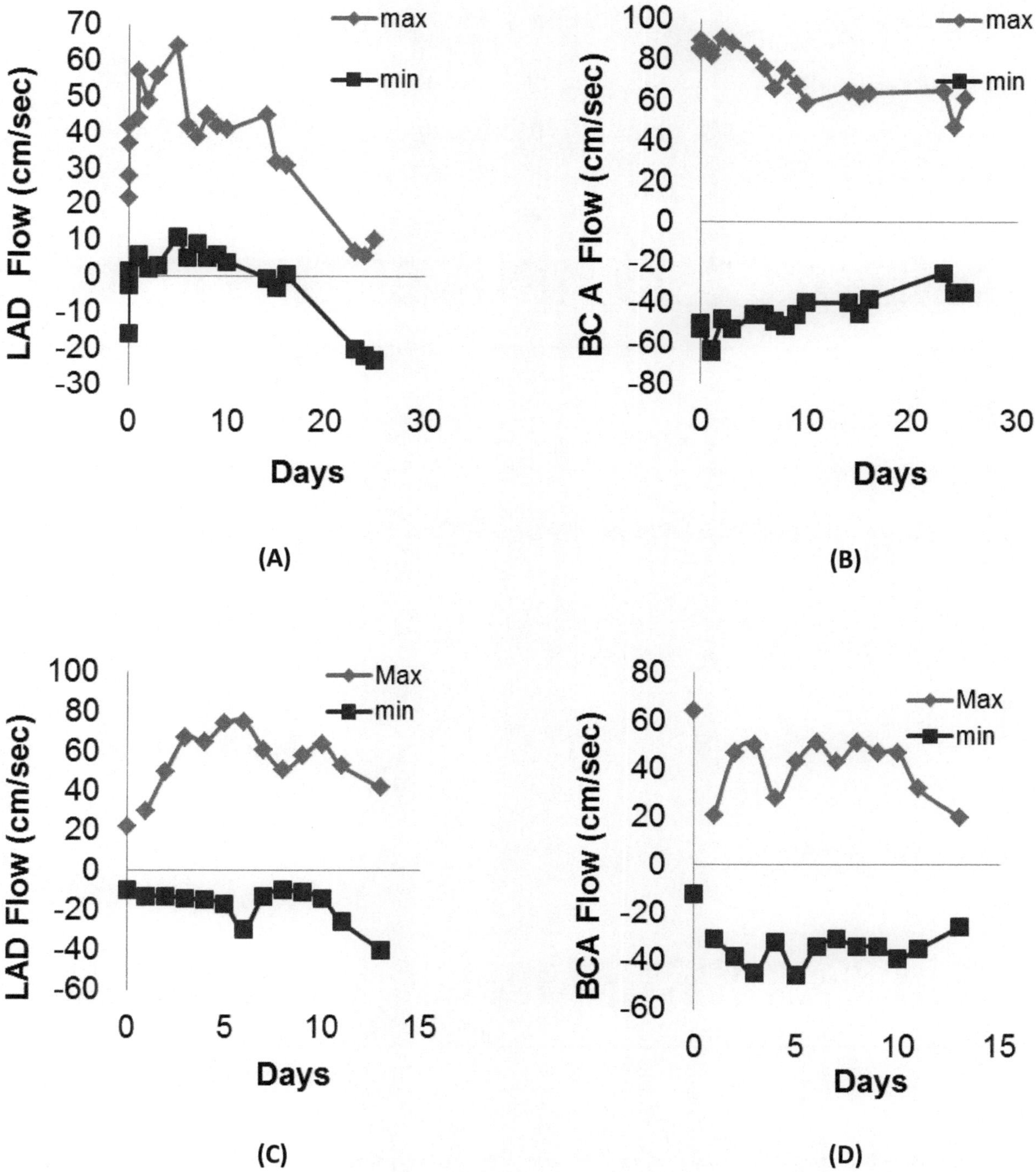

Figure 5. Blood flow velocity measurements in A) the left anterior descending (LAD) artery and B) the brachiocephalic artery in animals with volume overload (A-V fistula). Velocity measurements in C) the LAD artery and D) the brachiocephalic artery in animals with pressure overload (aortic banding).

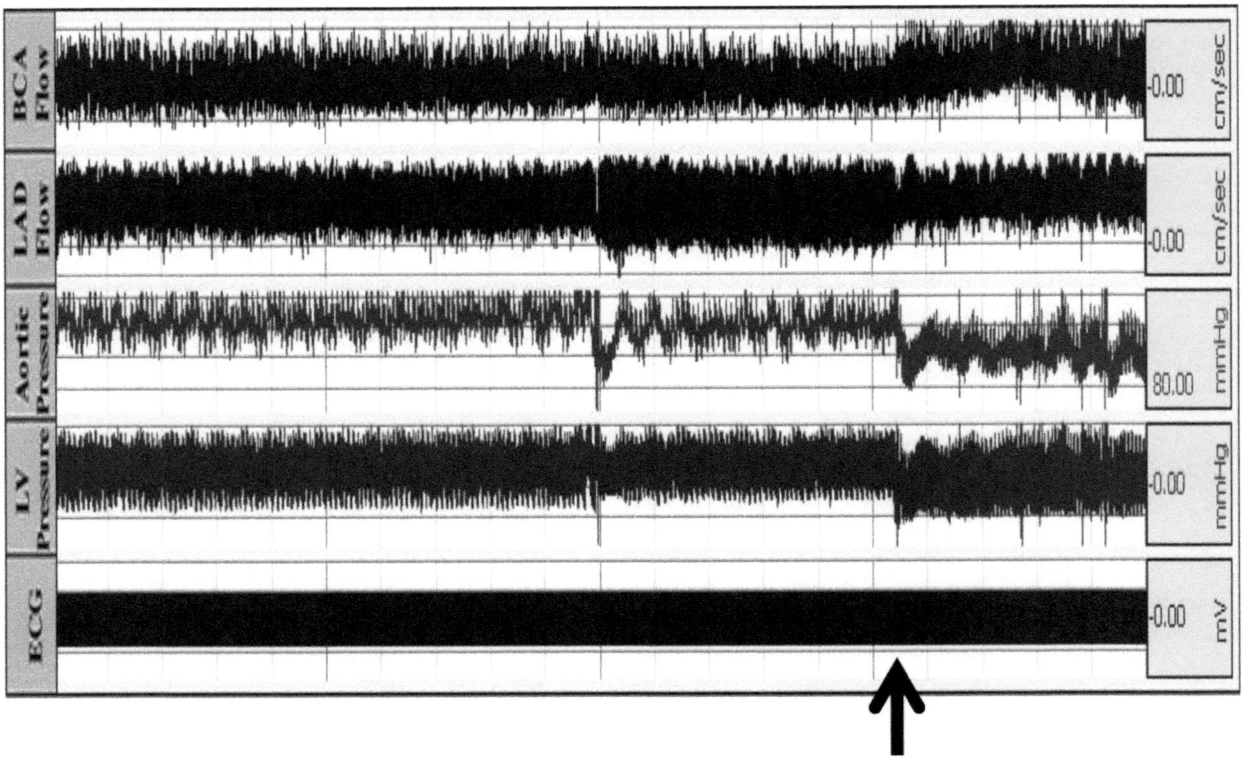

(A)

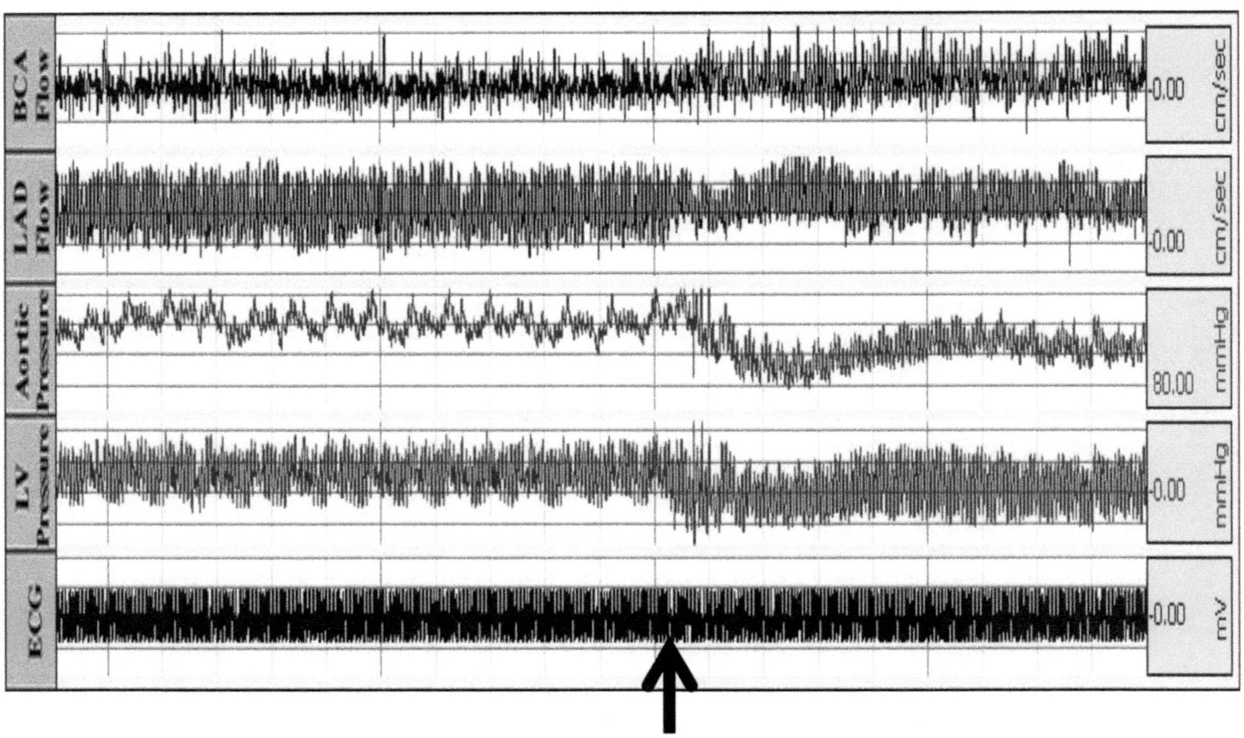

(B)

Figure 6. Representative tracings of telemetric recordings in a pacing-induced tachycardia animal (A) where an abrupt and transitory change (arrows) is observed in all cardiac parameters. A magnification of the tracings (B).

date a variety of Doppler probe applications and smaller piezoelectric sensors, which are useful in blood vessels <1 mm diameter. The new software-based Doppler decoding algorithm allows significantly lower power consumption (reduction of ~35%) and overall space saving. Other advantages are a PC-based control software that allows integration of the bidirectional control of the device and the data acquisition system for easier use and programmability. Finally, the transmission distance between the implanted animal and the base station decoder can be extended by adding additional remote transceivers, a useful capability when the animals are housed in larger enclosures.

The heart failure models used in this study are well established in both small and large animals, and the telemetry system implanted in the swine reliably detected hemodynamic changes during progression of the disease. The data collected was used to analyze LVESP and LVEDP as markers of heart failure, blood pressure as a marker of systemic circulation, and coronary flow for myocardial perfusion. The aortic banding animals showed a progressive increase of the systemic blood pressure (Figure 4C), which is in agreement with previous reports of hypertension in aortic coarctation [15]. The left ventricular pressure increased immediately after banding due to the increased resistance in the outflow tract (Figure 4A). It is well described in the literature [13] that a state of hypertension exists during the progression of disease, but interestingly, we found that after two weeks of progressive increase, the pressure dropped significantly during the third week, and increased again during the remainder of the study (i.e., non-monotonic pattern that may represent some compensatory response). The telemetry system was able to capture these fluctuations and compensatory responses, which otherwise would have been missed. It is also interesting to note the presence of flow reversal in the LAD and brachiocephalic arteries, which has been described in patients with LV hypertrophy in conditions such as aortic stenosis and systemic hypertension [1].

In the A-V fistula animals, the LV pressure also showed a non-monotonic pattern, with a drastic increase (more than double) at the end of the study (Figures 4A and 4B). Furthermore, the pulse flow (Figures 5A and 5B) that represents the difference between maximum and minimum flow velocity progressively decreased with the development of heart failure. This was more noticeable in the brachiocephalic artery (Figure 5B).

In pacing-induced tachycardia animals, there was a transient decrease of the aortic pressure during the first 2 weeks of rapid pacing, which then progressively increased for the remainder of the study (Figure 4C). The continuous recordings of the aortic pressure using telemetry allowed detection of those transient changes during the development of heart failure, which otherwise may have been missed [17,28]. We found that the left ventricular pressure did not change significantly over time (Figures 4A and 4B) as has been reported by other investigators [19,27]. Interestingly, a transient decrease in both left ventricular and aortic pressures as well as transient increase in the LAD flow velocity was observed (Figure 6). Ventricular diastolic suction with increased negative ventricular pressure has been reported in different animal models of heart failure, including pacing-induced tachycardia [4,5,20], which could explain the reason for increased coronary blood flow.

Study limitations

First, careful placement of the flow probe around the vessel is necessary to ensure that blood flow does not become restricted when the vessel remodels (enlarges) as the disease progresses. This can be avoided by placing the probe loosely around the vessel wall. Eventually, the connective tissue will cover the flow probe and help secure the position around the vessel.

Second, the time acquisition mode is a concern. During the approximately 4 weeks of telemetric measurements, we used a combination of continuous data recording and automated timed-acquisition mode data recording (20 min of data recording followed by 100 min power-down period). The timed-acquisition mode prolongs the battery life and reduces the amount of data collected, but this poses a risk of missing some meaningful and interesting data. Future improvements can be made by introducing internal trigger sensors.

In summary, this novel implantable telemetry system is capable of collecting high quality data over extended periods of time. To our knowledge, this is the first telemetry system implanted in a large animal model of heart failure. The system can monitor blood pressure, blood flow and ECG signals simultaneously in free-ranging animals. The compact size and high reliability of the implant provide significant utility for the long-term measurement of cardiovascular vitals in health and disease.

Author Contributions

Performed the experiments: JSC ZDZ. Analyzed the data: JSC ZDZ. Wrote the paper: JSC GSK. Designed the experiments: JSC. Contributed with materials: KP MS. Conceived the experiments: GSK.

References

1. Akasaka T, Yoshikawa J, Yoshida K, Maeda K, Takagi T, et al (1994) Phasic coronary flow characteristics in patients with hypertrophic cardiomyopathy: a study by coronary Doppler catheter. J Am Soc Echocardiogr 7(1):9–19.
2. Anderson NH, Devlin AM, Graham D, Morton JJ, Hamilton CA, et al (1999) Telemetry for cardiovascular monitoring in a pharmacological study: new approaches to data analysis. Hypertension 33(1 Pt 2):248–255.
3. Axelsson M, Dang Q, Pitsillides K, Munns S, Hicks J, et al (2007) A novel, fully implantable, multichannel biotelemetry system for measurement of blood flow, pressure, ECG, and temperature. J Appl Physiol 102(3):1220–1228.
4. Bell SP, Nyland L, Tischler MD, McNabb M, Granzier H, et al (2000) Alterations in the determinants of diastolic suction during pacing tachycardia. Circ Res 87(3):235–240.
5. Brecher GA (1958) Critical review of recent work on ventricular diastolic suction. Circ Res 6(5):554–566.
6. Cardon AD, Bailey MR, Bennett BT (2012) The Animal Welfare Act: from enactment to enforcement. J Am Assoc Lab Anim Sci 51(3):301–5.
7. Claude JP, Knutti JW, Allen HV, Meindl JD (1979) Applications of totally implantable telemetry systems to chronic medical research. Biotelem Patient Monit 6(3):160–71.
8. Dang CQ, Nenadic Z, Kassab GS (2008) A comparative analysis of coronary and aortic flow waveforms. Ann Biomed Eng 36(6):933–46.
9. DePasquale MJ, Ringer LW, Winslow RL, Buchholz RA, Fossa AA (1994) Chronic monitoring of cardiovascular function in the conscious guinea pig using radio-telemetry. Clin Exp Hypertens 16(2):245–260.
10. Franklin DL, Kemper WS, Van Citters RL, Watson NW (1970) Radio telemetry techniques for measurement of blood pressure and flow in unrestrained animals. UCLA Forum Med Sci 10:377–382.
11. Franklin DL, Watson NW, Vancitters RL (1964) Blood Velocity Telemertered from Unththered Animals. Nature 203:528–30.
12. Fryer TB, Sandler H, Freund SW, McCutcheon EP, Carlson EL (1975) A multichannel implantable telemetry system for flow, pressure, and ECG measurements. J Appl Physiol 39(2):318–326.
13. Gilson N, el Houda Bouanani N, Corsin A, Crozatier B (1990) Left ventricular function and beta-adrenoceptors in rabbit failing heart. Am J Physiol 258(3 Pt 2):H634–641.
14. Committee for the Update of the Guide for the Care and Use of Laboratory Animals, National Research Council (US) (2011) Guide for the Care and Use of Laboratory Animals. 8th edition. Washington (DC): National Academies Press (US); 2011.
15. Hollander W, Kramsch DM, Farmelant M, Madoff IM (1968) Arterial wall metabolism in experimental hypertension of coarctation of the aorta of short duration. J Clin Invest 47(5):1221–1229.
16. Huetteman DA, Bogie H (2009) Direct blood pressure monitoring in laboratory rodents via implantable radio telemetry. Methods Mol Biol 573:57–73.

17. Kawai H, Mohan A, Hagen J, Dong E, Armstrong J, et al (2000) Alterations in cardiac adrenergic terminal function and beta-adrenoceptor density in pacing-induced heart failure. Am J Physiol Heart Circ Physiol 278(5):H1708–1716.
18. Kvetnansky R, Sun CL, Lake CR, Thoa N, Torda T, et al (1978) Effect of handling and forced immobilization on rat plasma levels of epinephrine, norepinephrine, and dopamine-beta-hydroxylase. Endocrinology 103(5):1868–1874.
19. Lionetti V, Guiducci L, Simioniuc A, Aquaro GD, Simi C, et al (2007). Mismatch between uniform increase in cardiac glucose uptake and regional contractile dysfunction in pacing-induced heart failure. Am J Physiol Heart Circ Physiol 293(5):H2747–2756.
20. Nakatani S, Beppu S, Nagata S, Ishikura F, Tamai J, et al (1994) Diastolic suction in the human ventricle: observation during balloon mitral valvuloplasty with a single balloon. Am Heart J 127(1):143–147.
21. Nemeth S, Vigas M, Kvetnansky R, Orlicky, Mikulaj J (1997) The effect of repeated immobilization on the level of plasma corticosterone and on the activity of several liver enzymes in rats. Endokrinologie 69(1):87–93.
22. Rader RD, Meehan JP, Henriksen JK (1973) An implantable blood pressure and flow transmitter. IEEE Trans Biomed Eng 20(1):37–43.
23. Smith TL, Hutchins PM (1980) Anesthetic effects on hemodynamics of spontaneously hypertensive and Wistar-Kyoto rats. Am J Physiol 238(4): H539–544.
24. Stehlin E, Malpas SC, Budgett DM, Barrett CJ, McCormick D, et al (1985) Chronic measurement of left ventricular pressure in freely moving rats. J Appl Physiol 115(11):1672–82.
25. Taylor GL, Patel B, Sullivan AT (2007) Evaluation of blood flow parameters in addition to blood pressure and electrocardiogram in the conscious telemetered beagle dog. J Pharmacol Toxicol Methods 56(2):212–217.
26. van den Buuse M (1994) Circadian rhythms of blood pressure, heart rate, and locomotor activity in spontaneously hypertensive rats as measured with radio-telemetry. Physiol Behav 55(4):783–787.
27. Wilson JR, Douglas P, Hickey WF, Lanoce V, Ferraro N, et al (1987) Experimental congestive heart failure produced by rapid ventricular pacing in the dog: cardiac effects. Circulation 75(4):857–867.
28. Zhang Y, Popovic ZB, Bibevski S, Fakhry I, Sica DA, et al (2009) Chronic vagus nerve stimulation improves autonomic control and attenuates systemic inflammation and heart failure progression in a canine high-rate pacing model. Circ Heart Fail 2(6):692–699.

15

Endoplasmic Reticulum Stress Induces Different Molecular Structural Alterations in Human Dilated and Ischemic Cardiomyopathy

Ana Ortega[1], Esther Roselló-Lletí[1], Estefanía Tarazón[1], Maria Micaela Molina-Navarro[1], Luis Martínez-Dolz[2], José Ramón González-Juanatey[3], Francisca Lago[3], Jose David Montoro-Mateos[1], Antonio Salvador[2], Miguel Rivera[1], Manuel Portolés[1]*

1 Cardiocirculatory Unit, Health Research Institute of La Fe University Hospital, Valencia, Spain, **2** Heart Failure and Transplantation Unit, Cardiology Department, La Fe University Hospital, Valencia, Spain, **3** Cellular and Molecular Cardiology Research Unit, Department of Cardiology and Institute of Biomedical Research, University Clinical Hospital, Santiago de Compostela, Spain

Abstract

Background: The endoplasmic reticulum (ER) is a multifunctional organelle responsible for the synthesis and folding of proteins as well as for signalling and calcium storage, that has been linked to the contraction-relaxation process. Perturbations of its homeostasis activate a stress response in diseases such as heart failure (HF). To elucidate the alterations in ER molecular components, we analyze the levels of ER stress and structure proteins in human dilated (DCM) and ischemic (ICM) cardiomyopathies, and its relationship with patient's functional status.

Methods and Results: We examined 52 explanted human hearts from DCM (n = 21) and ICM (n = 21) subjects and 10 non-failing hearts as controls. Our results showed specific changes in stress (IRE1, $p<0.05$; p-IRE1, $p<0.05$) and structural (Reticulon 1, $p<0.01$) protein levels. The stress proteins GRP78, XBP1 and ATF6 as well as the structural proteins RRBP1, kinectin, and Nogo A and B, were upregulated in both DCM and ICM patients. Immunofluorescence results were concordant with quantified Western blot levels. Moreover, we show a novel relationship between stress and structural proteins. RRBP1, involved in procollagen synthesis and remodeling, was related with left ventricular function.

Conclusions: In the present study, we report the existence of alterations in ER stress response and shaping proteins. We show a plausible effect of the ER stress on ER structure in a suitable sample of DCM and ICM subjects. Patients with higher values of RRBP1 had worse left ventricular function.

Editor: David Long, UCL Institute of Child Health, United Kingdom

Funding: This work was supported by grants from the NIH "Fondo de Investigaciones Sanitarias del Instituto de Salud Carlos III". [RETICS 12/0042/0003, FIS Project PI10/00275]. The funders had no role in study design, data collection and analysis, decision to publish, or preparation of the manuscript.

Competing Interests: The authors have declared that no competing interests exist.

* Email: portoles_man@gva.es

Introduction

Heart failure (HF) is a syndrome with high morbidity and mortality in industrialized countries. This syndrome is usually associated with left ventricular (LV) systolic dysfunction, although diastolic impairment at rest is a frequent if not universal accompaniment [1]. HF is the end stage of many heart diseases [2] including dilated (DCM) and ischemic cardiomyopathies (ICM).

Several studies have associated HF with cellular and molecular alterations in cardiac tissue, including abnormal calcium handling [3]; changes in mitochondria [4,5], nuclear components [6–8], cytoskeletal proteins [9,10], and also alterations in the endoplasmic reticulum (ER) [11]. In particular, disruption of ER homeostasis has been linked to several processes of cardiovascular diseases including ischemia/reperfusion injury [12], DCM [13] and HF [14].

The ER is the primary site of secretory protein synthesis and maturation, calcium storage, and lipid biosynthesis. Various factors can disrupt ER homeostasis and alter its functions (ER stress), provoking the accumulation of unfolded and misfolded proteins in the ER lumen and leading to cellular and pathological dysfunctions. ER stress triggers a cellular response in which different pathways are implicated in maintaining ER homeostasis through attenuation of protein synthesis, transcriptional induction of ER chaperone genes and ER-associated degradation component genes, and finally, the induction of apoptosis to safely ensure the survival of the whole organism [11,15]. In all of these pathways, lumen and transmembrane proteins such as inositol-requiring protein-1 (IRE1) and glucose-related protein 78 (GRP78), and transcription factors such as X-box binding protein 1 (XBP1), activating transcription factor 6 (ATF6), ATF4 and eukaryotic initiation factor 2 alpha (eIF2α), act together to produce the ER stress response [16].

ER stress promotes the synthesis and expression of molecules implicated in the unfolded protein response (UPR), and this alteration could also occur at the structural level of the ER, leading to changes in the expression of proteins (e.g., scaffolding proteins and curvature stabilizing proteins) that stabilize the multiple folds that shapes the ER. These changes could impair the function of the ER and have undesirable consequences.

In this study, we hypothesize that patients with HF may display changes in proteins involved in the ER stress response and that these changes could differ between the DCM and ICM pathologies. Furthermore, we aim to establish a new link between these alterations and changes of structural proteins of the ER. Therefore, our objective was to analyze levels of highly representative ER stress proteins and ER structural proteins in LV tissue from patients with DCM and ICM. Moreover, we studied the relationship between these proteins and changes in LV function.

Materials and Methods

Ethics statement

All patients gave written informed consent to participate in the study. The project was approved by the Ethics Committee (Biomedical Investigation Ethics Committee of La Fe University Hospital of Valencia, Spain) and conducted in accordance with the principles of the current version of the Declaration of Helsinki [17].

Collection of samples

A total of 42 pathological human hearts were obtained from 21 patients with DCM and 21 with ICM undergoing cardiac transplantation. Clinical history, ECG, Doppler echocardiography, hemodynamic studies, and coronary angiography data were available on all of these patients. All patients were functionally classified according to the New York Heart Association (NYHA) criteria and were receiving medical treatment following the guidelines of the European Society of Cardiology [18]. Non-ischemic DCM was diagnosed when patients had intact coronary arteries on coronary angiography and LV systolic dysfunction [ejection fraction (EF) <40%] with a dilated non-hypertrophic left ventricle [LV end-diastolic diameter (LVEDD) >55 mm] on echocardiography. Furthermore, patients showed no more than mild valvular disease.

As control (CNT) samples, 10 non-diseased donor hearts were used. The cause of death was cerebrovascular accident or motor vehicle accident. All donors had normal LV function and no history of myocardial disease. The hearts were initially considered for cardiac transplantation but were subsequently deemed unsuitable either because of blood type or size incompatibility.

LV samples were taken from near the apex of the left ventricle and were flushed with 0.9% NaCl and stored at 4°C for a mean of 4.4 h from the time of coronary circulation loss. Samples were then placed at −80°C until the protein extraction procedure.

Homogenization of samples and protein determination

Twenty-five milligrams of frozen left ventricle was transferred into Lysing Matrix D tubes designed for use with the FastPrep-24 homogenizer (MP Biomedicals, USA) in a total protein extraction buffer (2% SDS, 10 mM EDTA, 6 mM Tris–HCl, pH 7.4) with protease inhibitors (25 μg/mL aprotinin and 10 μg/mL leupeptin). The homogenates were centrifuged at 16100× *g*, and the supernatant was aliquoted. The protein content of the aliquot was determined using Peterson's modification of the micro Lowry method with bovine serum albumin (BSA) as the standard [19].

Polyacrylamide gel electrophoresis and Western blot analysis

Protein samples for detection of IRE1, IRE1 phosphorylated (p-IRE1), GRP78, XBP1, ATF6, ATF4, eIF2α phosphorylated (p-eIF2α), Reticulon 1, ribosomal receptor-binding protein 1 (RRBP1), kinectin, and cytoskeleton-associated protein 4 (CKAP4) were separated using Bis-Tris Midi gel electrophoresis with 4–12% polyacrylamide. Tris-acetate 3–8% polyacrylamide gel was used for Nogo (Reticulon 4) A and B isoforms separation. After electrophoresis, the proteins were transferred from the gel to a PVDF membrane using the iBlot Dry Blotting System (Invitrogen Ltd, UK) for Western blot analyses. The membranes were blocked overnight at 4°C with 1% BSA in Tris buffer solution containing 0.05% Tween 20 and, after blocking, were incubated for 2 h with the primary antibody in the same buffer. The primary detection antibodies used were anti-IRE1 mouse monoclonal antibody (1:400), anti-p-IRE1 rabbit monoclonal antibody (1:200), anti-GRP78 rabbit polyclonal antibody (1:600), anti-XBP1 mouse monoclonal antibody (1:400), anti-ATF6 rabbit polyclonal antibody (1:1000), anti-ATF4 mouse monoclonal antibody (1:400), anti-p-eIF2α rabbit monoclonal antibody (1:250), anti-Reticulon 1 rabbit polyclonal antibody (1:500), anti-RRBP1 rabbit polyclonal antibody (1:250), anti-kinectin rabbit polyclonal antibody (1:500), anti-CKAP4 rabbit polyclonal antibody (1:1000), and anti-Nogo A+B rabbit polyclonal antibody (1:250). Anti-GAPDH mouse monoclonal antibody (1:1000) was used as a loading control. All antibodies were from Abcam (Cambridge, UK) except for p-IRE1 and p-eIF2α that were from EMD Millipore Corporation (Billerica, MA, USA).

The bands were then visualized using an acid phosphatase-conjugated secondary antibody and nitro blue tetrazolium/5-bromo-4-chloro-3-indolyl phosphate (NBT/BCIP, Sigma-Aldrich, St. Louis, USA) substrate system. Finally, the bands were digitalized using an image analyzer (DNR Bio-Imagining Systems, Israel) and quantified with the GelQuant Pro (v. 12.2) program.

Fluorescence microscopy analysis

Cardiac LV muscle samples were fixed in 4% formalin, embedded in paraffin blocks and sectioned into 5 μm using a microtome Microm HM 340E (Thermo Fisher Scientific Inc., Walldorf, Germany). Sections were transferred to glass slides and were kept at 60°C overnight, deparaffinized with xylol followed by washing in 100%, 96%, 80%, and 70% ethanol. Samples were then fixed in pure methanol for 4 min at −20°C. Sections were then blocked with PBS containing 1% BSA for 15 min at room temperature (RT). After blocking, sections were incubated for 2 h at RT with the primary antibodies for RRBP1 (1:200 dilution), kinectin (1:150 dilution), and Nogo A+B (1:200 dilution) (described in preceding section) in the same buffer solution and then with Alexa-conjugated secondary antibody (Invitrogen, USA) for 1 h at RT [20]. Then, sections were rinsed in PBS, mounted in Vectashield with DAPI for identifying nuclei (Vector, Burlingame, CA, USA), and observed with an Olympus BX50 fluorescence microscope (Tokyo, Japan). Finally, the images were processed using ImageJ (v. 1.46 r; National Institutes of Health, Bethesda, MD, USA) software.

Statistical methods

Data are presented as mean values ± standard deviation. The Kolmogorov–Smirnov test was used to analyze the distribution of variables. Comparisons of clinical characteristics were performed using the Student's *t*-test for continuous variables and the Fisher's exact test for discrete variables. Comparisons of protein expression levels between different groups were performed using the Student's *t*-test for variables with a normal distribution and the Mann–Whitney U test for variables with non-normal distribution. RRBP1 levels exhibited a non-normal distribution and were log transformed (and proved to be normalized) before parametric correlation analysis. Finally, Pearson's correlation coefficient was performed to analyze the association between variables. Significance was assumed at $p<0.05$. All statistical analyses were performed using SPSS software v. 20 for Windows (IBM SPSS Inc., Chicago, IL, USA).

Results

Clinical characteristics of patients

We analyzed 52 human hearts, including 42 explanted human hearts from patients diagnosed with HF (21 DCM and 21 ICM) undergoing cardiac transplantation and 10 non-diseased donor hearts as CNT samples. Most of the patients were men (79%) with a mean age of 53±11 years, a mean NYHA functional classification of III–IV, and previous diagnosis of significant comorbidities including hypertension, hypercholesterolemia, and diabetes mellitus. The clinical characteristics and echocardiographic parameters of HF patients according to etiology are shown in Table 1. The DCM group was significantly younger than ICM patients ($p<0.05$) and showed reduced levels of total cholesterol ($p<0.01$). Significant differences were also found in LV end-systolic diameter (LVESD) ($p<0.05$), LVEDD ($p<0.05$), and LV mass index (LVMI) ($p<0.05$), with higher values in the DCM group. The CNT group was comprised mainly of men (70%) with a mean age of 46±18 years.

HF etiology related changes in ER stress protein levels

We focused our study on the stress proteins IRE1, p-IRE1, GRP78, XBP1, ATF6, ATF4 and p-eIF2α that are highly representative in the activation of the UPR during ER stress process. When we compared stress protein levels between the pathological groups and our 10 CNT hearts, we found that IRE1 was significantly reduced in ICM [82±19 *vs.* 100±23 arbitrary units (AU), $p<0.05$] (Fig. 1A), while p-IRE1 was upregulated in DCM patients (136±29 *vs.* 100±34 AU, $p<0.05$) (Fig. 1B). GRP78, XBP1 and ATF6 were significantly increased in both DCM (120±19 *vs.* 100±23 AU, $p<0.05$, 124±33 *vs.* 100±14 AU, $p<0.05$, and 149±53 *vs* 100±31 AU, $p<0.05$, respectively) and ICM samples (117±21 *vs.* 100±23 AU, $p<0.05$, 120±22 *vs.* 100±14 AU, and 161±40 *vs* 100±31 AU, $p<0.01$, respectively) (Fig. 1C, D and E). The levels of ATF4 (Fig. 1F) and p-eIF2α did not show any changes in both pathologies.

Levels of ER structural proteins according to HF etiology

We analyzed the protein levels of the structural proteins Reticulon 1, RRBP1, kinectin, CKAP4 and two Nogo (Reticulon 4) isoforms (A and B); which are important proteins shaping the ER. Western blot experiments revealed significant alterations in the amount of distinct structural proteins of the ER organelle. However, we found no statistically significant differences between levels of CKAP4 protein in the two HF etiologies compared to CNT group (Fig. 2A). Reticulon1 showed protein changes according to HF etiology. Whereas this protein was significantly reduced in the DCM group compared with levels in the CNT group (79±13 *vs.* 100±17 AU, $p<0.01$), we observed no significant alterations in the ICM group. On the other hand, when we compared the levels of Reticulon 1 in the DCM and ICM groups, we found significant differences (79±13 *vs.* 105±31 AU, $p<0.01$), (Fig. 2B).

Furthermore, RRBP1 was significantly increased in the DCM and ICM groups compared with levels in the CNT group (311±208 *vs.* 100±54 AU, $p<0.001$, and 203±75 *vs.* 100±54 AU, $p<0.01$, respectively) (Fig. 3A) as well as kinectin (140±76 *vs.* 100±25 AU, $p<0.05$, and 161±94 *vs.* 100±25 AU, $p<0.05$, respectively) (Fig. 3C), Nogo A (128±33 *vs.* 100±13 AU, $p<0.01$, and 149±38 *vs.* 100±13 AU, $p<0.001$, respectively) (Fig. 4A),

Table 1. Clinical characteristics of patients according to HF etiology.

	DCM (n = 21)	ICM (n = 21)
Age (years)	49±13	57±7*
Gender male (%)	79	79
NYHA class	3.4±0.4	3.3±0.5
BMI (kg/m^2)	25±6	25±3
Hemoglobin (mg/dL)	14±2	13±2
Hematocrit (%)	41±6	37±7
Total cholesterol (mg/dL)	142±42	185±40**
Prior hypertension (%)	25	46
Prior smoking (%)	63	75
Diabetes mellitus (%)	15	29
EF (%)	22±8	22±8
FS (%)	12±4	13±6
LVESD (mm)	65±11	56±9*
LVEDD (mm)	74±11	64±8*
Left ventricle mass index (g/cm^2)	204±64	147±46*

DCM, dilated cardiomyopathy; ICM, ischemic cardiomyopathy; NYHA class, New York Heart Association class; BMI, body mass index; EF, ejection fraction; FS, fractional shortening; LVESD, left ventricular end-systolic diameter; LVEDD, left ventricular end-diastolic diameter.
*$p<0.05$;
**$p<0.01$.

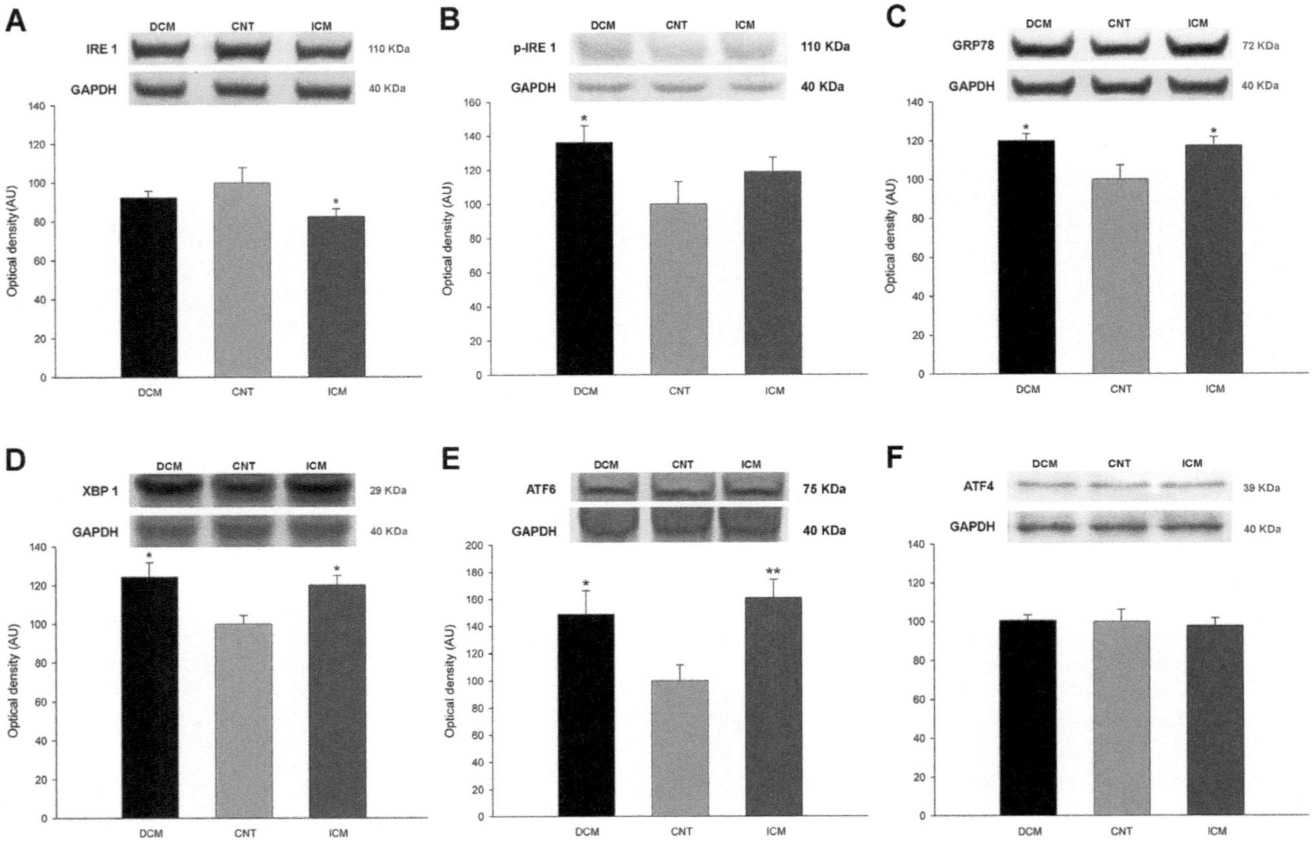

Figure 1. Protein expression levels of endoplasmic reticulum stress proteins in dilated (DCM) and ischemic (ICM) cardiomyopathy and control (CNT) groups. (**A**) Inositol-requiring protein-1 (IRE1). (**B**) Inositol-requiring protein-1 phosphorylated (p-IRE1) (**C**) Glucose-related protein 78 (GRP78). (**D**) X-box binding protein 1 (XBP1). (**E**) Activating transcription factor 6 (ATF6) (**F**) Activating transcription factor 4 (ATF4). The values are normalized to GAPDH and finally to the CNT group. Values from the CNT group are set to 100. The data are expressed as means ± standard error of the mean (SEM) in optical density, arbitrary units (AU), of six independent experiments. *$p<0.05$, **$p<0.01$ *vs.* the CNT group.

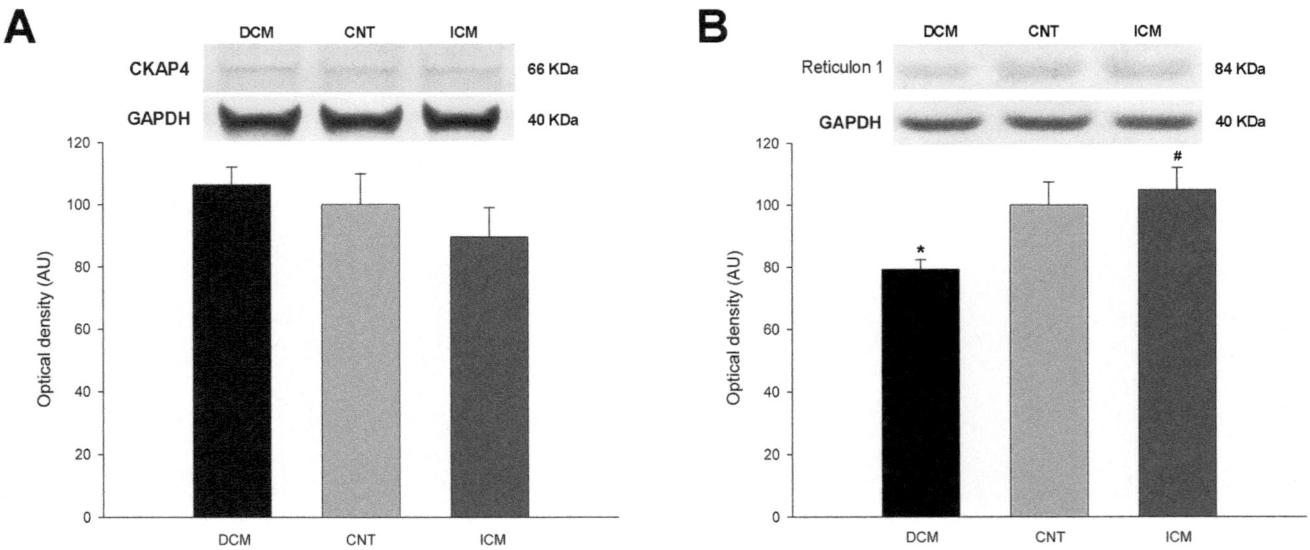

Figure 2. Western blot analysis of structural proteins of the endoplasmic reticulum in dilated (DCM) and ischemic (ICM) cardiomyopathy and control (CNT) groups. (**A**) Cytoskeleton-associated protein 4 (CKAP4). (**B**) Reticulon 1. The values are normalized to GAPDH and finally to the CNT group. Values from the CNT group are set to 100. The data are expressed as means ± standard error of the mean (SEM) in optical density, arbitrary units (AU), of two independent experiments. *$p<0.01$ *vs.* the CNT group. #$p<0.01$ DCM *vs.* the ICM group.

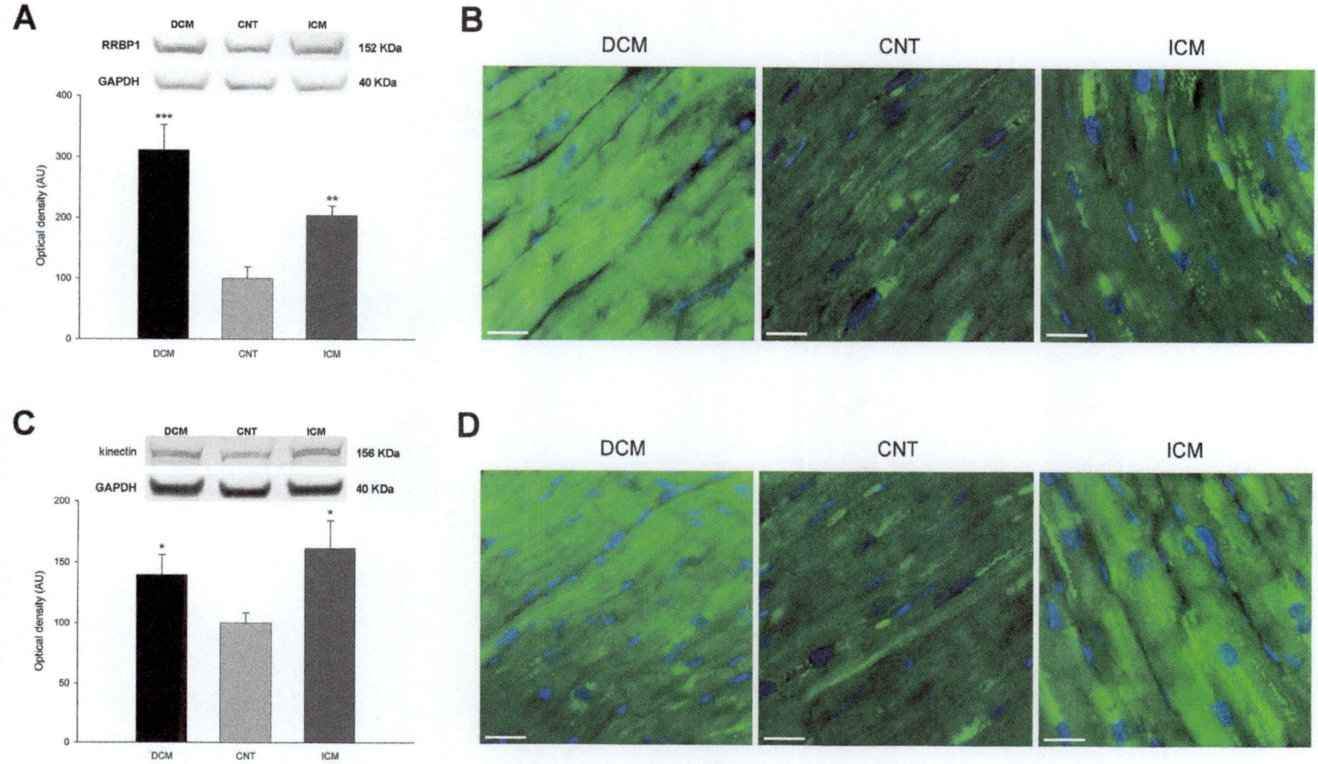

Figure 3. Western blot and immunofluorescence studies of cell distribution of some endoplasmic reticulum structural proteins in human left ventricular cardiomyocytes according to heart failure etiology and compared to a control (CNT) group. (**A**) Ribosomal receptor-binding protein (RRBP1) levels. (**B**) Immunofluorescence of RRBP1 protein. (**C**) Kinectin protein levels. (**D**) Immunofluorescence of kinectin. The values are normalized to GAPDH and finally to the CNT group. Values from the CNT group are set to 100. The data are expressed as means ± standard error of the mean (SEM) in optical density, arbitrary units (AU), of two independent experiments. *$p<0.05$, **$p<0.01$, ***$p<0.001$ *vs.* the CNT group. The bar represents 10 μm.

and Nogo B (177±76 *vs.* 100±52 AU, $p<0.01$, and 234±125 *vs.* 100±52 AU, $p<0.001$, respectively) (Fig. 4B). Our results also showed significant differences in Nogo A protein between the two pathological groups (128±33 *vs.* 149±38 AU, $p<0.05$) (Fig. 4A).

Effect of HF on distribution of ER structural proteins

Additionally, we studied the distribution of some ER structural proteins using immunofluorescence. The results were consistent with the increased levels observed by Western blot. The high levels observed in DCM and ICM patients of RRBP1 (Fig. 3B), kinectin (Fig. 3D), and Nogo A+B proteins (Fig. 4C), were distributed in the same diffuse pattern in the cytoplasm of the cardiomyocytes in both, patients and CNT group.

Relationship between stress and structural protein levels and with LV function

We further analyzed the relationships between proteins and we found significant relationships between the structural protein kinectin with Nogo A ($r=0.404$, $p=0.016$), Nogo B ($r=-0.390$, $p=0.017$) and with Reticulon1 ($r=0.362$, $p=0.042$) in both the DCM and ICM groups; and between stress proteins GRP78 and XBP1 ($r=-0.685$, $p=0.001$) in the DCM group. The structural protein RRBP1 and the stress protein XBP1 were related among them ($r=0.536$, $p=0.022$) in DCM.

Finally, we studied the relationship between these proteins and LV function. For 35 out of 42 samples, the LV function parameters were completely available. Of all the studied proteins, only RRBP1 was inversely related to EF ($r=-0.464$, $p=0.005$) (Fig. 5) and fractional shortening (FS) ($r=-0.463$, $p=0.005$) in DCM and ICM patients.

Discussion

The present study provides new data into the ER stress process that occurs in HF patients [21,22] and comprises not only alterations in stress-implicated molecules but also changes in ER structural proteins. We determined the levels of the most important proteins involved in these functions in the cardiac tissue of DCM and ICM patients. Our results revealed a general increase of these proteins in both pathological groups and some differences in protein levels between DCM and ICM. Furthermore, immunofluorescence images of structural proteins showed higher fluorescence intensity in DCM and ICM tissues compared with those in the CNT group, according to the observed protein expression levels.

Transcriptional induction of ER stress proteins in HF

The UPR pathway is activated when ER stress is produced to re-establish the homeostasis of the ER. This adaptive response triggers the activation of three signaling pathways that include transcriptional induction of ER chaperones and folding catalysts, transcriptional activation of genes encoding components of ER-associated degradation, and general translational attenuation. However, if ER stress is prolonged or severe, apoptosis is induced to eliminate unhealthy cells [23]. In these pathways, three ER transmembrane sensors [IRE1, protein kinase-like ER kinase

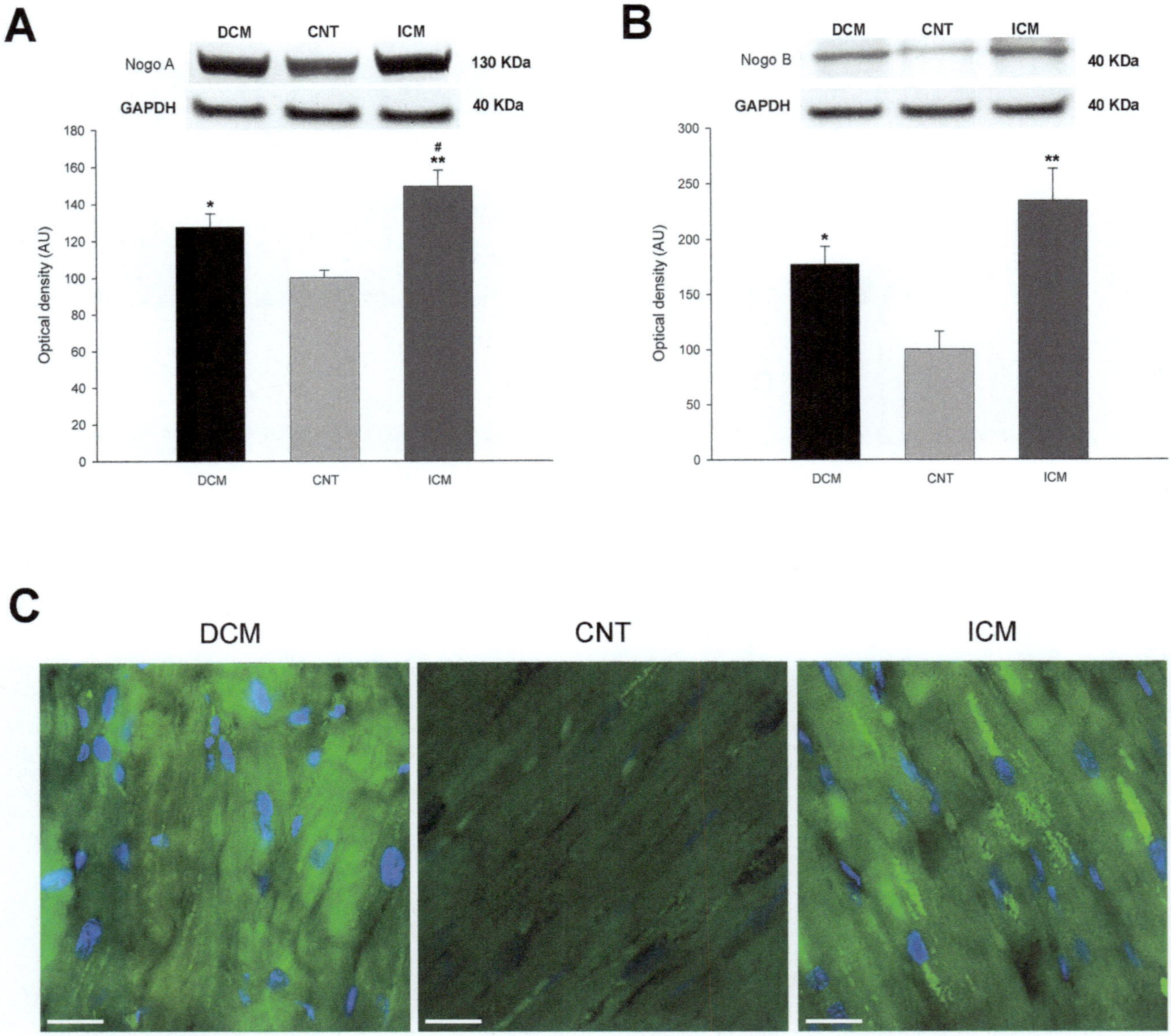

Figure 4. Western blot and immunofluorescence studies of Nogo A and B according to heart failure etiology and compared to a control (CNT) group. (**A**) Protein levels of Nogo A. (**B**) Protein levels of Nogo B. (**C**) Immunofluorescence of Nogo A+B. The values are normalized to GAPDH and finally to the CNT group. Values from the CNT group are set to 100. The data are expressed as means ± standard error of the mean (SEM) in optical density, arbitrary units (AU), of two independent experiments. DCM, dilated cardiomyopathy, ICM, ischemic cardiomyopathy. **p*<0.01, ***p*<0.001 *vs.* the CNT group. #*p*<0.05 DCM *vs.* the ICM group. The bar represents 10 μm.

(PERK), and ATF6] initiate the response to manage accumulated unfolded proteins by facilitating the activation of the transcription factors XBP1, ATF6, ATF4 and eIF2α, which mediate ER stress response induction [24].

GRP78 is an ER chaperone that is used as a marker for ER stress [25,26]. Under non-stressed conditions, GRP78 is bound to IRE1, PERK, and ATF6 and maintains them in an inactive state. In stress situations, GRP78 dissociates from these proteins, allowing their oligomerization to constitute an active form and triggering the UPR cascade [16,27]. Our results show an upregulation of GRP78 protein in DCM and ICM patients compared with levels in CNT subjects, in presence of a decrease in IRE1, especially in ICM patients, as discussed later. Most studies report an upregulation of this protein in animal models of HF [25,26,28]. Studies of human DCM patients have also demonstrated upregulation of this protein [14] and, in addition, this protein has been proposed as a therapeutic target for reducing the effects of ER stress [29]. So, we can infer that in HF the increase observed in the level of GRP78 may be a consequence of UPR activation in the presence of ER stress.

IRE1 is a transmembrane serine/threonine protein kinase receptor activated by dissociation of GRP78, and phosphorylation, is the most fundamental ER stress sensor that inhibits protein synthesis, it has an endonuclease activity that specifically cleaves an alternative spliced mRNA encoding the transcription factor XBP1 [30,31]. This transcription factor activates the transcription of genes involved in the ER stress response. IRE1 was downregulated in ICM patients in our work, and a similar tendency was found in the DCM group. We also analyzed the levels of the activated form of IRE1, p-IRE1, and we found that

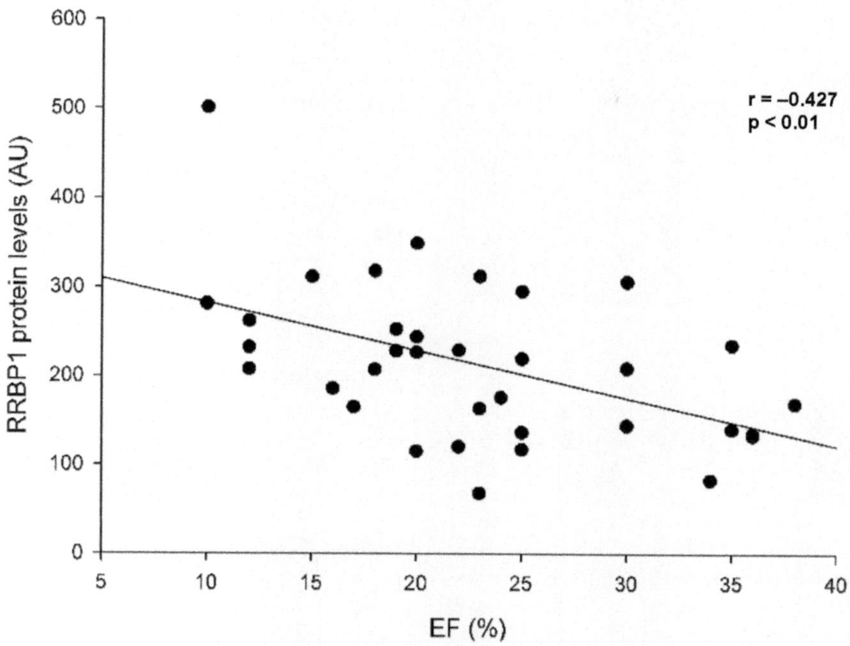

Figure 5. Scatter plots of correlation between RRBP1 and ejection fraction (EF) in dilated and ischemic cardiomyopathy human hearts. The values of RRBP1 are normalized to GAPDH.

this protein was upregulated in DCM patients and the same tendency was shown in ICM. Interestingly, XBP1 protein displayed increased levels in the two pathological groups studied. The decreased levels observed in IRE1 and the increased levels of p-IRE1 are also consistent with the activation of the UPR mechanism, since this not implies an increase in the protein levels but also the activation is possible through dimerization and autophosphorylation [32]. XBP1 upregulation has been reported in studies analyzing hypoxic effects in mouse culture cardiomyocytes [21]. All of these findings are consistent with the XBP1 activation in the UPR to increase the transcription of ER stress response genes.

ATF6 is a ER transmembrane signaling protein that together with IRE1 and PERK are the major sensors of unfolded proteins of the ER. ATF6 is activated by dissociation of GRP78 and its translocation to the Golgi and to the nucleus [24], is responsible for transcriptional regulation of pro-survival genes following ER stress, inducing the expression of ER stress genes [16]. We found that ATF6 was upregulated in both DCM and ICM patients, demonstrating that this ER stress pathway is highly important to activate the response during HF. All these results evidence the strong activation of UPR mechanism in HF patients that implies alterations in the levels of the majority of ER stress proteins.

ER structural protein levels in HF

Due to the ER stress process, is probably that a modification of the structure and shape of ER could occur in HF. The reticulons are a family of proteins that function mainly to stabilize the curvature of ER tubules [33]. In this work, we analyzed three members of this family, Reticulon 1 and two isoforms of Reticulon 4 (Nogo A and B). We found that Reticulon 1 is downregulated in DCM patients, whereas Nogo A and B were upregulated. Voeltz *et al.* have studied the effect of expression modification of reticulons *in vitro* and found that the downregulation of Reticulon 1 under stress conditions produces changes in the peripheral ER through the formation of membrane sheets; when the reticulons are overexpressed, tubule formation increases [34].

These changes in the protein levels of reticulons may alter the stabilization of the ER curvature, conferring it a different structure. Nevertheless, none studies have examined this relationship in heart disease; however the findings shown in this study strongly suggest that vital functions of the ER rely on its morphological integrity.

Other structural proteins analyzed were RRBP1 (also known as p180), kinectin, and CKAP4. A common feature of these proteins is their coiled-coil domains that form luminal bridges (in the case of CKAP4) and flat scaffolds (in RRPB1 and kinectin proteins). These proteins are implicated in shaping, cisternae stacking, and cytoskeletal interactions [35]. RRBP1 and kinectin are ER integral membrane proteins. The former plays a role in polysome assembly and therefore in protein biosynthesis as well as expansion of the Golgi complex [36]; also, it has been shown that is an inductor of membrane biogenesis [37,38]. Kinectin is a receptor for kinesin, which is involved in cellular component transport along microtubules [39].

Both RRBP1 and kinectin were upregulated in the pathological groups studied. These results could indicate that modeling of the ER structure occurs as a possible consequence of UPR activation in ER stress conditions. Moreover, the upregulation of RRBP1 may influence the enhancement of protein synthesis necessary in some UPR pathways. In addition, we found a direct relationship between this protein and the stress protein XBP1 in the DCM group, giving evidence about the existence of a specific relationship between stress and structure.

Besides, we found a solid inverse relationship between RRBP1 and LV function parameters EF and FS. These parameters are related to the ventricular remodeling that occurs in HF patients. This ventricular remodeling implies the activation of several pathways including inflammation and fibrosis that need a production of their related proteins. RRBP1 has a relevant role in protein synthesis and particularly it has been shown that is a crucial step in cardiac remodeling throughout increasing procollagen synthesis [40], necessary to develop the fibrosis processes in maladaptive cardiac remodeling.

In addition, there is evidence supporting structural modifications under stress conditions. Tumarovs'ka *et al.* reported the dilation of ER cisternae in induced ER stress in isolated cardiomyocytes [41]. Taking into account these findings and altogether with the results obtained in our study, we conclude that alterations in various UPR molecules as a consequence of ER stress may influence the architecture of the ER and alter its structure since we have observed changes in some of the proteins involved in forming and organizing the ER.

Study limitations

One limitation of this work is the inherent variability of the samples in disease etiology and treatment. However, to make our study etiologically homogenous, we chose DCM patients that reported no family history of the disease. Moreover, the patients selected in this study were on conventional therapy, and certain drugs may have influenced the levels of ER proteins. Furthermore, our tissue samples were confined to the transmural left ventricle apex, so our findings cannot be generalized to all layers and regions of the left ventricle. It is also noteworthy that this study was carried out using a high human sample size of both pathological and CNT hearts, making our results applicable for both DCM and ICM population.

Conclusions

We report the existence of new alterations in proteins related to ER stress response and shaping in HF. We show a plausible effect of ER stress on ER structure in a suitable sample of human hearts with DCM and ICM. Patients with higher values of RRBP1, linked to procollagen production, had worse LV function. Our results show a novel relationship between stress and structure of the ER and may be used to find specific therapeutic targets.

Acknowledgments

The authors thank the Transplant Coordination Unit (La Fe University Hospital, Valencia, Spain) for their help in obtaining the samples. Furthermore, we are grateful to Ana Villalba, Irene Valls, Julia Oto, and Mila Galiana, for their technical support in this work.

Author Contributions

Conceived and designed the experiments: AO ER ET. Performed the experiments: AO MM LM. Analyzed the data: AS JM. Contributed reagents/materials/analysis tools: JRG FL. Wrote the paper: AO ER ET. Supervised the study and corrected the writing: MR MP.

References

1. Remme WJ, Swedberg K (2002) Comprehensive guidelines for the diagnosis and treatment of chronic heart failure. Task force for the diagnosis and treatment of chronic heart failure of the European Society of Cardiology. Eur J Heart Fail 4: 11–22.
2. Davis RC, Hobbs FD, Lip GY (2000) ABC of heart failure. History and epidemiology. BMJ 320: 39–42.
3. Garcia-Rua V, Otero MF, Lear PV, Rodriguez-Penas D, Feijoo-Bandin S, et al. (2012) Increased expression of fatty-acid and calcium metabolism genes in failing human heart. PLoS One 7: e37505.
4. Rosca MG, Hoppel CL (2010) Mitochondria in heart failure. Cardiovasc Res 88: 40–50.
5. Rosca MG, Vazquez EJ, Kerner J, Parland W, Chandler MP, et al. (2008) Cardiac mitochondria in heart failure: decrease in respirasomes and oxidative phosphorylation. Cardiovasc Res 80: 30–39.
6. Cortes R, Rosello-Lleti E, Rivera M, Martinez-Dolz L, Salvador A, et al. (2010) Influence of heart failure on nucleocytoplasmic transport in human cardiomyocytes. Cardiovasc Res 85: 464–472.
7. Tarazon E, Rivera M, Rosello-Lleti E, Molina-Navarro MM, Sanchez-Lazaro IJ, et al. (2012) Heart failure induces significant changes in nuclear pore complex of human cardiomyocytes. PLoS One 7: e48957.
8. Molina-Navarro MM, Rosello-Lleti E, Tarazon E, Ortega A, Sanchez-Izquierdo D, et al. (2013) Heart failure entails significant changes in human nucleocytoplasmic transport gene expression. Int J Cardiol 2013;168:2837–2843.
9. Hein S, Kostin S, Heling A, Maeno Y, Schaper J (2000) The role of the cytoskeleton in heart failure. Cardiovasc Res 45: 273–278.
10. Pawlak A, Gil RJ, Grajkowska W, Nasierowska-Guttmejer AM, Rzezak J, et al. (2013) Significance of low desmin expression in cardiomyocytes in patients with idiopathic dilated cardiomyopathy. Am J Cardiol 111: 393–399.
11. Minamino T, Kitakaze M (2010) ER stress in cardiovascular disease. J Mol Cell Cardiol 48: 1105–1110.
12. Liu XH, Zhang ZY, Sun S, Wu XD (2008) Ischemic postconditioning protects myocardium from ischemia/reperfusion injury through attenuating endoplasmic reticulum stress. Shock 30: 422–427.
13. Hamada H, Suzuki M, Yuasa S, Mimura N, Shinozuka N, et al. (2004) Dilated cardiomyopathy caused by aberrant endoplasmic reticulum quality control in mutant KDEL receptor transgenic mice. Mol Cell Biol 24: 8007–8017.
14. Okada K, Minamino T, Tsukamoto Y, Liao Y, Tsukamoto O, et al. (2004) Prolonged endoplasmic reticulum stress in hypertrophic and failing heart after aortic constriction: possible contribution of endoplasmic reticulum stress to cardiac myocyte apoptosis. Circulation 110: 705–712.
15. Yoshida H (2007) ER stress and diseases. FEBS J 274: 630–658.
16. Chakrabarti A, Chen AW, Varner JD (2011) A review of the mammalian unfolded protein response. Biotechnol Bioeng 108: 2777–2793.
17. Macrae DJ (2007) The Council for International Organizations and Medical Sciences (CIOMS) guidelines on ethics of clinical trials. Proc Am Thorac Soc 4: 176–178, discussion 178–179.
18. Dickstein K, Vardas PE, Auricchio A, Daubert JC, Linde C, et al. (2010) 2010 Focused Update of ESC Guidelines on device therapy in heart failure: an update of the 2008 ESC Guidelines for the diagnosis and treatment of acute and chronic heart failure and the 2007 ESC Guidelines for cardiac and resynchronization therapy. Developed with the special contribution of the Heart Failure Association and the European Heart Rhythm Association. Europace 12: 1526–1536.
19. Winters AL, Minchin FR (2005) Modification of the Lowry assay to measure proteins and phenols in covalently bound complexes. Anal Biochem 346: 43–48.
20. Azorin I, Portoles M, Marin P, Lazaro-Dieguez F, Megias L, et al. (2004) Prenatal ethanol exposure alters the cytoskeleton and induces glycoprotein microheterogeneity in rat newborn hepatocytes. Alcohol Alcohol 39: 203–212.
21. Thuerauf DJ, Marcinko M, Gude N, Rubio M, Sussman MA, et al. (2006) Activation of the unfolded protein response in infarcted mouse heart and hypoxic cultured cardiac myocytes. Circ Res 99: 275–282.
22. Doroudgar S, Thuerauf DJ, Marcinko MC, Belmont PJ, Glembotski CC (2009) Ischemia activates the ATF6 branch of the endoplasmic reticulum stress response. J Biol Chem 284: 29735–29745.
23. Szegezdi E, Fitzgerald U, Samali A (2003) Caspase-12 and ER-stress-mediated apoptosis: the story so far. Ann N Y Acad Sci 1010: 186–194.
24. Doroudgar S, Glembotski CC (2013) New concepts of endoplasmic reticulum function in the heart: programmed to conserve. J Mol Cell Cardiol 55: 85–91.
25. Xin W, Li X, Lu X, Niu K, Cai J (2011) Involvement of endoplasmic reticulum stress-associated apoptosis in a heart failure model induced by chronic myocardial ischemia. Int J Mol Med 27: 503–509.
26. Arumugam S, Thandavarayan RA, Veeraveedu PT, Nakamura T, Arozal W, et al. (2012) Beneficial effects of edaravone, a novel antioxidant, in rats with dilated cardiomyopathy. J Cell Mol Med 16: 2176–2185.
27. Bertolotti A, Zhang Y, Hendershot LM, Harding HP, Ron D (2000) Dynamic interaction of BiP and ER stress transducers in the unfolded-protein response. Nat Cell Biol 2: 326–332.
28. Sun Y, Liu G, Song T, Liu F, Kang W, et al. (2008) Upregulation of GRP78 and caspase-12 in diastolic failing heart. Acta Biochim Pol 55: 511–516.
29. Fu HY, Minamino T, Tsukamoto O, Sawada T, Asai M, et al. (2008) Overexpression of endoplasmic reticulum-resident chaperone attenuates cardiomyocyte death induced by proteasome inhibition. Cardiovasc Res 79: 600–610.
30. Lee K, Tirasophon W, Shen X, Michalak M, Prywes R, et al. (2002) IRE1-mediated unconventional mRNA splicing and S2P-mediated ATF6 cleavage merge to regulate XBP1 in signaling the unfolded protein response. Genes Dev 16: 452–466.
31. Oikawa D, Kimata Y, Kohno K (2007) Self-association and BiP dissociation are not sufficient for activation of the ER stress sensor Ire1. J Cell Sci 120: 1681–1688.
32. Shamu CE, Walter P (1996) Oligomerization and phosphorylation of the Ire1p kinase during intracellular signaling from the endoplasmic reticulum to the nucleus. EMBO J 15: 3028–3039.
33. Hu J, Shibata Y, Voss C, Shemesh T, Li Z, et al. (2008) Membrane proteins of the endoplasmic reticulum induce high-curvature tubules. Science 319: 1247–1250.
34. Voeltz GK, Prinz WA, Shibata Y, Rist JM, Rapoport TA (2006) A class of membrane proteins shaping the tubular endoplasmic reticulum. Cell 124: 573–586.

35. Goyal U, Blackstone C (2013) Untangling the web: mechanisms underlying ER network formation. Biochim Biophys Acta 1833: 2492–2498.
36. Ueno T, Kaneko K, Sata T, Hattori S, Ogawa-Goto K (2012) Regulation of polysome assembly on the endoplasmic reticulum by a coiled-coil protein, p180. Nucleic Acids Res 40: 3006–3017.
37. Becker F, Block-Alper L, Nakamura G, Harada J, Wittrup KD, et al. (1999) Expression of the 180-kD ribosome receptor induces membrane proliferation and increased secretory activity in yeast. J Cell Biol 146: 273–284.
38. Benyamini P, Webster P, Meyer DI (2009) Knockdown of p180 eliminates the terminal differentiation of a secretory cell line. Mol Biol Cell 20: 732–744.
39. Toyoshima I, Yu H, Steuer ER, Sheetz MP (1992) Kinectin, a major kinesin-binding protein on ER. J Cell Biol 118: 1121–1131.
40. Ueno T, Tanaka K, Kaneko K, Taga Y, Sata T, et al. (2010) Enhancement of procollagen biosynthesis by p180 through augmented ribosome association on the endoplasmic reticulum in response to stimulated secretion. J Biol Chem 285: 29941–29950.
41. Tumanovs'ka LV, Nahibin VS, Dosenko V, Moibenko OO (2008) Ultrastructural changes in isolated cardiomyocytes in modeling of endoplasmic reticulum stress. Fiziol Zh 54: 10–21.

16

Validity of Heart Failure Diagnoses in Administrative Databases

Natalie McCormick[1,2], Diane Lacaille[2,3,4], Vidula Bhole[2,5], J. Antonio Avina-Zubieta[2,3,4]*

1 Faculty of Pharmaceutical Sciences, University of British Columbia, Vancouver, British Columbia, Canada, **2** Arthritis Research Centre of Canada, Richmond, British Columbia, Canada, **3** Division of Rheumatology, Department of Medicine, University of British Columbia, Vancouver, British Columbia, Canada, **4** Cardiovascular Committee of the Canadian Rheumatology Administrative Data Network, Richmond, British Columbia, Canada, **5** EpiSolutions Consultancy Services, Thane, India

Abstract

Objective: Heart failure (HF) is an important covariate and outcome in studies of elderly populations and cardiovascular disease cohorts, among others. Administrative data is increasingly being used for long-term clinical research in these populations. We aimed to conduct the first systematic review and meta-analysis of studies reporting on the validity of diagnostic codes for identifying HF in administrative data.

Methods: MEDLINE and EMBASE were searched (inception to November 2010) for studies: (a) Using administrative data to identify HF; or (b) Evaluating the validity of HF codes in administrative data; and (c) Reporting validation statistics (sensitivity, specificity, positive predictive value [PPV], negative predictive value, or Kappa scores) for HF, or data sufficient for their calculation. Additional articles were located by hand search (up to February 2011) of original papers. Data were extracted by two independent reviewers; article quality was assessed using the Quality Assessment of Diagnostic Accuracy Studies tool. Using a random-effects model, pooled sensitivity and specificity values were produced, along with estimates of the positive (LR+) and negative (LR−) likelihood ratios, and diagnostic odds ratios (DOR = LR+/LR−) of HF codes.

Results: Nineteen studies published from1999–2009 were included in the qualitative review. Specificity was ≥95% in all studies and PPV was ≥87% in the majority, but sensitivity was lower (≥69% in ≥50% of studies). In a meta-analysis of the 11 studies reporting sensitivity and specificity values, the pooled sensitivity was 75.3% (95% CI: 74.7–75.9) and specificity was 96.8% (95% CI: 96.8–96.9). The pooled LR+ was 51.9 (20.5–131.6), the LR− was 0.27 (0.20–0.37), and the DOR was 186.5 (96.8–359.2).

Conclusions: While most HF diagnoses in administrative databases do correspond to true HF cases, about one-quarter of HF cases are not captured. The use of broader search parameters, along with laboratory and prescription medication data, may help identify more cases.

Editor: Yiru Guo, University of Louisville, United States of America

Funding: This study was funded in part by the Canadian Arthritis Network (http://www.canradnetwork.ca). Natalie McCormick is supported by a Doctoral Research Award from the Canadian Institutes of Health Research. J. Antonio Avina-Zubieta held a salary award from the Canadian Arthritis Network and The Arthritis Society of Canada. He is currently the British Columbia Lupus Society Scholar and holds a Scholar Award from the Michael Smith Foundation for Health Research. Diane Lacaille holds the Mary Pack Chair in Arthritis Research from UBC and The Arthritis Society of Canada. The funders had no role in study design, data collection and analysis, decision to publish, or preparation of the manuscript.

Competing Interests: Vidula Bhole is the sole proprietor of a consulting company, EpiSolutions Consultancy Services. There are no patents, products in development or marketed products to declare.

* Email: azubieta@arthritisresearch.ca

Introduction

Heart failure (HF) is a chronic condition that affects about 26 million people worldwide [1] and imposes a tremendous burden on these individuals and their families. The typical 40 year-old faces a 20% lifetime risk of developing HF [2], and the incidence of HF amongst adults 65 years of age and older is approximately 12.5 per 1,000 person-years [3]. About half of new cases are expected to die within five years of diagnosis [2], and estimates of the annual economic burden of HF have recently exceeded $30 billion in the United States [2], and $108 billion worldwide [4].

The European Society of Cardiology describes HF as a disorder of cardiac structure or function where the heart is unable to deliver adequate levels of oxygen to the tissues [5]. Cases often have primary left systolic HF, which is characterized by "reduced contraction and emptying of the left ventricle" [5]. Still, many cases have left diastolic HF, in which ventricular compliance and filling are impaired [6] but the contractile function of the ventricle is preserved. HF has some 'classic' signs and symptoms, including ankle oedema, and exertional dyspnoea and fatigue [5,6]. However, HF is not considered to be a discrete condition but a "complex clinical syndrome" [6] that occurs in conjunction with other cardiovascular diseases such as coronary artery disease, valvular heart disease, hypertension, dilated cardiomyopathy [6], and conduction and rhythm disorders [5]. A significant source of morbidity on its own, HF frequently occurs in concordance with other chronic disorders such as renal disease [7–9], chronic obstructive pulmonary disease (COPD) [8,10–12], and diabetes [7–11]. Thus when evaluating treatments for these and other chronic conditions, it is essential to adjust for diagnoses of HF.

Administrative databases have become excellent resources for the study of HF by allowing for long-term evaluation of large numbers of patients at relatively low cost. Some examples are the Medicare databases in the United States (USA) and health ministry databases from countries such as Canada where healthcare is funded by provincial governments and available to all residents. These data sources allow the patient-level linkage of health resource utilization data (including hospital separations, outpatient encounters, and sometimes, dispensed prescriptions) to demographic and vital statistics data. When studying clinic-based populations, patients with severe HF are likely to be overrepresented, but administrative databases provide a means for identifying risk factors for HF, and quantifying the effects of treatment in unselected populations.

However, administrative databases are only useful for HF research if the diagnostic codes contained within are valid; that is, if they can be used to distinguish those who actually have HF from those who do not. Their validity can be assessed by comparing the administrative database diagnosis to an accepted 'gold standard' reference diagnosis. This diagnosis is typically obtained through more resource-intensive processes such as patient self-report, retrospective chart review, or prospective clinical examination. Principal measures of validity include sensitivity (how many HF cases in the population are actually coded for HF) and specificity (how many of the non-HF cases in the population are, in turn, *not* coded for HF). Unfortunately, there is some uncertainty surrounding the validity of diagnoses recorded in administrative databases since most databases are not established for research purposes. Validity is of particular concern when studying HF patients, as they tend to have high comorbidity burdens and be hospitalized for other cardiovascular and respiratory conditions [13,14]. While HF may have contributed to the need for these hospitalizations, this diagnosis may not be entered on the discharge record, leaving this potential confounding variable to go undetected in subsequent epidemiologic investigations. Although several assessments of the validity of HF codes in administrative databases have been published [15–17], there is considerable heterogeneity amongst them with regards to the clinical settings and reference standards used. Of note, many of these assessments were limited to specific populations (e.g. those diagnosed with atrial fibrillation [15] or myocardial infarction (MI) [16]) so may not be generalizable to the HF diagnoses recorded for other individuals.

As a part of a Canadian Rheumatology Network for establishing best practices in the use of administrative data for health research and surveillance (CANRAD) [18–22], we have conducted a systematic review of studies reporting on the validity of diagnostic codes for identifying cardiovascular diseases (CVD) in administrative data. Data from these studies were used to compare the validity of these codes, and to evaluate whether administrative health data can accurately identify CVD for the purpose of identifying these events as covariates, outcomes, or complications in future research. We recently reported our findings on the validity of codes for MI [23]. In the current paper, we focus on HF and undertake both a qualitative analysis, and for the first time, a quantitative synthesis of studies reporting on the validity of HF codes in administrative databases.

Methods

Literature Search

Comprehensive searches of the MEDLINE and EMBASE databases from inception (1946 and 1974, respectively) to November 2010 for all available peer-reviewed literature were conducted by an experienced librarian (M-DW). Two search strategies were employed: (1) All studies where administrative data was used to identify CVD; (2) All studies reporting on the validity of administrative data for identifying CVD. Our MEDLINE and EMBASE search strategies are available as (Text S1 and S2). To find additional articles, the authors hand-searched the reference lists of the key articles located through the database search. The Cited-By tools in PubMed and Google Scholar were also used to find relevant articles that had cited the articles located through the database search (up to February 2011). The titles and abstracts of each record were screened for relevance by two independent reviewers. No protocol for this systematic review has been published, though the review was conducted in accordance with the Preferred Reporting Items for Systematic Reviews and Meta-Analyses (PRISMA) [24] and Meta-Analysis of Observational Studies in Epidemiology (MOOSE) [25] statements; our completed checklists are provided as (Checklist S1 and S2).

Inclusion Criteria

We selected full-length, peer-reviewed articles published in English that used administrative data and reported validation statistics for the main International Classification of Diseases (ICD) codes for HF (ICD-8 and ICD-9 428, and ICD-10 I50), or provided sufficient data enabling us to calculate them. Any discrepancies were discussed until consensus was reached. When the conflict persisted a third reviewer (JAA-Z) was consulted.

Data Extraction

The full text of each selected record was examined by two independent reviewers (NM and VB) who abstracted data using a standardized collection form (a copy is provided in **Text S3**). While extracting data, particular attention was given to the study population, administrative data source, algorithm used to identify HF, validation method, and gold standard. Validation statistics comparing the HF codes to definite or possible cases were abstracted. These statistics included sensitivity, specificity, positive predictive value (PPV), negative predictive value (NPV), and kappa scores. Because hospital separations typically contain multiple diagnoses, with the primary or principal diagnosis in the first position followed by one or more secondary diagnoses, we abstracted statistics for each of these positions, where available. This was especially important given some recent studies of administrative databases that suggest hospitalizations with HF in the primary position are decreasing, while those with HF coded in secondary diagnostic positions are increasing [26,27]. Data were independently abstracted by each reviewer who subsequently compared their forms to correct any errors and resolve discrepancies.

Quality Assessment

The design and methods used by each study, including the rigour of the reference standard, can directly influence the validity statistics produced. Thus, all studies were evaluated for quality, and the validation statistics were stratified by level of study quality. This was done using the Quality Assessment of Diagnostic

Accuracy Studies (QUADAS) tool [28] (available as a part of **Text S3**), used previously by the CANRAD network in assessing the validity of codes for diabetes mellitus [21], osteoporosis and fractures [22], and myocardial infarction [23]. Briefly, it is a 14-item evidence-based quality assessment tool used in systematic reviews of diagnostic accuracy studies. Each item, phrased as a question, addresses one or more aspects of bias or applicability; however, there is no overall score. Instead, as done previously [22,23], items were independently answered by each reviewer and used to qualitatively assess each study as High, Medium, or Low quality. Any disagreements were resolved by consensus.

Statistical Analysis

All validation statistics were abstracted as reported. Where sufficient data were available we calculated 95% confidence intervals (95% CI) and additional validity statistics not directly reported in the original publication. These were evaluated on aggregate, and, as pre-specified, stratified by geographic region and time period of publication. In evaluating the HF codes in administrative data, we considered the diagnosis assigned during the validation process to be the diagnostic gold standard; this meant, for instance, that cases coded for HF and classified as HF during validation were true-positive cases, while cases coded for HF but classified during validation as no-HF were false-positives. Sensitivity (the ability of the codes to identify true positive HF cases) was equal to the number of true positives divided by the sum of true positives and false negatives (all those with HF). Specificity (the ability of the HF codes to exclude false-positive cases) was equal to the number of true negatives divided by the sum of true negatives and false positives (all those without HF). Sensitivity and specificity were also used to calculate the positive and negative likelihood ratios (LR+ and LR−) and diagnostic odds ratios (DOR). The DOR (the ratio of the odds that coded individuals will actually have HF compared to the odds that non-coded individuals will have HF) was equal to the LR+ divided by the LR−.

The positive likelihood ratio (LR+), the ratio of true-positives to false-positives amongst all those coded for HF, was equal to the sensitivity divided by 1 − specificity. The negative likelihood ratio (LR−), the ratio of false-negatives to true-negatives amongst all those not coded for HF, was equal to 1 − sensitivity divided by the specificity. Thus, higher LR+ values (those greater than 1) mean the presence of an HF code is more indicative of true HF and lower LR- values (those closer to 0 than 1) mean the absence of an HF code is more indicative of non-disease (no HF). Specificity values typically fall close to 1, such that the denominator for LR+ (1 − specificity) is usually much smaller than the denominator for LR−. As a result, the values for LR+ (which range from 1 to 10 or more) are usually much larger than those for LR− (which range from 0 to 1). An LR+ of 5 to 10 means the codes are moderately good for detecting HF, and an LR+>10 means the codes are very good. Similarly, with an LR− of 0.1 to 0.2, the absence of an HF code corresponds moderately to non-disease (no HF), while an LR− of <0.1 corresponds very well to non-disease [29].

Three other validation statistics of interest were PPV, NPV, and kappa score. The PPV (the likelihood that the HF code corresponds to a true-positive case) was equal to the number of true positives divided by the total number of cases coded for HF (true-positives and false-positives). NPV (the likelihood that an individual not coded for HF is a true-negative case) was equal to the number of true negatives divided by the total number of cases not coded for HF (true-negatives and false-negatives). Kappa (a measure of the agreement, beyond that expected by chance, between how cases are classified in the administrative database and by the validation process) was equal to the observed agreement (the percent of cases classified as either true-positives or true-negatives) minus that expected by chance, divided by [100% - the agreement expected by chance]. Kappa scores greater than 0.60 indicate substantial/almost perfect agreement, 0.41–0.60 is considered as moderate agreement, 0.21–0.40 as fair agreement, and those 0.20 or lower as light/poor agreement [30].

Where available, we abstracted statistics for definite and possible cases of HF, though the number of categories reported depended on the choice of reference standard. In some studies, the reference standard is the presence of any notation of an HF diagnosis in the medical chart, and cases are classified simply as HF or no HF. The Framingham criteria [31] also classify cases as either HF or no HF; at least two of the major Framingham criteria (which include neck vein distension, cardiomegaly, and acute pulmonary edema) or one major criterion and two minor criteria (which include ankle oedema, hepatomegaly, and plural effusion) must be met for the diagnosis of HF. Other sets of standard criteria do allow for further classification. The Carlson criteria [32] use a points system in which potential cases are evaluated in three categories (history, physical examination, and chest radiography), and allocated a maximum of four points in each category, and a maximum overall score of 12. A score of 8 or more is considered Definite HF while 5–7 points are considered Possible HF, and 4 or fewer points are classified as Unlikely HF [32]. Under the European Society of Cardiology criteria [33], for a case to be classified as HF there must be both signs and symptoms of HF, and objective evidence of cardiac dysfunction. Some investigators [17,34] have classified cases meeting both of these criteria as Definite HF, and those meeting only one of these criteria as Questionable, Possible, or Probable HF. It should be noted that while the New York Heart Association functional classification is used to measure the degree of functional limitation experienced by HF patients, and may assist in the selection of therapies [5], it is not used to make the initial diagnosis of HF.

Meta-Analysis

Studies that reported raw data for sensitivity and specificity were included in the meta-analysis. Forest plots and a summary receiver operating characteristic (ROC) curve were constructed, and pooled estimates (and 95% CI's) of the sensitivity and specificity values, LR+, LR−, and DORs were calculated. More informative diagnostic tests (in this case, being HF codes) - those with good sensitivity and good specificity - will produce ROC curves positioned in the top-left area of the ROC plane, well away from the positive diagonal line [35]. Two additional summary measures of test performance were determined from the ROC curve, the area under the curve (AUC) and Q*. The AUC ranges between 0 and 1, with 1 corresponding to a perfect test [36]. In the context of our research question, an AUC of 1 would mean that, given two cases, one with HF and one without, there is a 100% probability that the positive case will be coded for HF and the negative case will not. The Q*, the lower bound of the AUC, is the point at which the sensitivity and specificity are equal [36]. Higher Q* values indicate better-performing tests.

To assess for the presence of heterogeneity amongst the included studies, we visually inspected the forest plots and ROC curve, and calculated the χ^2 statistic, Cochran's Q [37] and I^2 [38] statistics. The I^2 index, a measure of the degree of inconsistency across study findings, is expressed as the percentage of variation between studies due to heterogeneity as opposed to chance [38]. A value of 0% indicates no observed heterogeneity, while 25% is indicative of low heterogeneity, 50% moderate, and 75% high heterogeneity [38]. When there are a small number of studies, the I^2 index is a preferred measure over Cochrane's Q [38]. In the absence of substantial heterogeneity, a fixed-effects model was to be applied. Otherwise, a random-effects model was to be applied, using the DerSimonian Laird method.

To assess the impact each individual study had on the pooled estimates, a jackknife sensitivity analysis [39] was performed in which one study was removed and all summary statistics were re-calculated. This process was repeated for all studies. The impact of publication bias was not evaluated as the common tests available to assess publication bias, including the Begg, Egger, and Macaskill tests, have been shown to be misleading for meta-analyses of test accuracy [40]. All analyses were conducted using Meta-Disc software, version 1.4 [41].

Results

Literature Search

After the removal of duplicates, 1,587 citations were identified through MEDLINE and EMBASE searches and screened for relevance to our study objectives. We then assessed 98 full-text articles for eligibility (**Figure 1**), of which 12 were selected for inclusion. We also assessed 30 full-text articles for eligibility that were identified from hand searches, and selected 7 additional articles therein. Thus, a total of 128 articles were assessed for eligibility, from which 109 were excluded, mainly because they reported on the validity of other CVD (n = 59), or did not actually validate HF diagnoses in administrative data (n = 20). Six articles were excluded because they were not published in English; their languages of publication were Danish, German, Italian, Japanese, Portuguese, and Spanish. Ultimately 19 articles were included for the qualitative systematic review of HF.

Study Characteristics

Of the 19 articles evaluating HF diagnoses that were included in the final review, nine (47%) were from the United States, six (32%) were from Canada, three (16%) from Europe, and one was from Australia. Characteristics of these studies are presented in **Table 1**. Validation was the primary objective in all but one [42] of these studies. Six studies [17,34,42–45] reported on the validity of HF exclusively, while 13 reported on the validity of other diagnoses as well. Overall, data were collected over a thirty-year period (1976–2005), though the studies were all published relatively recently (the earliest in 1999 [16]). PPV data were available from all but one [16] study, sensitivity and NPV data were available from 14 studies (74%), and specificity data from 13 studies (68%). Kappa scores were less frequently reported. Only four studies [17,46–48] reported on the validity of ICD-10 codes separately from ICD-9. Most of the administrative databases pertained to hospitalizations though diagnoses recorded for outpatient encounters were included in five studies [42,44,45,49,50]. None of the studies reported on the validity of HF as a cause-of-death.

Chart reviews, sometimes in conjunction with unspecified diagnostic criteria, formed the basis of the gold standard in nine (47%) studies [15,16,43,46–48,50–52], and patient self-report was used in one [49]. Cardiac disease registries were used in two studies [53,54], while a specific set of diagnostic criteria were incorporated in the reference standards of the seven remaining studies [17,34,42,44,45,55,56].

Study quality was evaluated based on the QUADAS tool [28], with 11 of 19 studies (58%) categorized as high quality, seven as medium (37%), and just one (5%) as low quality. A detailed breakdown of the quality assessment for each study is provided in **Table S1**. Of the seven medium-quality studies, two did not adequately describe the validation process [47,48], and five used a less-reliable gold standard than published diagnostic criteria (being patient self-report in one [49] and chart review by an individual other than a clinician or trained hospital coder in four [15,16,50,51]). The low-quality study [52] employed a very select source population (women at one institution undergoing vaginal hysterectomy), assessed only two potential cases of HF, and did not adequately describe the validation process.

Validity of Heart Failure Diagnoses

The validation statistics reported by each of the included studies are provided in **Table 2**. Sensitivity was reported by 14 studies, and was ≥69% in half of them (range: 0 to 87%). PPV was undefined (0/0) in one of the studies [52], but was at least 87% in nine of the 17 remaining studies (range: 34 to 100%). Specificity was ≥95% in all 13 studies reporting this statistic, and NPV was ≥88% in all but two of the 14 studies where this data was available. Kappa was only reported in six (32%) studies [43,46,47,51,53,55]. The values in three of the studies (which ranged from 0.43 to 0.58) indicated there was moderate agreement between the diagnostic codes and reference standard, while those in the other three (range 0.72 to 0.94) indicated there was substantial to almost perfect agreement.

The Framingham criteria were used in three studies, with the PPV's reported as 65% [45], 82% [42], and 94% [56]. One of these studies [56] used both the Framingham and Carlson criteria, and found higher accuracy with the Framingham (PPV = 94%) than with the Carlson (PPV = 89%). The European Society of Cardiology criteria were used in two studies; the PPV for definite HF was 82% in one [34] but just 65% in the other [17]. Sex-stratified statistics were provided by two studies; one [56] reported a slightly higher PPV for ICD-9 428 in females, and the other [43] found that the sensitivity of ICD-9 428 was significantly better in females than males (66% vs. 61%). In that study, the sensitivity was also significantly better amongst Mexican Americans than Non-Hispanic whites (66% vs. 59%) [43].

The studies in **Table 2** are ordered chronologically by publication year for the purpose of identifying any secular trends in the validity of HF codes. The nine-earliest studies included in this review were published between 1999 and 2004, with the ten remaining studies published from 2005 to 2009. However, no secular trends were observed for any of the validation statistics. Eleven (58%) of the studies included in this review were rated as high quality and seven (37%) as medium quality. Sensitivity ranged from 43% to 87% amongst the high quality studies, and from 58% to 87% amongst the medium quality. The PPV's for these two categories were also similar, ranging from 36% to 99% amongst the high quality studies, and from 34% to 100% amongst the medium quality. Any geographic comparisons were limited by the fact that 15 of the 19 studies were conducted in North America. The only difference observed was that the sensitivity values tended to be higher amongst the seven US studies than the five Canadian ones.

Meta-Analysis

Included in the quantitative synthesis were the 11 articles from which raw data on sensitivity and specificity were available. Forest plots of the pooled sensitivity and specificity values are illustrated in **Figure 2**. A random-effects model was used since the χ^2, Q*, and I^2 statistics indicated there was a high level of heterogeneity between studies. The pooled sensitivity was 75.3% (95% CI: 74.7–75.9) and the pooled specificity was 96.8% (95% CI: 96.8–96.9). The summary LR+ was 51.9 (95% CI: 20.5–131.6) and the summary LR- was 0.27 (95% CI: 0.20–0.37), giving a summary DOR of 186.5 (95% CI: 96.8–359.22). The summary ROC curve is illustrated in **Figure 3**, wherein the AUC was 0.93 (SE 0.0396) and the Q* was 0.86 (SE 0.0466).

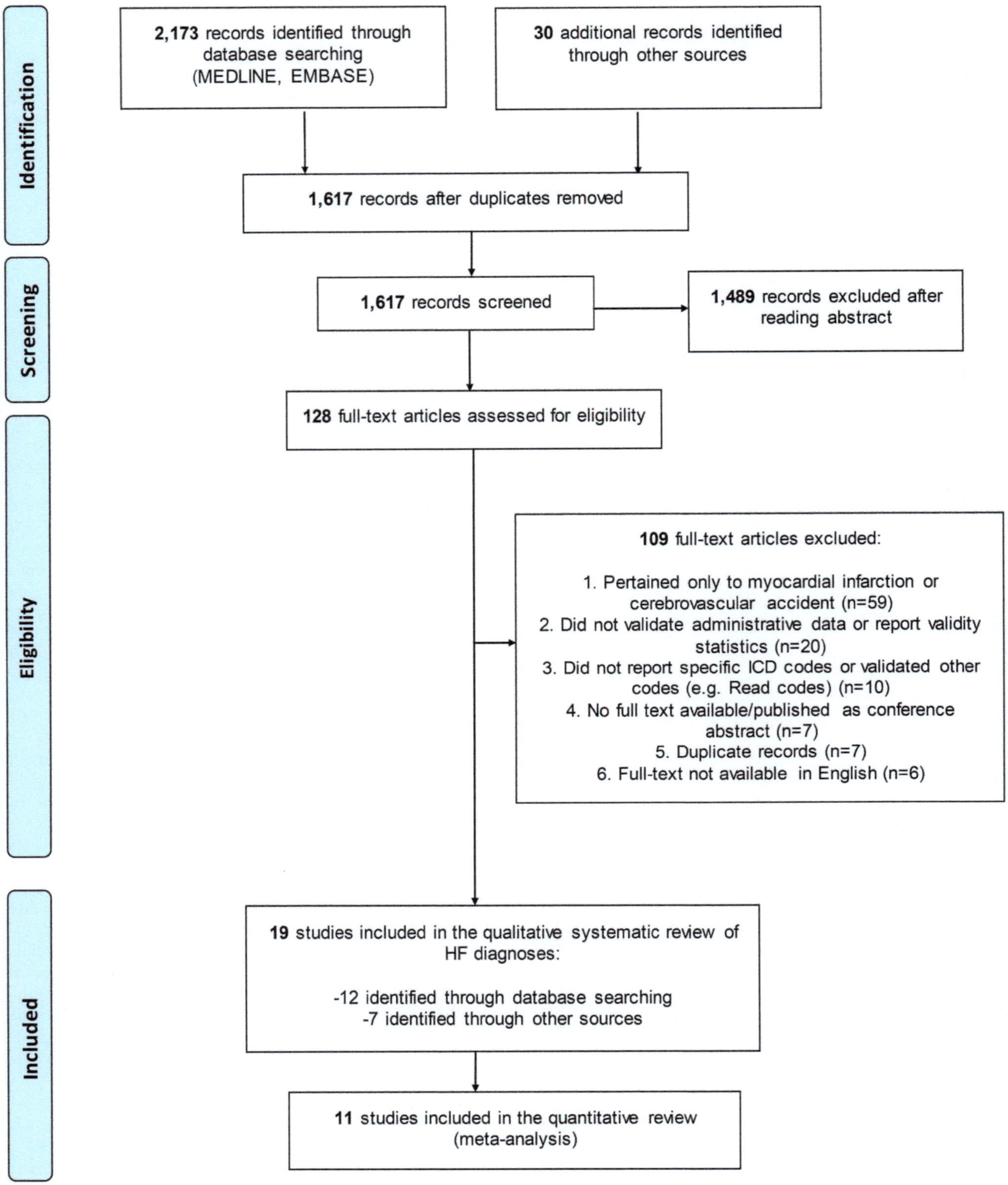

Figure 1. Preferred Reporting Items for Systematic Reviews and Meta-Analyses (PRISMA)-style Flowchart of Study Selection and Review. HF = heart failure; ICD = International Classification of Diseases

Results of the jackknife sensitivity analysis, wherein the pooled estimates were re-calculated after the removal of one study at a time, are shown in **Table 3**. The resulting pooled sensitivity estimates ranged mainly from 74% to 76%, and the specificities from 96.6% to 96.9%. The two most influential studies were those by Onofrei *et al* (sensitivity = 77.5% and specificity = 93.3% after

Table 1. Characteristics of Included Studies.

First Author, Year of Publication	Year(s) of Data Collection	Primary Validation Study?	Country	Records Evaluated (N)	Source Population	Type of Administrative Data	Gold Standard
Alqaisi [45], 2009	2004–2005	Yes	USA (Michigan)	400	enrollees in large HMO receiving care from large multi-specialty medical group	ICD-9 inpatient/ outpatient records	CRDC – Framingham criteria
Austin [53], 2002	1996–2000	Yes	Canada (Ontario)	58,816	consecutive patients ≥20 years old admitted to coronary care units from emergency room	ICD-9 inpatient records	disease registry - diagnosis of bedside nurse (as recorded in Fastrak II prospective acute coronary syndromes registry)
Birman-Deych [15], 2005	1998–1999	Yes	USA	23,657	Medicare beneficiaries (aged 20-105 years) hospitalized for atrial fibrillation	ICD-9 inpatient records	chart review
Chen [47], 2009	2003	Yes	Canada (Alberta)	4,008	general hospitalized population	ICD-10 inpatient records	chart review
Goff [43], 2000	1988–1994	Yes	USA (Texas)	5,083	general hospitalized population (participants in population-based Corpus Christi Heart Project, all residents 25-74 years of one Texas county)	ICD-9 inpatient records	chart review
Heckbert [55], 2004	1994–2000	Yes	USA	34,016	women participating in the Women's Health Initiative clinical and observational studies	ICD-9 inpatient records	CRDC – Women's Health Initiative criteria
Heisler [52], 2009	2004–2005	Yes	USA (Minnesota)	712	women undergoing vaginal hysterectomy for benign indication	ICD-9 inpatient records	chart review
Henderson [46], 2006	1998–1999, 2000–2001	yes	Australia	14,635	all hospitalized patients (excluding same-day chemotherapy and dialysis)	ICD-10 inpatient records	chart review: charts were re-coded by professional coders
Humphries [51], 2000	1994–1995	yes	Canada (British Columbia)	817	patients hospitalized for percutaneous coronary intervention	ICD-9 inpatient records	chart review
Ingelsson [34], 2005	1976–2001	yes	Sweden	317	men (aged 50 years at enrolment) in a cohort study aimed at identifying metabolic risk factors for cardiovascular disease	ICD-8,9,10 inpatient records	CRDC - European Society of Cardiology criteria
Khand [17], 2005	1997–1998	yes	UK	339	hospitalized patients	ICD-10 inpatient records	CRDC - European Society of Cardiology criteria
Lee [56], 2005	1997–1999	yes	Canada (Ontario)	1,808	general hospitalized population (<105 years)	ICD-9 inpatient records	CRDC - Framingham and Carlson criteria

Table 1. Cont.

First Author, Year of Publication	Year(s) of Data Collection	Primary Validation Study?	Country	Records Evaluated (N)	Source Population	Type of Administrative Data	Gold Standard
Levy [16], 1999	1994	yes	Canada	224	individuals ≥65 years hospitalized with myocardial infarction	ICD-9 inpatient records	chart review: mentioned in records
Merry [54], 2009	1987–2003	yes	Netherlands	21,110	residents of one region of the Netherlands, aged 20–59 years at registration, participating in two large monitoring projects	ICD-9 inpatient records	disease registry - diagnosis listed in Cardiology Information System (hospital cardiology service)
Onofrei [44], 2004	1998–2000	yes	USA (Oregon)	205,756	all patients attending a network of nine internal medicine and family practice clinics	ICD-9 inpatient/ outpatient records	CRDC - left ventricular ejection fraction value
Rector [49], 2004	1999–2000	yes	USA (Midwest and Northeast)	3,633	Medicare beneficiaries ≥65 years of age	ICD-9 inpatient/ outpatient records	patient self-report
Roger [42], 2004	1979–2000	no	USA (Minnesota)	7,298	population-based heart failure cohort	ICD-9 inpatient/ outpatient records	CRDC - Framingham criteria, and chart review – mentioned in chart
So [48], 2006	2003	yes	Canada (Alberta)	193	patients hospitalized for myocardial infarction	ICD-9,10 inpatient records	chart review
Szeto [50], 2002	1996–1998	yes	USA (California)	148	patients attending a Veterans Affairs general medicine clinic	ICD-9 outpatient records	chart review - mentioned in records/problem list

CRDC = Chart Review, Diagnostic Criteria – the charts of potential cases were reviewed, and a formal set of diagnostic criteria were applied when evaluating cases.

Table 2. Results of Studies Validating Diagnoses of Heart Failure (HF) in Administrative Data.

First Author, Year	Diagnostic Codes	Parameter	Sensitivity (95% CI)	Specificity (95% CI)	PPV (95% CI)	NPV (95% CI)	Kappa (95% CI)	LR+	LR-	DOR	Quality
Levy [16], 1999	ICD-9 402, 408, 425, 428, 429.3	HF as a comorbidity (secondary diagnosis) of MI	65 (59–72)			78 (72–83)		5.91 (3.47–10.05)	0.39 (0.30-0.51)	15.06 (7.47-30.37)	Medium
Goff [43], 2000	ICD-9 428	primary or secondary diagnosis	62.79 (60.17–65.34)	95.39 (94.65–96.03)	83.48 (81.04–85.66)	87.38 (86.28–88.35)		13.61 (11.69–15.85	0.39 (0.36-0.42)	34.90 (28.90-42.13)	High
	ICD-9 428 or 402	primary or secondary diagnosis	66.21 (63.63–68.69)	93.28 (92.42–94.06)	78.53 (76.04–80.84)	88.18 (87.09–89.19)		9.86 (8.69–11.18)	0.36 (0.34-0.39)	27.21 (22.95-32.26)	
	ICD-9 398.91, 402.x1, 404.x, 415.0, 416.9, 425.4, 428.x, 429.4, 514, 518.4, 786.0	primary or secondary diagnosis	67.08 (64.51–69.55)	92.61 (91.71–93.42)	77.11 (74.60–79.44)	88.34 (87.28–89.33)	0.72	9.08 (8.05–10.23)	0.36 (0.33-0.38)	25.53 (21.61-30.16)	
	ICD-9 428.x	females	66	95.3	86.3	86.2					
	ICD-9 428.x	males	60.5	95.7	81.9	88.2					
	ICD-9 428.x or 402.x	females	68.8	92.2	79.7	86.8					
	ICD-9 428.x or 402.x	males	64.6	93.2	75.5	89.0					
	ICD-9 398.91, 402.x1, 404.x, 415.0, 416.9, 425.4, 428.x, 429.4, 514, 518.4, 786.0	females	70.2	92.1	79.9	87.3					
	ICD-9 398.91, 402.x1, 404.x, 415.0, 416.9, 425.4, 428.x, 429.4, 514, 518.4, 786.0	males	65.0	93.2	75.5	89.1					
Humphries [51], 2000	ICD-9 428	as pre-admission comorbid diagnosis	66.1	94.8	50.6	97.2	0.53	12.71	0.36	35.28	Medium
Austin[a] [53], 2002	ICD-9 428	primary diagnosis	58.52 (57.20–59.83)	96.78 (96.63–96.93)	65.14 (63.78–66.46)	95.79 (95.61–95.95)	0.58	18.20 (17.29–19.17)	0.43 (0.42-0.44)	42.47 (39.51-45.65)	High
		primary or secondary	85.41 (84.44–86.33)	84.28 (83.97–84.59)	35.80 (34.98–36.63)	98.25 (98.13–98.37)	0.43	5.43 (5.31–5.56)	0.17 (0.16–0.19)	31.38 (29.01–33.94)	
Szeto [50], 2002	ICD-9 428.1, 428.0, 428.9	in administrative database	86.67 (58.39–97.66)	100.00 (96.50–100.00)	100.00 (71.66–100)	98.00 (94.21–99.74)		223.16 (14.1–3625.5)	0.16 (0.05–0.49)	1441.8 (65.77–31608.6)	Medium
Onofrei [50], 2004	ICD-9 402.01, 402.11, 402.91, 404.01, 404.03, 404.11, 404.13, 404.91, 404.93, 425.xx, 428.xx	HF defined as LVEF≤55%	43.9 (41.3–46.6)	99.5 (99.4–99.5)	35.6 (33.3–37.9)	99.6 (99.6–99.6)		80.40 (73.98–87.37)	0.56 (0.54–0.59)	142.54 (126.33–160.84)	High
		HF defined as LVEF≤40%	54.4 (50.8–57.9)	99.4 (99.3–99.4)	24.9 (22.9–27.0)	99.8 (99.8–99.8)		85.69 (78.81–93.17)	0.46 (0.43–0.50)	186.52 (160.54–216.71)	
Heckbert [55], 2004	ICD-9 428 or 425		78.99 (75.96–81.74)	97.72 (97.55–97.88)	45.34 (42.70–48.01)	99.49 (99.40–99.56)	0.56 (0.53–0.59)	34.67 (32.03–37.52)	0.22 (0.19–0.25)	161.27 (134.00–194.09)	High

Table 2. Cont.

First Author, Year	Diagnostic Codes	Parameter	Sensitivity (95% CI)	Specificity (95% CI)	PPV (95% CI)	NPV (95% CI)	Kappa (95% CI)	LR+	LR-	DOR	Quality
	ICD-9 428 only				48.59 (45.78–51.41)						
	ICD-9 425 only				17.36 (11.75–24.76)						
Rector[b] [49], 2004	ICD-9 398.91, 402.01, 402.11, 402.91, 404.01, 404.11, 404.91, 404.03, 404.13, 404.93, 428.xx	from 1 year of data, diagnosis on 1 claim	57.80 (50.93–64.38)	92.83 (91.90–93.66)	33.96 (29.20–39.06)	97.18 (96.54–97.71)		8.06 (6.83–9.51)	0.46 (0.39–0.53)	17.72 (13.15–23.89)	Medium
		from 1 year of data, diagnosis on ≥2 claims	46.79 (40.06–53.64)	94.67 (93.85–95.39)	35.92 (30.39–41.83)	96.54 (95.85–97.12)		8.78 (7.19–10.72)	0.56 (0.50–0.64)	15.62 (11.51–21.19)	
Roger [42], 2004	ICD-9 428, as primary diagnosis	against Framingham criteria			82 (81.09–82.87)						High
		against clinical diagnosis			90 (89.28–90.67)						
Khand [17], 2005	ICD-10 I50.1, I50.2, I11.0, I11.1, I25.5, I42.9	possible, probable, or definite; 1st-6th diagnostic positions			86.67 (82.41–90.05)						High
		probable or definite; 1st-6th diagnostic positions			77.27 (72.29–81.60)						
		definite; 1st-6th diagnostic positions			65.45 (60.02–70.53)						
Ingelsson [34], 2005	ICD-8 427.00, 427.10, 428.99; ICD-9 428; ICD-10 I50	overall definite			81.70 (76.91–85.71)						High
		overall definite or questionable			97.79 (95.31–99.03)						
		definite as primary diagnosis			95.00 (89.58–97.79)						
		definite or questionable as primary diagnosis			99.29 (95.49–99.96)						
Lee [56], 2005	ICD-9 428.x	vs. Framingham criteria, entire cohort; primary diagnosis			94.33 (93.07–95.38)						High
		vs. Framingham criteria, women; primary diagnosis			94.62 (92.81–96.01)						

Table 2. Cont.

First Author, Year	Diagnostic Codes	Parameter	Sensitivity (95% CI)	Specificity (95% CI)	PPV (95% CI)	NPV (95% CI)	Kappa (95% CI)	LR+	LR-	DOR	Quality
		vs. Framingham criteria, men; primary diagnosis			93.91 (91.97–95.42)						
		vs. Carlson criteria, entire cohort; primary diagnosis			88.60 (86.94–90.08)						
		vs. Carlson criteria, women; primary diagnosis			89.35 (87.02–91.32)						
		vs. Carlson criteria, men; primary diagnosis			87.83 (85.32–89.96)						
Birman-Deych [15], 2005	ICD-9 428.x, 398.91, 402.01, 402.11, 402.91, 404.01, 404.11, 404.91, 404.03, 404.13, 404.93	any diagnostic position (current or past event)	76.00 (75.19–76.80)	97.95 (97.69–98.19)	97.00 (96.61–97.34)	82.41 (81.79–83.02)		37.10 (32.87–41.87)	0.25 (0.24–0.25)	151.44 (132.90–172.57)	Medium
		primary position, during baseline hospitalization (current event)	33.00 (32.13–33.89)	99.41 (99.26–99.53)	97.98 (97.46–98.40)	63.15 (62.47–63.81)		55.97 (44.59–70.24)	0.67 (0.67–0.68)	83.04 (65.95–104.56)	
		any position, during baseline hospitalization (current event)	83.00 (82.29–83.70)	86.00 (85.38–86.60)	85.00						
		any position, all hospitalizations within past 12 months of baseline (current event)	86.00 (85.33–86.64)	82.01 (81.33–82.68)	80.64 (79.91–81.35)	87.05 (86.43–87.65)		4.78 (4.60–4.97)	0.17 (0.16–0.18)	28.01 (26.11–30.05)	
So [48], 2006	ICD-9 428.x	as a comorbidity of MI	81.8 (68.65–90.48)	96.4 (91.75–98.81)	90.0 (78.19–96.67)	93.0 (87.52–96.60)		22.58 (9.47–53.87)	0.19 (0.11–0.33)	119.70 (38.84–368.88)	Medium
	ICD-10 I09.9, I11.0, I13.0, I13.2, I25.5, I42.2, I42.5-I42.9, I43.x, I50.x, P29.0		80.0 (67.03–89.57)	97.8 (93.78–99.55)	93.6 (82.46–98.66)	92.5 (86.92–96.18)		36.80 (11.92–113.58)	0.20 (0.12–0.35)	180.00 (48.03–674.60)	
Henderson [46], 2006	ICD-10 I50	1998–1999	87.0 4 (83.13–90.17)	99.44 (99.22–99.60)	89.89 (86.22–92.69)	99.26 (99.02–99.45)	0.88	155.87 (112.77–215.44)	0.13 (0.10–0.17)	1195.7 (769.3–1858.4)	High
		2000–2001	86.25 (79.71–91.00)	99.71 (99.55–99.81)	86.25 (79.71–91.00)	99.71 (99.55–99.81)	0.86	292.90 (192.10–446.59)	0.14 (0.09–0.20)	2123.9 (1148.9-3926.4)	
Alqaisi[c] [45], 2009	ICD-9 428.xx, 398.91, 402.01, 402.11, 402.91				65.00 (60.08–69.63)						High

Table 2. Cont.

First Author, Year	Diagnostic Codes	Parameter	Sensitivity (95% CI)	Specificity (95% CI)	PPV (95% CI)	NPV (95% CI)	Kappa (95% CI)	LR+	LR-	DOR	Quality
Chen [47], 2009	ICD-10 I09.9, I11.0, I13.0, I13.2, I25.5, I42.0, I42.5- I42.9, I43.x, I50.x, P29.0	1st–16th diagnostic positions	68.56 (63.24–73.45)	99.32 (98.98–99.55)	90.16 (85.65–93.41)	97.20 (96.61–97.70)		100.76 (67.72–149.92)	0.32 (0.27–0.37)	318.33 (201.73–502.32)	Medium
		kappa					0.76				
		prevalence-adjusted, bias-adjusted kappa					0.94				
Heisler [52], 2009	ICD-9 428, 428.0, 428.1, 428.9		0.00 (0.00–80.21)	100.00 (99.32–100.0)	n/a (0/0)	99.72 (98.87–99.95)					Low
Merry [54], 2009	ICD-9 428		43.04 (35.27–51.15)	99.92 (99.86–99.95)	80.00 (69.64–87.60)	99.57 (99.45–99.64)		530.43 (319.19–881.47)	0.57 (0.50–0.65)	930.44 (525.99–1645.9)	High

[a]Validation was conducted amongst a coronary care unit population.
[b]Thirty-eight algorithms were evaluated in this study; the first parameter we selected achieved the highest sensitivity with specificity ≥90%, the second was chosen for comparison purposes.
[c]Sixteen algorithms were evaluated in this study; the validity of the primary algorithm is reported here 95% CI = 95% confidence interval; DOR = diagnostic odds ratio; HF = heart failure; LR+ = positive likelihood ratio; LR- = negative likelihood ratio; LVEF = left ventricular ejection fraction; MI = myocardial infarction; NPV = negative predictive value; PPV = positive predictive value.

its removal) and Austin *et al* (sensitivity = 71.8% and specificity = 99.1% after its removal).

Discussion

To our knowledge this is the first systematic review and meta-analysis on the validity of HF diagnoses in administrative data. Findings from this review suggest that the sensitivity of these codes is suboptimal, as sensitivity was ≤69% in 8 of the 14 studies reporting this statistic. However, the specificity and PPV of these codes appears much better: specificity was at least 95% in the 13 studies where this statistic was reported, and, in the majority of studies, the PPV was at least 87%. Further support was provided by the results of the meta-analysis, as the pooled specificity of HF codes was 97%, and the pooled LR+ was 52. This means an individual coded for HF is fifty-two-times more likely to actually have HF than someone not coded. However, the pooled sensitivity was modest, at just 75%, and the summary LR- value of 0.27 suggests that the absence of an HF code can rule out the diagnosis of HF only moderately.

The PPV's and NPV's amongst the studies included in this review were generally good, being at least 87% in the majority of studies reporting these statistics. A recently-published qualitative review of the validity of HF codes in North American databases also found the PPV to be generally high (>90% in most) [57]. However, it must be kept in mind that PPV and NPV are both dependent on the prevalence of the condition in the study population [35], and will be lower for rare conditions than for common conditions. This is important for HF because this condition differentially affects older individuals: for example, HF is reported to affect approximately 7.8% of US males aged 60–79 years, but only 1.5% of US males aged 40–59 years [2]. A higher baseline risk of HF in the study population may explain why several studies included in this review reported exceptionally high PPV's. For example, in the study by Szeto *et al* [50], which was conducted amongst a cohort of patients attending a Veteran's Affairs clinic, the prevalence of HF was 10%, and the PPV was 100%. So *et al* [48] examined the charts of patients hospitalized for MI, amongst whom the prevalence of HF was 29%, and the PPV in that study was 94%. Similarly, the prevalence of HF was 47% amongst the atrial fibrillation cohort studied by Birman-Deych *et al* [15], and the PPV was 97%. Consequently, if the exclusion of false-positive HF cases is of upmost priority for a particular study, the age and disease history of the study population must be taken into account when evaluating how accurately these codes will identify true HF cases.

Findings from our review suggest that administrative data codes are less-than-optimal for capturing HF cases, and this is consistent with another qualitative review of the validity of HF codes in which the sensitivity of HF diagnoses was highly-variable [58]. Instead of HF itself, some authors have suggested there is a tendency to list the underlying cause of the HF (such as MI or atrial fibrillation [17]), or another cardiac condition [53], in the primary position of the hospital discharge summary. Moreover, hospital coders generally report active conditions [51] such as MI, but may leave out chronic conditions such as HF if they were deemed not to have impacted the treatments provided in hospital or length-of-stay [47,58]. Similarly, the study by Birman-Deych *et al*, where sensitivity for HF increased with disease severity (from 80% for mild cases to 94% for severe [15]), suggested that severe cases of HF may be recorded more often in administrative databases than mild ones. Thus, to maximize the capture of HF cases, authors are advised to broaden their search parameters by examining all diagnostic positions of the hospital record,

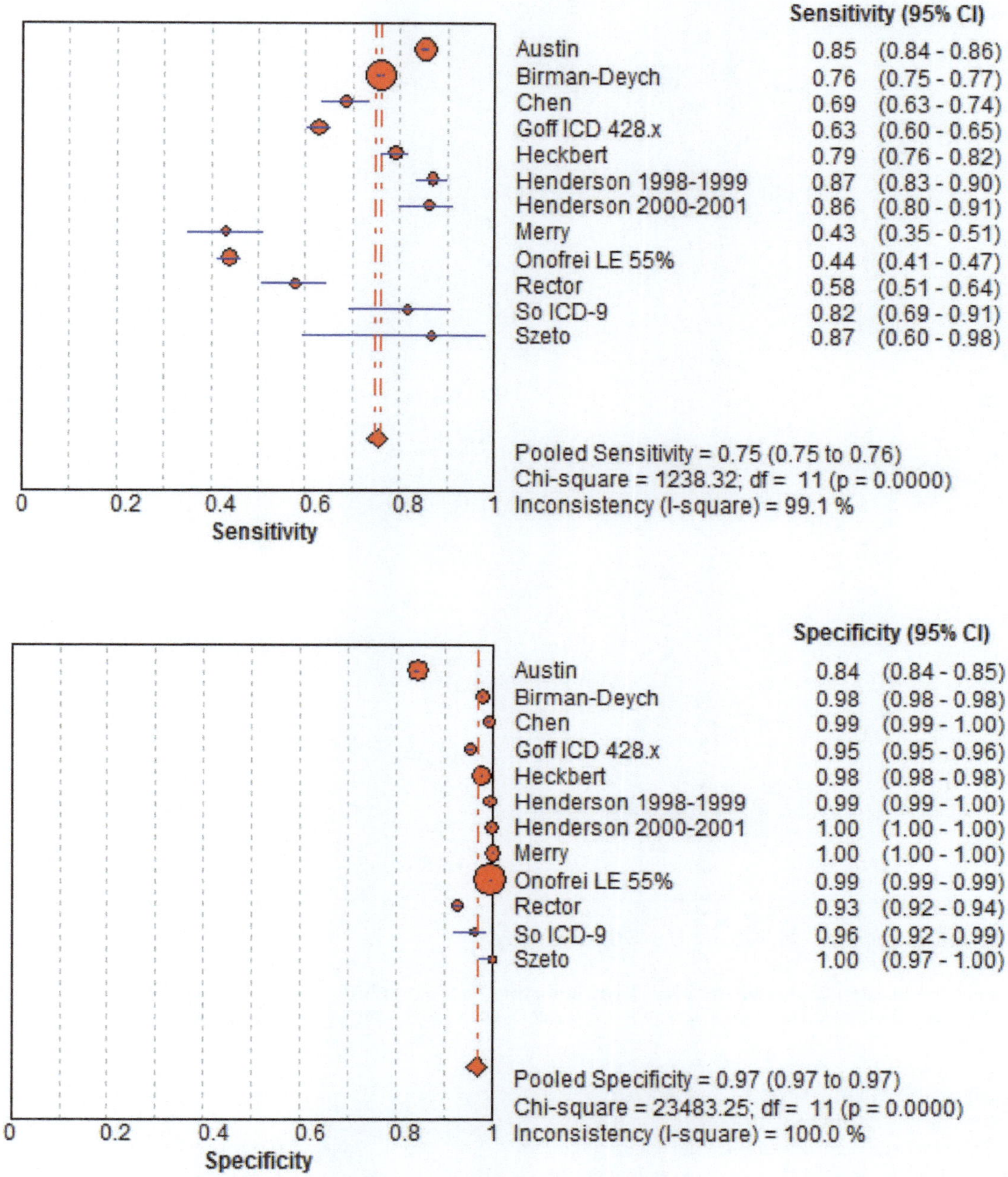

Figure 2. Forest Plots of Sensitivities and Specificities of Heart Failure Codes as Reported by Included Studies. 95% CI = 95% confidence interval; DF = degrees of freedom.

considering the inclusion of more HF-related codes (other than ICD-9 428 or ICD-10 I50) in the search algorithm, and, where available, searching for HF cases in both hospitalization and outpatient databases.

Sources of Administrative Data

While the improvements were not substantial, some studies we reviewed suggested HF cases could be identified more accurately if algorithms combining hospital codes with prescription data were applied. For example, Rector *et al* [49] tested several algorithms to identify HF, some of which incorporated prescription claims for an angiotensin converting enzyme (ACE) inhibitor, angiotensin-II receptor antagonist, loop diuretic, or digoxin. When using an algorithm that required a healthcare encounter and HF-related prescription, the specificity was high (92%), though the sensitivity was modest (53%) [49]. While further research is needed in this area, findings from that study also suggested that HF cases could be identified from prescription data alone, as the specificity of an algorithm that included a single HF-related prescription, but no healthcare encounters, was 78% [49]. This occurred despite the fact that many medications used in the treatment of HF are also used to treat other conditions [49]. Hence, prescription medication data could be used to validate HF cases first identified from hospital or outpatient data, or used alone to identify HF cases in a sensitivity analysis. Requiring that cases be dispensed a combination of medications - for example, each of a diuretic, ACE

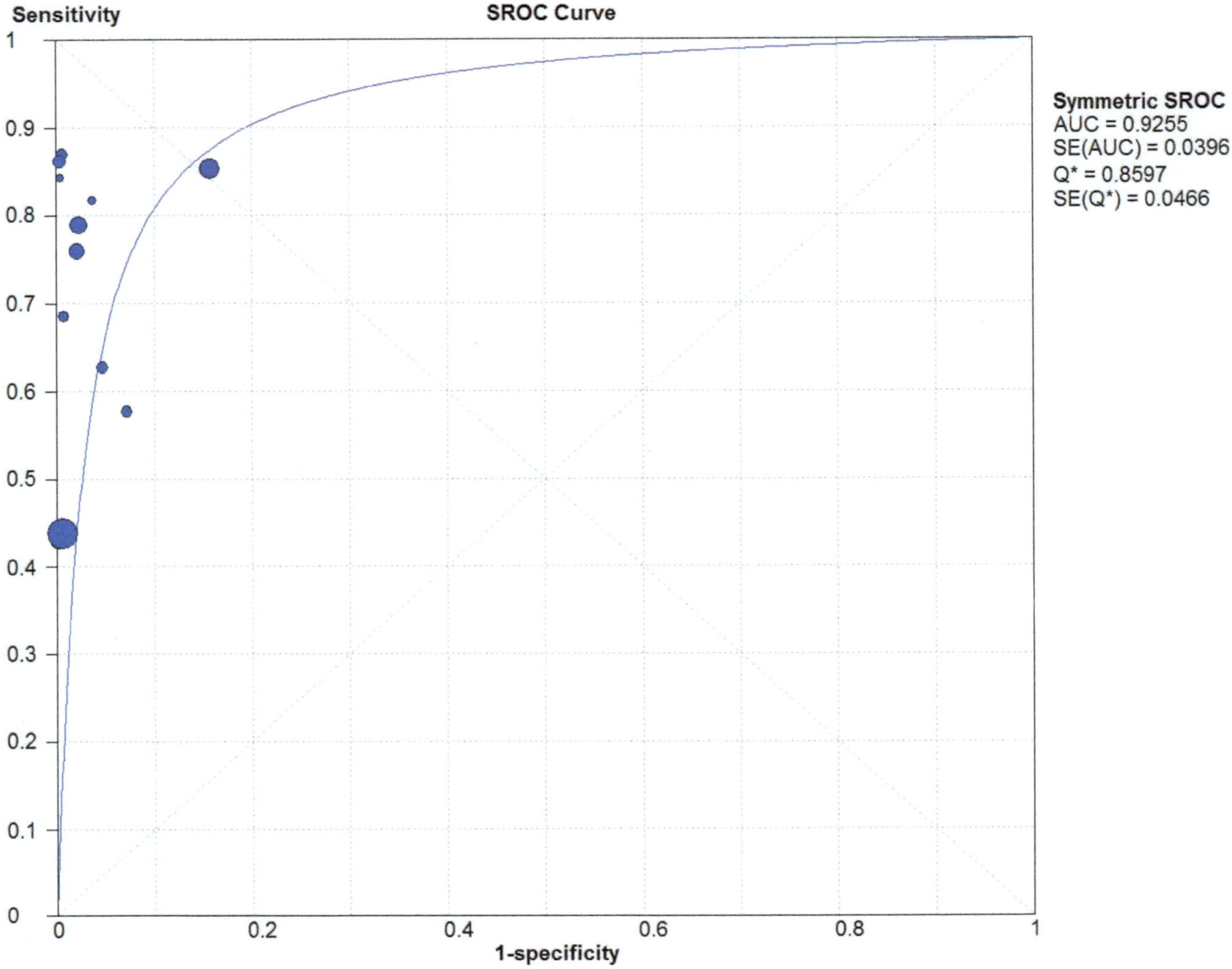

Figure 3. Receiver Operating Characteristic Curve Describing the Diagnostic Performance of Heart Failure Codes in Administrative Databases. AUC = Area Under the Curve; SROC = Summary Receiver Operating Characteristic; SE = standard error.

inhibitor or angiotensin-II receptor antagonist, and beta blocker - may improve specificity. At this time the prescription databases in many countries only include government-subsidized prescriptions, limiting the potential of this data source for identifying cases. Thus, prescription medication data should only be used if the database contains records on all community-dispensed prescriptions, regardless of payer, or at least all prescriptions dispensed to senior citizens.

Laboratory databases may also be a useful source for identifying HF. Specifically, levels of B-type natriuretic peptide(BNP) are often elevated in patients with left ventricular HF [6], so individuals with high BNP values could be identified as HF cases. One study in this review, by Alqaisi *et al* [45], compared the accuracy of different algorithms for identifying HF, some of which included BNP levels, and the highest-sensitivity algorithm in that study was ≥2 outpatient encounters for HF, or ≥1 hospitalizations for HF, or a BNP level of ≥200 pg/ml. That algorithm achieved a sensitivity of 76% and a specificity of 75%. BNP levels can be elevated in conditions other than HF, such as pulmonary embolism and chronic obstructive pulmonary disease [6], which may limit the specificity of BNP levels for identifying HF. However, additional findings from the Alqaisi *et al* study [45], where the specificities of BNP levels of ≥100 pg/ml, 200 pg/ml, and 500 pg/ml (without considering any diagnoses from healthcare encounters) were 76%, 88%, and 95%, respectively, suggest this test is reasonably specific for HF. Any potential increases in sensitivity will be limited by the fact that BNP levels tend to be elevated more in HF patients with left systolic dysfunction than diastolic dysfunction [6]. Another caveat is that BNP is less sensitive a test in non-acute HF [5]. Where laboratory data are available, we suggest researchers incorporate BNP levels into their case definition and, in a sensitivity analysis, compare the HF cases identified with- and without BNP levels.

Reference Standards

Findings from our meta-analysis suggested a high degree of heterogeneity amongst the included studies; thus, a random-effects model was used to produce the summary measures. Part of this heterogeneity can be attributed to differences in the characteristics of the study populations. Some studies were community-based or conducted on a general hospitalized population while others were conducted on select populations (i.e. elderly people or those with a history of MI) in whom HF is more prevalent. Variations in the size of the study population may also have contributed, as there

Table 3. Results of Sensitivity Analysis Using a Jackknife Approach.

Omitted Study: First Author, Year of Publication	Records Evaluated (N)	Pooled Sensitivity (95% CI)	Pooled Specificity (95% CI)	Pooled LR+ (95% CI)	Pooled LR- (95% CI)	Pooled Diagnostic OR (95% CI)
All studies included	371,055	75.3 (74.7–75.9)	96.8 (96.8–96.9)	51.9 (20.5–131.6)	0.27 (0.20–0.37)	186.5 (96.8–359.22)
Austin [53], 2002	58,816	71.8 (71.1–72.5)	99.1 (99.1–99.1)	62.1 (35.2–109.6)	0.28 (0.21–0.38)	220.2 (119.1–407.3)
Birman-Deych [15], 2005	23,657	74.6 (73.7–75.4)	96.8 (98.7–96.9)	53.4 (21.2–134.7)	0.27 (0.18–0.40)	193.3 (90.0–415.2)
Chen [47], 2009	4,008	75.4 (74.8–76.0)	96.8 (96.8–96.9)	48.8 (18.6–128.1)	0.26 (0.19–0.37)	176.9 (89.4–350.0)
Goff [43], 2000	5,083	76.2 (75.6–76.8)	96.9 (96.8–96.9)	59.2 (21.5–162.9)	0.26 (0.18–0.37)	221.9 (108.3–454.7)
Heckbert [55], 2004	34,016	75.2 (74.6–75.8)	96.8 (96.7–96.8)	54.5 (18.3–162.3)	0.28 (0.20–0.38)	189.9 (93.8–384.6)
Henderson [46], 2006: 1998–1999	7,004	75.1 (74.5–75.7)	96.8 (96.7–96.8)	46.7 (17.9–121.8)	0.29 (0.21–0.40)	154.4 (80.5–296.0)
Henderson [46], 2006: 2000–2001	7,631	75.2 (74.6–75.8)	96.8 (96.7–96.8)	44.1 (16.9–115.2)	0.29 (0.21–0.39)	147.8 (76.6–285.3)
Merry [54], 2009	21,110	75.6 (75.0–76.1)	96.6 (96.6–96.7)	41.8 (16.0–109.2)	0.25 (0.18–0.34)	159.7 (81.8–311.6)
Onofrei [44], 2004	205,756	77.5 (76.9–78.1)	93.2 (93.0–93.3)	49.8 (19.0–130.0)	0.25 (0.20–0.32)	193.56 (92.4–405.3)
Rector [49], 2004	3,633	75.5 (74.9–76.1)	96.9 (96.8–96.9)	62.2 (22.7–170.8)	0.26 (0.18–0.35)	235.5 (118.8–467.1)
So [48], 2006	193	75.3 (74.7–75.9)	96.8 (96.8–96.9)	55.9 (21.2–147.6)	0.28 (0.20–0.38)	193.1 (97.6–381.9)
Szeto [50], 2002	148	75.3 (74.7–75.9)	96.8 (96.8–96.9)	48.1 (18.6–124.9)	0.28 (0.20–0.38)	174.9 (89.9–340.3)

95% CI = 95% confidence interval; LR+ = positive likelihood ratio; LR- = negative likelihood ratio; OR = odds ratio.

were changes, though not substantial, in the pooled sensitivity and specificity estimates after each of the two largest studies (n = 205,755 and n = 58,816) were removed.

More importantly, there was much heterogeneity in the reference standards used by different studies. This was not surprising as there is no single accepted gold standard for the diagnosis of HF, and a definitive diagnosis of HF is often difficult [53,58], especially in elderly patients with multiple complications [34]. The reference standards used included patient self-report, chart reviews by clinicians and non-clinicians, two distinct disease registries, and the application of several sets of standard diagnostic criteria including the Framingham, Carlson, and European Society of Cardiology (ESC). One study included in our review, by Onofrei *et al* [44], reported both low sensitivity (44%) and low PPV (36%) for HF codes, which could be explained, in part, by their choice of reference standard. It consisted of a single measurement, left ventricular ejection fraction (LVEF) of either ≤55% or ≤40%. The LVEF is not typically used for HF diagnosis, but instead for classifying HF patients with left ventricular systolic or diastolic dysfunction [59]. Although the thresholds vary, an LVEF below 40% or 50% is usually indicative of systolic dysfunction, while higher LVEF values in HF patients are usually indicative of diastolic dysfunction but preserved systolic function [59]. It is possible that some of the false-positive cases in that study (coded for HF but whose LVEF measurement did not fall below the thresholds) exhibited other signs and symptoms that would fulfill the criteria for HF under the less-restrictive Framingham, Carlson, or ESC definitions. Thus, this choice of reference standard may have attenuated the PPV.

Furthermore, although the Framingham and Carlson criteria have been shown to be 100% sensitive to cases of definite HF [60], especially severe cases [61], the Framingham criteria are considered by some to be insensitive for detecting early HF [62,63]. Therefore, the application of standard diagnostic criteria may also attenuate the PPV. In this review, we did observe a trend towards greater PPV (80-100%) when simply a physician's written confirmation of HF diagnosis or other notation in the medical chart was used as a gold standard [15,42,50]. In fact, Roger *et al* [42] compared two gold standards, physician diagnosis (as written in the chart) and the Framingham criteria, and found that the PPV from physician diagnosis was higher compared with the Framingham criteria (90% vs. 82%). Although the physician diagnosis may be more subjective, it may better reflect the diagnoses made in day-to-day clinical practice and thus be more meaningful to health researchers.

In addition to prescription medication and laboratory data, a third resource that could be used in conjunction with conventional administrative (billing) data to capture more HF cases is the electronic medical record (EMR), or electronic health record (EHR). The EMR or EHR is a digital file used by healthcare providers for patient care [64]. Though some authors use EMR when referring to the digital file maintained by a single practitioner, and EHR when referring to a digital file containing inpatient and outpatient data from multiple practitioners, for simplicity we will employ a single term, EMR, in this discussion. The materials available in the EMR can vary, but generally include clinical notes (similar to those recorded in a paper medical chart), prescription records, and laboratory and radiology reports [64]. With access to EMRs, researchers can identify HF cases by searching for an ICD code for HF amongst the patient's Problem List, a list maintained by the practitioner of all current and active diagnoses. In addition, researchers can also search for the term 'heart failure' amongst the entire free-text areas of the clinical notes, laboratory and radiological reports, and any correspondence from specialists. For example, the Mayo Clinic has used a natural language processing (NLP) algorithm containing the terms 'cardiomyopathy', 'heart failure', 'congestive heart failure', 'pulmonary edema', 'decompensated heart failure', 'volume overload' and 'fluid overload', along with 426 synonyms for these terms [65]. A potential case is eliminated if a negative term (such as 'no' or 'unlikely'), or sometimes even a speculative term (such as 'rule-out' or 'suspected') is found within close proximity of the HF term [65,66]. For chronic conditions like HF that may be superseded by other diagnoses on reimbursement claims, this EMR-based search strategy may be more sensitive than relying on the diagnostic codes in claims-based administrative databases, and may aid in capturing milder cases.

However, the EMR also has some limitations, many of which stem from the fact that, similar to most administrative databases, the EMR was not established for research purposes [64]. For example, when searching the free-text notes and reports, computer programs may have difficulty processing whether ambiguous phrases like "cannot be ruled out" [67] correspond to a positive case. In addition, while the information contained in administrative databases is already de-identified, the EMR does contain personally-identifying information. US law stipulates that, unless each patient provides consent [68], researchers cannot use data collected from the EMR without it undergoing a de-identification process [69]. Thus, it may be costly and time-consuming for researchers to access this data, especially as many hospitals do not use de-identification tools at present [68]. A lack of standardization across EMR systems [64] and challenges in linking EMRs from different hospitals or provider networks [70] may also limit the use of EMR. Finally, just as with ICD codes, the validity of the HF cases identified from the free-text areas of the EMR must be assessed before EMRs can be used for HF research. While the results of some validation studies [65,67] have been promising, more validation studies conducted in different settings, and using different EMR platforms, are needed to confirm these findings.

Limitations

We acknowledge some limitations to our systematic review. There is the potential for a language bias as we could not consider articles whose full-texts were not available in English; articles published after the conclusion of our search period (February 2011) could not be considered either. Another potential limitation stems from the fact that, even though our database searches were conducted by an experienced librarian, administrative databases are not well catalogued in MEDLINE and EMBASE (e.g. no MeSH term pertaining to "administrative database"). Although most of the included studies were located through database searches, our subsequent hand search turned up several more relevant articles, most of which had not been indexed under terms relating to Administrative Data or Validation. As a result, despite our extensive hand search, we may have missed some relevant articles if they were not indexed in MEDLINE or EMBASE under a term relating to administrative data or validation. Our findings are also subject to publication bias, wherein reports of HF codes having poor validity may have been differentially withheld from publication. However, given the number of reports we located where the sensitivity of HF codes was suboptimal, we feel this is unlikely

Recommendations

After qualitative and quantitative analysis of the evidence, we conclude that the HF codes that do appear in administrative databases are highly predictive of true HF cases. At the same time, administrative databases fail to capture a non-negligible number of true cases, perhaps 25% to 30% of all diagnoses, and may differentially capture the most severe cases. Based on current evidence, we recommend several strategies for increasing the capture of HF cases in administrative data:

- Hospitalizations with HF in the primary position are decreasing, while those with HF in secondary positions are increasing [26,27]. Thus, researchers should search amongst all available diagnostic positions in hospitalization data for HF codes.
- With many HF patients treated exclusively on an outpatient basis, data from both inpatient and outpatient encounters should be searched.
- Where available, researchers should supplement their data with searches of laboratory databases (specifically BNP values) and/or prescription medication data.
- Searching the free-text areas of the EMR for mentions of 'heart failure' and related terms, as well as the Problem List, should help identify cases whose HF diagnosis has not been recorded on an inpatient or outpatient billing record. This may particularly aid in the capture of mild HF.

Conclusions

The chronic and syndromic nature of HF creates difficulties for researchers studying this condition at the population level. To guide their efforts, we conducted a systematic review and meta-analysis of articles reporting on the validity of HF diagnoses in administrative data. Our findings suggest that, although the HF diagnoses identified using administrative data frequently correspond to true HF cases, this data source may not capture all cases. Administrative databases are increasingly being used to study long-term patient outcomes and disease burden; thus, to maximize the sensitivity of these data sources for all conditions, physicians and hospital coders are encouraged to record diagnoses of all comorbidities that may have contributed to a given healthcare encounter. In the meantime, the use of broader case definitions, potentially in combination with prescription medication and laboratory data, and searches of electronic medical records, may increase the sensitivity of this data source for HF, and in turn, its application in population-based health outcomes and economics research.

Supporting Information

Table S1 Item-by-Item QUADAS Breakdown for Each Study.

Text S1 MEDLINE Search Strategy.

Text S2 EMBASE Search Strategy.

Text S3 Data Collection Form.

Checklist S1 PRISMA Checklist.

Checklist S2 MOOSE Checklist.

Acknowledgments

The authors wish to thank members of the CANRAD network, librarian Mary-Doug Wright (B.Sc., M.L.S.) for conducting the literature search, Reza Torkjazi, and Kathryn Reimer for their help during their administrative support and editing the manuscript.

Author Contributions

Conceived and designed the experiments: DL JAAZ. Analyzed the data: NM DL VB JAAZ. Contributed to the writing of the manuscript: NM DL VB JAAZ. Final approval of the version of the manuscript to be published: NM DL VB JAAZ.

References

1. Ambrosy AP, Fonarow GC, Butler J, Chioncel O, Greene SJ, et al. (2014) The global health and economic burden of hospitalizations for heart failure: lessons learned from hospitalized heart failure registries. J Am Coll Cardiol 63: 1123–1133. doi:10.1016/j.jacc.2013.11.053.
2. Go AS, Mozaffarian D, Roger VL, Benjamin EJ, Berry JD, et al. (2014) Heart disease and stroke statistics—2014 update: a report from the American Heart Association. Circulation 129: e28–e292. doi:10.1161/01.cir.0000441139.02102.80.
3. Chen Y-T, Vaccarino V, Williams CS, Butler J, Berkman LF, et al. (1999) Risk factors for heart failure in the elderly: a prospective community-based study. Am J Med 106: 605–612. doi:10.1016/S0002-9343(99)00126-6.
4. Cook C, Cole G, Asaria P, Jabbour R, Francis DP (2014) The annual global economic burden of heart failure. Int J Cardiol 171: 368–376. doi:10.1016/j.ijcard.2013.12.028.
5. McMurray JJV, Adamopoulos S, Anker SD, Auricchio A, Bohm M, et al. (2012) ESC Guidelines for the diagnosis and treatment of acute and chronic heart failure 2012: The Task Force for the Diagnosis and Treatment of Acute and Chronic Heart Failure 2012 of the European Society of Cardiology. Developed in collaboration with the Heart Failure Association (HFA) of the ESC. Eur Heart J 33: 1787–1847. doi:10.1093/eurheartj/ehs104.
6. Hunt SA, Abraham WT, Chin MH, Feldman AM, Francis GS, et al. (2009) 2009 focused update incorporated into the ACC/AHA 2005 Guidelines for the Diagnosis and Management of Heart Failure in Adults: a report of the American College of Cardiology Foundation/American Heart Association Task Force on Practice Guidelines: developed in collaboration with the International Society for Heart and Lung Transplantation. Circulation 119: e391–479. doi:10.1161/CIRCULATIONAHA.109.192065.
7. Van Deursen VM, Urso R, Laroche C, Damman K, Dahlström U, et al. (2014) Co-morbidities in patients with heart failure: an analysis of the European Heart Failure Pilot Survey. Eur J Heart Fail 16: 103–111. doi:10.1002/ejhf.30.
8. Wong CY, Chaudhry SI, Desai MM, Krumholz HM (2011) Trends in comorbidity, disability, and polypharmacy in heart failure. Am J Med 124: 136–143. doi:10.1016/j.amjmed.2010.08.017.
9. Cleland JGF, Swedberg K, Follath F, Komajda M, Cohen-Solal A, et al. (2003) The EuroHeart Failure survey programme— a survey on the quality of care among patients with heart failure in Europe. Part 1: patient characteristics and diagnosis. Eur Heart J 24: 442–463.
10. Van Deursen VM, Damman K, van der Meer P, Wijkstra PJ, Luijckx G-J, et al. (2014) Co-morbidities in heart failure. Heart Fail Rev 19: 163–172. doi:10.1007/s10741-012-9370-7.
11. Braunstein JB, Anderson GF, Gerstenblith G, Weller W, Niefeld M, et al. (2003) Noncardiac comorbidity increases preventable hospitalizations and mortality among Medicare beneficiaries with chronic heart failure. J Am Coll Cardiol 42: 1226–1233.
12. Hawkins NM, Jhund PS, Simpson CR, Petrie MC, Macdonald MR, et al. (2010) Primary care burden and treatment of patients with heart failure and chronic obstructive pulmonary disease in Scotland. Eur J Heart Fail 12: 17–24. doi:10.1093/eurjhf/hfp160.
13. Dunlay SM, Redfield MM, Weston SA, Therneau TM, Hall Long K, et al. (2009) Hospitalizations after heart failure diagnosis a community perspective. J Am Coll Cardiol 54: 1695–1702. doi:10.1016/j.jacc.2009.08.019.
14. Dai S, Walsh P, Wielgosz A, Gurevich Y, Bancej C, et al. (2012) Comorbidities and mortality associated with hospitalized heart failure in Canada. Can J Cardiol 28: 74–79. doi:10.1016/j.cjca.2011.05.002.
15. Birman-Deych E, Waterman AD, Yan Y, Nilasena DS, Radford MJ, et al. (2005) Accuracy of ICD-9-CM codes for identifying cardiovascular and stroke risk factors. Med Care 43: 480–485.
16. Levy AR, Tamblyn RM, Fitchett D, McLeod PJ, Hanley JA (1999) Coding accuracy of hospital discharge data for elderly survivors of myocardial infarction. Can J Cardiol 15: 1277–1282.
17. Khand AU, Shaw M, Gemmel I, Cleland JG (2005) Do discharge codes underestimate hospitalisation due to heart failure? Validation study of hospital discharge coding for heart failure. Eur J Heart Fail 7: 792–797.
18. Bernatsky S, Lix L, O'Donnell S, Lacaille D, CANRAD Network (2013) Consensus statements for the use of administrative health data in rheumatic disease research and surveillance. J Rheumatol 40: 66–73.
19. Widdifield J, Labrecque J, Lix L, Paterson JM, Bernatsky S, et al. (2013) Systematic review and critical appraisal of validation studies to identify rheumatic diseases in health administrative databases. Arthritis Care Res 65: 1490–1503. doi:10.1002/acr.21993.
20. Barber C, Lacaille D, Fortin PR (2013) Systematic review of validation studies of the use of administrative data to identify serious infections. Arthritis Care Res 65: 1343–1357. doi:10.1002/acr.21959.
21. Leong A, Dasgupta K, Bernatsky S, Lacaille D, Avina-Zubieta A, et al. (2013) Systematic review and meta-analysis of validation studies on a diabetes case definition from health administrative records. PloS One 8: e75256. doi:10.1371/journal.pone.0075256.
22. Hudson M, Avina-Zubieta A, Lacaille D, Bernatsky S, Lix L, et al. (2013) The validity of administrative data to identify hip fractures is high—a systematic review. J Clin Epidemiol 66: 278–285. doi:10.1016/j.jclinepi.2012.10.004.
23. McCormick N, Lacaille D, Bhole V, Avina-Zubieta JA (2014) Validity of myocardial infarction diagnoses in administrative databases: a systematic review. PloS One 9: e92286. doi:10.1371/journal.pone.0092286.
24. Moher D, Liberati A, Tetzlaff J, Altman DG, PRISMA Group (2009) Preferred reporting items for systematic reviews and meta-analyses: the PRISMA statement. PLoS Med 6: e1000097. doi:10.1371/journal.pmed.1000097.
25. Stroup DF, Berlin JA, Morton SC, Olkin I, Williamson GD, et al. (2000) Meta-analysis of observational studies in epidemiology: a proposal for reporting. Meta-analysis Of Observational Studies in Epidemiology (MOOSE) group. JAMA 283: 2008–2012.
26. Blecker S, Paul M, Taksler G, Ogedegbe G, Katz S (2013) Heart failure–associated hospitalizations in the United States. J Am Coll Cardiol 61: 1259–1267. doi:10.1016/j.jacc.2012.12.038.
27. Fang J, Mensah GA, Croft JB, Keenan NL (2008) Heart failure-related hospitalization in the U.S., 1979 to 2004. J Am Coll Cardiol 52: 428–434. doi:10.1016/j.jacc.2008.03.061.
28. Whiting P, Rutjes AW, Reitsma JB, Bossuyt PM, Kleijnen J (2003) The development of QUADAS: a tool for the quality assessment of studies of diagnostic accuracy included in systematic reviews. BMC Med Res Methodol 3: 25.
29. Jaeschke R (1994) Users' Guides to the Medical Literature: III. How to Use an Article About a Diagnostic Test B. What Are the Results and Will They Help Me in Caring for My Patients? JAMA 271: 703. doi:10.1001/jama.1994.03510330081039.
30. Landis JR, Koch GG (1977) The measurement of observer agreement for categorical data. Biometrics 33: 159–174.
31. McKee PA, Castelli WP, McNamara PM, Kannel WB (1971) The Natural History of Congestive Heart Failure: The Framingham Study. N Engl J Med 285: 1441–1446. doi:10.1056/NEJM197112232852601.
32. Carlson KJ, Lee DC, Goroll AH, Leahy M, Johnson RA (1985) An analysis of physicians' reasons for prescribing long-term digitalis therapy in outpatients. J Chronic Dis 38: 733–739.
33. Dickstein K, Cohen-Solal A, Filippatos G, McMurray JJV, Ponikowski P, et al. (2008) ESC Guidelines for the diagnosis and treatment of acute and chronic heart failure 2008: the Task Force for the Diagnosis and Treatment of Acute and Chronic Heart Failure 2008 of the European Society of Cardiology. Developed in collaboration with the Heart Failure Association of the ESC (HFA) and endorsed by the European Society of Intensive Care Medicine (ESICM). Eur Heart J 29: 2388–2442. doi:10.1093/eurheartj/ehn309.
34. Ingelsson E, Arnlov J, Sundstrom J, Lind L (2005) The validity of a diagnosis of heart failure in a hospital discharge register. Eur J Heart Fail 7: 787–791.
35. Kramer M (1988) Chapter 16: Diagnostic Tests. Clinical Epidemiology and Biostatics: A Primer for Clinical Investigators and Decision Makers. Berlin: Springer. pp. 236–253.
36. Walter SD (2002) Properties of the summary receiver operating characteristic (SROC) curve for diagnostic test data. Stat Med 21: 1237–1256. doi:10.1002/sim.1099.
37. Cochran WG (1954) The Combination of Estimates from Different Experiments. Biometrics 10: 101. doi:10.2307/3001666.
38. Higgins JPT, Thompson SG, Deeks JJ, Altman DG (2003) Measuring inconsistency in meta-analyses. BMJ 327: 557–560. doi:10.1136/bmj.327.7414.557.
39. Miller RG (1974) The jackknife-a review. Biometrika 61: 1–15. doi:10.1093/biomet/61.1.1.
40. Deeks JJ, Macaskill P, Irwig L (2005) The performance of tests of publication bias and other sample size effects in systematic reviews of diagnostic test accuracy was assessed. J Clin Epidemiol 58: 882–893. doi:10.1016/j.jclinepi.2005.01.016.
41. Zamora J, Abraira V, Muriel A, Khan K, Coomarasamy A (2006) Meta-DiSc: a software for meta-analysis of test accuracy data. BMC Med Res Methodol 6: 31. doi:10.1186/1471-2288-6-31.
42. Roger VL, Weston SA, Redfield MM, Hellermann-Homan JP, Killian J, et al. (2004) Trends in heart failure incidence and survival in a community-based population. JAMA 292: 344–350.
43. Goff DJ, Pandey DK, Chan FA, Ortiz C, Nichaman MZ (2000) Congestive heart failure in the United States: is there more than meets the I(CD code)? The Corpus Christi Heart Project. Arch Intern Med 160: 197–202.
44. Onofrei M, Hunt J, Siemienczuk J, Touchette DR, Middleton B (2004) A first step towards translating evidence into practice: heart failure in a community practice-based research network. Inform Prim Care 12: 139–145.
45. Alqaisi F, Williams LK, Peterson EL, Lanfear DE (2009) Comparing methods for identifying patients with heart failure using electronic data sources. BMC Health Serv Res 9: 237–6963–9–237.
46. Henderson T, Shepheard J, Sundararajan V (2006) Quality of diagnosis and procedure coding in ICD-10 administrative data. Med Care 44: 1011–1019.
47. Chen G, Faris P, Hemmelgarn B, Walker RL, Quan H (2009) Measuring agreement of administrative data with chart data using prevalence unadjusted and adjusted kappa. BMC Med Res Methodol 9: 5–2288–9–5.
48. So L, Evans D, Quan H (2006) ICD-10 coding algorithms for defining comorbidities of acute myocardial infarction. BMC Health Serv Res 6: 161.

49. Rector TS, Wickstrom SL, Shah M, Greeenlee NT, Rheault P, et al. (2004) Specificity and sensitivity of claims-based algorithms for identifying members of Medicare+Choice health plans that have chronic medical conditions. Health Serv Res 39: 1839–1857.
50. Szeto HC, Coleman RK, Gholami P, Hoffman BB, Goldstein MK (2002) Accuracy of computerized outpatient diagnoses in a Veterans Affairs general medicine clinic. Am J Manag Care 8: 37–43.
51. Humphries KH, Rankin JM, Carere RG, Buller CE, Kiely FM, et al. (2000) Co-morbidity data in outcomes research: are clinical data derived from administrative databases a reliable alternative to chart review? J Clin Epidemiol 53: 343–349.
52. Heisler CA, Melton LJ 3rd, Weaver AL, Gebhart JB (2009) Determining perioperative complications associated with vaginal hysterectomy: code classification versus chart review. J Am Coll Surg 209: 119–122.
53. Austin PC, Daly PA, Tu JV (2002) A multicenter study of the coding accuracy of hospital discharge administrative data for patients admitted to cardiac care units in Ontario. Am Heart J 144: 290–296.
54. Merry AH, Boer JM, Schouten LJ, Feskens EJ, Verschuren WM, et al. (2009) Validity of coronary heart diseases and heart failure based on hospital discharge and mortality data in the Netherlands using the cardiovascular registry Maastricht cohort study. Eur J Epidemiol 24: 237–247.
55. Heckbert SR, Kooperberg C, Safford MM, Psaty BM, Hsia J, et al. (2004) Comparison of self-report, hospital discharge codes, and adjudication of cardiovascular events in the Women's Health Initiative. Am J Epidemiol 160: 1152–1158. doi:10.1093/aje/.
56. Lee DS, Donovan L, Austin PC, Gong Y, Liu PP, et al. (2005) Comparison of coding of heart failure and comorbidities in administrative and clinical data for use in outcomes research. Med Care 43: 182–188.
57. Saczynski JS, Andrade SE, Harrold LR, Tjia J, Cutrona SL, et al. (2012) A systematic review of validated methods for identifying heart failure using administrative data. Pharmacoepidemiol Drug Saf 21: 129–140. doi:10.1002/pds.2313.
58. Quach S, Blais C, Quan H (2010) Administrative data have high variation in validity for recording heart failure. Can J Cardiol 26: 306–312.
59. Gaasch WH (1994) Diagnosis and treatment of heart failure based on left ventricular systolic or diastolic dysfunction. JAMA 271: 1276–1280.
60. Mosterd A, Deckers JW, Hoes AW, Nederpel A, Smeets A, et al. (1997) Classification of heart failure in population based research: an assessment of six heart failure scores. Eur J Epidemiol 13: 491–502.
61. Remes J, Reunanen A, Aromaa A, Pyörälä K (1992) Incidence of heart failure in eastern Finland: a population-based surveillance study. Eur Heart J 13: 588–593.
62. Marantz PR, Alderman MH, Tobin JN (1988) Diagnostic heterogeneity in clinical trials for congestive heart failure. Ann Intern Med 109: 55–61.
63. Senni M, Tribouilloy CM, Rodeheffer RJ, Jacobsen SJ, Evans JM, et al. (1999) Congestive heart failure in the community: trends in incidence and survival in a 10-year period. Arch Intern Med 159: 29–34.
64. Dean BB, Lam J, Natoli JL, Butler Q, Aguilar D, et al. (2009) Review: use of electronic medical records for health outcomes research: a literature review. Med Care Res Rev 66: 611–638. doi:10.1177/1077558709332440.
65. Pakhomov S, Weston SA, Jacobsen SJ, Chute CG, Meverden R, et al. (2007) Electronic medical records for clinical research: application to the identification of heart failure. Am J Manag Care 13: 281–288.
66. Friedman C, Hripcsak G, Shagina L, Liu H (1999) Representing information in patient reports using natural language processing and the extensible markup language. J Am Med Inform Assoc 6: 76–87.
67. Friedlin J, McDonald CJ (2006) A natural language processing system to extract and code concepts relating to congestive heart failure from chest radiology reports. AMIA Annu Symp Proc: 269–273.
68. Liu F, Weng C, Yu H (2012) Chapter 16: Natural Language Processing, Electronic Health Records, and Clinical Research. Clinical Research Informatics. Health Informatics. Springer.pp. 305–306.
69. Guidance Regarding Methods for De-identification of Protected Health Information in Accordance with the Health Insurance Portability and Accountability Act (HIPAA) Privacy Rule (n.d.). Available: http://www.hhs.gov/ocr/privacy/hipaa/understanding/coveredentities/De-identification/guidance.html. Accessed 21 May 2014.
70. Bradley CJ, Penberthy L, Devers KJ, Holden DJ (2010) Health Services Research and Data Linkages: Issues, Methods, and Directions for the Future. Health Serv Res 45: 1468–1488. doi:10.1111/j.1475-6773.2010.01142.x.

The Effects of Comorbidity on the Benefits and Harms of Treatment for Chronic Disease

Terri R. Fried[1,2*], John O'Leary[1,3], Virginia Towle[3], Mary K. Goldstein[4,5], Mark Trentelange[3], Deanna K. Martin[1,3]

1 Clinical Epidemiology Research Center, VA Connecticut Healthcare System, West Haven, Connecticut, United States of America, **2** Department of Medicine, Yale School of Medicine, New Haven, Connecticut, United States of America, **3** Program on Aging, Yale School of Medicine, New Haven, Connecticut, United States of America, **4** Palo Alto Geriatrics Research Education and Clinical Center (GRECC), VA Palo Alto Health Care System, Palo Alto, Connecticut, 94304, United States of America, **5** Center for Primary Care and Outcomes Research, Stanford University School of Medicine, Stanford, California, 94305, United States of America

Abstract

Background: There are concerns about the potential for unintentional harms when clinical practice guidelines are applied to patients with multimorbidity. The objective was to summarize the evidence regarding the effect(s) of comorbidity on the outcomes of medication for an index chronic condition.

Methods: A systematic review was conducted of studies published in MEDLINE and Cochrane Trials before May 2012. The search strategy was constructed to identify articles indexed with "comorbidity" or a related term or by a given condition and one or more additional specified comorbid conditions. The search yielded 3252 articles, of which 37 passed the title/abstract screening process, and 22 were included after full-text review. An additional 23 articles were identified by screening the reference lists for included articles. Information was extracted on study design; population; therapy; comparison groups; outcome(s); main findings.

Findings: Indexing of articles was inconsistent, with no term for "multimorbidity," and rare use of "comorbidity". Only one article examined the effects of comorbidity *per se,* finding no benefit of tight control of DM among persons with high comorbidity, defined using a comorbidity index. The remainder examined pairs of conditions, the majority of which were post-hoc analyses of randomized controlled trials and which found no difference in outcomes according to whether a comorbid condition was present. Several demonstrated no difference or an increased risk of adverse outcome among persons with DM and tight control of HTN as compared to usual control. Several demonstrated lack of benefit of statins among persons with end-stage renal disease.

Conclusions: There is limited evidence regarding the effects of multiple comorbidities on treatment outcomes. The majority of studies demonstrated no effect of a single comorbid condition on outcomes. Additional studies examining a broad range of comorbidity are required, along with clear and consistent indexing to allow for improved synthesis of the evidence.

Editor: Olaf M. Dekkers, Leiden University Medical Centre, Netherlands

Funding: This project was supported by grant DF11-303 from the Donaghue Foundation (www.donaghue.org) and by grant P30 AG021342 from the NIH/NIA (www.nih.nia.gov). The funders had no role in study design, data collection and analysis, decision to publish, or preparation of the manuscript.

Competing Interests: The authors have declared that no competing interests exist.

* Email: terri.fried@yale.edu

Introduction

Multimorbidity, or the co-existence of multiple diseases, is the most common chronic condition among adults. [1] There is increasing concern about the appropriateness of disease-based clinical practice guidelines to the care of the patient with multimorbidity. When applied to a theoretical patient, the many medications recommended by these guidelines result in the potential for adverse drug-drug and drug-disease interactions. [2] The likelihood of adverse drug events increases with the number of medications, [3] leading to questions about altered benefit/harm ratios associated with the prescription of multiple medications for patients with multimorbidity. [4] In addition, evidence about the benefits and harms of interventions from randomized controlled trials (RCTs) may not be generalizable to patients with multimorbidity. These patients are frequently excluded from the trials that form the evidence base for practice guidelines, and the trials have incomplete ascertainment of harms [4].

We sought to determine the extent of the evidence regarding the treatment of persons with multimorbidity by performing a systematic literature review. Although RCTs are generally considered to provide the highest quality evidence regarding treatment benefits, we elected to include both RCTs and observational studies because of the limitations of RCTs as applied to this population of patients and because of evidence that rigorously conducted observational studies provide accurate estimates of treatment effects [5].

Materials and Methods

Data Sources and Searches

Because "multimorbidity" is not a MeSH terms, the search was constructed around the concept of "comorbidity" to address the following question: "Among persons age 65 years and older, what effect does the presence of comorbid conditions have on the benefits and/or harms of medical treatment for a specific index chronic condition?" The following databases were searched for relevant studies: MEDLINE (OvidSP 1946–May Week 5 2012, April 13, 2012); MEDLINE In-Process & Other Non-Indexed Citations (OvidSP, April 13, 2012); Cochrane Trials (Wiley, April 11, 2012). While there are medical subject headings (MeSH) for comorbidity, when we examined four key articles, we found that only one of the four articles was indexed using these terms. We therefore had to create search strategies to capture the concept of comorbidity. We did this by using search terms that consisted of a given condition and at least one other of a list of additional conditions (heart failure [HF], coronary artery disease [CAD], angina pectoris, stable angina, hypertension [HTN], chronic obstructive pulmonary disease, osteoarthritis, hyperlipidemias, chronic kidney disease [CKD], diabetes mellitus [DM]). We repeated this process, with each condition becoming the index condition, and the rest considered together as comorbid conditions, using controlled vocabulary terms and synonymous free text words. The search strategy was limited to cohort studies, randomized controlled trials, or decision support techniques (Appendix S1). We specified older age in our question because of the increasing prevalence of multimorbidity with age, [6] with the goal of identifying study populations with the broadest possible range of comorbid conditions.

Because of the large number of references resulting from this search, the first 100 abstracts were reviewed to determine whether the search strategy could be made more specific. We found that we had captured a large number of studies that examined appropriateness of a given therapy, with appropriateness determined according to whether the patient had a given condition rather than according to the outcome of therapy. We therefore reran the analysis excluding these studies. Because of our interest in medical therapies, we also excluded studies that focused on surgical interventions. The full strategy is shown in appendix S1.

Study Selection

We included articles that examined the outcomes of treatment for an index condition in the presence and absence of comorbidity. We also included articles that examined the outcomes associated with different intensity of treatment of an index condition in the presence of comorbidity, regardless of whether the treatment was explicitly defined. For example, we included articles examining outcomes according to different HgbA1C levels, regardless of whether the diabetic treatment was specified. We included articles that examined only the effect of a treatment for a given condition in the presence of comorbidity (e.g. there were no participants without the comorbid condition) when the effect of the treatment in the absence of the comorbidity is well established.

We excluded articles that examined surrogate outcomes, such as lab values. This exclusion was based on evidence that surrogate outcomes are frequently not accurate markers for clinically relevant outcomes and that studies examining surrogate outcomes may not capture relevant harms. [7] We did not exclude any clinically relevant outcomes, and planned to include studies examining quality of life outcomes, such as symptoms and function. In addition, it became apparent that the search strategy resulted in many articles with persons under the age of 65. Articles were therefore included if the study population included persons age 65 years or older, even if they also included younger persons. A total of 50 titles and/or abstracts were reviewed independently by three of the investigators (TRF, JRO, VT) to confirm uniformity in the process of excluding articles. The titles and/or abstracts of the remaining references were initially reviewed by one of two investigators (JRO, VT), and articles that were not excluded were re-reviewed by a third investigator (TRF) to achieve consensus regarding inclusion. Full text review was performed for these articles. The reference lists for the final set of articles identified by this search were also examined to identify additional articles meeting inclusion criterion.

Data Extraction and Quality Assessment

For each of the included studies, we extracted the following data elements: 1) study design; 2) study population, including index condition; 3) intervention; 4) comparison groups; 5) outcome; 6) main findings.

We did not perform quality assessments for the articles based on two considerations. First, for the reasons provided above, we included both RCTs and observational studies. This posed a challenge for doing quality assessment, since, on the one hand, observational studies are generally considered to provide lower quality evidence than are randomized controlled trials, [8] but, as discussed above, in the case of multimorbidity, randomized controlled trials may not enroll patients with representative comorbidity burden. It is therefore difficult to apply metrics across the two types of study design that reflect their relative quality as specifically related to the study question. Second, many studies consisted of post-hoc analyses of RCTs, so that the initial randomization no longer applied, and there are no established criteria to evaluate the extent to which this affects the quality of the study. Given these considerations, we concluded that the best representation of study quality was a description of the study design, as extracted from each of the studies.

Data Synthesis and Analysis

Because the large majority of studies examined treatment for an index condition among persons with or without a single comorbid condition, we organized studies according to the pairs of conditions being examined. Even within these groups, the heterogeneity in design, population, and interventions precluded combining the results in a meta-analysis.

Results

Identification of Articles

The literature search yielded 3252 articles. A total of 38 articles passed the title/abstract screening process. Full-text review resulted in the exclusion of 16 articles. Review of the reference lists for the remaining 22 articles resulted in the identification of an addition 23 articles, for a total of 45 (Figure 1).

Types of Studies Identified

Table 1 provides a description of the types of studies identified in the systematic review, including the approach to the analysis of comorbidity, conditions and outcomes examined, and study design. Only one of the studies examined the effect of comorbidity *per se*. [9] This study examined the cardiovascular outcomes associated with tight diabetic control among persons with different levels of comorbidity. The remaining 44 studies examined the

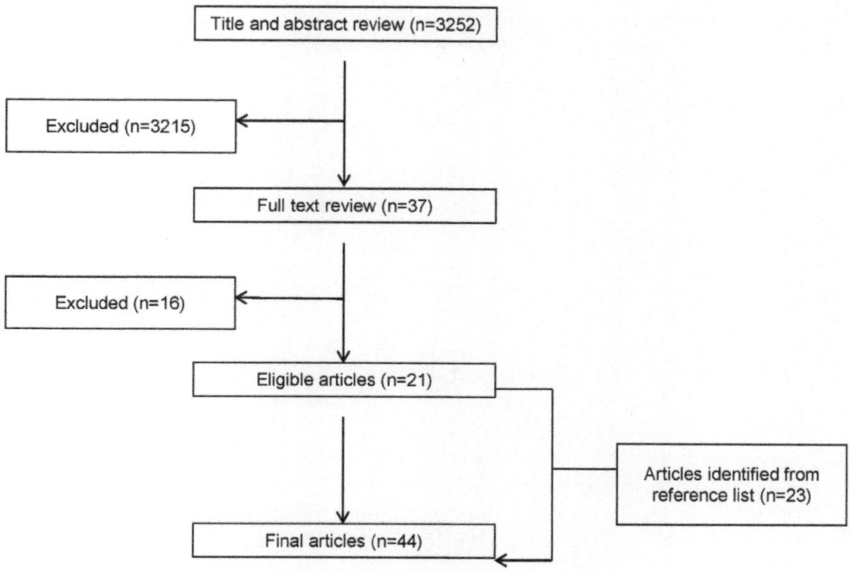

Figure 1. Summary of literature search and selection.

effects of treating an index condition in the presence or absence of a single other condition. The vast majority of these studies included DM as either the index or comorbid condition. The most common combinations of conditions examined were HF and DM (10 studies), [10–19] HTN and DM (9 studies), [20–28] and DM and CKD (10 studies) [29–38]. The studies examining HF and DM focused primarily on all-cause mortality among patients with HF who received treatment with beta blockers according to the presence or absence of DM. The majority of studies examining HTN and DM compared outcomes according to different intensities of HTN treatment, measured as the desired or achieved systolic and/or diastolic blood pressure. The studies examining CKD and DM primarily compared outcomes according to different intensities of diabetes treatment, measured as the achieved HgbA1C. An additional 5 studies examined DM and cardiovascular disease other than HF; these studies varied in terms of which was considered the index condition and which the comorbidity, the interventions, and outcomes [39–43].

A total of eight studies examined cardiovascular disease (HF, ischemic heart disease, or hyperlipidemia) and CKD [14,44–50]. A total of four studies examined a variety of miscellaneous disease combinations [41,51–53].

Across the different disease combinations, over one-half (55%) were conducted as post-hoc analyses of randomized controlled trials, in which patients with and without the comorbid condition were identified after study randomization, and the effect of the treatment was compared in these two groups. There were two studies that included only patients with both the index condition of hyperlipidemia or high cardiovascular disease risk and the comorbidity of CKD. These were randomized controlled trials in which patients were assigned to treatment with a statin versus a placebo. These studies assumed a well-established benefit of statins among patients with the index condition who did not have CKD. Only two studies examined differences in the likelihood of harm according to whether a comorbid condition was present; the remainder of the studies examined the likelihood of benefit. Of the studies examining benefit, only one examined functional outcomes; the remainder examined reduction in risk of mortality, hospitalization, or disease-specific outcomes, such as cardiovascular events.

Study Findings

The majority of studies found no effect of comorbidity on the benefits or harms of therapy for an index condition. Of the 25 studies examining the benefit of therapy for a given condition according to whether comorbidity was present or absent, 23 found no difference or a greater benefit in the presence of the comorbidity (Table 2). The two studies examining the harm of therapy according to whether comorbidity was present or absent found no difference in harms. Results were more mixed for the 15 studies examining the benefit of tighter versus less tight control of one condition in the presence of a second. Of these, seven found tighter control was more beneficial than less tight control, six found tighter control was of no greater benefit or was harmful compared to less tight control, one found a U-shaped relationship, and one had different findings for different outcomes.

Table 3 provides a detailed description of the study results according to the study population, study design, intervention(s) examined, and comparison groups. The single study examining comorbidity *per se* and its effects on the treatment of DM demonstrated that for persons with low to moderate comorbidity, measured with a validated comorbidity index, achieving a HgbA1C $\leq$6.5% was associated with a decreased risk of cardiovascular events, but for persons with high comorbidity, achieving this HgbA1C level was not associated with decreased risk [9].

All but two of the ten studies examining the effect of DM on the treatment of HF with beta blockers concluded that there were no differences in outcomes according to the presence or absence of DM or greater risk reduction among patient with DM [10–17,19]. Figure 2 provides a graphical summary of the results for those studies presenting their outcomes in terms of a form of relative risk. One study reported a significant benefit of beta-blockers on all-cause mortality and cardiovascular outcomes among patients without DM with a hazard ratio (HR) of.78 (95% confidence interval [CI].65, .93) but no benefit among patients with DM with a HR of 1.04 (.80, 1.35). [11] The second study concluding that

Table 1. Description of studies identified in systematic review.

Approach to analysis of comorbidity:	
Comorbidity index	1
Pairwise combinations of conditions	44
Combinations of conditions*:	
Heart failure and diabetes mellitus	10
Diabetes mellitus and hypertension	9
Cardiovascular disease and diabetes	5
Diabetes mellitus and renal disease	10
Cardiovascular disease and chronic kidney disease	8
Study design:	
Randomized controlled trial	6
Randomized controlled trial with post-hoc subgroup analysis	25
Observational cohort study	14
Miscellaneous combinations	5
Outcome(s) examined*:	
Mortality	35
Disease-specific outcome (e.g. stroke, cardiovascular event)	24
Hospitalization	5
Function/symptoms	1
Adverse effect	2

* Total >45 because some articles examined more than one combination of conditions and/or more than one outcome.

there was a difference in all-cause mortality reported a non-significant effect of beta-blockers among patients with DM with a hazard ratio (HR) of.79 (95% confidence interval [CI].50, 1.20) and a borderline significant effect among patients without DM with a HR of.60 (.35, 1.01). [18] While another study also showed a significant effect among patients without DM and a non-significant effect among patients with DM, it concluded that there was no difference in benefit because of a non-significant "heterogeneity test for interaction." [14].

Among the six studies examining intensity of HTN treatment in patients with DM, the definition of tight control changed over time, as did the study results. The United Kingdom Prospective

Table 2. Main study findings according to approach of article.

Examination of benefit of therapy in presence or absence of comorbidity (n = 25):	
No difference in benefit	19
Benefit greater in presence of comorbidity	4
Benefit smaller or absent in presence of comorbidity	2
Examination of harm of therapy in presence or absence of comorbidity (n = 2):	
No difference in harm	2
Harm smaller or absent in presence of comorbidity	0
Harm great in presence of comorbidity	0
Examination of benefit of tighter versus less tight control of one condition when second condition present (n = 15):	
Tighter control more beneficial versus less tight control	7
Tighter control of no greater benefit or harmful versus less tight control	6
U-shaped relationship, or different relationship for different outcomes	2
Examination of benefit of intervention established as standard of care when comorbidity absent in the presence of comorbidity (n = 3):	
Intervention beneficial	1
Intervention not beneficial	2

Table 3. Studies identified in systematic review.

Author, Year	Study Design & N	Population	Intervention/ Comparison Groups	Outcome/Main Findings (Differences between Groups)
Diseases: HEART FAILURE AND DIABETES MELLITUS				
Bobbio, 2003	Cohort N = 2,843	Italian patients w/HF, mean ages 63–66	Beta-blockers/with and w/o DM	All-cause mortality: no difference.
deBoer, 2010	Post-hoc RCT N = 2,128	Dutch patients ≥70 w/HF	Nebivolol (BB)/with and w/o DM	All-cause mortality and CV hospital admission: risk reduction greater in patients with DM.
Deedwania, 2005	Post-hoc RCT N = 3,991	European patients, ages 40–80 w/HF	Metoprolol CR/XL (BB)/with and w/o DM	All-cause mortality and hospitalization due to HF: no difference
Domanski, 2003	Post-hoc RCT N = 2,708	US patients, ages 19–93 w/HF	Bucindolol (BB)/with and w/o DM.	Death or HF hospitalizations: no difference.
Erdmann, 2001	Post-hoc RCT N = 2,647	European patients w/HF, mean age 61	Bisoprostol/with and w/o DM	All-cause mortality: no difference.
MacDonald, 2008	Post-hoc RCT N = 7,599	European patients w/HF, mean ages 65–67	Candesartan/with and w/o DM	All-cause mortality, CV morbidity and mortality: no difference.
Nodari, 2003	Cohort N = 193	Italian patients w/HF, mean ages 60 (w/DM) and 55 (w/o DM)	Carvedilol/with and w/o DM	NYHA functional class, exercise tests, and other hemodynamic parameters: no difference.
Ryden, 2000	Post-hoc RCT N = 3,164	International patients >55 w/HF	Lisinopril high vs. low dose/with and w/o DM	All-cause mortality: no difference.
Subramanian 2009	Cohort N = 412	Veterans w/HF, mean ages 66–70	Beta-blockers (cardioselective CSB)/with and w/o DM	All-cause mortality: no benefit for patients with DM; borderline significant benefit for patients without DM.
Torp-Pedersen, 2007	Post-hoc RCT N = 3,029	European patients w/HF, mean ages 61–64	Carvedilol vs. metoprolol/with and w/o DM	All-cause mortality: no difference.
Diseases: DIABETES AND HYPERTENSION				
ACCORD, 2010 (Cushman)	Factorial RCT N = 4,733	DM pts ≥40 w/CVD or ≥55 w/atherosclerosis, albuminuria, LVH, or ≥2 risk factors for CVD	BP therapy/tight (<120 SBP) vs less tight (<140 SBP) BP control	Major cardiovascular event: no difference. All-cause or cardiovascular mortality: no difference Significantly higher rate SAE (3.3% vs. 1.29%, p<.001), hyperkalemia, and elevated Cr in tight control group vs less tight group.
Berl, 2005	Post-hoc RCT N = 1,715	US patients, ages 30–70 w/DM, HTN, proteinuria	BP therapy/observed SBP≤120 vs >120; DBP 10 mm Hg increments	All-cause mortality: increased risk with SBP<120. MI: increased risk with lower DBP. Stroke: decreased risk with lower DBP.
Cooper-DeHoff, 2010	Post-hoc RCT N = 6,400	US patients, ≥50 w/stable CAD and DM	BP control/observed tight (SBP<130), usual (SBP 130–139), uncontrolled (≥140)	All-cause mortality: no difference during study f/u. 5-yr mortality: higher in tight control.
Curb, 1996	Post-hoc RCT N = 4,736	US patients, ≥60 w/HTN	Chlorthalidone (+atenolol or reserpine as needed)/with and w/o DM	All-cause mortality, non-fatal plus fatal stroke, nonfatal MI plus fatal CHD, major CHD events, major CVD events: risk reduction as great if not greater for persons with DM (no formal test for interaction)
Estacio, 2000	RCT N = 470	US patients, ages 40–74 w/DM	Stepped BP therapy/DBP≤70 vs. DBP 80–89	CrCl, retinopathy, neuropathy: no difference. All-cause mortality: lower in tight control.
Hansson, 1998	Stratified RCT N = 1,501	European patients, ages 50–80 w/DM	Stepped BP therapy/DBP≤90 vs. ≤85 vs. ≤80	Major CV events: lower in tight control (significant difference ≤80 vs. ≤90).
Tuomilehto, 1999	Post-hoc RCT N = 4,695	European patients, ≥60 with HTN	Nitrendipine (+others as needed)/with and w/o DM	All-cause mortality, mortality from cardiovascular disease, all cardiovascular events: greater risk reduction in patients with DM
UKPDS, 1998	RCT N = 1,148	UK patients, ages 25–65 w/HTN & DM	BP therapy/tight (<150 SBP) vs. less tight (<180 SBP) BP control	All-cause mortality, MI: no difference. Any DM-related endpoints, DM-related deaths, stroke, microvascular disease: lower in tight control.
Wang, 2000	Post-hoc RCT N = 2,394	Chinese patients, ≥60 w/HTN	Nitrendipine (+others as needed)/with and w/o DM	All-cause mortality, CV mortality, stroke, all cardiovascular events: no difference
Diseases: CARDIOVASCULAR DISEASE AND DIABETES				
Berthet, 2004	Post-hoc RCT N = 6,105	International patients w/hx of CVA or TIA, mean ages 63–64	ACE-inhibitor (+indapamide as needed)/with and w/o DM	Recurrent stroke: no difference.
Collins, 2003	Post-hoc RCT N = 20,536	UK patients, ages 40–80 w/CAD, PAD, or HTN.	Simvastatin/with and w/o DM	Coronary events and vascular events: no difference.
Komajda, 2010	Post-hoc RCT N = 4,447	International patients w/DM	Rosiglitazone/with and w/o CVD	Heart failure: no difference

Table 3. Cont.

Author, Year	Study Design & N	Population	Intervention/ Comparison Groups	Outcome/Main Findings (Differences between Groups)
Shinohara, 2008	Post-hoc RCT N = 1,095	Japanese patients w/prior CVA or TIA	Cilostazol/with and w/o DM, HTN	Recurrent stroke: no difference.
Wernicke, 2009	Post-hoc RCTs (pooled analysis) N = 1,024	US patients ≥18 with diabetic peripheral neuropathy	Duloxetine/with and w/o CVD	Adverse events: no difference.
Diseases: DIABETES AND RENAL DISEASE				
Hayashino, 2007	Cohort N = 1,569	Japanese patients w/ESRD on HD, mean ages 58–64	Glycemic control during stable, regular HD/Quintile of HgbA1C	All-cause mortality: top quintile of HgbA1C assoc w/increased risk compared to lowest quintile.
Kalantar-Zadeh, 2007	Cohort N = 23,618	US patients w/ESRD on HD, mean ages 60–63	Glycemic control during stable regular HD/HgbA1C level	All-cause mortality: unadjusted analysis demonstrated lower HR with higher HgbA1C; adjustment resulted in higher HR as HgbA1c increased.
Lambers Heerspink, 2010	Post-hoc RCT N = 10,640	European patients with DM, mean age 65–68	Perindopril-indapamide/w/o CKD and w/3 stages of CKD	Macrovascular events, cardiovascular death, all-cause mortality, cerebrovascular events, new or worsening nephropathy, renal death: no difference.
Mann, 2001	Post-hoc RCT N = 980	International patients >55 w/DM and cardiac risk factor	Ramipril/with and w/o CRI	CV death, MI or CVA (combined outcome): no difference. CV mortality, all-cause mortality, heart failure–related hospitalization: risk reduction greater in patients with CRI.
Morioka, 2001	Cohort N = 150	Japanese patients w/ESRD on HD, ages 29–85, mean age 60.5	Glycemic control prior to start of dialysis/HgbA1C level	1, 3, and 5-year mortality: Risk increased with higher HgbA1C.
Okada, 2007	Cohort N = 78	Japanese patients w/type 2 DM and ESRD, age ≥20, mean age 58	Glycemic control prior to start of dialysis and during dialysis/HgbA1C level	All-cause mortality: no difference.
Oomichi, 2006	Cohort N = 114	Japanese patients w/ESRD on HD, ages 33–80, mean age 60.8	Glycemic control during stable, regular dialysis/Good, fair, poor HgbA1C	5-year mortalty: Higher in those w/poor HgbA1C (≥8) than in those with fair (6.5–8) or good (<6.5) HgbA1C.
Shurraw, 2010	Cohort N = 1,484	Canadian patients receiving hemodialysis, mean age 66	Glycemic control/HgbA1C level	All-cause mortality: no difference.
Shurraw, 2011	Cohort N = 23,296	Canadian patients w/DM and CKD, mean age 65–73	Glycemic control/HgbA1C level	All-cause mortality: U-shaped association: increased risk with <6.5% and >8.0%.
Williams, 2006	Cohort N = 24,744	US patients w/ESRD on HD, mean age 63.7	Glycemic control during stable, regular dialysis/HgbA1C level	All-cause mortality: no difference.
Diseases: CARDIOVASCULAR DISEASE AND CHRONIC KIDNEY DISEASE				
Baigent, 2011	RCT N = 9,270	European patients, ≥40 with moderate-severe CKD	Simvastatin+ezetimibe vs. placebo*	17% decrease in major CVD events with treatment; no difference in effect comparing patients with ESRD on dialysis and those with less severe CKD
Cohen-Solal, 2009	Post-hoc RCT (prespecified group) N = 2,112	European patients, >70 w/HF	Nebivolol/Tertiles of eGFR	All-cause mortality and CV hospitalizations: no difference.
Erdmann, 2001	Post-hoc RCT N = 2,647	European patients w/HF, mean age 61	Bisoprostol/with and w/o CKD.	All-cause mortality: no difference.
Fellström, 2009	RCT N = 2,776	European patients, ages 50–80 w/ESRD on HD	Rosuvastatin vs. placebo*	CV death, non-fatal MI, or non-fatal stroke: no risk reduction with rosuvastatin
McAlister, 2004	Cohort N = 754	Canadian patients w/HF, median age 69	ACE-inhibitors and beta-blockers/with and w/o CKD (GFR <60)	All-cause mortality: no difference
Nakamura, 2009	Post-hoc RCT N = 7,195	Japanese patients, ages 40–70 w/HL	Pravastatin/with and w/o moderate CKD	CHD, stroke, CVD, all-cause mortality: risk reduction greater in moderate CKD than without moderate CKD.
Tonelli, 2004	Post-hoc RCT N = 19,700	International patients w/CAD or at high risk for CAD, mean ages 50–65	Pravastatin/with and w/o moderate CKD	MI, coronary death, PTCA/surgical revascularization: no difference.
Wanner, 2005	RCT N = 1,255	European patients, ages 18–80 w/Type II DM w/ESRD on HD	Atorvastatin vs. placebo*	Composite of cardiac death, nonfatal MI, and stroke: no risk reduction with atorvastatin
MISCELLANEOUS DISEASE COMBINATIONS				
Bavry, 2010	Post-hoc RCT N = 22,576	International patients, ≥50 w/HTN and stable CAD	BP lowering/with and w/o PAD	All-cause mortality, nonfatal MI and nonfatal CVA: more pronounced J-shaped curve for relationship of HTN and outcome among PAD compared to no PAD.

Table 3. Cont.

Author, Year	Study Design & N	Population	Intervention/ Comparison Groups	Outcome/Main Findings (Differences between Groups)
Du, 2009	Post-hoc RCT N = 11,140	International patients, ≥55 w/DM and 1 additional CV risk	Perindopril+indapamide/with and w/o AF	All-cause mortality, CV deaths, major coronary events, major cerebrovascular events, HF: no difference.
Greenfield, 2009	Cohort N = 2,613	UK patients w/DM, mean ages 61–64	Glycemic control/w/low-to-mod comorbidity (TIBI <12) vs. high comorbidity (TIBI ≥12)	CV events: HbA1c ≤6.5 associated with reduced risk in low CM but not mod-high CM.
Shinohara, 2008	Post-hoc RCT N = 1,095	Japanese patients w/prior CVA or TIA	Cilostazol/with and w/o HTN	Recurrent stroke: no difference.
Sin, 2002	Cohort N = 11,942	Canadian patients ≥65 w/HF	Beta-blockers/With and w/o IHD	All-cause mortality: no difference.

RCT = randomized controlled trial.
w/o = without.
HF = heart failure.
DM = diabetes mellitus.
CV = cardiovascular.
NYHA = New York Heart Association.
LVH = left ventricular hypertrophy.
CVD = cardiovascular disease.
BP = blood pressure.
HTN = hypertension.
SBP = systolic blood pressure.
SAE = serious adverse event.
DBP = diastolic blood pressure.
MI = myocardial infarction.
CAD = coronary artery disease.
CHD = coronary heart disease.
CrCl = creatinine clearance.
UK = United Kingdom.
ACE = angiotensin converting enzyme.
PAD = peripheral arterial disease.
CVA = cerebrovascular accident.
AF = atrial fibrillation.
IHD = ischemic heart disease.
ESRD = end = stage renal disease.
HD = hemodialysis.
CKD = chronic kidney disease.
PTCA = percutaneous transluminal coronary angioplasty.
TIBI = Total Illness Burden Index.
*No inclusion of patients without CKD and therefore no comparison between patients with and without CKD; study assumed established benefit of therapy in the absence of CKD.

Diabetes study (UKPDS), defining tight control as a systolic blood pressure (SBP) of <150 mmHg, versus less tight control as SBP< 180 mmHg, demonstrated no difference in overall mortality associated with tight control but a decrease in any DM-related endpoints, DM-related deaths, stroke, or microvascular disease. [27] Later studies defining tight control as SBP<130 or < 120 mmHg demonstrated either no difference in outcome or an increased risk of adverse outcome associated with tight control. [20,21,23] The results were less consistent when tight control was defined on the basis of diastolic blood pressure (DBP). Two studies defining tight control as DBP<80 mmHg and as <70 mmHg demonstrated benefits in terms of lower all-cause mortality and major cardiovascular events, [24,25] whereas a third study examining DBP in 10 mm increments demonstrated a decreased risk of stroke but increased risk of myocardial infarction associated with tighter control [20].

Of the five studies examining patients with cardiovascular disease and diabetes, three examined the effects of medications to reduce risk of vascular outcomes (ACE-inhibitor, simvastatin, and cilostazol) and found no differences according to the presence or absence of DM [39–41]. The remaining two studies examined the likelihood of harm associated with medication use among persons with DM with and without cardiovascular disease. These studies found no difference in adverse effects associated with duloxetine and no difference in the likelihood of heart failure associated with rosiglitazone.

The eight studies examining outcomes in patients with renal disease according to control of blood sugar in DM showed conflicting results. A total of three studies demonstrated an increased risk of mortality associated with higher HgbA1C levels, [29,33,35] whereas three other studies demonstrated no difference in survival, [34,37,38] and one study demonstrated a U-shaped association. [36] In one study, the unadjusted analysis demonstrated a lower risk of mortality with higher HgbA1C levels but the adjusted analysis demonstrated a higher risk, suggesting that HgbA1C levels may be a marker of underlying health status. [30] The two studies examining the effects of ACE-inhibitors on cardiovascular outcomes among patients with DM demonstrated either no differences according to the presence or absence of CKD [31] or greater risk reduction among patients with renal disease [32].

Of the five studies examining a variety of medications among patients with cardiovascular disease, four demonstrated no difference in outcomes according to the presence or absence of

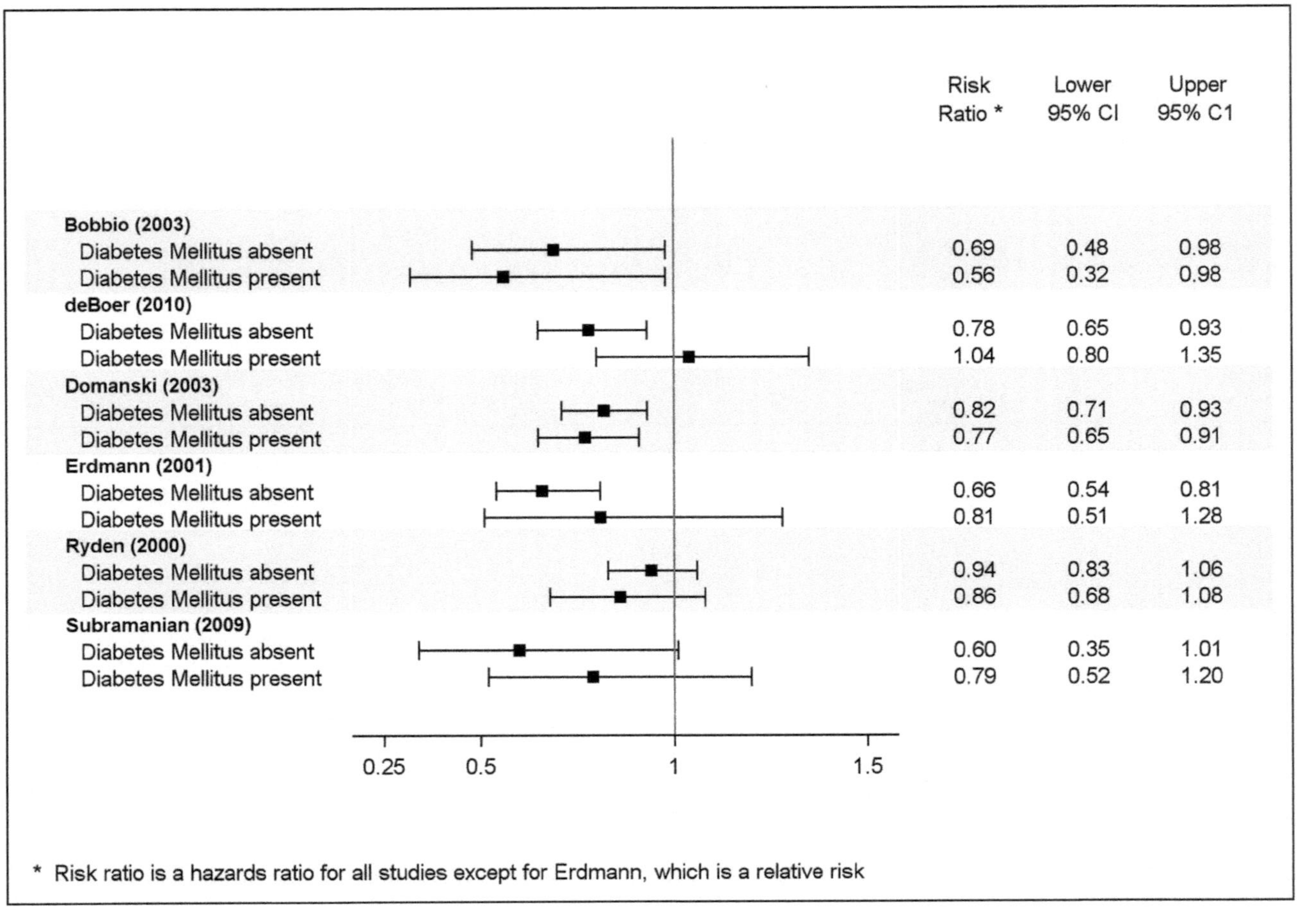

Figure 2. Risk Reduction Associated with Medication for Treatment of Heart Failure.

CKD. [14,45,47,49] The fifth, a study of pravastatin, demonstrated a decreased risk of a number of different outcomes among persons with moderate CKD but no decreased risk among persons with normal renal function or mild CKD, suggesting increased efficacy of the medication in the presence of CKD. [48] (Figure 3). Of the three studies examining the efficacy of statins among persons with CKD without a comparison group of persons without CKD, one demonstrated a decreased risk of major cardiac events with treatment and found no difference when comparing patients with end-stage renal disease (ESRD) and those with less severe CKD. [44] The two other studies demonstrated no decreased risk of major cardio/cerebrovascular events with treatment among patients with ESRD receiving hemodialysis [46,50].

Of the four studies examining miscellaneous combinations of conditions, three demonstrated no difference in the efficacy of treatment according to the presence or absence of the comorbid condition. This included the use of perindopril-indapamide among persons with DM and one additional cardiovascular risk factor in the presence or absence of AF, [52] the use of cilostazol in persons with prior cerebrovascular accident or transient ischemic attack in the presence or absence of HTN, [41] and the use of beta blockers in persons with HF in the presence or absence of ischemic heart disease. [53] The final study examined the effect of the intensity of treatment of HTN in persons with CAD in the presence or absence of PAD. This study found a J-shaped relationship between blood pressure and outcomes among persons with PAD, such that lower blood pressure was associated with increased risk, but no such relationship among persons without PAD [51].

Discussion

This systematic review was undertaken to address the question of how the presence of comorbid conditions affects the benefits and harms of medical treatment for an index chronic condition. The process of the review revealed that there is virtually no evidence regarding the effect of comorbidity *per se*, as the review identified only one study that characterized patients according to their burden of comorbid illnesses. Instead, the evidence consists of studies of pairs of conditions, in which investigators examine the effect of therapy in the presence or absence of a single comorbid condition. There is also little evidence regarding harms of treatment, as the vast majority of studies focused on examining benefit only. In addition, benefit was narrowly defined in terms of reducing the risk of mortality and other major disease-specific outcomes. Studies focused on a limited range of pairs, consisting of a combination of cardiovascular disease (HF and HTN), DM, and CKD. Few studies were originally designed to address the question of the effect of comorbidity on treatment of an index condition. The majority of studies demonstrated that the presence of a comorbid condition did not reduce the benefits associated with treatment of the index condition. The exceptions to this were the findings that patients with a high burden of comorbidity do not derive the same benefit from tight diabetic control as patients with a lower comorbidity burden, that patients with DM do not benefit

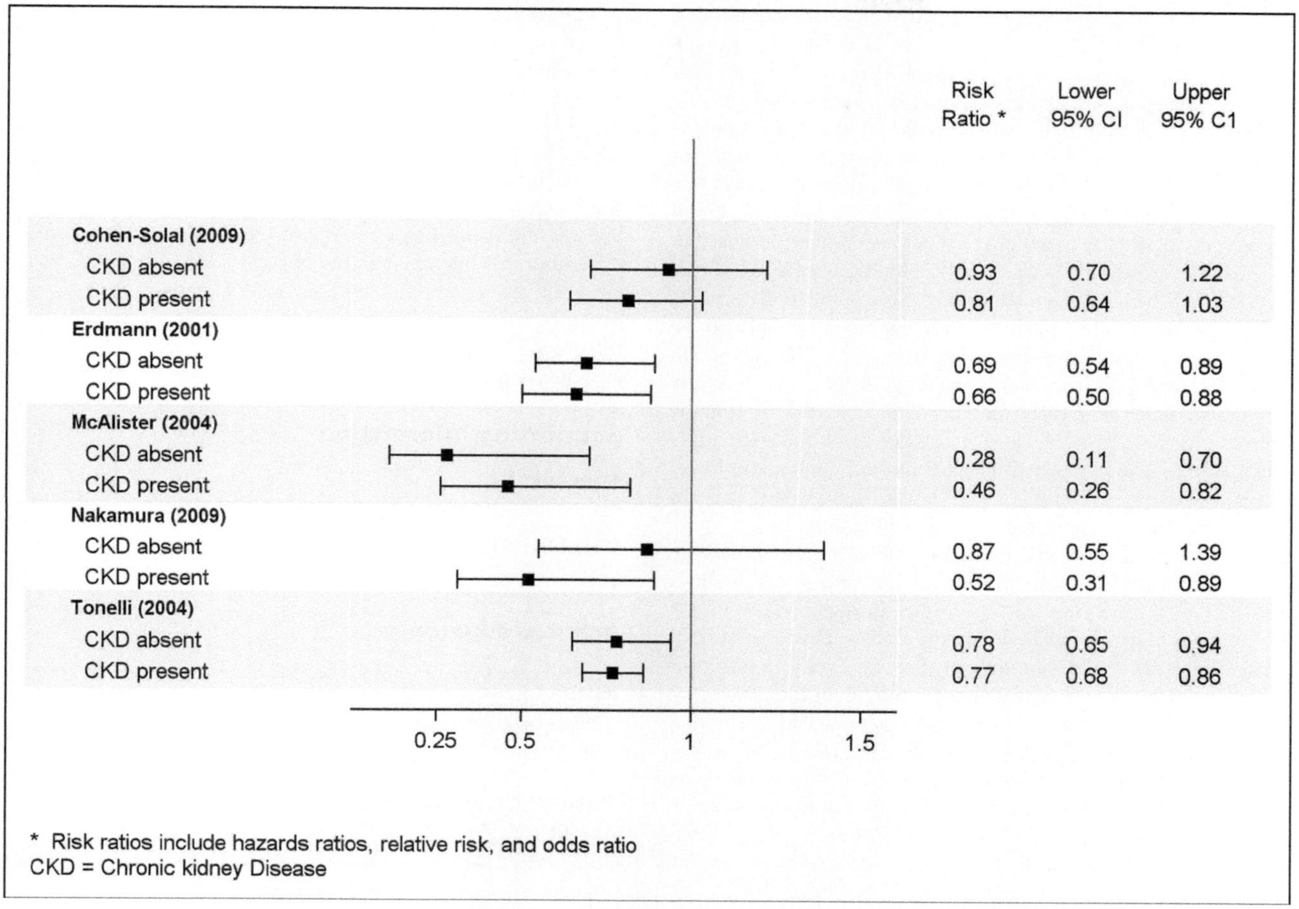

Figure 3. Risk Reduction Associated with Medication for Treatment of Cardiovascular Disease.

from tight control of HTN, and that patients with ESRD do not derive the same benefit from treatment with statin therapy as patients without ESRD.

This systematic review was motivated by concern raised in the literature about the unintended adverse consequences of treating patients with multimorbidity. This concern arises from the finding that treating patients with multimorbidity according to current disease-specific guidelines can result in polypharmacy with the potential for numerous drug-drug and drug-disease interactions. [2] Moreover, polypharmacy itself has been associated with adverse outcomes, including falls, [54] weight loss and balance impairment, [55] and hospitalization. [56] However, the existing literature does not address this patient population. Despite an extensive search, we found only one study that examined burden of comorbidity as a potential modifier of the effect of treatment. "Multimorbidity" is not an indexing term, and, while "comorbidity" is a term, it was infrequently used, so that it proved difficult to construct a search addressing our question of interest. With the growing attention being paid to the study of multiple medical conditions, there is a need for a clear and consistent approach to indexing future studies in order to facilitate the ability to synthesize evidence as it becomes available.

The great majority of studies examined either mortality or disease-specific outcomes, such as cardiovascular events. Disease-specific outcomes cannot be applied across individual diseases to facilitate treatment decision making that takes into account the net effect of an intervention on the health of a patient with multimorbidity, and universal outcomes that are applicable across diseases such as quality of life, physical function, or symptom reduction may be more important to these patients. [57,58] Moreover, studies did not examine time to benefit, a parameter particularly important for patients with multimorbidity because of their competing mortality risks [57].

The studies conducted as post-hoc analyses of randomized controlled trials are subject to the same limitations of their patient population as the original studies. The patients eligible for and participating in cardiovascular intervention studies are generally healthier and with fewer comorbid conditions than are patients who do not enroll in these studies. [59,60] There is evidence that these differences influence the benefits and harms of therapies. For example, the RALES RCT demonstrating the effectiveness of spironolactone in reducing hospitalization and mortality among patients with advanced HF had very low rates of adverse events. [61] The publication of the trial was followed by a marked increase in the use of spironolactone, and, among older persons who were taking ACE-inhibitors, this increase was accompanied by a substantial rise in the rates of hospitalization and mortality from hyperkalemia [62].

Because of the lack of studies examining comorbidity, our review ended up addressing the question of whether, among a limited spectrum of diseases, the presence of a second condition affects the benefits or harms of treatment for a first. While, for many pairs of conditions (DM and HF, DM and CKD, DM and CVD), the answer to this question appears to be "no," there was some evidence to suggest that the presence of a second condition can alter the outcomes of therapy. The finding of an increased risk of adverse outcome among patients with DM receiving tight blood pressure control illustrates an evolution in the approach to the treatment of HTN among diabetic patients. Recommendations published in 2003 included the statement that "there is no threshold value for blood pressure, and risk continues to decrease well into the normal range," [63] suggesting the lower the blood pressure, the better the outcomes. Recommendations published in 2013 call for treatment to a systolic blood pressure of <140, reserving treatment to lower targets for select populations, such as younger patients. [64] While these recommendations appear to be supported by the results of this systematic review, it is also worth noting that many disease management guidelines for DM also recommend different targets for HgbA1C according to comorbidities, ranging from 7% to 8%. Aside from the one study demonstrating a lack of benefit for patients with high comorbidity burden achieving a HgbA1C of <6.5%, our review did not identify any studies supporting these recommendations.

Our review has several limitations. First, because of the difficulty in constructing an effective search strategy, we found a relatively large proportion of our studies through review of the reference lists of articles identified in the search. This suggests that we may have missed relevant articles. Second data to inform our study question may exist that was not available in the articles we reviewed. For example, we identified two meta-analyses of studies examining the effect of DM on the treatment of HF. In our review of the articles referenced in the meta-analyses, we failed to find any subgroup analysis examining outcomes according to the presence or absence of DM. This suggests that the authors of the meta-analyses obtained additional data from the investigators of the original studies.

The conduct of this systematic review designed to address the question of how comorbid conditions affect the benefits and harms of treatment for an index chronic disease demonstrated that the evidence was difficult to find because of a lack of clear indexing. Moreover, few studies were designed to answer this question optimally. There was little evidence examining comorbidity *per se*, but rather studies examining pairs of conditions. Because many studies were derived from RCTs, their participants may not have had the full range of comorbidities present in unselected patient populations. While the majority of studies did not demonstrate an effect of the comorbid condition on outcomes, there is some evidence to support the notion that "less is more" [65] when treating patients with multiple chronic conditions. However, more evidence is needed to inform the care of these patients.

Supporting Information

Appendix S1.

Checklist S1 PRISMA checklist.

Acknowledgments

We would like to thank Janis Glover, MLS, for her assistance in designing and conducting the Medline search.

Views expressed are those of the authors and not necessarily those of the Department of Veterans Affairs.

Author Contributions

Conceived and designed the experiments: TRF. Performed the experiments: TRF JRO VT. Analyzed the data: TRF MG MT DKM. Contributed to the writing of the manuscript: TRF MG DKM.

References

1. Tinetti ME, Fried TR, Boyd CM (2012) Designing health care for the most common chronic condition-multimorbidity. JAMA 307: 2493–2494.
2. Boyd CM, Darer J, Boult C, Fried LP, Boult L, et al. (2005) Clinical practice guidelines and quality of care for older patients with multiple comorbid diseases: implications for pay for performance. JAMA 294: 716–724.
3. Gandhi TK, Weingart SN, Borus J, Seger AC, Peterson J, et al. (2003) Adverse drug events in ambulatory care. N Engl J Med 348: 1556–1564.
4. Tinetti ME, Bogardus ST Jr, Agostini JV (2004) Potential pitfalls of disease-specific guidelines for patients with multiple conditions. N Engl J Med 351: 2870–2874.
5. Concato J, Shah N, Horwitz RI (2000) Randomized, controlled trials, observational studies, and the hierarchy of research designs. N Engl J Med 342: 1887–1892.
6. Vogeli C, Shields A, Lee T, Gibson T, Marder W, et al. (2007) Multiple chronic conditions: prevalence, health consequences, and implications for quality, care management, and costs. J Gen Intern Med 22: 391–395.
7. D'Agostino RB (2000) Debate: The slippery slope of surrogate outcomes. Curr Control Trials Cardiovasc Med 1: 76–79.
8. Guyatt GH, Oxman AD, Vist GE, Kunz R, Falck-Ytter Y, et al. (2008) GRADE: an emerging consensus on rating quality of evidence and strength of recommendations. BMJ 336: 924–926.
9. Greenfield S, Billimek J, Pellegrini F, Franciosi M, De Berardis G, et al. (2009) Comorbidity affects the relationship between glycemic control and cardiovascular outcomes in diabetes: a cohort study. Ann Intern Med 151: 854–860.
10. Bobbio M, Ferrua S, Opasich C, Porcu M, Lucci D, et al. (2003) Survival and hospitalization in heart failure patients with or without diabetes treated with beta-blockers. J Card Fail 9: 192–202.
11. de Boer RA, Doehner W, van der Horst ICC, Anker SD, Babalis D, et al. (2010) Influence of diabetes mellitus and hyperglycemia on prognosis in patients> or = 70 years old with heart failure and effects of nebivolol (data from the Study of Effects of Nebivolol Intervention on Outcomes and Rehospitalization in Seniors with heart failure [SENIORS]). Am J Cardiol 106: 78–86.e71.
12. Deedwania PC, Giles TD, Klibaner M, Ghali JK, Herlitz J, et al. (2005) Efficacy, safety and tolerability of metoprolol CR/XL in patients with diabetes and chronic heart failure: experiences from MERIT-HF. Am Heart J 149: 159–167.
13. Domanski M, Krause-Steinrauf H, Deedwania P, Follmann D, Ghali JK, et al. (2003) The effect of diabetes on outcomes of patients with advanced heart failure in the BEST trial. J Am Coll Cardiol 42: 914–922.
14. Erdmann E, Lechat P, Verkenne P, Wiemann H (2001) Results from post-hoc analyses of the CIBIS II trial: effect of bisoprolol in high-risk patient groups with chronic heart failure. Eur J Heart Fail 3: 469–479.
15. MacDonald MR, Petrie MC, Varyani F, Östergren J, Michelson EL, et al. (2008) Impact of diabetes on outcomes in patients with low and preserved ejection fraction heart failure An analysis of the Candesartan in Heart failure: Assessment of reduction in mortality and morbidity (CHARM) programme. Eur Heart J 29: 1377–1385.
16. Nodari S, Metra M, Dei Cas A, Dei Cas L (2003) Efficacy and tolerability of the long-term administration of carvedilol in patients with chronic heart failure with and without concomitant diabetes mellitus. Eur J Heart Fail 5: 803–809.
17. Ryden L, Armstrong PW, Cleland J, Horowitz JD, Massie B, et al. (2000) Efficacy and safety of high-dose lisinopril in chronic heart failure patients at high cardiovascular risk, including those with diabetes mellitus. Results from the ATLAS trial. Eur Heart J 1 21: 1967–1978.
18. Subramanian U, Kamalesh M, Temkit Mh, Eckert GJ, Sawada S (2009) Do cardioselective beta-adrenoceptor antagonists reduce mortality in diabetic patients with congestive heart failure? Am J Cardiovasc Drugs 9: 231–240.
19. Torp-Pedersen C, Metra M, Charlesworth A, Spark P, Lukas MA, et al. (2007) Effects of metoprolol and carvedilol on pre-existing and new onset diabetes in patients with chronic heart failure: data from the Carvedilol Or Metoprolol European Trial (COMET). Heart 93: 968–973.
20. Berl T, Hunsicker LG, Lewis JB, Pfeffer MA, Porush JG, et al. (2005) Impact of achieved blood pressure on cardiovascular outcomes in the irbesartan diabetic nephropathy trial. J Am Soc Nephrol 16: 2170–2179.
21. Cooper-DeHoff RM, Gong Y, Handberg EM, Bavry AA, Denardo SJ, et al. (2010) Tight blood pressure control and cardiovascular outcomes among hypertensive patients with diabetes and coronary artery disease. JAMA 304: 61–68.
22. Curb JD, Pressel SL, Cutler JA, Savage PJ, Applegate WB, et al. (1996) Effect of diuretic-based antihypertensive treatment on cardiovascular disease risk in older diabetic patients with isolated systolic hypertension. Systolic Hypertension in the Elderly Program Cooperative Research Group. JAMA 276: 1886–1892.
23. Cushman WC (2010) Effects of Intensive blood-pressure control in type 2 diabetes mellitus. New Engl J Med 362: 1575–1585.

24. Estacio RO, Jeffers BW, Gifford N, Schrier RW (2000) Effect of blood pressure control on diabetic microvascular complications in patients with hypertension and type 2 diabetes. Diabetes Care 23 Suppl 2: B54–64.
25. Hansson L, Zanchetti A, Carruthers SG, Dahlöf B, Elmfeldt D, et al. (1998) Effects of intensive blood-pressure lowering and low-dose aspirin in patients with hypertension: principal results of the Hypertension Optimal Treatment (HOT) randomised trial. The Lancet 351: 1755–1762.
26. Tuomilehto J, Rastenyte D, Birkenhager WH, Thijs L, Antikainen R, et al. (1999) Effects of calcium-channel blockade in older patients with diabetes and systolic hypertension. Systolic Hypertension in Europe Trial Investigators. N Engl J Med 340: 677–684.
27. U. K. Prospective Diabetes Study Group (1998) Tight blood pressure control and risk of macrovascular and microvascular complications in type 2 diabetes: UKPDS 38. BMJ 317: 703–713.
28. Wang JG, Staessen JA, Gong L, Liu L (2000) Chinese trial on isolated systolic hypertension in the elderly. Systolic Hypertension in China (SYST-CHINA) Collaborative Group. Arch Intern Med 160: 211–220.
29. Hayashino Y, Fukuhara S, Akiba T, Akizawa T, Asano Y, et al. (2007) Diabetes, glycaemic control and mortality risk in patients on haemodialysis: the Japan Dialysis Outcomes and Practice Pattern Study. Diabetologia 50: 1170–1177.
30. Kalantar-Zadeh K, Kopple JD, Regidor DL, Jing J, Shinaberger CS, et al. (2007) A1C and survival in maintenance hemodialysis patients. Diabetes Care 30: 1049–1055.
31. Lambers Heerspink HJ, Ninomiya T, Perkovic V, Woodward M, Zoungas S, et al. (2010) Effects of a fixed combination of perindopril and indapamide in patients with type 2 diabetes and chronic kidney disease. Eur Heart J 31: 2888–2896.
32. Mann JFEMD, Gerstein HCMD, Pogue JM, Bosch JMA, Yusuf SMD, et al. (2001) Renal insufficiency as a predictor of cardiovascular outcomes and the impact of ramipril: the HOPE randomized trial. Ann Intern Med 134: 629–636.
33. Morioka T, Emoto M, Tabata T, Shoji T, Tahara H, et al. (2001) Glycemic control is a predictor of survival for diabetic patients on hemodialysis. Diabetes Care 24: 909–913.
34. Okada T, Nakao T, Matsumoto H, Shino T, Nagaoka Y, et al. (2007) Association between markers of glycemic control, cardiovascular complications and survival in type 2 diabetic patients with end-stage renal disease. Intern Medicine 46: 807–814.
35. Oomichi T, Emoto M, Tabata T, Morioka T, Tsujimoto Y, et al. (2006) Impact of glycemic control on survival of diabetic patients on chronic regular hemodialysis: a 7-year observational study. Diabetes Care 29: 1496–1500.
36. Shurraw S, Hemmelgarn B, Lin M, Majumdar SR, Klarenbach S, et al. (2011) Association between glycemic control and adverse outcomes in people with diabetes mellitus and chronic kidney disease: a population-based cohort study. Arch Intern Med 171: 1920–1927.
37. Shurraw S, Majumdar SR, Thadhani R, Wiebe N, Tonelli M, et al. (2010) Glycemic control and the risk of death in 1,484 patients receiving maintenance hemodialysis. Am J Kidney Dis 55: 875–884.
38. Williams ME, Lacson E Jr, Teng M, Ofsthun N, Lazarus JM (2006) Hemodialyzed type I and type II diabetic patients in the US: Characteristics, glycemic control, and survival. Kidney Int 70: 1503–1509.
39. Berthet K, Neal BC, Chalmers JP, MacMahon SW, Bousser M-G, et al. (2004) Reductions in the risks of recurrent stroke in patients with and without diabetes: the PROGRESS Trial. Blood Press 13: 7–13.
40. Collins R, Armitage J, Parish S, Sleigh P, Peto R (2003) MRC/BHF Heart Protection Study of cholesterol-lowering with simvastatin in 5963 people with diabetes: a randomised placebo-controlled trial. Lancet 361: 2005.
41. Shinohara Y, Gotoh F, Tohgi H, Hirai S, Terashi A, et al. (2008) Antiplatelet cilostazol is beneficial in diabetic and/or hypertensive ischemic stroke patients. Subgroup analysis of the cilostazol stroke prevention study. Cerebrovasc Dis 26: 63–70.
42. Wernicke JF, Prakash A, Kajdasz DK, Houston J (2009) Safety and tolerability of duloxetine treatment of diabetic peripheral neuropathic pain between patients with and without cardiovascular conditions. J Diabetes Complications 23: 349–359.
43. Komajda M, McMurray JJV, Beck-Nielsen H, Gomis R, Hanefeld M, et al. (2010) Heart failure events with rosiglitazone in type 2 diabetes: data from the RECORD clinical trial. Eur Heart J 31: 824–831.
44. Baigent C, Landray MJ, Reith C, Emberson J, Wheeler DC, et al. (2011) The effects of lowering LDL cholesterol with simvastatin plus ezetimibe in patients with chronic kidney disease (Study of Heart and Renal Protection): a randomised placebo-controlled trial. Lancet 377: 2181–2192.
45. Cohen-Solal A, Kotecha D, van Veldhuisen DJ, Babalis D, Böhm M, et al. (2009) Efficacy and safety of nebivolol in elderly heart failure patients with impaired renal function: insights from the SENIORS trial. Eur J Heart Fail 11: 872–880.
46. Fellstrom BC, Jardine AG, Schmieder RE, Holdaas H, Bannister K, et al. (2009) Rosuvastatin and cardiovascular events in patients undergoing hemodialysis. N Engl J Med 360: 1395–1407.
47. McAlister FA, Ezekowitz J, Tonelli M, Armstrong PW (2004) Renal insufficiency and heart failure: prognostic and therapeutic implications from a prospective cohort study. Circulation 109: 1004–1009.
48. Nakamura H, Mizuno K, Ohashi Y, Yoshida T, Hirao K, et al. (2009) Pravastatin and cardiovascular risk in moderate chronic kidney disease. Atherosclerosis 206: 512–517.
49. Tonelli M, Isles C, Curhan GC, Tonkin A, Pfeffer MA, et al. (2004) Effect of pravastatin on cardiovascular events in people with chronic kidney disease. Circulation 110: 1557–1563.
50. Wanner C, Krane V, März W, Olschewski M, Mann JFE, et al. (2005) Atorvastatin in patients with type 2 diabetes mellitus undergoing hemodialysis. N Engl J Med 353: 238–248.
51. Bavry AA, Anderson RD, Gong Y, Denardo SJ, Cooper-Dehoff RM, et al. (2010) Outcomes Among hypertensive patients with concomitant peripheral and coronary artery disease: findings from the INternational VErapamil-SR/Trandolapril STudy. Hypertension 55: 48–53.
52. Du X, Ninomiya T, de Galan B, Abadir E, Chalmers J, et al. (2009) Risks of cardiovascular events and effects of routine blood pressure lowering among patients with type 2 diabetes and atrial fibrillation: results of the ADVANCE study. Eur Heart J 30: 1128–1135.
53. Sin DD, McAlister FA (2002) The effects of beta-blockers on morbidity and mortality in a population-based cohort of 11,942 elderly patients with heart failure. Am J Med 113: 650–656.
54. Tinetti ME (2003) Preventing falls in elderly persons. N Engl J Med 348: 42–49.
55. Agostini JV, Han L, Tinetti ME (2004) The relationship between number of medications and weight loss or impaired balance in older adults. J Am Geriatr Soc 52: 1719–1723.
56. Beer C, Hyde Z, Almeida OP, Norman P, Hankey GJ, et al. (2011) Quality use of medicines and health outcomes among a cohort of community dwelling older men: an observational study. Br J Clin Pharmacol 71: 592–599.
57. American Geriatrics Society Expert Panel on the Care of Older Adults with Multimorbidity (2012) Patient-Centered Care for Older Adults with Multiple Chronic Conditions: A Stepwise Approach from the American Geriatrics Society. J Am Geriatr Soc 60: 1957–1968.
58. Fried TR, Tinetti ME, Iannone L, O'Leary JR, Towle V, et al. (2011) Health outcome prioritization as a tool for decision making among older persons with multiple chronic conditions. Arch Intern Med 171: 1854–1856.
59. Bahit MC, Cannon CP, Antman EM, Murphy SA, Gibson CM, et al. (2003) Direct comparison of characteristics, treatment, and outcomes of patients enrolled versus patients not enrolled in a clinical trial at centers participating in the TIMI 9 Trial and TIMI 9 Registry. Am Heart J 145: 109–117.
60. Hordijk-Trion M, Lenzen M, Wijns W, de Jaegere P, Simoons ML, et al. (2006) Patients enrolled in coronary intervention trials are not representative of patients in clinical practice: results from the Euro Heart Survey on Coronary Revascularization. Eur Heart J 27: 671–678.
61. Pitt B, Zannad F, Remme WJ, Cody R, Castaigne A, et al. (1999) The effect of spironolactone on morbidity and mortality in patients with severe heart failure. N Engl J Med 341: 709–717.
62. Juurlink DN, Mamdani MM, Lee DS, Kopp A, Austin PC, et al. (2004) Rates of hyperkalemia after publication of the randomized aldactone evaluation study. N Engl J Med 351: 543–551.
63. (2003) Treatment of hypertension in adults with diabetes. Diabetes Care 26: s80–s82.
64. (2013) Executive Summary: Standards of medical care in diabetes–2013. Diabetes Care 36: S4–S10.
65. Grady D, Redberg RF (2010) Less is more: How less health care can result in better health. Arch Intern Med 170: 749–750.

Cardiac Health Risk Stratification System (CHRiSS): A Bayesian-Based Decision Support System for Left Ventricular Assist Device (LVAD) Therapy

Natasha A. Loghmanpour[1], Marek J. Druzdzel[2,3], James F. Antaki[1]*

1 Department of Biomedical Engineering, Carnegie Mellon University, Pittsburgh, Pennsylvania, United States of America, **2** Decision Systems Laboratory, School of Information Sciences, University of Pittsburgh, Pittsburgh, Pennsylvania, United States of America, **3** Faculty of Computer Science, Bialystok University of Technology, Bialystok, Poland

Abstract

This study investigated the use of Bayesian Networks (BNs) for left ventricular assist device (LVAD) therapy; a treatment for end-stage heart failure that has been steadily growing in popularity over the past decade. Despite this growth, the number of LVAD implants performed annually remains a small fraction of the estimated population of patients who might benefit from this treatment. We believe that this demonstrates a need for an accurate stratification tool that can help identify LVAD candidates at the most appropriate point in the course of their disease. We derived BNs to predict mortality at five endpoints utilizing the Interagency Registry for Mechanically Assisted Circulatory Support (INTERMACS) database: containing over 12,000 total enrolled patients from 153 hospital sites, collected since 2006 to the present day, and consisting of approximately 230 pre-implant clinical variables. Synthetic minority oversampling technique (SMOTE) was employed to address the uneven proportion of patients with negative outcomes and to improve the performance of the models. The resulting accuracy and area under the ROC curve (%) for predicted mortality were 30 day: 94.9 and 92.5; 90 day: 84.2 and 73.9; 6 month: 78.2 and 70.6; 1 year: 73.1 and 70.6; and 2 years: 71.4 and 70.8. To foster the translation of these models to clinical practice, they have been incorporated into a web-based application, the Cardiac Health Risk Stratification System (CHRiSS). As clinical experience with LVAD therapy continues to grow, and additional data is collected, we aim to continually update these BN models to improve their accuracy and maintain their relevance. Ongoing work also aims to extend the BN models to predict the risk of adverse events post-LVAD implant as additional factors for consideration in decision making.

Editor: Yiru Guo, University of Louisville, United States of America

Funding: Funding was provided by the 1R41 HL120428-01, 1R01HL086918, and U01HL101066-01 National Institutes of Health grants. The funders had no role in study design, data collection and analysis, decision to publish, or preparation of the manuscript.

Competing Interests: The authors have declared that no competing interests exist.

* Email: antaki@cmu.edu

Introduction

Cardiac transplantation currently represents the most definitive treatment for end-stage heart failure (ESHF) with 90% 1-year survival and a 70% 5-year survival. However, there is a need for alternate therapies due to the limited supply of donor organs. For those ineligible for a heart transplant, or unable to wait, an alternative life-sparing therapy is to implant a left ventricular assist devices (LVAD). These devices have been used for nearly 25 years to support ESHF patients while awaiting transplant and have been consistently shown to improve mortality. The technology has now progressed to the point where they are offered as permanent or so-called Destination Therapy (DT). According to current estimates, the number of ESHF patients who may benefit from LVAD therapy is between 80,000 and 200,000 annually. [1]

LVAD Risk Scores

Optimal and responsible use of LVAD therapy requires a procedure for selecting patients who are most likely to benefit, and less likely to suffer adverse complications. In general, as a patient's disease progresses, the probability of poor outcomes increases. It is therefore important to identify candidates early in the progression of their disease so as not to miss the optimal window of opportunity [2,3]. The window is considered between INTERMACS level 7 and 3, where 7 is clinically stable but history of previous decompensation and 3 is stable but Inotrope dependent [4]. This has motivated the development of risk scores to stratify patients based on the factors that have historically been associated with outcomes, such as patient characteristics, advances in mechanical circulatory support technology and surgical experience.

The most commonly cited score is the Lietz-Miller Destination Therapy Risk Score (DTRS), which was derived from a patient cohort with first generation pumps [5]. The first generation LVADs were pulsatile flow pumps, which attempted to mimic the physiological conditions. One-year survival in subjects undergoing the first generation pulsatile flow HeartMate XVE implantation for DT in the Randomized Evaluation of Mechanical Assistance for the Treatment of Congestive Heart failure (REMATCH) trial was 52% [6]. Enrollment criteria of initial studies emphasized hemodynamic variables. The DTRS analyzed 45 baseline parameters and outcomes in 280 DT patients in the post-REMATCH era. The most important determinants of in-hospital mortality were poor nutrition, hematological abnormalities, markers of end-organ and RV dysfunction and lack of inotropic support. Patients were stratified into low, medium, high and very high risk based on a score calculated from these predictors to correspond with 1-year survival [5]. The DTRS, however, has many limitations. The majority of patients in the derivation cohort were ambulatory, older men with large body surface area. Co-morbidities such as diabetes, cardiac cachexia or obesity were under-represented, while psychosocial factors or echocardiographic parameters were not considered.

Since the DTRS was derived, there has been major advances in the technology. In particular, second generation (continuous flow) pumps have become available that are smaller in size, have simpler technique for implantation, longer durability and present reduced risk of thromboembolism, infection and malfunction. Consequently, the frequency of adverse events has diminished, which has further expanded the candidacy pool for LVAD therapy. This has rendered the DTRS less accurate [7]. Other risk scores have been introduced, but are limited for a variety of reasons, such as limited independent variables or limited training data (e.g. from a single center.) For example, a recently introduced HeartMate II Risk Score (HMRS) relies on only five preoperative variables for predicting 90 day survival; the long-term (1 year) model only contained two: age and implant center experience [8].

Clinical Decision Support Systems

The transition from paper to electronic medical records provides both a challenge and great opportunity for clinical decision making. On the one hand, the ever increasing quantity of information collected on a typical LVAD patient can overwhelm a clinical team, and arguably may introduce more uncertainty due to data incompleteness and noisiness. On the other hand, the wealth of information embedded in these data are ideal for computer-based Clinical Decision Support Systems (CDSS) [9,10]. This is the motivation for developing the Cardiac Health Risk Stratification System (CHRiSS). CHRiSS is a web-enabled decision support tool that provides patient-specific predictions of mortality at 5 endpoints post-implant: 30 day, 90 day, 6 month, 1 year and 2 year. It offers several advantages over traditional LVAD risk scores. Since it is based on a Bayesian machine learning algorithm, it can better represent the influence of large sets of interrelated variables as compared to traditional Cox model multivariate predictors [11,12]. Unlike most risk scores which compute survival at one time point, CHRiSS provides predictions of both short-term and long-term mortality. Since CHRiSS is implemented as an interactive software application, it also permits the user to explore various "what if" scenarios.

The purpose of this study is to evaluate the accuracy and sensitivity of the Bayesian Networks (BNs) in the CHRiSS tool. Accuracy is evaluated both in terms of True Negative (ability to predict survival) and True Positive (ability to predict mortality), which is also depicted by the receiver operating characteristics (ROC) curve. Sensitivity analysis was performed to identify the strongest predictive variables that are associated with either increased or decreased chance of survival post-LVAD.

Methods

This study was conducted with a comprehensive dataset, known as the Interagency Registry for Mechanically Assisted Circulatory Support (INTERMACS). This is the largest national registry for U.S. Food and Drug Administration (FDA) approved mechanical circulatory support devices that is jointly sponsored by the National Heart, Lung, and Blood Institute (NHLBI), Centers for Medicare and Medicaid Services (CMS), FDA and industry. The registry has over 12,000 total enrolled patients (over 8,000 continuous flow LVADs) from 153 hospital sitesand has been collecting data since 2006 to the present day. The dataset consists of over 300 pre-implant clinical variables, subdivided into six main categories: demographics, co-morbidities and limitations from transplant listing, laboratory values, hemodynamics, medications and quality of life questionnaires and surveys. A co-morbidity in this context is defined as a medical condition or disease that exists simultaneously with another condition or disease. They can either be independent or related conditions or diseases.

Patient Cohort

Institutional Review Board approval was obtained through hospitals participating within INTERMACS. The study described in this submission was approved by the INTERMACS Data, Access, Analysis, and Publication Committee (DAAP). Written informed consent was acquired from participants before being enrolled in INTERMACS. The Data Coordinating Center at University of Alabama at Birmingham provided us the data once it was de-identified. The data used in the present study was anonymized and de-identified prior to analysis. Inclusion criteria for this study was: use of a continuous flow LVAD as the primary implant and age>19, thus excluding pediatric patients. Patients who ultimately received an Right Ventricular Assist Device (RVAD) were included as long as the initial implant was an LVAD and an RVAD was placed thereafter. The specific type of RVAD was not considered. Total Artificial Heart recipients were excluded from this study. This translated to 8,050 patients from year 2006 to 2013 in the initial dataset. Data from patients whose LVAD was electively removed (e.g., due to transplantation or recovery) were censored at the time of event (See Table 1).

Pre-processing

The raw data from the registry was pre-processed to transform continuous data into discrete bins (required by the Bayesian algorithm) and to fill in missing data, described below.

Discretization. Discretization was done based on a balance of equal frequency binning and published upper and lower limits of clinically normal values [13,14]. Table S1 provides the list of variables with their respective formats and input values. Clinical scenarios and outcomes, such as events during hospitalization, adverse events prior to implant and interventions within 48 hours of implant, were defined using the INTERMACS definitions.

Missing data. The patient records provided by the INTERMACS data set were found to be routinely incomplete (see Table S1 for percentages missing). Missing data was separated into two categories: *missing at random* (MAR), and *missing not at random* (MNAR) [15]. Missing demographics and lab values, for example, were considered to be either MAR, in which case we assumed the most probable values (i.e. BMI between 24–27 since it is considered normal). The method of using normal values has been cited in previous studies to produce superior results compared to

Table 1. Mortality statistics, censored for explant and transplant.

Endpoint	Survival No. (%)	Death No. (%)	Total	Survival SMOTE No. (%)	Death SMOTE No. (%)	Total SMOTE No. (%)
30 Day	7620 (95.2)	387 (4.8)	8007	7620 (90.8)	774 (9.2)	8394
90 Day	7024 (90.5)	737 (9.5)	7761	7024 (82.6)	1474 (17.3)	8498
6 Month	6245 (86.1)	1007 (13.9)	7252	6245 (75.6)	2014 (24.4)	8259
1 Year	5241 (79.7)	1334 (20.3)	6575	5241 (66.2)	2668 (33.7)	7909
2 Year	4432 (72.7)	1667 (27.3)	6099	4432 (57.1)	3334 (42.9)	7766

SMOTE: synthetic minority oversampling technique.

listwise deletion and other methods [16]. Missing co-morbidities, on the other hand were considered MNAR, in which case we assumed that it was not a concern for that patient. This is standard procedure for handling MNAR data in medical datasets. For example, if a patient has no record of a chest x-ray then the doctor probably did not feel the need to order one. In these cases, it is common to assume a "normal" value, which in the case of the x-ray would be *not ordered* as opposed to *unknown*, or simply *missing*. Additional data in the MAR category were missing laboratory and hemodynamic values were designated as *not ordered*. Missing medication data was considered MNAR, in which we assumed that no such medication was prescribed. Finally, missing quality of life metrics were considered MNAR, and designated as *unknown*. This was justified based on voluntary and sporadic participation in the two quality of life surveys, the EuroQoL [17] (offered since the beginning of the registry)and the Kansas City Cardiomyopathy Questionnaire (KCCQ) [18] implemented after 2012.

Synthetic Minority Oversampling Technique (SMOTE)

A common challenge in data mining that inhibits the predictive ability of the model, is an uneven distribution of the outcome (survival post-LVAD). In medicine, there is often a larger portion of the cohort that are free of death or adverse event as compared to the number of events. The 30-day mortality rate in INTERMACS is 4.8%, compared to a 95.2% survival rate. With such a discrepancy, the model will always predict the majority class (survival) if uncertain how to classify a new patient. This will pose a setback clinically, as it is most important to identify the high-risk patients (early mortality).

One of the most frequently cited methods for addressing this bias is SMOTE [19], which is used when the minority class is increased by creating synthetic examples rather than by over-sampling with replacement. The minority class (mortality) is over-sampled by taking each minority class sample and introducing synthetic examples along the line segments joining any or all of the k minority class nearest neighbors. For this study we increased the minority class by 100%, which would essentially double the mortality number at each endpoint, while the survival number remained unchanged. The 100% was identified by incrementally increasing the percentage from 0% to 100% and identifying the best performing percentage. We set the cut off at 100% to ensure there would be at least an even number of actual and synthetic cases, as opposed to more synthetic compared to actual cases. Synthetic samples are generated by taking the difference between the instance (or patient) under consideration and its nearest neighbor. This difference was multiplied by a random number between 0 and 1, and added to the feature vector under consideration. (This causes the selection of a random point along the line segment between two specific features.) SMOTE effectively forces the decision region of the minority class to become more general. Table 1 juxtaposes the dataset before and after application of SMOTE.

Bayesian Networks

The machine learning methods used for the present study were built upon Bayesian techniques used previously by our group for multiple decision support studies, including: optimal VAD weaning [20], the need for right ventricular support due to right ventricular failure [21–23] and a two-center study to predict 90-day survival for continuous flow LVADs [24,25]. Bayesian networks (BNs) [26] are acyclic directed graphs in which nodes represent random variables and directed arcs (represented as arrows) between pairs of variables represent influences between them. In addition to the graph structure, a BN is equipped with conditional probability tables (CPT), associated with each node, and describes the probability distribution over the variable's values conditional on all combinations of values of its immediate predecessors (parents) in the graph. A BN is a representation of a factorization of the joint probability distribution over its variables. Independence between a pair of variables is represented by absence of a directed arrow between these variables. Explicit representation of independences results in significant savings in the number of parameters necessary to represent the complete joint probability distribution, making BNs highly practical even in very complex domains.

The joint probability distribution represented by a BN can be updated in the light of new evidence by means of Bayes theorem. Efficient algorithms exist that given observed values of some of the variables, produce the new joint (conditional) probability distribution over the remaining variables. While the quality of the results rests on the quality of the underlying representation of the joint probability distribution, BNs have been shown to be very robust to precision of their parameters [27] and there are indications that possible errors in structure (i.e., incorrect independences) have also limited influence on the quality of the results [28].

To illustrate, one may consider a simple BN model in Figure S1, modeling risk factors related to LVAD survival. The network models the joint probability distribution over the four factors and the survival variable. Not all variables need to be known. For example, we could derive from the network the average survival probability for a center with limited LVAD experience.

For this study, we evaluated four BNs: *Näive Bayes*, *Tree-Augmented Näive Bayes*, *Bayesian Search* and the *Greedy Thick Thinning Algorithm* [29]. We ultimately chose the *Greedy Thick Thinning Algorithm* as the final model based on a tradeoff between complexity and accuracy. The model starts with an empty graph and iteratively adds and removes arcs as it builds the

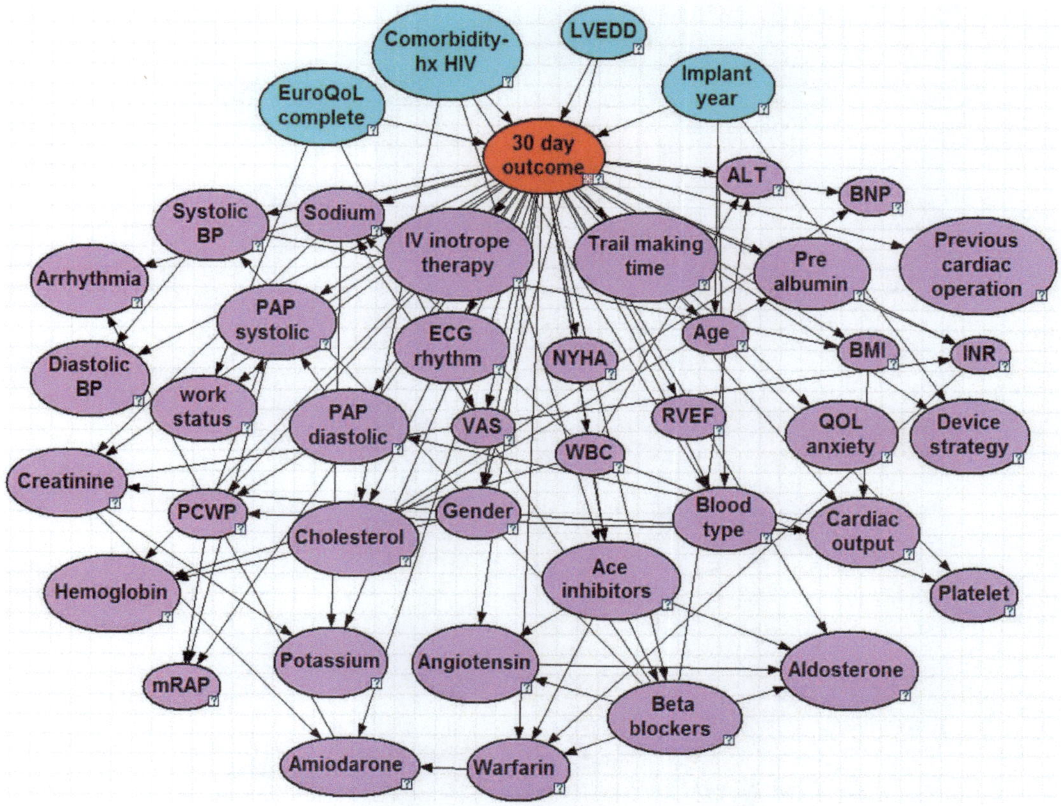

Figure 1. 30 Day Bayesian Model. Node colors: red = class, blue = parent, purple = child. Question marks identify nodes that do not have specific evidence set and use the population distribution as the prior distribution. LVEDD = left ventricle end diastolic diameter, ALT = alanine transaminase, BP = blood pressure, mRAP = mean right atrial pressure, PCWP = pulmonary capillary wedge pressure, VAS = visual analog scale, BNP = B-type natriuretic peptide, WBC = white blood cell, NYHA = New York Heart Association functional class, RVEF = right ventricle ejection fraction, INR = international normalized ratio, BMI = body mass index, ECG = Electrocardiography, QOL = quality of life, hx HIV = history of human immunodeficiency virus.

network, incrementally increasing the Bayesian scoring metric: in this case, the K2 prior distribution over the parameters [30].

Markov Blanket

We applied the Markov Blanket to simplify the network and reduce the likelihood of over-fitting the model to the dataset (i.e. performs well only on the training data, but unable to generalize to other datasets). It has been shown in previous studies that using the Markov Blanket is one of the most effective and efficient methods of feature selection [31]. The Markov Blanket for each of the BN models was comprised of the class node and the family of nodes that make it conditionally independent of all other nodes in the network. This includes the parents, the children and the parents of the children, or spouses [26].

Evaluation

Ten-fold cross validation was the vehicle for model derivation and optimization. The BN classifiers were evaluated on an independent testing/holdout dataset comprised of a training set of approximately 90% of the data records and a testing set from the remaining approximate 10%. The models were derived, built and implemented using two open-source machine learning software libraries: The GeNIe modeling environment developed by the Decision Systems Laboratory of the University of Pittsburgh [32] and the machine learning library WEKA (Waikato Environment for Knowledge Analysis) [33]. Performance metrics included: Accuracy, True Positive, True Negative and area under the ROC curve (AUC). A sensitivity analysis was also performed, where all variables are kept constant and a single parameter is changed to observe the direct affects. This is then expanded to change additional parameters to visualize their additive affects.

Results

The optimized BNs can be seen in Figures 1–5, and a summary of their performance can be found in Table 2. Accuracy was greatest for the 30 day model with 95% and lowest for the 2 year model with 71%. The True Positive (proportion of patients who were correctly predicted to not survive) was greatest for the 2 year at 65% and lowest for the 90 day model at 23%. The True Negative (proportion of patients who were correctly predicted to survive past the endpoint) was greatest for the 30 day model at nearly 100% and lowest for the 2 year model at 76%. The ROC % was greatest for the 30 day model at 93% and lowest for the 6 month, 1 year and 2 year models (all 71%).

30 Day Model

The 30-day mortality model consisted of 44 nodes and 93 arcs. There are four parent nodes for 30 day mortality: whether or not a patient completed the EuroQoL survey, a history of HIV, implant year, and left ventricular end diastolic dimension (LVEDD), an indicator of dilated cardiomyopathy. Positive HIV was the strongest predictive node, followed by the implant year. When a

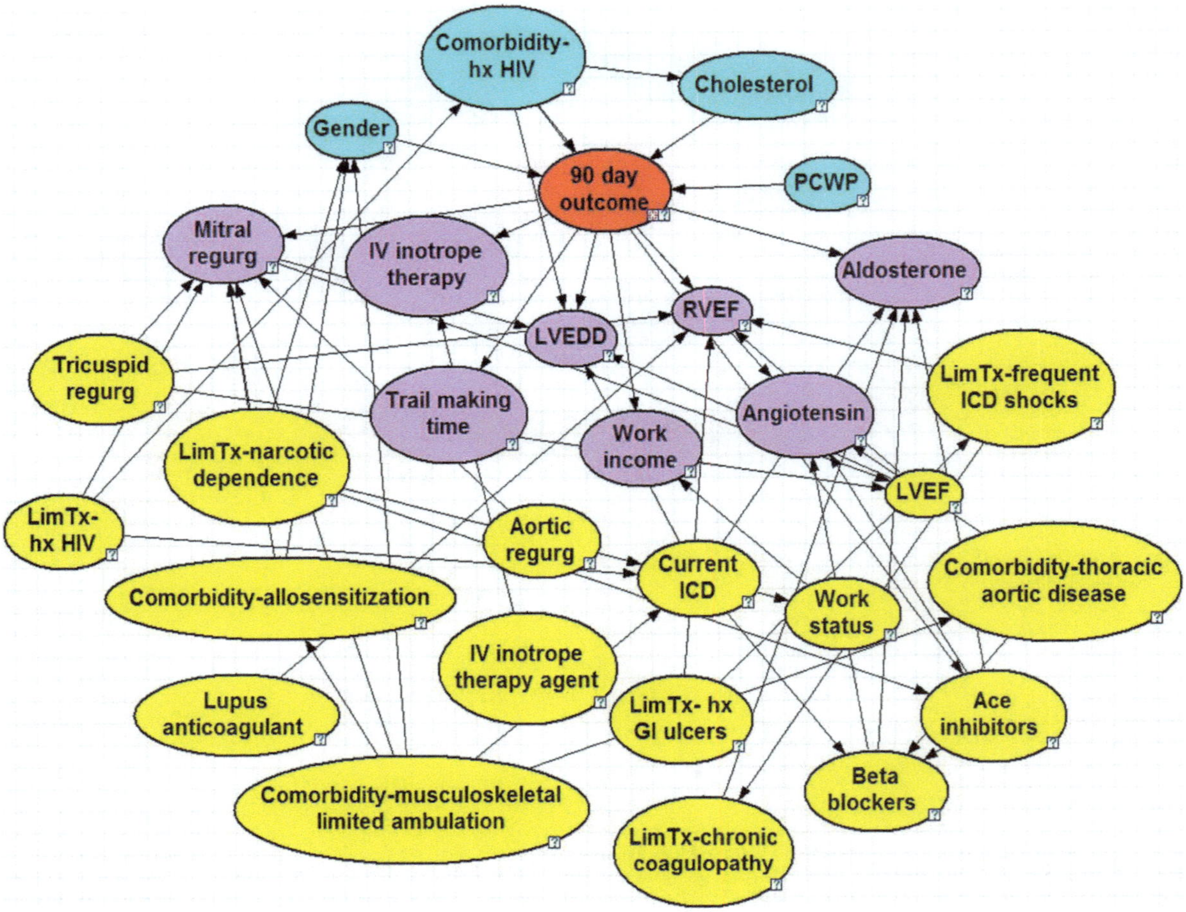

Figure 2. 90 Day Bayesian Model. Node colors: red = class, blue = parent, purple = child, yellow = spouse. Question marks identify nodes that do not have specific evidence set and use the population distribution as the prior distribution. LVEDD = left ventricle end diastolic diameter, PCWP = pulmonary capillary wedge pressure, RVEF = right ventricle ejection fraction, LVEF = left ventricle ejection fraction, hx HIV = history of human immunodeficiency virus, ICD = implantable cardioverter defibrillator, Lim tx = limitation for transplant listing, GI = gastrointestinal, IV = intravenous.

patient is indicated to have a history of HIV, then the baseline likelihood of survival drops from 95% (when no patient-specific evidence is specified) to 53% and drops further to 43% chance of survival when the LVEDD is above 75 mm. The children nodes includes a combination of laboratory values (sodium, BNP and platelets), hemodynamics (mean right arterial pressure, diastolic blood pressure and ECG rhythm), demographics (age and gender) and pre-implant medication (beta blockers, aldosterone and amiodarone). This model was the one exception to using the Markov Blanket, as it would approach nearly 150 nodes with the inclusion of the spousal nodes and would be more prone to over-fitting the dataset. For the model, we simply used the parents and children nodes, which put it at a comparable size as the other endpoint Bayesian models.

90 Day Model

The 90-day model consisted of 30 nodes and 56 arcs. There are four parent nodes: gender, co-morbidity of HIV, cholesterol and pulmonary capillary wedge pressure. History of HIV decreased 90-day chance of survival from 87% to 52% and, when combined with elevated cholesterol (above 150 mg/dL), further decreases to 47%. The chance of survival increases (as compared to the baseline) to 91% if a patient's cholesterol is below 110 mg/dL and they do not have HIV. The children nodes include variables such as mitral regurgitation, right ventricular ejection fraction and work income. Spouse nodes include tricuspid and aortic regurgitation, pre-implant beta blockers, pre-implant ace inhibitors, and left ventricular ejection fraction.

6 Month Model

The 6-month model consisted of 34 nodes and 70 arcs. There are five parent nodes: limitation for transplant due to thoracic aortic disease, creatinine, number of cardiac hospitalizations within the 12 months prior to LVAD implant, cholesterol and HIV. Compared to the baseline chance of survival at 6 months of 76%, the limitation for transplant reduces to 48%, and when combined with creatinine levels below 1.1 mg/dL further reduces to 37%. The children nodes include variables such as BMI, work income and angiotensin. Spouse nodes include presence of an implantable cardioverter defibrillator (ICD), admission reason before implant, history of gastrointestinal bleeding, limitation for transplant listing due to advanced age, and the INTERMACS profile (from level 1 critical cardiogenic shock to level 7 resting heart failure symptoms but stable).

1 Year Model

The 1-year model consisted of 39 nodes and 76 arcs. There are six parent nodes: co-morbidity of HIV, limitation for transplant

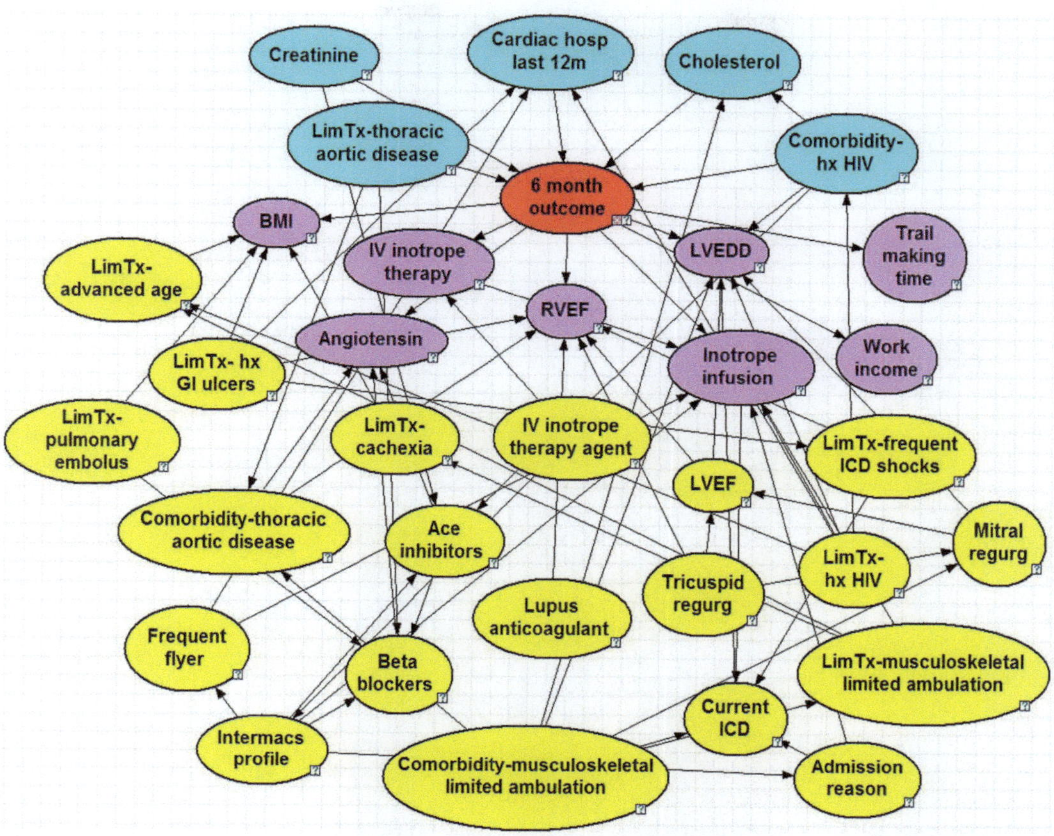

Figure 3. 6 Month Bayesian Model. Node colors: red = class, blue = parent, purple = child, yellow = spouse. Question marks identify nodes that do not have specific evidence set and use the population distribution as the prior distribution. LVEDD = left ventricle end diastolic diameter, RVEF = right ventricle ejection fraction, LVEF = left ventricle ejection fraction, hx HIV = history of human immunodeficiency virus, BMI = body mass index, ICD = implantable cardioverter defibrillator, Lim tx = limitation for transplant listing, GI = gastrointestinal, IV = intravenous.

listing due to thoracic aortic disease, gender, implant year, limitation for transplant listing due to pulmonary hypertension and cholesterol. The baseline chance of survival at 1 year post-implant is 75%, and more recent implants (2013) have higher chances of survival (86%) compared to implants done between 2008–2010 (64–66%). Although this is likely due to shorter follow up times for the more recent implants, it may also reflect advances in implant techniques and changes in the patient post-VAD management. Similar to the other models, both a history of HIV and thoracic aortic disease have major impacts on the chance of 1 year survival. The children nodes include age, right ventricular ejection fraction, BMI, ace inhibitors and diastolic blood pressure. Spouse nodes include admission reason, systolic blood pressure, the INTERMACS profile, temporary mechanical circulatory device, current ICD and co-morbidity due to cachexia (malnutrition).

2 Year Model

The model for 2-year mortality consisted of 45 nodes and 78 arcs. There are eight parent nodes: pro-BNP, BNP, co-morbidity of solid organ cancer, implant year, gender, limitation for transplant listing due to limited social support, patient refusal for transplant listing, and limitation for transplant listing due to large BMI. The baseline 2-year chance of survival is 69%, which increases by 5% if the patient's BNP levels are below 540 pg/dL and increases further to 84% if the implant was done more recently. The chance of survival falls below the baseline (to 62%) if BNP is elevated above 1200 pg/dL, drops further to 58% if the patient declines transplant listing and drops even further to 50% if the patient also has limited social support. The children nodes included age, trail making time (a neuro-psychological test of visual attention and task switching), co-morbidity due to a history of illicit drug use and blood type. Spousal nodes included limitation for transplant listing due to peripheral vascular disease, the INTERMACS profile, being a so-called *frequent flyer* (patients who are repeatedly in and out of the hospital emergency room), the IV inotrope therapy agent and age.

HMRS

The HMRS was derived and validated for 90-day and 1-year mortality and identifies patients as either low risk (4–8% mortality), medium risk (11–16% mortality) or high risk (25–29% mortality). When applied to the INTERMACS database, 93.1% of patients were predicted as low risk with a 9% morality rate, 4.4% were predicted as medium risk with a 16% mortality rate, and 2.3% were predicted as high risk with a 14.6% mortality rate. The ROC for the 90-day HMRS score was 60.3% compared to 73.9% for the 90-day CHRiSS model and the 1-year HMRS score 57.4% compred to 70.9% for the 1-year CHRiSS model.

Discussion

The decision to refer a patient for LVAD therapy entails processing numerous, dynamically evolving and inter-related

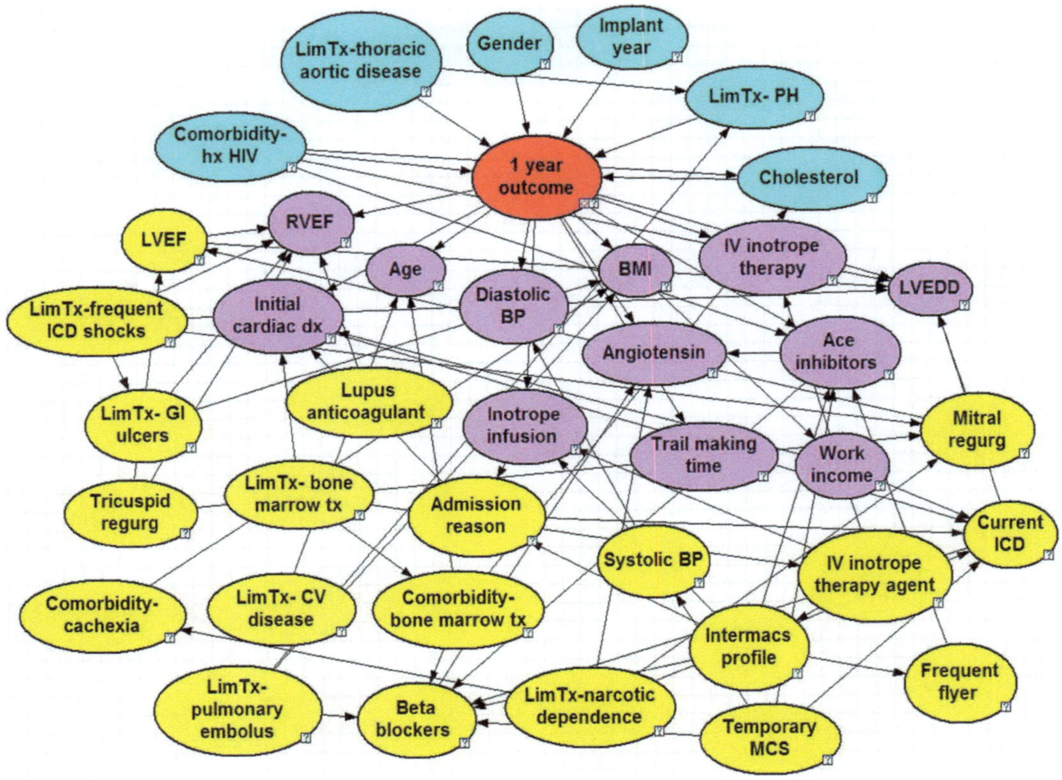

Figure 4. 1 Year Bayesian Model. Node colors: red = class, blue = parent, purple = child, yellow = spouse. Question marks identify nodes that do not have specific evidence set and use the population distribution as the prior distribution. LVEDD = left ventricle end diastolic diameter, RVEF = right ventricle ejection fraction, BMI = body mass index, lim tx PH = limitation for transplant listing due to pulmonary hypertension, IV = intravenous, ICD = implantable cardioverter defibrillator, CV = cardiovascular, GI = gastrointestinal, BP = blood pressure, hx HIV = history of human immunodeficiency virus, MCS = mechanical circulatory support.

clinical variables, which is a complex task filled with uncertainty. The trajectory by which a patient may be offered the option to receive a LVAD involves multiple specialties and decision points. The extensive volume of information and data that must be considered (demographics, labs, history, family support, insurance, etc.) is at odds with the rapidity with which some decisions must be made. Deferring a decision to implant an LVAD, may allow the severity of ESHF to progress thereby increasing the likelihood of an adverse event. Lietz and Miller describe an "optimal window" for LVAD implantation, beyond which the operative risk may deem the intervention futile. However, the key to successful and timely implementation of LVAD therapy is the proper identification of the patient who will benefit from this type of therapy: before clinical instability occurs, which has a major impact on the downstream morbidity and mortality with this intervention.

The advanced heart failure team must evaluate risk in terms of both immediate complications as well as likelihood of repeated readmissions due to longer-term complications. Hence there is a need for a CDSS to aid the physicians in pre-LVAD candidate assessment, by providing personalized risk predictions to ultimately encourage earlier intervention in the appropriate patients. We envision two steps (with iteration) when using CHRiSS: the clinician would first input the variables available for that patient and calculate their initial risk and then adjust actionable variables to perform the "what if" scenarios. For example, a clinician assessing a patient who is initially malnourished (has lower levels of albumin), could then adjust the albumin to the normal range and see if the prognosis improves and by how much.

Such a dynamic CDSS does not exist for advanced HF patients and the BNs offer several advantages over the traditional statistical methods used to derive risk scores such as the HMRS or DTRS. Current risk scores are limited by their: (1) simplistic four to nine variable summed scoring system; (2) inability to co-evolve with the changing HF risk factors and emerging treatment options; and (3) requirement to know a fixed set of variables and inability to be computed when any are missing. BNs address these limitations, as they are able to: (1) account for hundreds of inter-related variables in a single model; (2) dynamically update as risk factors change and different drugs are created; and (3) compute predictions with missing values by using the prior probabilities encoded within each variable node. The current study demonstrated the potential for developing advanced CDSS based on these models in the domain of HF, as well as other medical applications.

For example, in the absence of any decision tool, expert judgment resulted in the correct prognosis of survival at 1 year 79.7% (n = 5241 patients) of the time (true survival rate, see Table 1). This translates to 20.3% (n = 1334 patients) frequency of incorrect judgment of survival. (Presuming that the decision to implant an LVAD in these patients was predicated on positive 1-year survival prognosis.) With the added contribution of CHRiSS in decision-making, 85.3% (see True Negative in Table 2) of these 79.7% (actual survival from Table 1) would be corroborated by the prognostic model. Thereby denying an LVAD from 14.7% of these patients who would have survived, had the physician followed CHRiSS recommendation. On the other hand, the expert incorrectly predicted survival in 20.3% (n = 1334, mortality

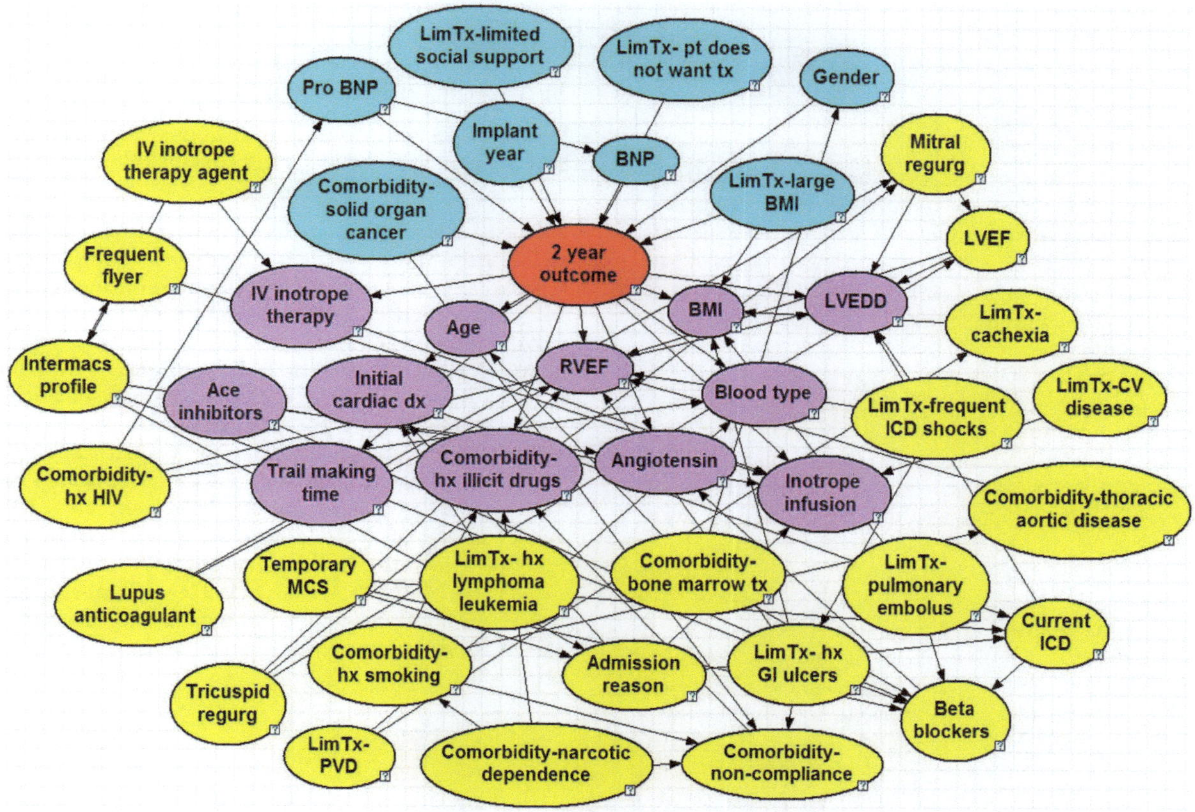

Figure 5. 2 Year Bayesian Model. Node colors: red = class, blue = parent, purple = child, yellow = spouse. Question marks identify nodes that do not have specific evidence set and use the population distribution as the prior distribution. LVEDD = left ventricle end diastolic diameter, BNP = B-type natriuretic peptide, LVEF = left ventricle ejection fraction, GI = gastrointestinal, IV = intravenous, ICD = implantable cardioverter defibrillator, PVD = peripheral vascular disease, hx HIV = history of human immunodeficiency virus, BMI = body mass index, MCS = mechanical circulatory support, CV = cardiovascular.

% from Table 1). CHRiSS would have predicted almost half of these patients, hence sparing 667 patients from a suboptimal outcome. Although there is no way of knowing, retrospectively, how long these LVAD patients would have survived if they did not receive a LVAD, the additional insight provided by CHRiSS would assist the patient and physician in weighing the risks and benefits of the various courses of treatment. For example, these patients may be prioritized for cardiac transplantation, thereby making better use of limited organ supply for those who would not otherwise survive on a LVAD (in exchange for a transplant patient who would have done just as well on a LVAD.)

The 2-year CHRiSS model correctly identified 65% of patients who would not survive past the endpoint, which would be very important to know for DT patients to decide if they wish to accept this risk considering chance of surviving (and thriving) for many years with this end of life treatment. Following the same logic for predicting short-term outcomes, CHRiSS would spare half of the 387 patients from undergoing a major surgery who would do very poorly during the recovery post-implant. The 30-day model could aid in vetting potential high risk DT and bridge to transplant (BTT) candidates. Paradoxically, the performance of the 90-day and 6-month models were not as good as the 30-day, 1-year, and 2-year models. This may be attributable to the heterogeneity in causes of death, which may confound the Bayesian Network to identify specific predictive variables.

Table 2. Summary of Bayesian Model Performance.

Endpoint	Accuracy (%)	True Positive (Dead) (%)	True Negative (Alive) (%)	ROC (%)
30 Day	94.9	51.0	99.4	92.5
90 Day	84.2	22.9	97.1	73.9
6 Month	78.2	30.3	93.7	70.6
1 Year	73.1	49.1	85.3	70.6
2 Year	71.4	65.0	76.2	70.8

ROC = receiver operating characteristic curve.

We had also conducted a sensitivity analysis to observe the direct effects of each variable on the outcome, as well as the additive effects of several variables. The variables that created the greatest effect on the outcome were presented in the results section for each model. For the short-term outcome, positive HIV increased likelihood of mortality by 42% at 30-days and 35% at 90-days. Each of these percentages were further increase by 5–10% when adding an enlarged LVEDD (dilated cardiomyopathy) or elevated cholesterol, respectively. When considering long-term predictors (2-year model), one of the parent nodes was BNP, which had bi-modal effects: normal levels lead to reduced chance of mortality by 5% and elevated levels increased mortality by 7%.

The use and acceptance of Bayesian methodology are becoming increasingly prevalent in the medical community (see, for example [34–42]). For example, in 2010, the FDA released a guidance for the use of Bayesian statistics in medical device clinical trials [43]. In 2013, the United Network for Organ Sharing (UNOS) proposed the adoption of a new Bayesian methodology to better identify those transplant programs that may be underperforming in the area of patient and graft survival.

Although the methods described in this study are more advanced than the current risk scores used in HF prognosis, the results are far from perfect. There are several limitations that may adversely affect performance, including inherent retrospective bias, imbalance of the outcome variable, and extensive missing data. We aim to address these limitations in our ongoing prospective studies. It is also important to clarify that the CHRiSS models are able to discern likelihood of mortality for patients receiving an LVAD and does not allude to any predictions for patients not receiving the device. We plan to perform a follow up study that will derive BN models based on both INTERMACS data, as well as a HF cohort for those who do not receive an LVAD. Nevertheless, the current models are able to provide decision support to the HF clinicians regarding potential future LVAD recipients.

This study was the first application of the Bayesian Network algorithm to a cohort of LVAD recipients. Although the current models outperform the current LVAD risk scores, there is an opportunity to improve them yet further as additional prospective data is collected, and additional risk factors are added to the model. Most certainly, the Bayesian models better represent the complex inter-variable relationships between clinical variables, better emulating human logic, which in turn makes them more appealing to end users.

Supporting Information

Figure S1 A simple Bayesian network model modeling risk factors related to LVAD survival.

Table S1 Many = not all format options listed, DT = destination therapy, BTT = bridge to transplant, BTR = bridge to recovery, CPB = cardiopulmonary bypass, MI = myocardial infarction, ECMO = extracorporeal membrane oxygenator, CABG = coronary artery bypass graft, IABP = intra-aortic balloon pump, INR = international normalized ratio, ICD = implantable cardioverter defibrillator, BNP = B-type natriuretic peptide, WBC = white blood cell, ALT = alanine transaminase, AST = aspartate aminotransferase, CRP = C-Reactive Protein, LVEF = left ventricle ejection fraction, LVEDD = left ventricle end diastolic diameter, RVEF = right ventricle ejection fraction, PCWP = pulmonary capillary wedge pressure, NYHA = New York Heart Association functional class, HF = heart failure, GI = gastrointestinal, HIV = human immunodeficiency virus.

Acknowledgments

We would like to thank Dr. Manreet Kanwar, Dr. Srinivas Murali and Dr. Raymond Benza at Allegheny General Hospital for their clinical insight and expertise. We thank Dr. James Kirklin, Dr. Francis Pagani and Dr. David Naftel of INTERMACS for allowing us to use their registry for the study. We would lastly like to thank Susan Meyers and Grant Studdard for their administrative, database, and statistical assistance with INTERMACS. Models described in this paper have been constructed using GeNIe, a modeling environment for graphical probabilistic models available at http://genie.sis.pitt.edu/.

Author Contributions

Conceived and designed the experiments: NAL JFA MJD. Performed the experiments: NAL. Analyzed the data: NAL. Contributed reagents/materials/analysis tools: MJD. Wrote the paper: NAL JFA. Created the software used in analysis: MJD. Provided technical insight: MJD. Provided funding: JFA.

References

1. Lietz K, Miller LW (2008) Destination therapy: current results and future promise. In: Seminars in thoracic and cardiovascular surgery. Elsevier, volume 20, pp. 225–233.
2. Miller LW (2011) Left ventricular assist devices are underutilized. Circulation 123: 1552–1558.
3. Stewart GC, Stevenson LW, Miller LW (2011) Keeping left ventricular assist device acceleration on track. Circulation 123: 1559–1568.
4. Peura JL, Colvin-Adams M, Francis GS, Grady KL, Hoffman TM, et al. (2012) Recommendations for the use of mechanical circulatory support: Device strategies and patient selection a scientific statement from the american heart association. Circulation 126: 2648–2667.
5. Lietz K, Long JW, Kfoury AG, Slaughter MS, Silver MA, et al. (2007) Outcomes of left ventricular assist device implantation as destination therapy in the post-rematch era implications for patient selection. Circulation 116: 497–505.
6. Rose EA, Moskowitz AJ, Packer M, Sollano JA, Williams DL, et al. (1999) The rematch trial: rationale, design, and end points. The Annals of thoracic surgery 67: 723–730.
7. Teuteberg JJ, Ewald GA, Adamson RM, Lietz K, Miller LW, et al. (2012) Risk assessment for continuous flow left ventricular assist devices: does the destination therapy risk score work? an analysis of over 1,000 patients. Journal of the American College of Cardiology 60: 44–51.
8. Cowger J, Sundareswaran K, Rogers JG, Park SJ, Pagani FD, et al. (2013) Predicting survival in patients receiving continuous flow left ventricular assist devicesthe heartmate ii risk score. Journal of the American College of Cardiology 61: 313–321.
9. Brahnam S, Jain LC (2011) Intelligent Decision Support Systems in Healthcare. Springer.
10. Musen MA, Middleton B, Greenes RA (2014) Clinical decision-support systems. In: Biomedical informatics, Springer. pp. 643–674.
11. Berry DA (2006) Bayesian clinical trials. Nature Reviews Drug Discovery 5: 27–36.
12. Ibrahim JG, Chen MH, Sinha D (2005) Bayesian survival analysis. Wiley Online Library.
13. Kratz A, Ferraro M, Sluss PM, Lewandrowski KB (2004) Laboratory reference values. New England Journal of Medicine 351: 1548–1564.
14. Parameters NH (2009) Laboratory values. Edwards Lifesciences website: www edwards com.
15. Lin JH, Haug PJ (2008) Exploiting missing clinical data in bayesian network modeling for predicting medical problems. Journal of biomedical informatics 41: 1–14.
16. Oniœko A, Druzdzel MJ, Wasyluk H (2002) An experimental comparison of methods for handling incomplete data in learning parameters of bayesian networks. In: Intelligent Information Systems 2002, Springer. pp. 351–360.
17. EuroQol G (1990) Euroqol–a new facility for the measurement of health-related quality of life. Health policy (Amsterdam, Netherlands) 16: 199.
18. Faller H, Steinbüchel T, Schowalter M, Spertus JA, Störk S, et al. (2004) [the kansas city cardiomyopathy questionnaire (kccq)–a new disease-specific quality

of life measure for patients with chronic heart failure]. Psychotherapie, Psychosomatik, medizinische Psychologie 55: 200–208.
19. Chawla NV, Bowyer KW, Hall LO, Kegelmeyer WP (2011) Smote: synthetic minority over-sampling technique. arXiv preprint arXiv:11061813.
20. Santelices LC, Wang Y, Severyn D, Druzdzel MJ, Kormos RL, et al. (2010) Development of a hybrid decision support model for optimal ventricular assist device weaning. The Annals of thoracic surgery 90: 713–720.
21. Wang Y, Simon MA, Bonde P, Harris BU, Teuteberg JJ, et al. (2012) Decision tree for adjuvant right ventricular support in patients receiving a left ventricular assist device. The Journal of Heart and Lung Transplantation 31: 140–149.
22. Wang Y, Simon M, Bonde P, Harris BU, Teuteberg JJ, et al. (2012) Prognosis of right ventricular failure in patients with left ventricular assist device based on decision tree with smote. Information Technology in Biomedicine, IEEE Transactions on 16: 383–390.
23. Wang Y, Rosé CP, Ferreira A, McNamara DM, Kormos RL, et al. (2010) A classification approach for risk prognosis of patients on mechanical ventricular assistance. In: Machine Learning and Applications (ICMLA), 2010 Ninth International Conference on. IEEE, pp. 293–298.
24. Loghmanpour N, Kanwar M, Wang Y, Snyder T, Horstmanshof D, et al. (2013) A novel, risk stratification model using bayesian networks for continuous flow left ventricular assist device 90-day survival. The Journal of Heart and Lung Transplantation 32: S232.
25. Kanwar M, Loghmanpour N, Wang Y, Snyder T, Horstmanshof D, et al. (2013) A novel, risk stratification model using bayesian networks for continuous-flow left ventricular assist device 90-day survival. Journal of the American College of Cardiology 61.
26. Pearl J (1988) Probabilistic reasoning in intelligent systems: networks of plausible inference. Morgan Kaufmann.
27. Oniœko A, Druzdzel MJ (2013) Impact of precision of bayesian network parameters on accuracy of medical diagnostic systems. Artificial intelligence in medicine 57: 197–206.
28. Oniœko ADM (2014) Impact of bayesian network model structure on the accuracy of medical diagnostic systems. 13th International Conference on Artificial Intelligence and Soft Computing (ICAISC-2014).
29. Heckerman D (1998) A tutorial on learning with Bayesian networks. Springer.
30. Cooper GF, Herskovits E (1991) A bayesian method for constructing bayesian belief networks from databases. In: Proceedings of the Seventh conference on Uncertainty in Artificial Intelligence. Morgan Kaufmann Publishers Inc., pp. 86–94.
31. Koller D, Sahami M (1996) Toward optimal feature selection.
32. Druzdzel MJ (1999) Genie: A development environment for graphical decision-analytic models. In: Proceedings of the AMIA Symposium. American Medical Informatics Association, p. 1206.
33. Witten IH, Frank E (2005) Data Mining: Practical machine learning tools and techniques. Morgan Kaufmann.
34. Hoot N, Aronsky D (2005) Using bayesian networks to predict survival of liver transplant patients. In: AMIA annual symposium proceedings. American Medical Informatics Association, volume 2005, p. 345.
35. Lucas P (2001) Bayesian networks in medicine: a model-based approach to medical decision making. In: Proceedings of the EUNITE workshop on Intelligent Systems in patient Care. pp. 73–97.
36. Eom JH, Kim SC, Zhang BT (2008) Aptacdss-e: A classifier ensemble-based clinical decision support system for cardiovascular disease level prediction. Expert Systems with Applications 34: 2465–2479.
37. Sadeghi S, Barzi A, Sadeghi N, King B (2006) A bayesian model for triage decision support. International Journal of Medical Informatics 75: 403–411.
38. Gevaert O, De Smet F, Timmerman D, Moreau Y, De Moor B (2006) Predicting the prognosis of breast cancer by integrating clinical and microarray data with bayesian networks. Bioinformatics 22: e184–e190.
39. Charitos T, Van Der Gaag LC, Visscher S, Schurink KA, Lucas PJ (2009) A dynamic bayesian network for diagnosing ventilator-associated pneumonia in icu patients. Expert Systems with Applications 36: 1249–1258.
40. Austin RM, Onisko A, Druzdzel MJ (2010) The pittsburgh cervical cancer screening model: a risk assessment tool. Archives of pathology & laboratory medicine 134: 744–750.
41. Cao C, Leong TY, Leong AP, Seow FC (1998) Dynamic decision analysis in medicine: a data-driven approach. International journal of medical informatics 51: 13–28.
42. Diez FJ, Mira J, Iturralde E, Zubillaga S (1997) Diaval, a bayesian expert system for echocardiography. Artificial Intelligence in Medicine 10: 59–73.
43. FDA (2010). Guidance for the use of bayesian statistics in medical device clinical trials.

Aerobic Exercise Training Prevents Heart Failure-Induced Skeletal Muscle Atrophy by Anti-Catabolic, but Not Anabolic Actions

Rodrigo W. A. Souza[1], Warlen P. Piedade[1], Luana C. Soares[1], Paula A. T. Souza[1], Andreo F. Aguiar[4], Ivan J. Vechetti-Júnior[1], Dijon H. S. Campos[2], Ana A. H. Fernandes[3], Katashi Okoshi[2], Robson F. Carvalho[1], Antonio C. Cicogna[3], Maeli Dal-Pai-Silva[1]*

1 Department of Morphology, São Paulo State University, Botucatu, São Paulo, Brazil, **2** Department of Internal Medicine, São Paulo State University, Botucatu, São Paulo, Brazil, **3** Department of Biochemistry, São Paulo State University, Botucatu, São Paulo, Brazil, **4** Centre of Biological and Health Sciences, North University of Paraná, Londrina, Paraná, Brazil

Abstract

Background: Heart failure (HF) is associated with cachexia and consequent exercise intolerance. Given the beneficial effects of aerobic exercise training (ET) in HF, the aim of this study was to determine if the ET performed during the transition from cardiac dysfunction to HF would alter the expression of anabolic and catabolic factors, thus preventing skeletal muscle wasting.

Methods and Results: We employed ascending aortic stenosis (AS) inducing HF in Wistar male rats. Controls were sham-operated animals. At 18 weeks after surgery, rats with cardiac dysfunction were randomized to 10 weeks of aerobic ET (AS-ET) or to an untrained group (AS-UN). At 28 weeks, the AS-UN group presented HF signs in conjunction with high TNF-α serum levels; soleus and plantaris muscle atrophy; and an increase in the expression of TNF-α, NFκB (p65), MAFbx, MuRF1, FoxO1, and myostatin catabolic factors. However, in the AS-ET group, the deterioration of cardiac function was prevented, as well as muscle wasting, and the atrophy promoters were decreased. Interestingly, changes in anabolic factor expression (IGF-I, AKT, and mTOR) were not observed. Nevertheless, in the plantaris muscle, ET maintained high PGC1α levels.

Conclusions: Thus, the ET capability to attenuate cardiac function during the transition from cardiac dysfunction to HF was accompanied by a prevention of skeletal muscle atrophy that did not occur via an increase in anabolic factors, but through anti-catabolic activity, presumably caused by PGC1α action. These findings indicate the therapeutic potential of aerobic ET to block HF-induced muscle atrophy by counteracting the increased catabolic state.

Editor: Junichi Sadoshima, Rutgers New Jersey Medical School, United States of America

Funding: This study was supported by the São Paulo Research Foundation, Brazil, (FAPESP 2010/50332-1 and 2010/10583-5) and the National Council for Scientific and Technological Development, Brazil (CNPq 141120/2010-0). The funders had no role in study design, data collection and analysis, decision to publish, or preparation of the manuscript.

Competing Interests: The authors have declared that no competing interests exist.

* Email: maeli@ibb.unesp.br

Introduction

Cardiac dysfunction precedes heart failure (HF) and is typically characterized by enlargement of the heart and increased myocyte cell volume [1]. Pathological hypertrophy of the myocardium temporarily preserves its pump function, although prolongation of this state is a leading predictor of HF [1]. HF is the main cause of hospitalization and death worldwide. In the terminal phase of HF, a complex metabolic syndrome called cardiac cachexia, which is characterized by a loss of muscle and fat mass that is unresponsive to nutritional supplementation alone and which has been identified as a strong independent risk factor for mortality, is often observed [2]. However, the process leading to the progressive muscle atrophy that ultimately results in cardiac cachexia is still not completely understood.

Skeletal muscle atrophy is related to endocrine disorders and inflammatory conditions that can induce hypertrophy and atrophy-related gene/protein expression. Considerable evidence suggests that neurohormonal and immune mechanisms may play a central role in the pathogenesis of HF by controlling the balance between pro- and anti-growth signals in the skeletal muscle. Several factors have been demonstrated to be responsible for muscle wasting during HF, including reduced local insulin-like growth factor I (IGF-I) expression [3], increased muscular tumor necrosis factor alpha (TNF-α) [4], increased myostatin expression [5], and overexpression of the E3-ligases Muscle RING Finger 1 (MuRF-1) and atrogin-1/Muscle Atrophy F-Box (MAFbx), which activate the ubiquitin–proteasome system [6]. However, a direct effect of humoral factors on muscle-mass regulators during HF has not been well established.

In HF, alterations in multiple anabolic and catabolic systems result in progressive catabolism, which leads to skeletal muscle atrophy in advanced stages of the disease [7,8]. IGF-I/AKT/mTOR is an essential regulator of skeletal muscle capacity for protein synthesis and degradation [9]. In the canonical IGF-I/AKT/mTOR pathway, AKT activation of mTOR and the subsequent phosphorylation of p70S6K and 4E-BP1 induce protein synthesis. In the early stages, chronic HF-related muscle atrophy is associated with reduced expression of IGF-I [10]. In addition to protein synthesis, the IGF-I pathway inhibits protein degradation through the sequestration of the forkhead box O (FoxO) family of transcription factors in the cytoplasm, where they are transcriptionally inactive [11]. In skeletal muscle, FoxO1 and 3 activation have been observed under conditions of muscle atrophy, such as cachexia [12] and HF [13], thereby promoting the transcription of atrophy-related genes. However, FoxO-induced muscle atrophy activity is also modulated by other intracellular signaling molecules, such as peroxisome proliferator-activated receptor-γ coactivator-1α (PGC1α), a regulator of skeletal muscle mass, particularly in conditions of muscle atrophy [14]. Significant evidence has demonstrated that increased PGC1α expression is sufficient to inhibit *in vivo* FoxO3-induced muscle fiber atrophy and that transgenic muscle-specific PGC1α overexpression protects against denervation- and fasting-induced atrophy, an effect associated with a reduction of the expression of MAFbx, MuRF1, and cathepsin L [14].

Exercise training (ET) is a widely accepted and widely proposed nonpharmacological intervention to minimize the symptoms of HF [15]. In humans, ET has been shown to directly improve metabolic and functional abnormalities of the peripheral muscles without changing cardiac performance [16]. In addition, ET has anti-inflammatory effects, with the potential to reduce local cytokine expression (e.g., TNF-α, IL-1β, and IL-6) [4] and increase the expression of anti-apoptotic factors (e.g., myostatin) [17], indicating that this type of intervention could partially reverse the catabolic state in skeletal muscle.

While the potential beneficial effects of ET on the loss of muscle mass in HF are clear, the exact molecular mechanisms by which ET might delay the onset of cardiac cachexia in the HF remain unclear. Therefore, the aim of the present study was to examine the effects of ET during the transition from cardiac dysfunction to HF on the expression of muscle mass-related anabolic and catabolic factors. We hypothesized that ET would increase anabolic factor expression and decrease catabolic factor expression, thus preventing muscle wasting during the transition from cardiac dysfunction to HF.

Materials and Methods

Animal Care and Experimental Design

All experiments and procedures were performed in accordance with the Guide for the Care and Use of Laboratory Animals published by the U.S. National Institute of Health and were approved by the Animal Ethics Committee, São Paulo State University (#198). Three- to four-week-old male Wistar rats weighing 90–100 g were anesthetized with a mixture of ketamine (50 mg/kg, i.p.) and xylazine (10 mg/kg, i.p.). A total of 16 rats was submitted to aortic stenosis (AS) surgery, which involved placing a 0.6-mm-i.d. stainless steel clip on the ascending aorta via a thoracic incision [1]. A total of 16 age-matched control animals underwent left thoracotomy without clip placement (Sham group). The rats were housed in collective polypropylene cages (2 animals per cage) covered with metallic grids in a temperature-controlled room (22–24°C) under a reverse light cycle (the dark cycle began at 7:00 a.m., and the light cycle began at 7:00 p.m.). The animals were given standard rat chow (Labina; Purina, SP, Brazil) and water *ad libitum*.

At 18 weeks after surgery, when the AS animals presented a cardiac dysfunction as measured by echocardiography, both groups (Sham and AS) were randomly redistributed in either sedentary untrained groups (Sham-UN, n = 8, and AS-UN, n = 8) and groups that underwent to 10 weeks of aerobic ET protocol (Sham-ET, n = 8, and AS-ET, n = 8). The ET protocol is described in detail below. Our laboratory has previously demonstrated that rats with AS start to exhibit evidence of HF approximately 21–25 weeks after surgery [18,19]. Thus, after 28 weeks, all 4 groups underwent another echocardiogram and were then euthanized. The experimental design is shown in Figure 1. At the time of euthanasia, the rats were weighed and anesthetized with intraperitoneal pentobarbital sodium (50 mg/kg). The heart was removed via thoracotomy, and the atria and ventricles were separated and weighed. The soleus and plantaris muscles, which were chosen because of their contrasting structural and metabolic characteristics (i.e., fiber type distribution and prevalent metabolism), were harvested, rapidly frozen in isopentane cooled by liquid nitrogen, and subsequently stored at −80°C. For the HF examination, 2 observers determined the presence or absence of clinical and pathological HF features at the time of euthanasia. The clinical finding suggestive of HF was tachypnea and labored respiration. The pathological assessment of cardiac decompensation included left atrial thrombi, pulmonary congestion (lung weight/body weight ratio>2 SD above the mean for the Sham-UN group), right ventricular hypertrophy, ascites, and hepatic congestion [20]. In this study, rats with atrial thrombi, pulmonary congestion, and/or right ventricular hypertrophy were considered to have HF [21].

Lactate Threshold Determination

To determine their lactate threshold and the velocity at which the lactate threshold occurred, the animals allocated into the exercise training study were subjected to incremental exercise testing on a motor treadmill adapted to experimental models [22]. The lactate threshold was defined as the running velocity that could be maintained without a lactate increase of 1.0 mmol/L above the blood lactate concentration obtained at the previous speed [23]. The protocol used for the incremental load test was adapted from that previously described by Carvalho et al. [24] and was performed at the end of Week 1 (week of adaptation), Week 4, and Week 7.

After a 1-week (10 min/day) adaption to the treadmill exercises, the rats were submitted to exercise testing. The treadmill speed started at 6 m/min and was progressively increased by 3 m/min every 3 min at 0% grade until exhaustion, which was defined as the point at which the rats could no longer maintain a running speed over 3 min. After each load increase, the animal was manually removed from the treadmill for 1 min for blood collection. Blood samples were taken from the tail vein and was pipetted evenly onto a test strip, which was inserted into a portable lactate analyzer (Accutrend Lactate, Boehringer-Mannheim) [25,26]. The equipment was calibrated with a code strip specific to each lactate determination package.

Aerobic Exercise Training

Rats in the training groups, Sham-ET and AS-ET, performed an aerobic ET program for 10 weeks (5 days/week). The program

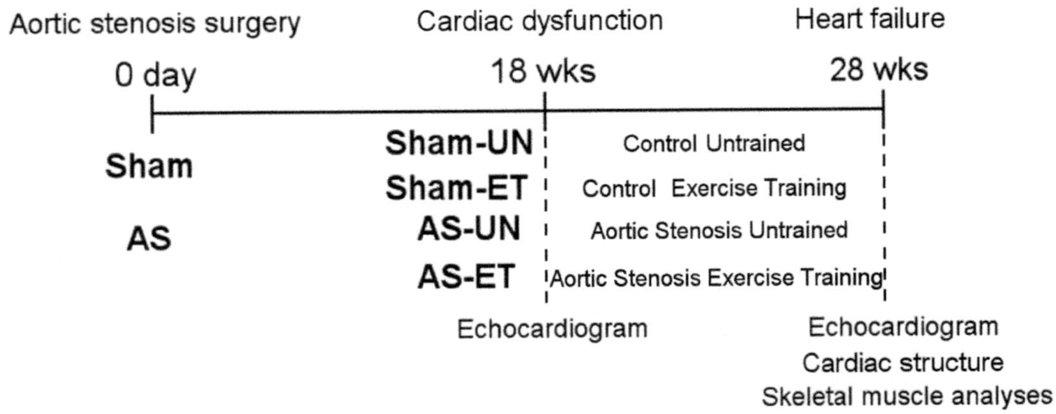

Figure 1. Experimental design. Sham, control group; AS, animals submitted to aortic stenosis surgery; Sham-UN, control untrained group; Sham-ET, control exercise training group; AS-UN, aortic stenosis untrained group; AS-ET, aortic stenosis exercise training group.

was modified from those previously described by De Souza et al. [27] and Siu et al. [28]. The duration and intensity of the training sessions progressively increased from 5 min, 5 m/min (Sham-ET and AS-ET, 1st week) to 10, 12, and 14 min, 9 m/min (Sham-ET) and 6 m/min (AS-ET, 2nd to 4th week); 16, 18 and 20 min, 18 m/min (Sham-ET) and 12 m/min (AS-ET, 5th to 7th week); 20, 22 and 22 min, 21 m/min (Sham-ET) and 15 m/min (AS-ET, 8th to 10th week). The running speed corresponded to the lactate threshold, which was determined by the incremental exercise test (described above) performed at the end of Weeks 1, 4, and 7 to adjust the training velocities. The training sessions were performed at the same time of day, between 2 and 4 p.m.

Echocardiographic Study

Echocardiographic measurements were performed before and after aerobic ET using a commercially available echocardiograph (General Electric Medical Systems, Vivid S6, Tirat Carmel, Israel) equipped with a 5–11.5 MHz multifrequency transducer. Rats were anesthetized by intramuscular injection of a mixture of ketamine (50 mg/kg) and xylazine (0.5 mg/kg) and positioned in supine position and ultrasound transmission gel was applied to the precordium. A two-dimensional parasternal short-axis view of the left ventricle (LV) was obtained at the level of the papillary muscles. M-mode tracings were obtained from short-axis views of the LV at or just below the tip of the mitral-valve leaflets, and at the level of the aortic valve and left atrium. All LV structures were manually measured by the same observer according to the leading-edge method of the American College of Echocardiography [29]. The measurements obtained were the mean of at least five cardiac cycles on the M-mode tracings. The following structural variables were measured: left atrium (LA) diameter, LV diastolic and systolic dimensions (LVDD and LVSD, respectively), LV diastolic posterior wall thickness (PWT), LV relative thickness in diastole (RWT; calculated as 2*PWT/LVDD), and aortic diameter (AO). Left ventricular function was assessed by the following parameters: heart rate (HR), endocardial fractional shortening (FS), LV ejection fraction (EF), posterior wall shortening velocity (PWSV), and early-to-late diastolic mitral inflow ratio (E/A ratio).

Muscles and Histochemical Procedures

Serial histological sections (12 μm thick) from soleus and plantaris muscles were obtained in a cryostat (JUNG CM1800, Leica Germany) at −24°C to histochemical analysis. To determine muscle fiber-type frequency and cross sectional area (CSA) myofibrillar adenosine triphosphatase (mATPase) histochemistry was performed after preincubation at pH 4.2, 4.5 and 10.6 [30]. Muscle fibers (Type I, IIA, IID, and IIB) were identified based on their staining intensities [31] (Figure 2). The stained sections were used for photographic documentation of 4 histological fields (400 random fibers; 20×lens) from soleus and plantaris muscles of each animal. Fiber type frequency and CSA (used as an index of type-specific fiber atrophy) were analyzed using an Image Analysis System Software (Leica QWin Plus, Germany).

Serum TNF-α and IGF-I Levels

TNF-α and IGF-I levels were analyzed by enzyme-immunometric using a commercially available kits (Quantikine Rat TNF-α Immunoassay, and Quantikine Mouse/Rat IGF-I Immunoassay, R & D Systems, Minneapolis, MN) and the procedures were performed according to manufacturer's instructions. All the samples were run in duplicate and the average values are reported.

Biochemical Assay Procedures

Soleus and plantaris muscle samples (200 mg) were homogenized in 5 ml cold phosphate buffer (0.1 mmol/L, pH 7.4) using a motor-driven Teflon glass Potter-Elvehjem (1 min, 100×g). The whole homogenate was centrifuged at 10,000×g for 15 min, and the supernatant was used for determination of lactate dehydrogenase (LDH; E.C.1.1.1.27) and citrate synthase (CS; E.C.4.1.3.7). CS was measured in a medium containing 50 mmol/L Tris-HCl pH 8.1, 0.3 mmol/L acetyl-CoA, 0.1 mmol/L DTNB (5,5′ dithiobia-2-nitrobenzoic acid), and 0.5 mmol/L oxaloacetate, according to Bass and colleagues [32]. The assay medium for LDH contained 50.0 mmol/L Tris-HCl buffer pH 7.5, 0.15 mmol/L nicotinamide adenine dinucleotide reduced form (NADH), and 1 mmol/L pyruvate, as previously described [33]. Enzyme activities were performed at 25°C using a microplate reader (μQuant-MQX 200 with Kcjunior software to computer system control, Bio-Tec Instruments, Winooski, Vermont, USA). All chemicals and solvents were from Sigma (St. Louis, Missouri, USA).

Quantitative Real-time PCR

Total RNA was extracted from soleus and plantaris muscles using Trizol Reagent (Life Technologies, CA, USA), solubilized in nuclease-free water and quantified (NanoVue Plus; GE HealthCare, Little Chalfont, UK). After assessment of RNA concentration (ng/μl), purity (ensured by 260/280 nm ratio of ~2.0) and

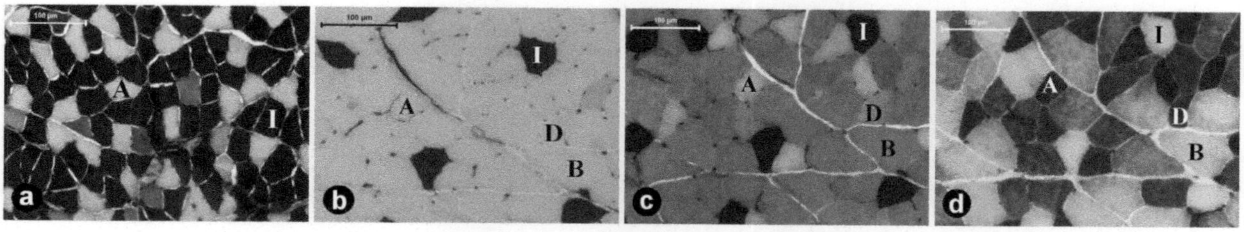

Figure 2. Serial cross sections of the rat hindlimb muscles. Soleus (a) and plantaris (b, c and d) muscles taken from a Sham-UN group rat demonstrating fiber-type delineation as determined by the myofibrillar adenosine triphosphatase (mATPase) reaction after preincubation at pH 4.2 (b), 4.5 (a, c), and 10.6 (d). (I, type I; A, type IIA; D, type IID; and B, type IIB).

integrity (RNA integrity number >8; RNA 6000 Nano assay; Agilent, Waldbronn, Germany), the RNA was treated with Amplification Grade Deoxyribonuclease I (Life Technologies, Carlsbad, CA, USA) to remove any genomic DNA contamination. cDNA was synthesized using High Capacity cDNA Reverse Transcription Kit (Life Technologies, Carlsbad, CA, USA) according to the manufacturer's protocols, and the genes involved in atrophic system, as TNF-α (Rn00562055_m1), NFκB (Rn01502266_m1), MAFbx (Rn00591730_m1), MuRF1 (Rn00590197_m1), FoxO1 (Rn01494868_m1) and myostatin (Rn00569683_m1); hypertrophic system IGF-I (Rn00710306_m1), AKT1 (Rn00583646_m1) and mTOR (Rn00571541_m1) and anti-proteolytic PGC1α (Rn00580241_m1) were analyzed. All genes were measured by real-time quantitative PCR (RT-qPCR) using microfluidic TaqMan Low Density Array (TLDA; Life Technologies, Carlsbad, CA, USA) cards. Five control genes were tested 18S rRNA (Hs99999901_s1), Actb (Rn00667869_m1), Gapdh (Rn01775763_g1), Hprt1 (Rn01527840_m1) and Tbp (Rn01455648_m1) and Hprt1, Actb and Tbp were used as reference genes to normalize the data as they recorded the highest stability. A total of 100 μl reaction mixture with 50 μl of cDNA template (200 ng mRNA) was added to 50 μl of TaqMan Universal PCR Master Mix (Applied Biosystems, Foster City, CA, USA) and was dispensed into loading wells on the TLDA card. The cards were centrifuged twice at 1,200 rpm for 1 min each time, sealed, and placed in the thermal cycler. The following cycling conditions were used for all TLDA applications: 50°C for 2 min, 95°C for 10 min, and 40 cycles of 95°C for 15 s followed by 60°C for 1 min and thermal cycling and fluorescence detection was performed on Applied Biosystems ABI Prism ViiA7 Sequence Detection System with ABI Prism ViiA7 SDS Software 2.4. TLDAs data were analyzed using the DataAssist software 2.0 (Life Technologies).

Western blot

Protein levels of TNF-α, NFκB (p65), MAFbx, MuRF1, FoxO1, Phospho-FoxO1 (Ser^{256}), myostatin, IGF-I, AKT, Phospho-AKT (Ser^{473}), mTOR, Phospho-mTOR (Ser^{2448}), PGC1α and Gapdh were quantified by Western blot assays in soleus and plantaris muscle extracts. Muscle samples were homogenised in lysis buffer (1% Triton X-100, 10 mM sodium pyrophosphate, 100 mM NaF, 10 μg/mL aprotinin, 1 mM phenylmethylsulfonylfluoride (PMSF), 0.25 mM Na_3VO_4, 150 mM NaCl and 50 mM Tris-HCl pH 7.5). The samples were centrifuged and 50 μL of the homogenate fraction were resuspended in 25 μL of Laemmli loading buffer (2% SDS, 20% glycerol, 0.04 mg/mL bromophenol blue, 0.12 M Tris-HCl pH 6.8, and 0.28 M b-mercaptoethanol). Fifty micrograms of total protein were separated by one-dimensional SDS-PAGE, stained with Ponceau S red (Sigma Chemical) to confirm equal loading of each sample. As a second approach to verify similar loading between the lanes, gels were loaded in duplicate, and one gel was stained with Coomassie blue. Proteins were transferred from a gel to a nitrocellulose membrane (Bio-Rad Laboratories, Hercules, CA, USA). Using a vacuum-enhanced detection system (SNAP i.d., Millipore, Billerica, MA, USA) nonspecific binding sites were blocked with a 3% bovine serum albumin (BSA) solution in phosphate-saline buffer (PBS-T: 0.1 M $NaH_2PO_4 \cdot H_2O$, 0.1 M $Na_2HPO_4 \cdot 7H_2O$, 0.15 M NaCl, 0.1% Tween-20, pH 7.4) for 10 minutes. Following blocking, the membranes were incubated with specific primary antibodies against TNF-α (Santa Cruz, California, USA; #sc-1349), NFκB - p65 (Santa Cruz, California, USA; #sc-8008), MAFbx (Santa Cruz, California, USA; #sc-27644), MuRF1 (Santa Cruz, California, USA; #sc-27642), FoxO1 (Cell Signaling, Beverly, USA; #9454), myostatin (Santa Cruz, California, USA; #sc-6884), Phospho-FoxO1 (Cell Signaling, Beverly, USA; #9461), IGF-I (Santa Cruz, California, USA; #sc-7144), AKT (Cell Signaling, Beverly, USA; #9272), Phospho-AKT (Cell Signaling, Beverly, USA; #4060), mTOR (Cell Signaling, Beverly, USA; #2972), Phospho-mTOR (Cell Signaling, Beverly, USA; #5536), PGC1α (Abcam, Cambridge, UK; ab-106814) and Gapdh (Cell Signaling, Beverly, USA; #2118) in a 1% BSA solution for 10 min. After four wash steps with PBS-T, membranes were incubated in a 1:2,000 dilution of specific secondary antibodies (Santa Cruz Biotechnology, Santa Cruz, CA, USA) conjugated with horseradish peroxidase for 10 min. Finally, immunoreactive protein signals were detected using SuperSignal West Pico Chemiluminescent Substrate Kit (Thermo Fisher Scientific, Rockford, IL, USA), according to the manufacturer's instructions. The chemiluminescent signal was visualized and quantified by densitometry using the image analyzer ImageQuant 350 (GE Healthcare, Little Chalfont, UK). The values were normalized by the values obtained for Gapdh protein.

Statistical Analysis

Data are expressed as mean ± SD. Shapiro-Wilk normality test was used to verify data normal distribution. Differences in echocardiographic parameters before aerobic ET between Sham and AS animals were tested with unpaired Student's t test. The muscle fiber type frequency data were analyzed using Kruskal-Wallis test. One-way analysis of variance (ANOVA) followed by *a posteriori* Tukey multiple comparison test was used to analyze circulating TNF-α, CSA, CS, LDH, mRNA and protein expression data after ET among the groups. To analyze the involvement of exercise on cardiac parameters between before and after aerobic ET, echocardiographic values were probed with two-way ANOVA for repeated measures with a Bonferroni's *post test.* Linear regression was used to assess the relationship between PGC1α - FoxO1 mRNA and protein expression in the plantaris muscle. Statistical significance was considered achieved when the value of p was <0.05.

Results

Clinical and Anatomical Parameters

Relevant anatomical data are summarized in Table 1. At 18 weeks post-surgery and before the aerobic ET period, all the AS rats displayed deterioration of cardiac structure and function but did not present HF signs. In this study, an HF diagnosis was based on the presence of tachypnea and labored respiration and confirmed by pathological *post mortem* findings, such as right ventricular hypertrophy, pulmonary congestion, left atrial thrombus, and ascites. At 28 weeks after surgery, six of 8 AS-UN animals showed severe ascites, moderate tachypnea and atrial thrombi; however, the AS-ET animals presented a reduced intensity and frequency of these signs. Of the 8 AS-ET rats, three had mild ascites and tachypnea and only one presented atrial thrombi. Although the LV weight and LV/BW ratio were increased in both of the AS groups, the ET period attenuated the presence of cardiac thrombi and the increase in the atria, right ventricle, and lung weights in both absolute and BW-normalized values.

Cardiac Geometry, Function and Running Performance

To evaluate cardiac function, all the animals were submitted to an echocardiographic study before and after the aerobic ET protocol (Table 2). Before ET, AS groups showed pathological cardiac remodeling evidenced by increased PWT and RWT, while cardiac dysfunction was demonstrated by a decrease in PWSV and an elevation of the mitral E/A wave and LA/AO ratios. No change in heart rate (HR) under anesthesia was observed, indicating that the depth of anesthesia was similar among the groups during the echocardiographic examination. At the end of the experiment, the AS-UN group displayed a deterioration of cardiac dysfunction compared with the AS group at 18-weeks as shown by significant LV dilation at systole (LVSD) and diastole (LVDD) and accompanied by an increased PWT and E/A wave ratio. Furthermore, after 10 weeks of the training period, the left ventricular PWSV, endocardial FS and EF deteriorated even further in the AS-UN group compared with the preprotocol 18-week AS rats.

The echocardiographic parameters remained unchanged in the AS-ET group after aerobic ET. Moreover, in the AS-ET the ET protocol prevented contractile dysfunction (decreased FS) and ejection fraction (EF) and avoided increases in the LV diameter at systole and diastole compared with the AS-UN group. In addition, we observed improved exercise tolerance and performance, as demonstrated by a significant increase in velocity at the lactate threshold in the Sham-ET and AS-ET groups between the Week 1 and Week 7 tests (Figure 3).

Citrate Synthase and Lactate Dehydrogenase Activities

The activities of the enzymes citrate synthase (CS) (an indicator of cellular aerobic metabolism) and lactate dehydrogenase (LDH) (an indicator of anaerobic metabolism) were measured in soleus and plantaris muscle samples obtained from all groups after aerobic ET. HF induced a significant decrease (25%) in CS activity in both muscles in the AS-UN group compared with the Sham-UN group. CS maximal activity was similar within ET rats studied (Sham-ET and AS-ET), moreover, CS activity was preserved in AS-ET group when compared with AS-UN, suggesting that oxidative metabolism was improved, enhancing the muscle performance (Figure 4, A and C). LDH activity in the plantaris muscle was significantly increased in the AS-UN group compared with the Sham-UN group (Figure 4D), while the AS-ET group remained unchanged. In the soleus muscle, no significant difference was observed in LDH enzyme activity among the groups (Figure 4B).

Muscle Fiber Type Frequency and Cross-Sectional Area

Using the histochemical reaction of myofibrillar ATPase (m-ATPase), we observed that aerobic ET performed between cardiac dysfunction and HF prevented in 16% the reduction in the percentage of slow-twitch fibers (i.e., Type I) and Type I-to-Type IIA fiber conversion in the soleus muscle of the AS-ET rats (Figure 5A). In the plantaris muscle, ET attenuated the decrease in Type IIA fibers to approximately 22%, and it decreased the Type IIA-to-Type IID fiber conversion in AS-ET compared to AS-UN group (Figure 5B). To determine if the aerobic ET subjected

Table 1. Anatomical data after exercise training.

	Sham-UN (n = 8)	Sham-ET (n = 8)	AS-UN (n = 8)	AS-ET (n = 8)
BW (g)	489±29	475±48	464±36	440±45
LV (g)	0.77±0.07	0.65±0.07	1.15±0.15*	1.06±0.13#
LV/BW (mg/g)	1.57±0.18	1.37±0.20	2.53±0.23*	2.45±0.22#
RV (g)	0.25±0.05	0.24±0.03	0.46±0.10*	0.35±0.09
RV/BW (mg/g)	0.52±0.09	0.51±0.04	1.00±0.26*	0.86±0.25
Atria (g)	0.11±0.03	0.10±0.01	0.40±0.08*	0.28±0.09#†
Atria/BW (mg/g)	0.23±0.06	0.20±0.02	0.87±0.17*	0.64±0.22#†
Incidence of cardiac thrombi	0%	0%	56%	11%
Lung (g)	1.92±0.44	1.89±0.20	3.25±0.62*	2.52±0.59†
Lung/BW (mg/g)	3.92±0.93	4.00±0.54	7.16±1.53*	5.49±1.17†

Sham and aortic stenosis rats that remained untrained (UN) or were submitted to aerobic exercise training (ET) during the 10 weeks of training protocol; AS-ET, aortic stenosis rats that BW, body weight; LV, left ventricle; RV, right ventricle. Data are expressed as mean ± SD, except for the percentage of animals that displayed cardiac thrombi.

*$p<0.05$ vs. Sham-UN;

#$p<0.05$ vs. Sham-ET;

†$p<0.05$ vs. AS-UN.

Table 2. Echocardiografic data before and after exercise training.

	Before exercise training (18 wks)				After exercise training (28 wks)			
	Sham-UN	Sham-ET	AS-UN	AS-ET	Sham-UN	Sham-ET	AS-UN	AS-ET
HR, bpm	290±29	294±30	272±26	296±40	301±26	296±31	282±49	282±55
LVDD, mm	8.13±0.42	8.05±0.51	8.31±0.57	8.15±0.87	8.40±0.66	8.42±0.38	9.14±0.32*‡	8.19±0.77†
LVSD, mm	3.49±0.59	3.72±0.55	3.91±0.73	3.45±0.62	3.82±0.63	3.84±0.36	5.08±0.57*‡	3.41±1.01†
PWT, mm	1.45±0.11	1.42±0.04	2.09±0.16*	2.02±0.24#	1.46±0.06	1.43±0.07	2.29±0.20*‡	2.15±0.25#
RWT	0.36±0.04	0.36±0.03	0.48±0.05*	0.52±0.04#	0.35±0.03	0.34±0.02	0.51±0.05*	0.53±0.08#
LA/AO	1.43±0.16	1.50±0.17	1.93±0.36*	1.85±0.14#	1.44±0.10	1.56±0.18	2.21±0.26*	2.08±0.24#
FS, %	57.27±5.73	53.70±5.81	53.03±7.94	55.93±11.29	55.33±4.40	54.37±4.02	43.78±6.68*‡	58.84±10.72†
PWSV, mm/s	40.40±2.62	38.61±5.56	25.93±2.89*	28.75±7.38#	37.72±4.81	37.17±3.51	23.30±3.91*‡	29.18±5.17#†
E/A	1.49±0.23	1.44±0.32	5.15±1.95*	4.97±1.36#	1.33±0.32	1.36±0.23	7.93±1.75*‡	4.24±2.23#†
EF, %	92±3	90±4	89±6	90±8	90±3	90±3	82±6*‡	92±6†

HR, heart rate; LVDD and LVSD, LV diastolic and systolic diameters, respectively; PWT, LV posterior wall thickness; RWT, LV relative wall thickness in diastole; LA, left atrium diameter; AO, aortic diameter; FS, LV endocardial fractional shortening; PWSV, LV posterior wall shortening velocity; E/A, early-to-late diastolic mitral inflow ratio; EF, ejection fraction. n = 8 per group. Data are expressed as mean ± SD.

*$p<0.05$ vs. Sham-UN and,

#$p<0.05$ vs. Sham-ET at the same time (18 wk or 28 wk);

†$p<0.05$ vs. AS-UN;

‡$p<0.05$ vs. AS; t test, one-way or 2-way ANOVA with Bonferroni *post hoc* test as appropriate.

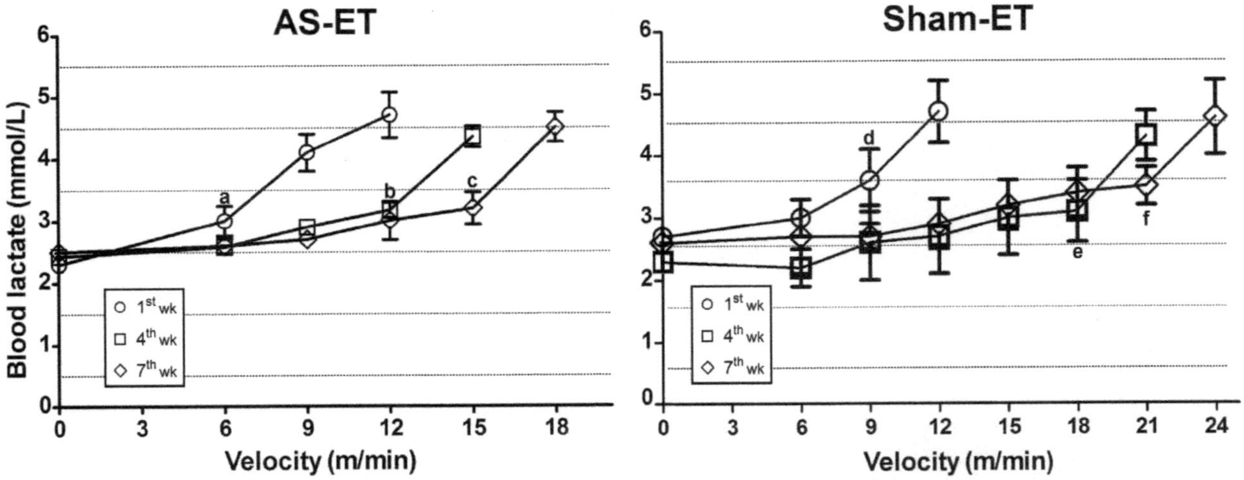

Figure 3. Blood lactate concentration in the AS-ET and Sham-ET groups assessed on the 1st, 4th and 7th weeks by incremental load test. Values are expressed as the mean ± SD. Significant differences ($p<0.05$) at the same time were in AS-ET group: a. vs. 9 m/min; b. vs. 15 m/min; and c. vs. 18 m/min. Sham-ET: d. vs. 12 m/min; e. vs. 21 m/min; and f. vs. 24 m/min.

between cardiac dysfunction and HF was able to prevent atrophy of the soleus and plantaris muscles, we used the m-ATPase reaction to measure the skeletal muscle fiber cross-sectional area (CSA). At the end of the experiment, the AS-UN group presented a significant reduction in the CSA of Type I and IIA fibers in the soleus muscle (Table 3). Moreover, in this muscle, aerobic ET attenuated the reduction of fibers CSA in AS-ET animals. On the other hand, Type I and IIA fibers of plantaris muscle were not affected by AS and ET stimuli. However, a significant decrease in the CSA of plantaris Type IID and IIB fibers was observed in the AS-UN group, indicating that ET prevented the atrophy of plantaris Type IID and IIB fibers (Table 4).

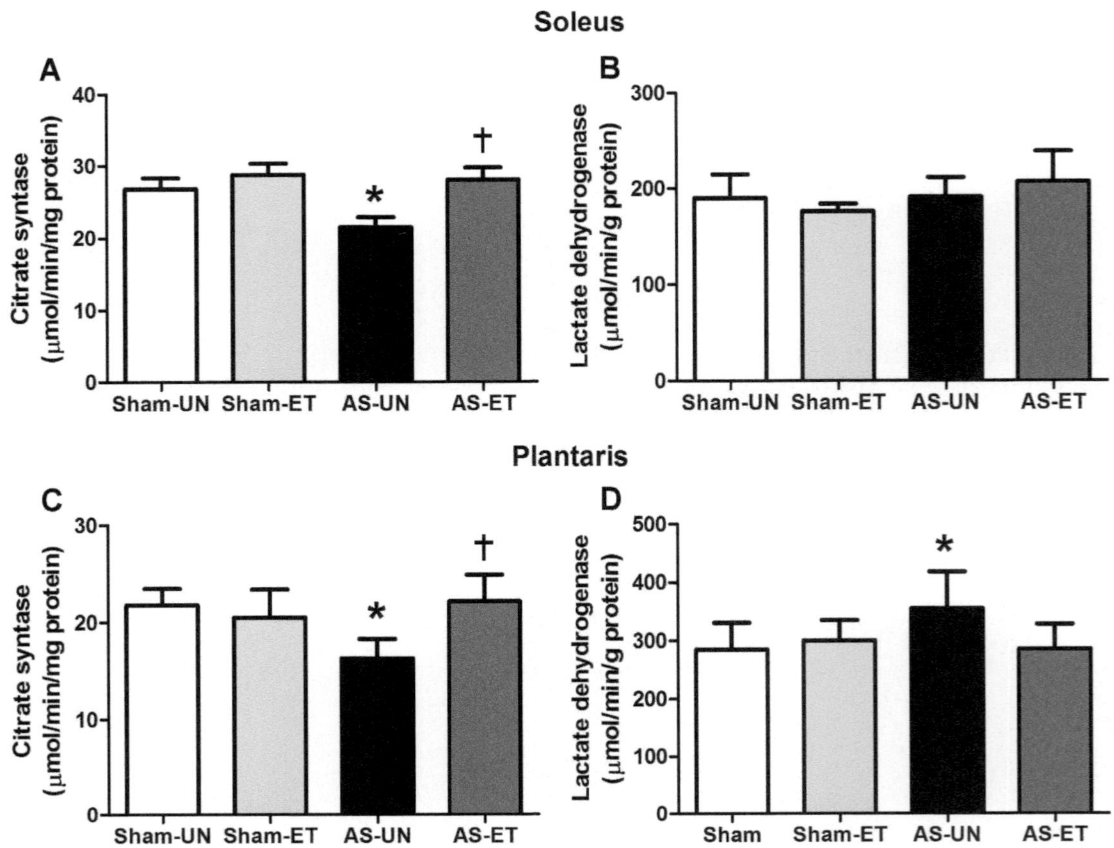

Figure 4. CS and LDH activities. Soleus (A and B) and plantaris (C and D) muscles of the Sham-UN, Sham-ET, AS-UN, and AS-ET groups. Data are presented as the mean ± SD. *$p<0.05$ vs. Sham-UN; †$p<0.05$ vs. AS-UN.

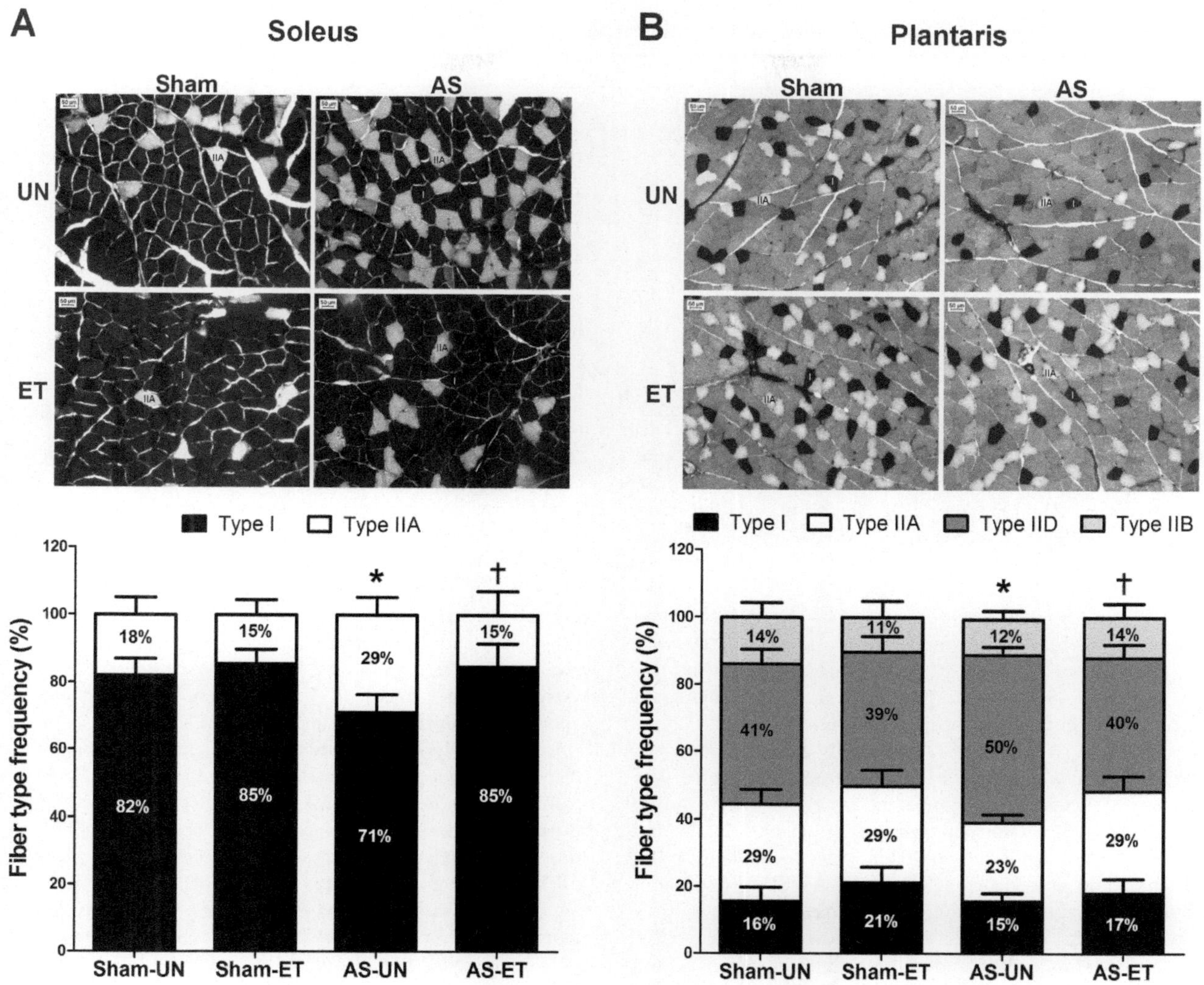

Figure 5. Soleus (A) and plantaris (B) muscle fiber-type frequencies. Representative photographs of mATPase reaction after preincubation at pH 4.5 and the data of the muscle fiber-type frequencies in Sham-UN, Sham-ET, AS-UN, and AS-ET groups. (Type I; type IIA; type IID; and type IIB). Soleus (A), type I and IIA *p<0.05 vs. Sham-UN; †p<0.05 vs. AS-UN. Plantaris (B), type IIA and IID, *p<0.05 vs. Sham-UN; †p<0.05 vs. AS-UN.

Systemic Concentration of TNF-α and IGF-I

The serum concentration of TNF-α showed a significant increase only between the non-trained HF animals (AS-UN group) and Sham-UN group (AS-UN: 18.04±3.96 pg/mL vs. Sham-UN: 12.07±1.67 pg/mL; p<0.05). However, AS-ET group still remained not significantly lower than of the AS-UN group (Figure 6A). On the other hand, the serum concentration of IGF-I was significantly lower in the non-trained rats (AS-UN group) as compared to Sham-UN (AS-UN: 918.7±123.2 pg/mL vs. Sham-UN: 1328.0±143.7 pg/mL, p<0.05); the trained rats (AS-ET) remained not significantly higher than the sedentary rats (Figure 6B).

Skeletal Muscle Gene and Protein Expression

Proteolytic system. To investigate the effects of ET on changes in the skeletal muscle proteolytic system in HF animals,

Table 3. Cross sectional area (μm^2) of the two major soleus muscle fiber types after ET.

	Sham-UN (n = 8)	Sham-ET (n = 8)	AS-UN (n = 8)	AS-ET (n = 8)
I	3564.09±307.87	3582.96±204.80	3056.92±281.86*	3565.18±376.28†
IIA	3485.77±232.03	3755.20±359.61	2950.67±223.70*	3976.28±408.96†

Data are expressed as mean ± SD.
*p<0.05 vs. Sham-UN;
†p<0.05 vs. AS-UN.
One-way ANOVA + Tukey test.

Table 4. Cross sectional area (μm²) of plantaris muscle fiber types after ET.

	Sham-UN (n = 8)	Sham-ET (n = 8)	AS-UN (n = 8)	AS-ET (n = 8)
I	2317.28±247.10	2223.10±231.19	2270.52±426.69	2158.09±378.18
IIA	2229.72±165.23	2222.16±186.57	2141.53±298.37	2246.69±282.28
IID	2703.84±272.88	2716.39±184.22	2307.12±276.74*	2679.91±303.61†
IIB	4159.27±397.15	4357.31±405.12	3508.91±228.85*	4273.55±490.45†

Data are expressed as mean ± SD.
*$p<0.05$ vs. Sham-UN;
†$p<0.05$ vs. AS-UN.
One-way ANOVA + Tukey test.

we measured the mRNA and protein levels of TNF-α, NFκB (p65), MAFbx, MuRF1, FoxO1, and myostatin in the soleus and plantaris muscles (Figure 7). Furthermore, the catabolic effect of HF on skeletal muscle was assessed by the phosphorylation status of FoxO1^{Ser256} in Sham-UN, Sham-ET, AS-UN and AS-ET rats. In the soleus muscle, there was a significant ($p<0.05$) increase in TNF-α, NFκB (p65), FoxO1, and myostatin gene (Figure 7A) and protein (Figure 7B and C) expression in the AS-UN group compared to the Sham-UN group (Figure 7B and C). Interestingly, this upregulation in catabolic factor expression was attenuated in the AS-ET group (Figure 7A and B) in conjunction with an increase in the phosphorylation levels of FoxO1^{Ser256}. In addition, MAFbx mRNA was significantly increased, and the increases in MAFbx and MuRF1 protein content in the AS-UN group were significantly attenuated in the AS-ET group (Figure 7B and C). In the plantaris muscle (Figure 7D, E, and F), we observed a significant ($p<0.05$) increase in TNF-α and FoxO1 gene and protein expression in the AS-UN group and a decrease in the ratios of phosphorylated FoxO1 protein to total protein expression and a significant attenuation in the AS-ET group. Furthermore, a significant increase in myostatin gene and protein expression was observed in the AS-UN group, and attenuation of this increase at the protein level was observed in the AS-ET group. In addition, MAFbx gene and protein expression were increased in the AS-UN group compared with the Sham-UN group, but no significant effect of ET was observed in the AS-ET group. NFκB (p65) mRNA expression was increased in the AS-UN group and attenuated in the AS-ET group. Moreover, AS-UN group showed not significantly higher in MuRF1 gene and protein expression and attenuated protein levels in the AS-ET group.

Hypertrophy Pathway. To determine if ET stimulates the hypertrophic pathway and attenuates the atrophic effect observed in skeletal muscles in our HF model, we measured IGF-I expression and its downstream AKT and mTOR. Our results indicated that there were no differences ($p>0.05$) in IGF-I mRNA and protein levels in the soleus (Figure 8A and B) and plantaris (Figure 8D and E) muscles among the groups. Similarly, no changes in AKT and mTOR mRNA and the ratios of phosphorylated protein to total protein expression occurred among the groups in either muscle type (Figure 8).

Anti-Proteolytic Component. To explore additional aspects of the prevention of skeletal muscle loss in HF via ET, PGC1α expression was investigated. As shown in Figure 9, although no statistically significant differences were observed in the soleus muscle, in the plantaris muscles, we observed a decrease in PGC1α mRNA levels in approximately 62% of the AS-UN animals (Figure 9D); furthermore, PGC1α protein levels were approximately 55% lower in the AS-UN animals compared with the other groups (Figure 9E and F). Interestingly, the AS-ET rats displayed significant attenuation of the reduction in PGC1α mRNA and protein levels, which remained at the same levels as in the Sham-ET group. In addition, linear regression analysis of the plantaris muscle results revealed a significant negative correlation between FoxO1 and PGC1α mRNA expression (Pearson's $r = -0.69$, $p = 0.003$) and FoxO1 and PGC1α protein levels (Pearson's $r = -0.90$, $p<0.0001$), based on an analysis of the individual data points for the AS-UN and AS-ET groups (Figure 10).

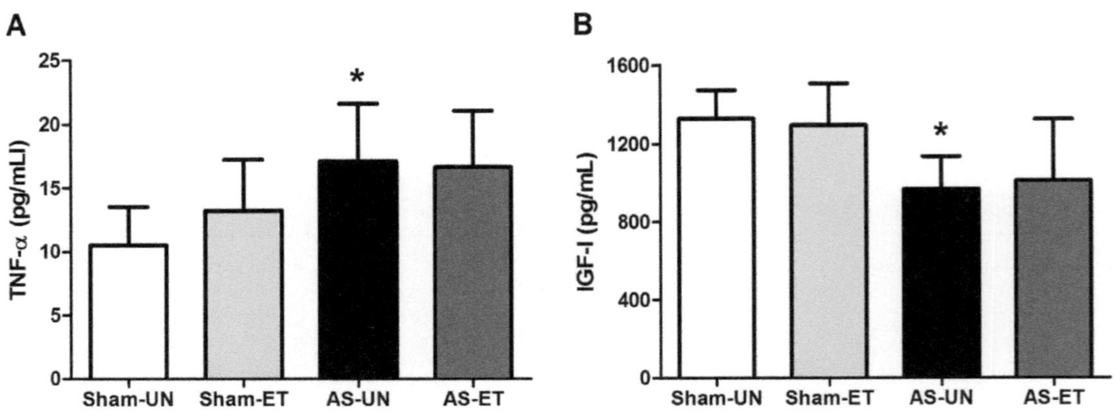

Figure 6. Serum concentration. Proinflammatory cytokine TNF-α (A) and growth factor IGF-I (B) in AS-UN, AS-ET, Sham-UN, and Sham-ET groups. Data are presented as the mean ± SD. *$p<0.05$ vs. Sham-UN.

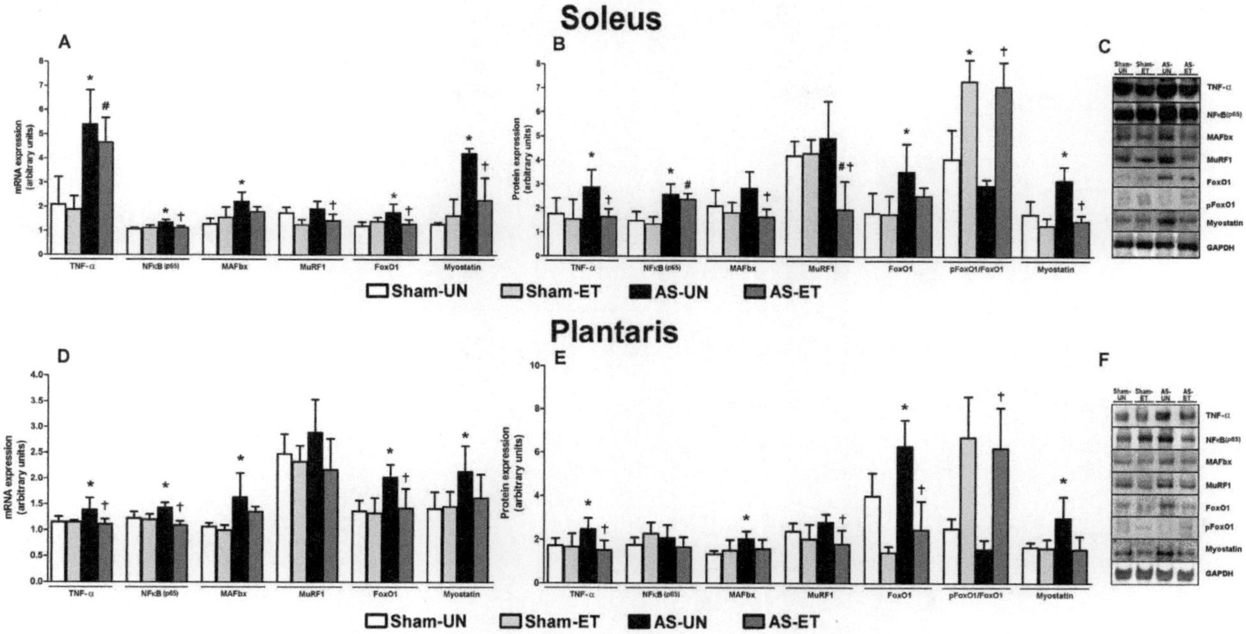

Figure 7. mRNA and protein levels of the skeletal muscle proteolytic system. A and D: mRNA levels in the soleus (A) and plantaris (D) muscles; protein content in the soleus (B) and plantaris (E) muscles; representative blots of soleus (C) and plantaris (F) muscles in Sham-UN, Sham-ET, AS-UN, and AS-ET groups. Data are expressed as the mean ± SD; *Significant difference from the Sham-UN group, $p<0.05$; #$p<0.05$ vs. Sham-ET; †$p<0.05$ vs. AS-UN group.

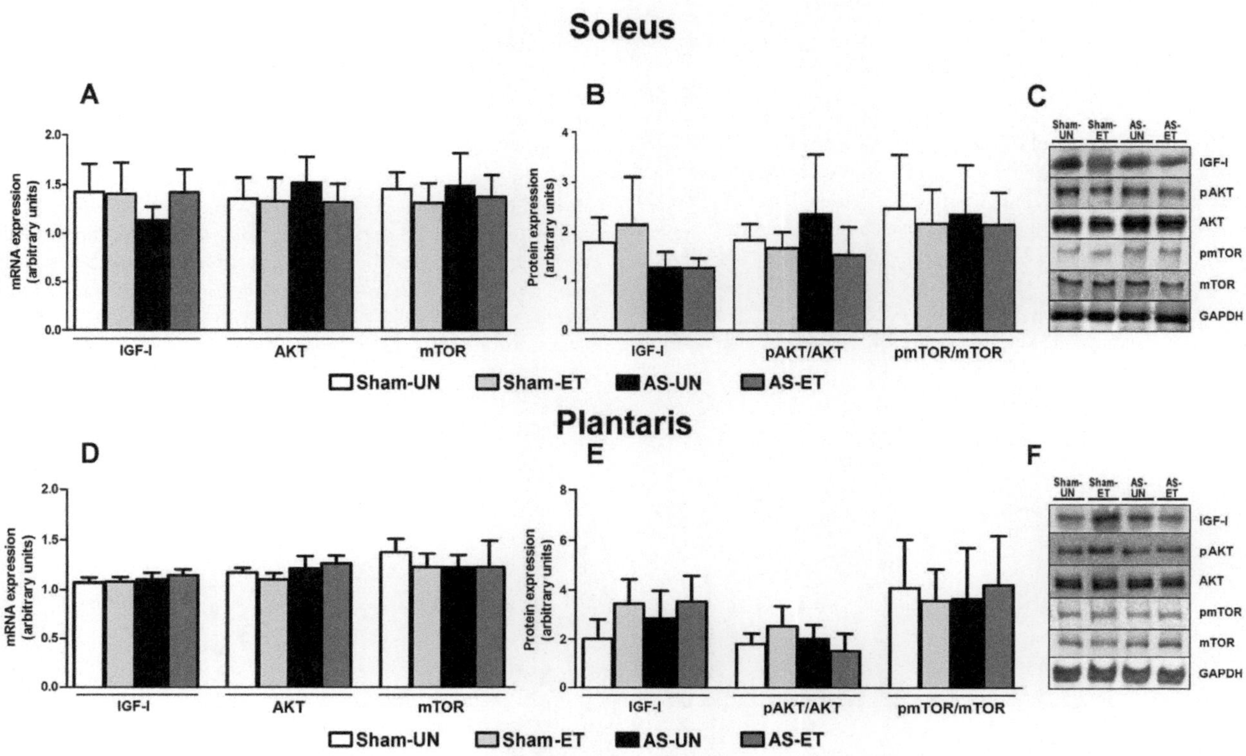

Figure 8. mRNA and protein levels of skeletal muscle hypertrophy components. A and D: mRNA levels in the soleus (A) and plantaris (D) muscles; protein content in the soleus (B) and plantaris (E) muscles; representative blots of soleus (C) and plantaris (F) muscles from Sham-UN, Sham-ET, AS-UN, and AS-ET groups. Data are expressed as the mean ± SD; *Significant difference from the Sham-UN group, $p<0.05$; #$p<0.05$ vs. Sham-ET; †$p<0.05$ from the AS-UN group.

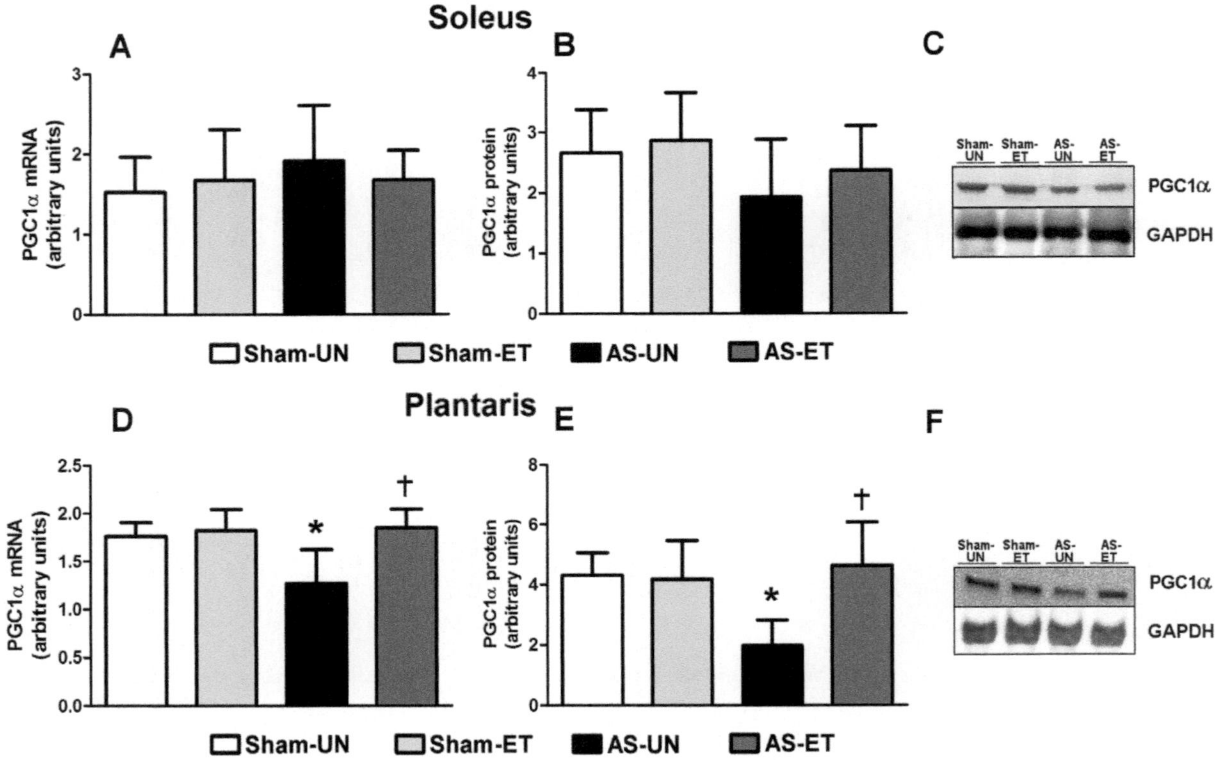

Figure 9. mRNA and protein levels of the skeletal muscle proteolysis inhibitor PGC1α. A and D: mRNA levels in the soleus (A) and plantaris (D) muscles; protein content in the soleus (B) and plantaris (E) muscles; representative blots of soleus (C) and plantaris (F) muscles in Sham-UN, Sham-ET, AS-UN, and AS-ET groups. Data are presented as the mean ± SD; *Significant difference from the Sham-UN group, $p<0.05$; †$p<0.05$ from the AS-UN group.

Discussion

Metabolic abnormalities resulting in a progressive catabolic state have been observed in various chronic diseases [34,35]. Since skeletal muscle dysfunction and loss of lean muscle mass have been described in HF [36,37], a number of studies have focused on identifying therapies that could improve clinical outcomes. Studies of HF have reported that ET is an effective non-pharmacological therapy for improving exercise capacity and quality of life and confers survival benefits [38]. Moreover, recent reports have demonstrated that ET has beneficial effects against HF-induced skeletal myopathy [39,40]. However, the molecular mechanisms by which ET attenuates or reverses skeletal muscle myopathy, which would become attractive targets for heart failure therapy, remain elusive.

In the present study, we used the ascending aortic stenosis (AS) model to promote a gradual development of left ventricular hypertrophy and posterior HF in rats [1]. In this model, animals develop cardiac remodeling that is associated, in the short term, with diastolic dysfunction and improved systolic function, followed by depressed systolic performance and HF. After 18 weeks of supra-aortic stenosis and before the training intervention, cardiac

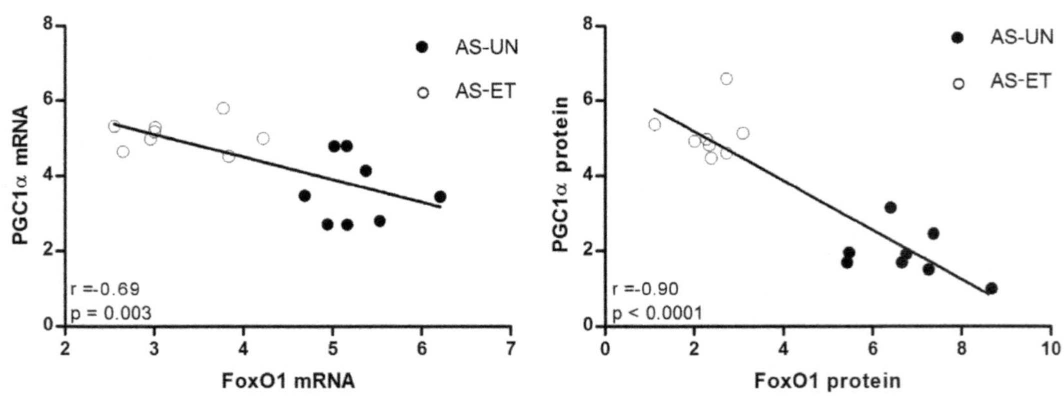

Figure 10. Relationship between PGC1α - FoxO1 mRNA and protein expression in the plantaris muscle. There were significant negative correlations between the PGC1α and FoxO mRNA/protein levels. For all correlations, individual data points from the AS-UN and AS-ET groups ($n=8$ rats per group) were used.

remodeling was noted on an echocardiographic assessment, although the animals did not show signs of HF. After 10 weeks of aerobic ET, the AS-ET animals presented an improved in structure and function in the systole and diastole compared with AS-UN. In addition, ET prevented the deterioration of cardiac structure and function in AS animals, when we compared the AS-ET group and the 18-week AS rats. Our data support previous findings that ET had a beneficial effect on the left ventricular function of individuals with HF [41,42] and indicates that ET can be an important clinical intervention for improving cardiac structure and function during the transition from cardiac dysfunction to HF.

Animal [10] and human [39] studies have demonstrated skeletal muscle abnormalities in HF, including changes in morphology, function, and depressed skeletal muscle aerobic capacity. In our model of HF, we also observed changes in oxidative and glycolytic skeletal muscle metabolic enzymes. The reduction of CS enzyme activity in both the soleus and plantaris muscles in the AS-UN group, suggests a decrease in aerobic metabolism. After 10 weeks of aerobic ET, a significant attenuation in the decreasing CS activity in AS-ET rats was evident. Although, our aerobic ET protocol did not change this enzyme in the Sham-ET group, probably due to the low training intensity used, CS was clearly detected in the AS-ET animals. This prevention in the reduction of CS activity in the AS-ET group may participate in de novo ATP synthesis during ET in HF rats; therefore, the higher citrate synthase activity in AS-ET rats than in AS-UN rats suggests aerobic metabolism improvements. Furthermore, we observed an increase in LDH enzyme in the AS-UN group, indicating higher anaerobic metabolic activity in the skeletal muscle, which was attenuated by ET. The changes in LDH activity were more evident in the plantaris muscles of the AS-UN group, most likely because this muscle has a higher frequency of Type II fibers (glycolytic) than the soleus muscle. The increased percentage of Type I fibers (oxidative metabolism) in the soleus and Type IIA fibers (more oxidative compared with the IID and IIB fiber types) in the plantaris muscle in the AS-ET group was further evidence that ET attenuated the decrease in aerobic metabolism in these muscles, because studies have shown that ET promotes a fiber type transition and a myosin heavy chain content shift from a fast-to-slow twitch [43,44]. Our findings regarding the fiber-type transition during HF corroborate a report by Moreira et al. [45] that moderate aerobic training increased the number of slow-twitch fibers in the soleus and plantaris muscles. Thus, our data strongly suggest that aerobic ET prevented the modulation of the fiber type toward the more glycolytic metabolic pattern.

There is a striking association between skeletal muscle atrophy and chronic HF [46]. Decreased muscle fiber CSA is a major aggravator in HF syndrome and has been observed in experimental HF studies [8,47,48]. However, the atrophy is dependent on the model used and the type of muscle examined. Oxidative muscles (e.g., the soleus) are more susceptible to damage caused by inactivity or unloading, whereas glycolytic muscles (e.g., the plantaris) tend to be more affected in diseased conditions [49,50]. Therefore, we decided to evaluate both the soleus and plantaris muscles because of their contrasting metabolic properties. Soleus atrophy in the AS-UN rats was correlated with a reduced CSA of Type I and Type IIA muscle fibers. These findings are consistent with a previous study by Moreira et al. [45], who also observed a decrease in both fiber types (I and IIA) in the soleus muscle. Moreover, in the plantaris muscle Moreira et al. [45] observed atrophy only in the glycolytic-type fibers, similarly to our results, which the plantaris muscle presented only IID and IIB glycolytic fiber-type atrophy in the AS-UN rats. This result suggests that only the glycolytic fiber types were more damaged under HF conditions and might exhibit a greater loss of blood perfusion, and increased damage from reactive oxygen species and local inflammation, compared with oxidative fiber types [34,39,51].

Abnormalities in HF affect various endocrine systems leading to an imbalance of catabolic and anabolic function. Skeletal muscle atrophy during HF may be induced by the activation of local and systemic markers of inflammation, most notably inflammatory cytokine, tumor necrosis factor (TNF-α), a proinflammatory secreted cytokine that was originally called "cachectin" [52]. In this study, similar to others [53,54], a significant increase in TNF-α level were observed in the serum and in the tissue in our AS-UN animals, while in the AS-ET animals, exercise attenuated the expression of this cytokine. An anti-inflammatory effect of physical exercise was recently proposed [55]; this effect may be mediated not only by a reduction in visceral fat mass, with a subsequent decrease in the production and release of proinflammatory cytokines such as IL-6 and TNF-α, but also by the induction of an anti-inflammatory environment with each bout of exercise [55]. Thus, our ET program in AS rats may have increased anti-inflammatory cytokines in skeletal muscle, indicating a potential mechanism for the anti-inflammatory effects of aerobic exercise in cardiovascular disease.

Since TNF-α exhibit catabolic effects in various tissues [56], the increased muscular expression of proinflammatory cytokine might further contribute to the local catabolic state with progressive atrophic alterations of the skeletal muscle in HF. The effects of TNF-α on HF-related muscle myopathy are mediated through the activation of a family of transcription factors known as nuclear factor kappa B (NFκB), which regulate ubiquitin-dependent proteosomal system activity (PDU) [57]. NFκB (p50/p65) activation leads to increased expression of the atrogenes MuRF1 and MAFbx [57], which results in sarcomeric protein proteolysis, promoting muscle atrophy. In our study, although there were slight variations in the gene and/or protein expression levels of NFκB, MuRF1, and MAFbx, the increased levels of these catabolic components in the AS-UN group may be at least partially responsible for the atrophy of the plantaris and soleus muscles. Indeed, we previously demonstrated marked muscle atrophy and a reciprocal increase in the components of the ubiquitin-proteasome system (e.g., MuRF1 and MAFbx) in rats in which HF was induced by monocrotaline [58]. These results indicate the possible involvement of these atrogenes in the HF-induced muscle atrophy process. Although several studies have investigated the muscle atrophy that occurs during HF [40,45,58], the effects of ET on the atrogene components have not been completely defined. The present finding that aerobic ET performed during the transition from cardiac dysfunction to HF prevents the overactivation of some proteasomal components is similar to that of Gielen et al. [59] that observed a attenuation of MuRF1 by exercise training and Campos et al. [6], who also observed a reduction of ubiquitin-proteasome system activation in response to ET. Campos et al. [6] also indicated that the possible attenuation of the ubiquitin-proteasome system by ET may be due to improvements in the redox balance driven by the increase in antioxidant enzymes and reduced levels of inflammatory cytokines, corroborating our finding of a decrease in TNF-α levels [4,6,54].

The transforming growth factor-β-related protein myostatin, a key regulator of muscle growth, has been considered an important mediator of cardiac-induced skeletal muscle wasting and cachexia in animal studies [5,60]. However, the effects of ET on myostatin expression in skeletal muscle remain inconclusive. Studies using swimming endurance training have shown a reduction in the myostatin mRNA content in skeletal muscle [61,62]. Lenk et al. [17] observed an increase in myostatin levels in the myocardium and the gastrocnemius muscle in a rat model of ischemic cardiomyopathy, and ET on a treadmill led to a significant reduction in myostatin protein expression in the skeletal muscle and myocardium of HF animals. Our results support these findings; we observed a significant increase in myostatin expression in the soleus and plantaris muscles in the AS-UN group and aerobic ET prevented the increase in myostatin expression in the AS-ET group in both muscles evaluated. Similar to Lenk et al. [17], we also demonstrated that aerobic ET decreased the expression of TNF-α. The significant reduction in myostatin levels in the soleus and plantaris muscles after ET could be linked to the reduction in the levels of the TNF-α; however, further experiments investigating TNF-α levels and myostatin should be performed to confirm the findings of the present study.

In chronic HF, alterations in multiple anabolic and catabolic systems result in progressive catabolism, which leads to cardiac cachexia in advanced stages of the disease [3]. As a key regulator of normal muscle growth and hypertrophy, the role of the IGF-I/AKT/mTOR signaling pathway has recently received increased attention as a potential means of suppressing protein breakdown while promoting muscle growth [9]. In patients with chronic HF [7,37] and in animal models of chronic left-ventricular dysfunction [10,63], reduced skeletal muscle expression of IGF-I is associated with muscle atrophy. In addition, in advanced stages of HF have been described low serum levels of IGF-I due to a growth hormone resistance and a loss of lean muscle mass [3]. In the present study, we observed low serum levels of IGF-I in AS-UN rats compared to Sham-UN, without difference in AS-ET vs. Sham-ET animals. In contrast, the tissue concentration of IGF-I was similar among the groups, indicating that AS-induced HF did not downregulate the IGF-I/AKT/mTOR pathway locally, and suggesting that the although aerobic ET counteracted muscle catabolism, aerobic ET did not enhance the muscle anabolic state. Although disease progression from mild-moderate to severe HF is likely multifactorial and is poorly understood, the available data suggest that GH/IGF-I may be implicated in this pathology. A possible explanation for these findings was suggested by Arcopinto et al. [64], who stated that during the gradual development of HF the IGF-I values are normal or slightly elevated in the beginning; in the intermediate stage, IGF-I levels tend to decrease or remain unaltered; and in advanced stages, IGF-I reduces and a markedly increase in GH circulating levels occur. Furthermore, the changes in skeletal muscle hypertrophy and atrophy turnover do not always proceed according to the balance between protein breakdown and protein synthesis [65]. Analyses of rat muscle growth by Li et al. [66] demonstrated that starvation causes decreased protein synthesis and increased protein degradation in both fast and slow rat muscles. However, in a model of muscle denervation, the authors observed an increase in protein degradation and an increase rather than decrease in protein synthesis [67]. Taken together, it is possible that in our experiment, the stage of HF greatly influenced the catabolic components without any change in the anabolic pathway and that the prevention of skeletal muscle atrophy by ET occurred independent of protein synthesis.

The members of the forkhead box O (FoxO) family are transcription factors responsible for the cross-talk between protein degradation and protein synthesis [9]. Similar to Reed et al. [68], who demonstrated that FoxO transcriptional activity is increased in skeletal muscles under 2 cachectic conditions, we also observed that HF-induced muscle atrophy is associated with an increase in the expression of FoxO in both muscles studied. By contrast, aerobic ET attenuated this change in FoxO expression; specifically, the effects of aerobic ET in phosphorylate FoxO1, contributing, at least in part, to the prevention of skeletal muscle atrophy. Here, we extend our findings to the preventive effect of aerobic ET on FoxO inhibition. FoxO activity is modulated by other intracellular signaling molecules, such as peroxisome proliferator-activated receptor gamma coactivator 1 alpha (PGC1α), a cofactor involved in mitochondrial biogenesis, fiber-type switching, and angiogenesis [69,70]. Low levels of PGC1α have been reported to contribute to muscle wasting during chronic HF [71]. We observed a decrease in the PGC1α levels only in the plantaris muscle, although HF-induced atrophy was observed in the soleus and plantaris muscles of the AS-UN animals. Considering that glycolytic muscles are more vulnerable to catabolic muscle wasting than are oxidative muscles [51,72] this result demonstrates the distinct responses to HF stimuli in the soleus and plantaris muscles, which in this case might be explained by 2 main factors. The first is a decrease in blood supply, which was likely more pronounced in the plantaris muscle than in the soleus muscle. This difference could occur because the plantaris muscle contains glycolytic fiber types, which receive less blood and, consequently, reduced antioxidant defense [71]. The second factor could be related to fiber-type modulation. The decrease in the percentage of type IIA and increase in the IID fibers in the plantaris muscle of AS-UN animals in our study, in association with a decrease in the PGC1α content, supports previous findings of Russell et al. [73], who showed that PGC-1 protein levels were higher in the type IIA fibers, lower in the type I fibers, and lowest in the type IID/X fibers in human skeletal muscle, thereby suggesting the idea that the increase in the IID fiber types in plantaris muscle in our experiment possibly induced the reduction in the PGC1α content of AS-UN animals. By contrast, the absence of changes in PGC1α levels in the soleus muscle could be related to the Type I-to-IIA fiber conversion, which occurred within fiber population in which PGC1α levels is already high [71,73]. In addition, although our ET did not altered PGC1α levels in Sham-ET group, moderate and intense aerobic ET is known to promote an oxidative phenotype, stimulates PGC1α expression in skeletal muscle [74], and by PGC1α overexpression prevents muscle atrophy through the inhibition of the transcriptional activity of the FoxO3, NFκB, and myostatin signaling pathways [9,75]. In the current study, we observed that aerobic ET during the transition from cardiac dysfunction to HF prevented the reduction in PGC1α expression levels in the plantaris muscle. Of particular interest, the expression levels of PGC1α and FoxO1 in this muscle were negatively correlated (mRNA, $r = -0.69$, $p = 0.003$; protein, $r = -0.90$, $p < 0.0001$). Although these results do not demonstrate a causal relationship between the anti-proteolytic component PGC1α and the atrophic factor FoxO1 in AS-induced HF, they confirm previous reports demonstrating a strong negative correlation between these proteins and provide insights into the functional role of PGC1α in the skeletal muscle in protection against catabolic muscle wasting [14,71,75].

Although much has already been achieved, there is a great deal more that we need to learn about ET applied during HF. Aerobic exercise training is now an integral part of the recommended treatment for stable New York Heart Association (NYHA) class I–III HF patients [76]. Nevertheless, the understanding of the molecular differences between beneficial vs. 'maladaptive' eccentric cardiac growth will instruct potential future therapy. Also, the precise definition of the molecular and cellular mechanisms mediating the beneficial effects of ET during HF should be elucidated to devise optimal treatment strategies that could in theory beneficially impact cardiovascular diseases and HF.

Limitations

Although the ascending AS is one of the more widely used surgical methods to induce pressure overload in rats [22,47,77,78] a limitation of this model is the evaluation of the grade of AS that could be done by the analyze of the aorta flow velocity. As this measurement is not reproducible technically in supravalvar AS in rats, this issue can be partially solved by using the left ventricular systolic pressure data [79] or by echocardiography parameters [18], as we used in the present study.

The beneficial effects of aerobic ET protocol attenuating the progression of the disease were evidenced in cardiac structure and function parameters. However, we cannot conclude whether the aerobic ET affected the skeletal muscles directly, or indirectly preventing the deterioration from cardiac dysfunction to HF. In addition, although we measured the degree of exercise tolerance and performance, we did not make a direct assessment of skeletal muscle force.

Finally, we used NFκB (p65) from nuclear and cytosolic fraction for assessment of ubiquitin proteosomal system activity (PDU). This protein does not allow us to verify the correct activity of the NFκB, but taken together with others downstream protein expression, this assay provides an important indicator of the PDU involvement in skeletal muscle during the transition from cardiac dysfunction to HF.

Conclusions

Collectively, our data provide evidence that aerobic ET performed during the transition from cardiac dysfunction to HF has beneficial effects on cardiac structure and function. Our results also show that muscle atrophy observed in HF due to an increase in catabolic pathways, was prevented by aerobic ET not via an increase in anabolic factors but by counteracting the catabolic activity, presumably by PGC1α expression.

Acknowledgments

We thank Dr. Frank Naya and his students Nelsa L. Estrella, Jose Medrano, Amanda Rice, and Cody Desjardins for valuable discussions.

Author Contributions

Conceived and designed the experiments: RWAS ACC MDPS. Performed the experiments: RWAS WPP LCS PATS DHSC AAHF KO. Analyzed the data: RWAS WPP LCS PATS ACC AAHF KO. Contributed to the writing of the manuscript: RWAS AFA IJVJ RFC MDPS.

References

1. Feldman AM, Weinberg EO, Ray PE, Lorell BH (1993) Selective changes in cardiac gene expression during compensated hypertrophy and the transition to cardiac decompensation in rats with chronic aortic banding. Circ Res 73: 184–192.
2. Evans WJ, Morley JE, Argilés J, Bales C, Baracos V, et al. (2008) Cachexia: a new definition. Clin Nutr 27: 793–799.
3. Hambrecht R, Schulze PC, Gielen S, Linke A, Möbius-Winkler S, et al. (2002) Reduction of insulin-like growth factor-I expression in the skeletal muscle of noncachectic patients with chronic heart failure. J Am Coll Cardiol 39: 1175–1181.
4. Gielen S, Adams V, Möbius-Winkler S, Linke A, Erbs S, et al. (2003) Anti-inflammatory effects of exercise training in the skeletal muscle of patients with chronic heart failure. J Am Coll Cardiol 42: 861–868.
5. Heineke J, Auger-Messier M, Xu J, Sargent M, York A, et al. (2010) Genetic deletion of myostatin from the heart prevents skeletal muscle atrophy in heart failure. Circulation 121: 419–425.
6. Cunha TF, Bacurau AVN, Moreira JBN, Paixão NA, Campos JC, et al. (2012) Exercise training prevents oxidative stress and ubiquitin-proteasome system overactivity and reverse skeletal muscle atrophy in heart failure. PLoS One 7: e41701.
7. Levine B, Kalman J, Mayer L, Fillit HM, Packer M (1990) Elevated circulating levels of tumor necrosis factor in severe chronic heart failure. N Engl J Med 323: 236–241.
8. Anker SD, Ponikowski P, Varney S, Chua TP, Clark AL, et al. (1997) Wasting as independent risk factor for mortality in chronic heart failure. Lancet 349: 1050–1053.
9. Bonaldo P, Sandri M (2013) Cellular and molecular mechanisms of muscle atrophy. Dis Model Mech 6: 25–39.
10. Schulze PC, Gielen S, Adams V, Linke A, Möbius-Winkler S, et al. (2003) Muscular levels of proinflammatory cytokines correlate with a reduced expression of insulin-like growth factor-I in chronic heart failure. Basic Res Cardiol 98: 267–274.
11. Sandri M, Sandri C, Gilbert A, Skurk C, Calabria E, et al. (2004) Foxo transcription factors induce the atrophy-related ubiquitin ligase atrogin-1 and cause skeletal muscle atrophy. Cell 117: 399–412.
12. Lecker SH, Jagoe RT, Gilbert A, Gomes M, Baracos V, et al. (2004) Multiple types of skeletal muscle atrophy involve a common program of changes in gene expression. FASEB J 18: 39–51.
13. Galasso G, De Rosa R, Piscione F, Iaccarino G, Vosa C, et al. (2010) Myocardial expression of FOXO3a-Atrogin-1 pathway in human heart failure. Eur J Heart Fail 12: 1290–1296.
14. Sandri M, Lin J, Handschin C, Yang W, Arany ZP, et al. (2006) PGC-1α protects skeletal muscle from atrophy by suppressing FoxO3 action and atrophy-specific gene transcription. Proc Natl Acad Sci U S A 103: 16260–16265.
15. Piña IL, Apstein CS, Balady GJ, Belardinelli R, Chaitman BR, et al. (2003) Exercise and heart failure: A statement from the American Heart Association Committee on exercise, rehabilitation, and prevention. Circulation 107: 1210–1225.
16. Minotti JR, Christoph I, Oka R, Weiner MW, Wells L, et al. (1991) Impaired skeletal muscle function in patients with congestive heart failure. Relationship to systemic exercise performance. J Clin Invest 88: 2077–2082.
17. Lenk K, Schur R, Linke A, Erbs S, Matsumoto Y, et al. (2009) Impact of exercise training on myostatin expression in the myocardium and skeletal muscle in a chronic heart failure model. Eur J Hear Fail J Work Gr Hear Fail Eur Soc Cardiol 11: 342–348.
18. Moreira VO, Castro AVB, Yaegashi MY, Cicogna AC, Okoshi MP, et al. (2006) Echocardiographic criteria for the definition of ventricular dysfunction severity in aortic banded rats. Arq Bras Cardiol 86: 432–438.
19. Moreira VO, Pereira CA, Silva MO, Felisbino SL, Cicogna AC, et al. (2009) Growth hormone attenuates myocardial fibrosis in rats with chronic pressure overload-induced left ventricular hypertrophy. Clin Exp Pharmacol Physiol 36: 325–330.
20. Cicogna AC, Robinson KG, Conrad CH, Singh K, Squire R, et al. (1999) Direct Effects of Colchicine on Myocardial Function: Studies in Hypertrophied and Failing Spontaneously Hypertensive Rats. Hypertension 33: 60–65.
21. Boluyt MO, Robinson KG, Meredith AL, Sen S, Lakatta EG, et al. (2005) Heart failure after long-term supravalvular aortic constriction in rats. Am J Hypertens 18: 202–212.
22. Mendes OC, Sugizaki MM, Campos DS, Damatto RL, Leopoldo AS, et al. (2012) Exercise tolerance in rats with aortic stenosis and ventricular diastolic and/or systolic dysfunction. Arq Bras Cardiol 100: 44–51.
23. Ferreira JCB, Rolim NPL, Bartholomeu JB, Gobatto CA, Kokubun E, et al. (2007) Maximal lactate steady state in running mice: effect of exercise training. Clin Exp Pharmacol Physiol 34: 760–765.
24. Carvalho JF, Masuda MO, Pompeu FAMS (2005) Method for diagnosis and control of aerobic training in rats based on lactate threshold. Comp Biochem Physiol A Mol Integr Physiol 140: 409–413.
25. Baldari C, Bonavolontà V, Emerenziani GP, Gallotta MC, Silva AJ, et al. (2009) Accuracy, reliability, linearity of Accutrend and Lactate Pro versus EBIO plus analyzer. Eur J Appl Physiol 107: 105–111.
26. Pérez EH, Dawood H, Chetty U, Esterhuizen TM, Bizaare M (2008) Validation of the Accutrend lactate meter for hyperlactatemia screening during antiretroviral therapy in a resource-poor setting. Int J Infect Dis 12: 553–556.
27. De Sousa E, Lechêne P, Fortin D, N'Guessan B, Belmadani S, et al. (2002) Cardiac and skeletal muscle energy metabolism in heart failure: beneficial effects of voluntary activity. Cardiovasc Res 56: 260–268.
28. Siu PM, Donley DA, Bryner RW, Alway SE (2004) Myogenin and oxidative enzyme gene expression levels are elevated in rat soleus muscles after endurance training. J Appl Physiol 97: 277–285.
29. Picard MH, Adams D, Bierig SM, Dent JM, Douglas PS, et al. (2011) American Society of Echocardiography recommendations for quality echocardiography laboratory operations. J Am Soc Echocardiogr 24: 1–10.
30. Brooke MH, Kaiser KK (1970) Muscle fiber types: how many and what kind? Arch Neurol 23: 369–379.
31. De Souza RWA, Aguiar AF, Carani FR, Campos GER, Padovani CR, et al. (2011) High-intensity resistance training with insufficient recovery time between bouts induce atrophy and alterations in Myosin heavy chain content in rat skeletal muscle. Anat Rec (Hoboken) 294: 1393–1400.
32. Bass A, Brdiczka D, Eyer P, Hofer S, Pette D (1969) Metabolic differentiation of distinct muscle types at the level of enzymatic organization. Eur J Biochem 10: 198–206.

33. Wilkinson JH (1965) Introducción al diagnostic enzimático. 3a ed. Ediciones Toray, editor Buenos Aires.
34. Yu Z, Li P, Zhang M, Hannink M, Stamler JS, et al. (2008) Fiber type-specific nitric oxide protects oxidative myofibers against cachectic stimuli. PLoS One 3: e2086.
35. Braun TP, Grossberg AJ, Krasnow SM, Levasseur PR, Szumowski M, et al. (2013) Cancer- and endotoxin-induced cachexia require intact glucocorticoid signaling in skeletal muscle. FASEB J 27(9): 3572–3582.
36. Harrington D, Anker SD, Chua TP, Webb-Peploe KM, Ponikowski PP, et al. (1997) Skeletal muscle function and its relation to exercise tolerance in chronic heart failure. J Am Coll Cardiol 30: 1758–1764.
37. Niebauer J, Pflaum CD, Clark AL, Strasburger CJ, Hooper J, et al. (1998) Deficient insulin-like growth factor I in chronic heart failure predicts altered body composition, anabolic deficiency, cytokine and neurohormonal activation. J Am Coll Cardiol 32: 393–397.
38. Piepoli MF, Davos C, Francis DP, Coats AJS (2004) Exercise training meta-analysis of trials in patients with chronic heart failure (ExTraMATCH). BMJ 328: 189.
39. Gielen S, Adams V, Linke A, Erbs S, Möbius-Winkler S, et al. (2005) Exercise training in chronic heart failure: correlation between reduced local inflammation and improved oxidative capacity in the skeletal muscle. Eur J Cardiovasc Prev Rehabil 12: 393–400.
40. Bacurau AVN, Jardim MA, Ferreira JCB, Bechara LRG, Bueno CR, et al. (2009) Sympathetic hyperactivity differentially affects skeletal muscle mass in developing heart failure: role of exercise training. J Appl Physiol 106: 1631–1640.
41. Giannuzzi P, Temporelli PL, Corrà U, Tavazzi L (2003) Antiremodeling effect of long-term exercise training in patients with stable chronic heart failure: results of the Exercise in Left Ventricular Dysfunction and Chronic Heart Failure (ELVD-CHF) Trial. Circulation 108: 554–559.
42. Smart NA, Steele M (2011) The effect of physical training on systemic proinflammatory cytokine expression in heart failure patients: a systematic review. Congest Heart Fail 17: 110–114.
43. Grondard C, Biondi O, Pariset C, Lopes P, Deforges S, et al. (2008) Exercise-induced modulation of calcineurin activity parallels the time course of myofibre transitions. J Cell Physiol 214: 126–135.
44. Sinoway LI, Li J (2005) A perspective on the muscle reflex: implications for congestive heart failure. J Appl Physiol 99: 5–22.
45. Moreira JBN, Bechara LRG, Bozi LHM, Jannig PR, Monteiro AWA, et al. (2013) High- versus moderate-intensity aerobic exercise training effects on skeletal muscle of infarcted rats. J Appl Physiol 114: 1029–1041.
46. Van Hees HWH, Li Y-P, Ottenheijm CAC, Jin B, Pigmans CJC, et al. (2008) Proteasome inhibition improves diaphragm function in congestive heart failure rats. Am J Physiol Lung Cell Mol Physiol 294: L1260–8.
47. Carvalho RF, Cicogna AC, Campos GER, De Assis JMF, Padovani CR, et al. (2003) Myosin heavy chain expression and atrophy in rat skeletal muscle during transition from cardiac hypertrophy to heart failure. Int J Exp Pathol 84: 201–206.
48. Santos DP, Okoshi K, Moreira VO, Seiva FRF, Almeida FLA, et al. (2010) Growth hormone attenuates skeletal muscle changes in experimental chronic heart failure. Growth Horm IGF Res 20: 149–155.
49. Riley DA, Bain JL, Thompson JL, Fitts RH, Widrick JJ, et al. (1998) Disproportionate loss of thin filaments in human soleus muscle after 17-day bed rest. Muscle Nerve 21: 1280–1289.
50. Wing SS, Haas AL, Goldberg AL (1995) Increase in ubiquitin-protein conjugates concomitant with the increase in proteolysis in rat skeletal muscle during starvation and atrophy denervation. Biochem J 307 Pt 3: 639–645.
51. Li P, Waters RE, Redfern SI, Zhang M, Mao L, et al. (2007) Oxidative phenotype protects myofibers from pathological insults induced by chronic heart failure in mice. Am J Pathol 170: 599–608.
52. Argilés JM, López-Soriano FJ (1999) The role of cytokines in cancer cachexia. Med Res Rev 19: 223–248.
53. Dalla Libera L, Sabbadini R, Renken C, Ravara B, Sandri M, et al. (2001) Apoptosis in the skeletal muscle of rats with heart failure is associated with increased serum levels of TNF-alpha and sphingosine. J Mol Cell Cardiol 33: 1871–1878.
54. Batista ML, Rosa JC, Lopes RD, Lira FS, Martins E, et al. (2010) Exercise training changes IL-10/TNF-alpha ratio in the skeletal muscle of post-MI rats. Cytokine 49: 102–108.
55. Petersen AMW, Pedersen BK (2005) The anti-inflammatory effect of exercise. J Appl Physiol 98: 1154–1162.
56. Charters Y, Grimble RF (1989) Effect of recombinant human tumour necrosis factor alpha on protein synthesis in liver, skeletal muscle and skin of rats. Biochem J 258: 493–497.
57. Acharyya S, Ladner KJ, Nelsen LL, Damrauer J, Reiser PJ, et al. (2004) Cancer cachexia is regulated by selective targeting of skeletal muscle gene products. J Clin Invest 114: 370–378.
58. Carvalho RF, Castan EP, Coelho CA, Lopes FS, Almeida FLA, et al. (2010) Heart failure increases atrogin-1 and MuRF1 gene expression in skeletal muscle with fiber type-specific atrophy. J Mol Histol 41: 81–87.
59. Gielen S, Sandri M, Kozarez I, Kratzsch J, Teupser D, et al. (2012) Exercise training attenuates MuRF-1 expression in the skeletal muscle of patients with chronic heart failure independent of age: the randomized Leipzig Exercise Intervention in Chronic Heart Failure and Aging catabolism study. Circulation 125: 2716–2727.
60. McPherron AC, Lawler AM, Lee SJ (1997) Regulation of skeletal muscle mass in mice by a new TGF-beta superfamily member. Nature 387: 83–90.
61. Matsakas A, Bozzo C, Cacciani N, Caliaro F, Reggiani C, et al. (2006) Effect of swimming on myostatin expression in white and red gastrocnemius muscle and in cardiac muscle of rats. Exp Physiol 91: 983–994.
62. Matsakas A, Friedel A, Hertrampf T, Diel P (2005) Short-term endurance training results in a muscle-specific decrease of myostatin mRNA content in the rat. Acta Physiol Scand 183: 299–307.
63. Brink M, Price SR, Chrast J, Bailey JL, Anwar A, et al. (2001) Angiotensin II induces skeletal muscle wasting through enhanced protein degradation and down-regulates autocrine insulin-like growth factor I. Endocrinology 142: 1489–1496.
64. Arcopinto M, Bobbio E, Bossone E, Perrone-Filardi P, Napoli R, et al. (2013) The GH/IGF-1 axis in chronic heart failure. Endocr Metab Immune Disord Drug Targets 13: 76–91.
65. Schiaffino S, Dyar KA, Ciciliot S, Blaauw B, Sandri M (2013) Mechanisms regulating skeletal muscle growth and atrophy. FEBS J 280: 4294–4314.
66. Li JB, Wassner SJ (1986) Protein synthesis and degradation in skeletal muscle of chronically uremic rats. Kidney Int 29: 1136–1143.
67. Argadine HM, Hellyer NJ, Mantilla CB, Zhan W, Sieck GC (2009) The effect of denervation on protein synthesis and degradation in adult rat diaphragm muscle. J Appl Physiol 107: 438–444.
68. Reed SA, Sandesara PB, Senf SM, Judge AR (2012) Inhibition of FoxO transcriptional activity prevents muscle fiber atrophy during cachexia and induces hypertrophy. FASEB J 26: 987–1000.
69. Lin J, Wu H, Tarr PT, Zhang C, Wu Z, et al. (2002) Transcriptional co-activator PGC-1 alpha drives the formation of slow-twitch muscle fibres. Nature 418: 797–801.
70. Arany Z (2008) PGC-1 coactivators and skeletal muscle adaptations in health and disease. Curr Opin Genet Dev 18: 426–434.
71. Geng T, Li P, Yin X, Yan Z (2011) PGC-1α promotes nitric oxide antioxidant defenses and inhibits FOXO signaling against cardiac cachexia in mice. Am J Pathol 178: 1738–1748.
72. Minnaard R, Drost MR, Wagenmakers AJM, van Kranenburg GP, Kuipers H, et al. (2005) Skeletal Muscle wasting and contractile performance in septic rats. Muscle Nerve 31: 339–348.
73. Russell AP, Feilchenfeldt J, Schreiber S, Praz M, Crettenand A, et al. (2003) Endurance training in humans leads to fiber type-specific increases in levels of peroxisome proliferator-activated receptor-gamma coactivator-1 and peroxisome proliferator-activated receptor-alpha in skeletal muscle. Diabetes 52: 2874–2881.
74. Baar K, Wende AR, Jones TE, Marison M, Nolte LA, et al. (2002) Adaptations of skeletal muscle to exercise: rapid increase in the transcriptional coactivator PGC-1. FASEB J 16: 1879–1886.
75. Ruas JL, White JP, Rao RR, Kleiner S, Brannan KT, et al. (2012) A PGC-1α isoform induced by resistance training regulates skeletal muscle hypertrophy. Cell 151: 1319–1331.
76. Piepoli MF, Conraads V, Corrà U, Dickstein K, Francis DP, et al. (2011) Exercise training in heart failure: from theory to practice. A consensus document of the Heart Failure Association and the European Association for Cardiovascular Prevention and Rehabilitation. Eur J Heart Fail 13: 347–357.
77. Weinberg EO, Schoen FJ, George D, Kagaya Y, Douglas PS, et al. (1994) Angiotensin-converting enzyme inhibition prolongs survival and modifies the transition to heart failure in rats with pressure overload hypertrophy due to ascending aortic stenosis. Circulation 90: 1410–1422.
78. Pacagnelli F, Okoshi K, Henrique DH, Campos S, Souza RWA, et al. (2014) Physical training attenuates cardiac remodeling in rats with supra-aortic stenosis. Exp Clin Cardiol 20: 3889–3905.
79. Bregagnollo EA, Mestrinel MA, Okoshi K, Carvalho FC, Bregagnollo IF, et al. (2007) Relative role of left ventricular geometric remodeling and of morphological and functional myocardial remodeling in the transition from compensated hypertrophy to heart failure in rats with supravalvar aortic stenosis. Arq Bras Cardiol 88: 225–233.

Defining Disease Phenotypes Using National Linked Electronic Health Records: A Case Study of Atrial Fibrillation

Katherine I. Morley[1,2,3*⊕], Joshua Wallace[1⊕], Spiros C. Denaxas[1], Ross J. Hunter[4], Riyaz S. Patel[1,5], Pablo Perel[1,6], Anoop D. Shah[1], Adam D. Timmis[4], Richard J. Schilling[4], Harry Hemingway[1]

1 Farr Institute of Health Informatics Research, University College London, London, United Kingdom, and Clinical Epidemiology, Department of Epidemiology and Public Health, University College London, London, United Kingdom, **2** Institute of Psychiatry, Psychology and Neuroscience, King's College London, London, United Kingdom, **3** Melbourne School of Global and Population Health, The University of Melbourne, Melbourne, Australia, **4** Barts NIHR Biomedical Research Unit, Queen Mary University London, London, United Kingdom, **5** The Heart Hospital, University College London NHS Trust, London, United Kingdom, **6** London School of Hygiene and Tropical Medicine, London, United Kingdom

Abstract

Background: National electronic health records (EHR) are increasingly used for research but identifying disease cases is challenging due to differences in information captured between sources (e.g. primary and secondary care). Our objective was to provide a transparent, reproducible model for integrating these data using atrial fibrillation (AF), a chronic condition diagnosed and managed in multiple ways in different healthcare settings, as a case study.

Methods: Potentially relevant codes for AF screening, diagnosis, and management were identified in four coding systems: Read (primary care diagnoses and procedures), British National Formulary (BNF; primary care prescriptions), ICD-10 (secondary care diagnoses) and OPCS-4 (secondary care procedures). From these we developed a phenotype algorithm via expert review and analysis of linked EHR data from 1998 to 2010 for a cohort of 2.14 million UK patients aged ≥30 years. The cohort was also used to evaluate the phenotype by examining associations between incident AF and known risk factors.

Results: The phenotype algorithm incorporated 286 codes: 201 Read, 63 BNF, 18 ICD-10, and four OPCS-4. Incident AF diagnoses were recorded for 72,793 patients, but only 39.6% (N = 28,795) were recorded in primary care and secondary care. An additional 7,468 potential cases were inferred from data on treatment and pre-existing conditions. The proportion of cases identified from each source differed by diagnosis age; inferred diagnoses contributed a greater proportion of younger cases (≤60 years), while older patients (≥80 years) were mainly diagnosed in SC. Associations of risk factors (hypertension, myocardial infarction, heart failure) with incident AF defined using different EHR sources were comparable in magnitude to those from traditional consented cohorts.

Conclusions: A single EHR source is not sufficient to identify all patients, nor will it provide a representative sample. Combining multiple data sources and integrating information on treatment and comorbid conditions can substantially improve case identification.

Editor: Stefan Kiechl, Innsbruck Medical University, Austria

Funding: This study was carried out on behalf of the ClinicAL research using LInked bespoke studies and Electronic health Records (CALIBER) programme. This study was supported by National Institute for Health Research (ADT, HH, RP-PG-0407-10314), Wellcome Trust (ADT, HH, 086091/Z/08/Z), and the Medical Research Council Prognosis Research Strategy (PROGRESS) Partnership (PP, ADT, HH, G0902393/99558; www.progress-partnership.org), and by awards to establish the Farr Institute of Health Informatics Research at UCL Partners (HH, SCD, ADT), from the Medical Research Council, Arthritis Research UK, British Heart Foundation, Cancer Research UK, Chief Scientist Office, Economic and Social Research Council, Engineering and Physical Sciences Research Council, National Institute for Health Research, National Institute for Social Care and Health Research, and Wellcome Trust (ADT, HH, grant MR/K006584/1). KIM and JW were supported by the PROGRESS Partnership while undertaking this research. SCD was supported by a UCL Provost's Strategic Development Fund Fellowship. ADS was supported by a clinical research training fellowship from the Wellcome Trust (0938/30/Z/10/Z). ADT was supported by Barts and The London NIHR Cardiovascular Biomedical Research Unit, funded by the National Institute for Health Research. The funders had no role in study design, data collection and analysis, decision to publish, or preparation of the manuscript.

Competing Interests: The authors have declared that no competing interests exist.

* Email: katherine.morley@ucl.ac.uk

⊕ These authors contributed equally to this work.

Introduction

One of the major challenges presented by the increasing use of electronic health record (EHR) data for research is the development of strategies for reliably identifying disease cases [1–4]. Hripcsak and Albers [5] argue that in order to improve the extraction of disease information from this type of data:

> *...[W]e need a better understanding of the EHR. The EHR is not a direct reflection of the patient and physiology, but a reflection of the recording process inherent in healthcare with noise and feedback loops. We must study the EHR as an object in itself, as if it were a natural system.*(p. 119)

This recommendation is particularly relevant to identification of chronic conditions in which patients may have multiple interactions with primary and secondary care, and undergo assessments and diagnostic tests, before ultimately receiving a diagnosis. Even after diagnosis, patients may receive follow-up care such as monitoring, prescriptions, or other medical interventions [6]. Consequently, one EHR data source rarely covers the full patient journey; usually data from different record sources (e.g. primary, secondary, and tertiary care; medication prescription and dispensing; mortality data) must be integrated to obtain a complete picture [7]. However, these data also encompass variation in patient measurement that may be context-dependent and thus effective integration requires an exploration of what is recorded in the EHR in relation to a particular condition, and how this compares to expectations based upon guidelines and preconceptions about clinical practice [4,8,9].

To highlight the challenges and complexities of identifying onset of a chronic condition in linked national EHR data, and how these can inform the development of strategies for identifying patients, we present a case study of atrial fibrillation (AF) using national linked EHR and administrative health data from the English National Health Service (NHS). AF is the most common cardiac arrhythmia, associated with increased risk of stroke, heart failure (HF), and premature mortality [10,11]. It presents many important challenges that may be encountered when developing strategies for case identification, or phenotypes, in EHR data including variability in symptoms and signs, different coding strategies and treatment options, and changes in clinical practice (for more in-depth discussion see [12]).

Clinical context of atrial fibrillation

Onset of AF often precedes diagnosis considerably; patients may be asymptomatic or experience paroxysmal AF (characterized by irregular, sudden symptoms) and clinical signs, such as irregular pulse, may be episodic. AF may also be diagnosed when a patient is admitted to hospital for another, potentially unrelated, condition. UK diagnostic guidelines and those from the European Society of Cardiology (ESC) recommend pulse palpation followed by an electrocardiogram if an irregular pulse is detected [13,14]. Opportunistic screening of patients over the age of 65 is recommended by the ESC, but not by North American organisations [15].

Confirming an AF diagnosis does not necessarily simplify documentation as recording and treatment may differ between primary and secondary care, which use different coding systems with different levels of granularity. Read codes, a subset of the Systematic Nomenclature Of Medicine - Clinical Terms (SNOMED-CT) clinical terminology, are used in primary care and permit specification of disease subtypes and differentiation of AF from atrial flutter. In contrast, the International Classification of Disease – 10th revision (ICD-10) terminology used in secondary care has one term for all categories. Treatment varies between patients depending upon symptoms, age and other clinical characteristics, and clinical context. Currently, most patients receive anti-thrombotic treatment to reduce stroke risk, although drugs for rate or rhythm control, and procedures such as cardioversion or catheter ablation, may also be used [14].

AF diagnostic and treatment practices have changed substantially over the last 10–15 years. This is due to increasing awareness of AF and recognition that, at least in the UK, it is more likely to be subject to under, rather than over, diagnosis [16,17]. Policy initiatives have been introduced in the UK to address this including: the 2004 Quality and Outcomes Framework (QOF), which financially rewards general practitioners for implementing treatment plans for chronic conditions, including AF [18]; the 2006 UK National Institute for Health and Care Excellence guidelines for AF diagnosis and management [19]; the English NHS Commissioning for Quality and Innovation (CQUIN) scheme, introduced in 2009 to provide financial incentives for quality improvements. Thus there may be temporal differences in coding practices for AF.

Identification of patients with atrial fibrillation

A consistent approach to integrating EHR and administrative health data to identify AF will facilitate transparent and reproducible research, but currently no universal method exists. Previous UK EHR studies have focused on primary care [20–23], but other studies used secondary care data. We reviewed research on AF risk factors and found substantial variation in the data sources used to identify AF cases; 21 of 27 studies identified used EHR data, with two using primary care [24,25], 15 using secondary care [26–40], and four using both [41–44]. However, many researchers are developing strategies for integrating EHR data for research and defining EHR phenotypes [2,45–51]. The USA-based eMERGE Consortium have developed an AF phenotype algorithm [52], but this was created for data from nine health care providers actively participating in research and focuses on clinical notes and electrocardiogram impressions. As these data are not available on a large scale to researchers in the UK, and elsewhere, using data from nationalised health services, our aims were to develop an understanding of EHR data relating to AF, and to use this to develop a phenotype algorithm applicable to linked, nationally collected data.

Thus we describe the development of the ClinicAl disease research using Linked Bespoke studies and Electronic Records (CALIBER) AF phenotype and use this to demonstrate how exploration of recording patterns in multiple data sources can inform the development of disease case identification strategies for EHR data. We investigated whether EHR data beyond diagnosis codes could be leveraged to refine date of disease onset; whether cases could be inferred on the basis of medical treatment; and whether changes in health care policy may have affected data collection. We evaluated the face validity of the phenotype by testing for associations with known risk factors. The strategies used and lessons learned are broadly applicable to all EHR phenotype development, particularly where the aim is to identify disease cases for longitudinal research.

Materials and Methods

Study population and linked electronic records

Anonymised patients were selected from the CALIBER cohort, which includes linked data from: (1) primary care EHR data: diagnoses coded using the Read system by general practitioners during consultation or by practice administrators from hospital discharge letters (from the Clinical Practice Research Datalink) and prescriptions; (2) secondary care administrative records: diagnoses and procedures recorded using the ICD terminology and Office of Population Censuses and Surveys Classification of Interventions and Procedures (OPCS-4, comparable to the American Medical Association Current Procedural Terminology medical classification system) by audit nurses after patient admission by abstracting data from hospital records (from Hospital Episode Statistics); (3) administrative mortality data from death certificates where cause(s) of death are recorded by a doctor and ICD-9 and ICD-10 codes added by trained non-clinical coders (from UK Office of National Statistics; ONS); (4) small-area patient social deprivation information from multiple administrative data sets (from ONS) [12]. CALIBER was approved by the Lewisham Local Research Ethics Committee (ref:09/H0810/16 date: 08/04/2009) and the Ethics and Confidentiality Committee (ECC) (ref: ECC 2-06(b)/2009 CALIBER dataset). CALIBER has been registered with the University College London Data Protection Officer (ref: Z6364106/2009/2/26). CALIBER EHR data are anonymized; individual informed consent was not sought from study participants.

Inclusion criteria were: age greater than 30, minimum one year of validated data prior to entry, and registration at a primary care provider with up-to-standard data. This defined a base cohort of 2,128,151 individuals in which to identify AF. Exclusion criteria were any records of AF diagnosis prior to cohort entry, or the first record of AF after entry being a term indicating monitoring of existing AF or a historical diagnosis of AF. Patients were included and followed-up from the date they met all inclusion criteria or January 1st, 1998, whichever was later. Follow-up ended on: the first of the administrative censoring date for primary care data (March 26th, 2010); last data collection date for a particular primary care provider; a patient leaving their primary care provider; or patient death as recorded in ONS. Risk factor analyses excluded patients with missing data for blood pressure (BP) measurements, body mass index (BMI), ethnicity or index of multiple deprivation score.

Strategy for EHR phenotype development

The CALIBER approach to EHR phenotype development iteratively cycles between expert discussion, review of codes and their semantic relations, and analysis of data (see Figure 1). An initial case definition listing codes, or combinations of codes, indicating diagnosis of a condition is drafted based on discussion with experts in the clinical phenotype, epidemiology, computer science, and bioinformatics. For AF, this preliminary definition only included diagnosis codes directly related to AF from primary or secondary care (extraction of data from free text or image processing is currently limited), but we also identified codes for medications and procedures used in AF treatment for further investigation (lists of all identified codes are available online on the CALIBER Data Portal at www.caliberresearch.org).

Initial examination of code usage. A test data set of 100,000 patients was used to investigate how frequently codes were used in practice, and the relationship between diagnosis codes and those for medications and procedures. We found, as have others [53], that although codes for AF subtypes exist within the Read system, they are infrequently used and most patients simply have an all-encompassing diagnosis of AF recorded. Codes indicating an existing condition (e.g. when taking a new patient's history) and monitoring of AF are used, but the main codes recorded relate to a diagnosis of AF. We examined procedure and prescription codes to see if they could assist in identifying additional cases. For procedure codes, the overall frequency was low and they were almost always recorded for patients with a pre-existing AF diagnosis. However, many patients had prescription records for warfarin or digoxin (medications used almost exclusively to treat AF during the time frame of the available data), but no AF diagnosis code.

Review of these results by the expert group led to three decisions: (i) due to the infrequent coding of AF subtypes in primary care, and the single ICD-10 code in secondary care, we should develop an AF phenotype algorithm combining all subtypes; (ii) the case definition should not include procedure codes; (iii) where AF-related prescriptions were made without recorded diagnoses, we should investigate whether a diagnosis of AF could be reasonably inferred. To pursue the latter aim, we developed case definitions based on clinical knowledge of treatment patterns strongly indicative of AF; warfarin prescriptions in the absence of prior deep vein thrombosis (DVT) or pulmonary embolism (PE), or digoxin prescriptions in the absence of heart failure (HF) were taken as evidence to support an "inferred" diagnosis of AF. These conditions were identified using previously defined CALIBER phenotype algorithms for DVT, PE, and HF (see CALIBER Data Portal at www.caliberresearch.org for details).

Exploration of the EHR

Refining disease onset. We investigated the time elapsed between incident AF diagnoses recorded using ICD-10 or Read codes in multiple data sources to see if combing data improved estimation of disease onset. We also investigated the utility of further refining onset using an indicator marker (irregular pulse), examining the frequency of these codes and the time that elapsed between the relevant code(s) being recorded and a subsequent coded diagnosis of AF.

Disease case identification. We investigated whether combining multiple sources of EHR data increased the overall number of disease cases identified by permitting us to infer AF diagnoses on the basis of patterns of medication use and comorbid conditions.

Characteristics of diagnosed patients

As the phenotype algorithm we developed was used to identify diagnoses from different data sources over an extended time period, we wanted to explore whether there were context-level and/or patient-level differences in the cases identified. We quantified the unique and non-unique AF cases identified in each source. We then investigated the relationship between the data source and (i) diagnosis context, specifically the year of diagnosis and whether AF was the primary or secondary reason for admission for secondary care diagnoses (HES provides up 15 secondary diagnosis codes); and (ii) individual patient characteristics at diagnosis including sex, age, and important comorbid conditions (HF, myocardial infarction, hypertension, stroke, diabetes, thyroid disease, renal failure, and chronic obstructive pulmonary disease).

Association with known risk factors

The face validity of the CALIBER AF phenotype was evaluated by conducting a pre-specified analysis of the association between AF diagnosis and factors for which there is strong prior evidence of

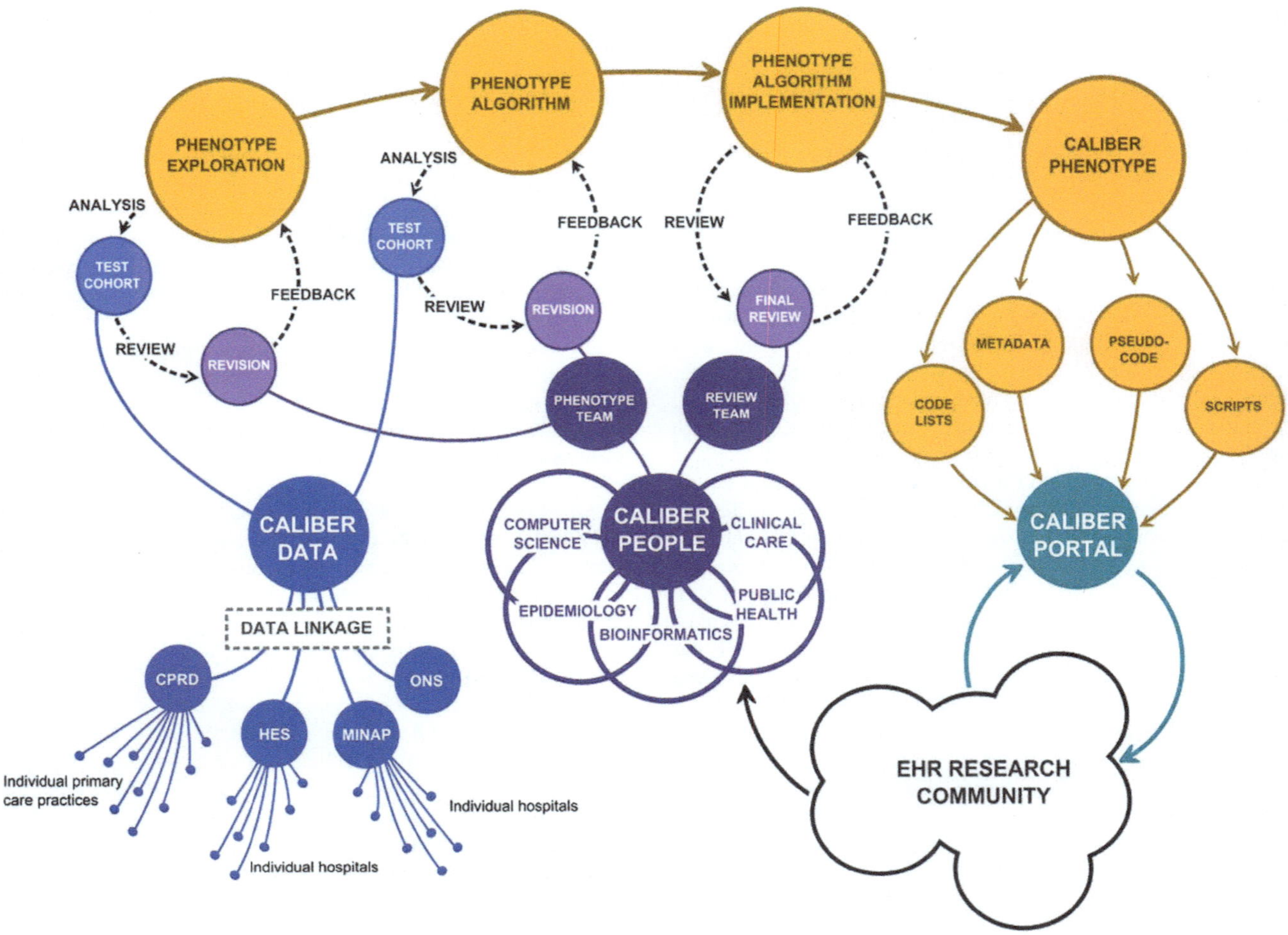

Figure 1. Illustration of phenotype algorithm developing using the Clinical Research Using Linked Bespoke Studies and Electronic health records (CALIBER) programme. CPRD represents the Clinical Practice Research Data link; HES represents Hospital Episode Statistics; MINAP is the Myocardial Ischaemia National Audit Registry; ONS is the UK Office of National Statistics (mortality and social deprivation data).

association with AF diagnosis from both clinical observations and multiple epidemiological studies: HF, hypertension, and myocardial infarction (MI) [11]. Cause specific Cox proportional hazards models were used to estimate hazard ratio and 95% confidence intervals for incident AF diagnosis associated with baseline measures of risk factors, adjusted for age, sex, and primary care practice [54,55]. All analyses excluded patients diagnosed with AF prior to study baseline. All statistical analyses were conducted in R version 15.2 for Mac and Linux [56].

Results

Sample characteristics

We identified 24 codes (23 Read codes and one ICD-10 code) relating to AF diagnosis. Ten codes refer to monitoring of pre-existing AF, three confirm a prior diagnosis of AF, and the remaining 11 indicate diagnosis by a current care provider. The CALIBER cohort of 2,128,151 participants included 33,383 individuals with an AF code in their record indicating diagnosis prior to cohort entry. Thus, at baseline, approximately 1.6% of the sample had already received a diagnosis of AF, which is similar to prevalence estimate of 2.0% (95% C.I. 1.6–2.4%) provided by the recent UK-based general population ECHOES study [57]. Of the remaining 2,094,768 patients without an AF diagnosis at baseline, 72,793 received their first recorded AF diagnosis code during the study period. A total of 22,939 (45.2%) of patients were initially diagnosed in primary care, with the remaining 39,863 (54.8%) initially diagnosed in secondary care (those diagnosed on the same date in two sources were attributed to secondary care).

Exploration of the EHR

Refining disease onset: Timeframe for diagnosis. To investigate whether combining data from primary and secondary care improved resolution of disease onset, we examined the data for 28,795 individuals with incident diagnoses recorded in both primary and secondary care. The time elapsed between AF diagnoses in the two sources depended on the source of the initial diagnosis. An AF diagnosis was first recorded in primary care for 13,707 individuals, and in secondary care for 10,380 individuals (for 4,708 individuals the dates were the same). The median time from primary care diagnosis to secondary care diagnosis was just over one year (367.0 days), while the mean was almost two years (724.4 days). In contrast, the median time from secondary to primary care AF diagnosis was 20 days (mean 212.6 days).

Refining disease onset: Irregular pulse. The primary care Read code system includes five codes for pulse palpation: two indicate a normal or "regular" pulse, and three indicate an "irregular" pulse. Only 1,252 (1.78%) of the 72,793 participants with an incident AF diagnosis had any pulse palpation recorded between study entry and AF diagnosis, with irregular pulse the record closest to AF diagnosis for 964 patients (77.1% of those with any pulse palpation recorded). The median time from first irregular pulse to AF diagnosis in patients where both were recorded after study entry was 71 days. Less than half (40.1%) of patients were diagnosed with AF by 30 days after the irregular pulse code, with 65.8% diagnosed by 12 months.

Disease case identification: Inferred diagnosis. Inferred diagnoses were identified based on a combination of 262 codes: 63 relating to prescriptions (36 for warfarin, 27 for digoxin) and 199 excluding conditions (97 for prior HF, 60 for prior DVT, 22 for prior PE) and procedures (20 for heart valve replacement). A total of 39,527 patients met the criteria for an inferred diagnosis of AF during the study period. Warfarin prescriptions accounted for 18,714 (47%) patient diagnoses, digoxin prescriptions for 10,592 (28%), and the remaining 10,221 (26%) had both prescription patterns. A small percentage of patients with an inferred diagnosis (3,754; 9.5%) received coded or historical diagnoses of AF prior to cohort entry. Of the remaining 35,773 individuals, 28,305 (71.6%) had an AF diagnosis code recorded during follow-up and 7,468 (18.9%) had no codes relating to AF diagnosis in their record.

Of the 28,305 individuals who met the inferred AF diagnosis criteria and had an AF diagnosis code within the study window, the majority (75.7%; 21,420 individuals) received the diagnosis code before meeting the criteria for an inferred diagnosis, and for a further 11.2% (3,167 individuals) this occurred on the same day. Thus only 13% of patients (3,718 individuals) met the inferred diagnosis criteria before an AF diagnosis was recorded. For these 3,718 individuals, the average time between an inferred diagnosis and receiving a diagnosis code was 19.8 months (median 6.54 months). Within 30 days of meeting inferred diagnosis criteria, 21.1% of these patients received a diagnosis code; 59.7% received a diagnosis code within one year. However, the temporal relationship between these diagnoses varied depending on the year of the initial inferred diagnosis; the proportion receiving a diagnosis code within 12 months increased gradually over time from 37.1% in 1998 to 92.3% in 2009. The proportion of AF cases based on inferred criteria also decreased over the study period, from just over 15% of cases in 1998 to less than 10% of cases from 2006 onwards.

EHR phenotype algorithm

The results above informed the development of the AF phenotype algorithm in two ways. First, as pulse palpation was only recorded for a small minority of patients we concluded it did not provide enough additional information to warrant inclusion in our current AF case definition. Second, although examining the pattern of treatments and co-existing conditions did identify additional disease cases, without additional information (e.g. review of free text) we could not confidently conclude that patients without a recorded AF diagnosis code should be considered as cases, or that medication prescriptions represent a diagnosis date. Consequently, we included individuals with only an inferred diagnosis in our EHR case definition as a separate category, and used date of recoded AF diagnosis code in preference to date of meeting inferred criteria.

The case definition for AF using the phenotype algorithm thus had three categories:

1. Historical: first recorded AF code indicates monitoring of an existing condition, or reference to a previous AF diagnosis.
2. Diagnosed: first record is a diagnosis code for AF; preference given to the earliest dated record rather than diagnosis source (i.e. no preference for primary *versus* secondary care).
3. Inferred: no diagnosis code is present, but the patient record includes a warfarin prescription in the absence of prior DVT or PE, or a digoxin prescription in the absence of HF.

The phenotype algorithm incorporates these definitions in a hierarchical, mutually exclusive manner (see **Figure 2**). If the earliest recorded AF codes relate to a historical diagnosis or monitoring, the patient is in category 1 which precludes inclusion in other categories. If these codes are absent, then the presence of a coded diagnosis from primary or secondary care places a patient in category 2. Finally, in the absence of a coded diagnosis, a patient may be allocated to category 3, depending on the combination of prescriptions and diagnoses in their record. Otherwise a participant is treated as undiagnosed.

Characteristics of diagnosed patients

Using the phenotype algorithm we identified 80,261 individuals with an incident coded or inferred AF diagnosis in the CALIBER cohort. Of these, 7,468 had no diagnosis code but met the inferred diagnosis criteria. Almost half the patients with a diagnosis code (39.6%; 28,795 individuals) had diagnoses recorded in both primary and secondary care (see **Figure 3**). All sources provided unique diagnoses, but substantially more were identified from secondary care, which provided almost three times the number of unique cases (32,930 cases compared to 11,068 from primary care). The proportion of AF cases identified in primary care or by inferred diagnosis decreased by year of diagnosis, whereas the proportion identified in secondary care increased, but no threshold effect was identified around the introduction of the QOF in 2004.

The proportion of cases contributed by each source differed by age at diagnosis; individuals identified by inferred diagnosis criteria made up a greater proportion of cases diagnosed at younger ages (≤60 years), while cases diagnosed at older ages (≥ 80 years) were mostly identified from secondary care data (see **Figure 4**). The proportion of cases identified in primary care was highest for ages 60–80 years, but for all age groups primary care contributed fewer cases than secondary care. For patients diagnosed in secondary care, AF was more likely to be the main diagnosis for the hospital episode when individuals were younger (≤50 years), whereas amongst those diagnosed at older ages AF was much more likely to be a secondary diagnosis made during admission for another condition. Patients with diagnoses recorded only in secondary care were slightly more likely to be female compared to those with diagnoses in both data sources, primary care only, or inferred diagnoses (51.3%, 48.2%, 48.8% and 47.6% female respectively).

The percentage of patients with comorbid conditions at the time that their AF diagnosis was recorded differed by source of diagnosis (see **Table 1**). Patients for which an AF diagnosis was drawn only from secondary care were more likely to have already received a diagnosis for all the conditions examined, with the exception of hypertension, than those with a diagnosis drawn from primary care or meeting the inferred diagnosis criteria. The difference between data sources was largest for renal failure; the percentage of patients with renal failure amongst those diagnosed with AF in secondary care only was twice that of patients with AF diagnoses recorded in the other data sources (22.4% *versus* 10.9%, 11.0%, and 10.0%). A similar, although less extreme, pattern was also observed for HF, MI, stroke, and diabetes (Type 2). This does not appear to be completely due to differences in the age of patients from each source as even within age groups the

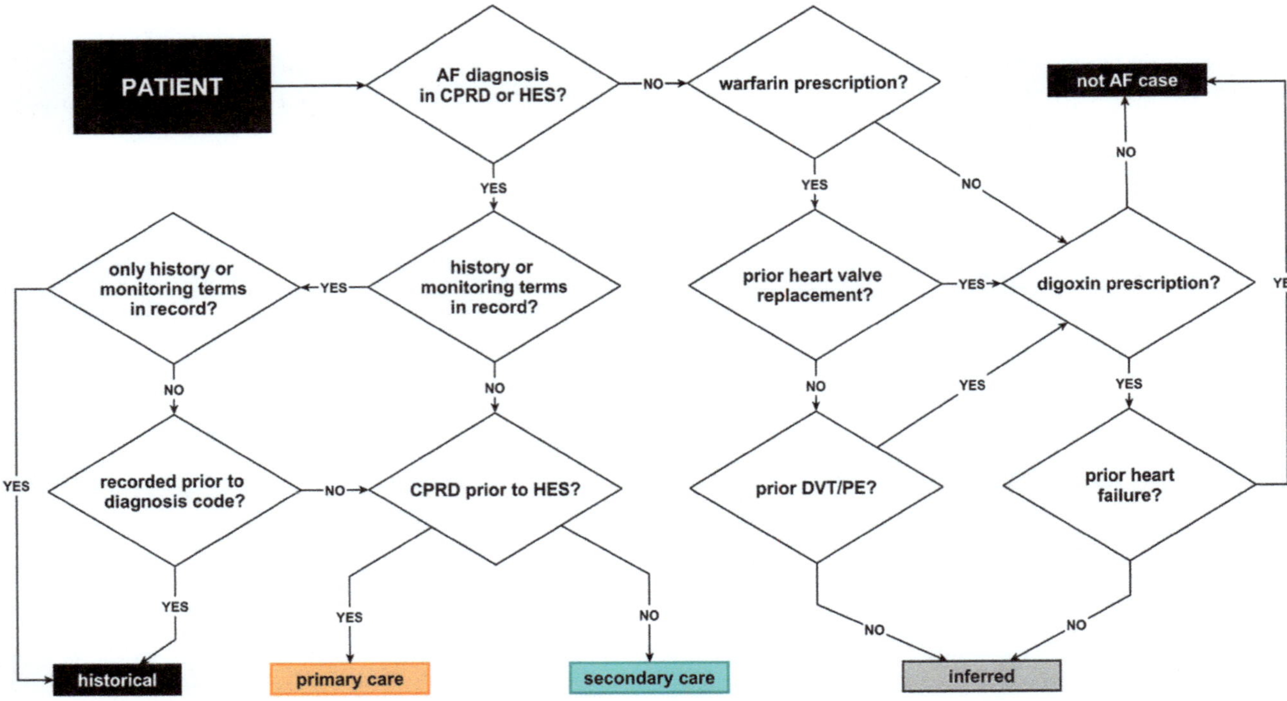

Figure 2. Flow diagram illustrating CALIBER phenotype for atrial fibrillation.

percentages of patients with pre-existing conditions were still higher for those diagnosed in secondary care, particularly for HF and diabetes. In contrast, the percentage of AF patients with hypertension was highest amongst those with a primary care diagnosis (86.0% for primary and secondary, 86.2% for primary only, compared to 83% for secondary only and 78% for inferred).

Associations with known risk factors

The associations between pre-specified risk factors and incident AF were consistent in magnitude across EHR sources and with estimates from traditional consented cohorts (see **Figure 5** and **Table S1**). For HF, the hazard ratio estimate was 2.07 (95% CI 1.95–2.19) using only primary care data for AF diagnosis, 2.31 (2.21–2.43) for secondary care data only, and 2.35 (2.25–2.46) for both sources combined (an inferred diagnosis could not be used for the HF analysis as this diagnosis is incorporated into the case definition). For hypertension, the hazard ratio estimates were 1.74 (95% CI 1.70–1.78) for primary care only, 1.80 (1.76–1.84) for secondary care only, 1.72 (1.68–1.77) for inferred diagnoses, and 1.80 (1.77–1.84) for the composite endpoint. The hazard ratio estimates for MI were 1.53 (1.46–1.60) for primary care only, 1.75 (1.68–1.82) for secondary care only, 1.69 (1.61–1.77) for inferred diagnoses, and 1.70 (1.64–1.76) for the composite endpoint.

The estimates for hypertension and MI were comparable to age and sex adjusted results from traditional cohort studies such as the Framingham Heart Study [58] (HR 1.80, 95% C.I. 1.48–2.18 for hypertension; HR 1.44, 95% C.I. 1.02–2.03 for MI) as well as those from the other EHR studies (see **Table S1**). The estimates for heart failure were towards the lower bound of those obtained from the Framingham Heart Study (HR 3.2, 95% C.I. 1.99–5.16) and EHR studies.

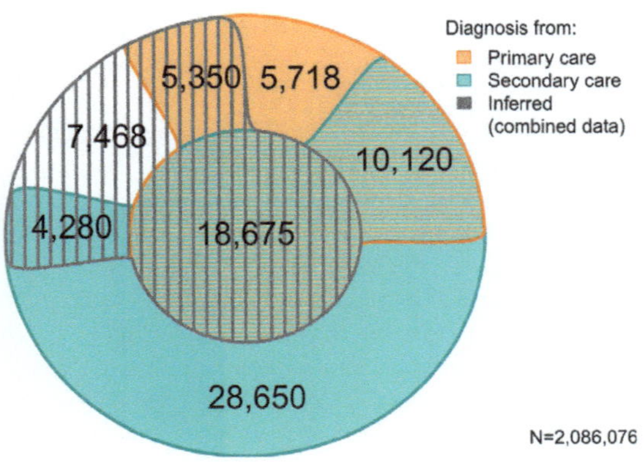

Figure 3. Euler diagram displaying the number of incident cases identified in the different sources, including overlap between multiple sources.

Discussion

We explored the characteristics of the information recorded around the diagnosis of a chronic condition, AF, in multiple linked data sources for a cohort of 2,128,151 individuals from the general population. This exploration highlighted a number of key findings with implications for EHR research on AF, and on chronic conditions more broadly. We found that: (i) refining the timing of disease onset can potentially be improved by the clinically-informed use of data that goes beyond diagnosis codes for the condition in question, but what is recorded as part of routine clinical practice may differ substantially from clinical guidelines; (ii) integrating data from multiple EHR sources and administrative data does improve case detection; (iii) the context in which data are collected may have an impact on the characteristics of the disease cases identified. We used this information to develop an EHR phenotype for identifying AF disease cases that was informed

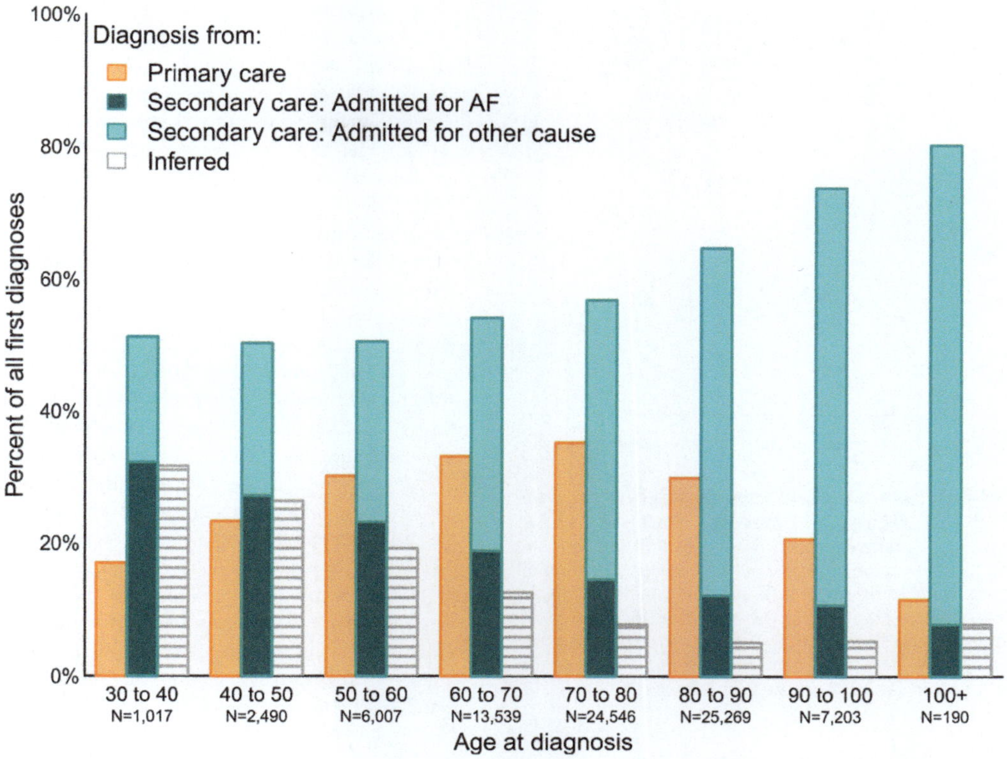

Figure 4. Proportion of incident atrial fibrillation cases identified in each source by age at diagnosis.

by an understanding of the patient record, and evaluated the face validity of it using epidemiological analyses.

Combining data from multiple sources to identify AF cases helped to refine estimates of disease onset in this sample. Using primary care data brought the date of diagnosis forward by one to two years for patients subsequently diagnosed in secondary care. Although there was a slight lag (median 20 days) from a diagnosis being recorded in secondary care to it being recorded in primary care, this more likely indicates a delay in transfer of diagnosis information from hospital to general practitioner than separate diagnoses. Pulse palpation records were investigated because this is recommended as a screening test for AF in primary care [11,14]. In our cohort, very few AF patients (just over 2%) had a record of pulse palpation prior to diagnosis and therefore these data had limited use for refining disease onset and were not incorporated into the phenotype algorithm. This underlines the importance of

Table 1. Percentage of patients with different comorbid conditions at date of atrial fibrillation diagnosis, by source of diagnosis.

Characteristic	Category	Source of diagnosis			
		Secondary only (N = 32930)	**Primary and secondary (N = 28795)**	**Primary only (N = 11068)**	**Inferred (N = 7468)**
HF		18.8	15.1	12.7	8.5
MI		13.2	10.0	8.3	14.1
Stroke		9.2	6.0	6.2	8.7
Diabetes	Type 1	0.62	0.39	0.49	0.90
	Type 2	14.73	10.79	9.40	9.53
	NOS	1.76	1.13	1.38	1.94
Hypertension		83.0	86.0	86.2	78.0
Thyroid disease	Hyper	1.7	1.5	1.6	1.0
	Hypo	8.5	7.1	6.8	5.6
Renal failure		22.4	10.9	11.0	10.0
COPD		46.9	44.7	40.9	38.7

Practice Research HF indicates heart failure, MI indicates myocardial infarction, COPD indicates chronic obstructive pulmonary disease, NOS indicates not otherwise specified. Note that some conditions may have been recorded on the same date as the atrial fibrillation diagnosis.

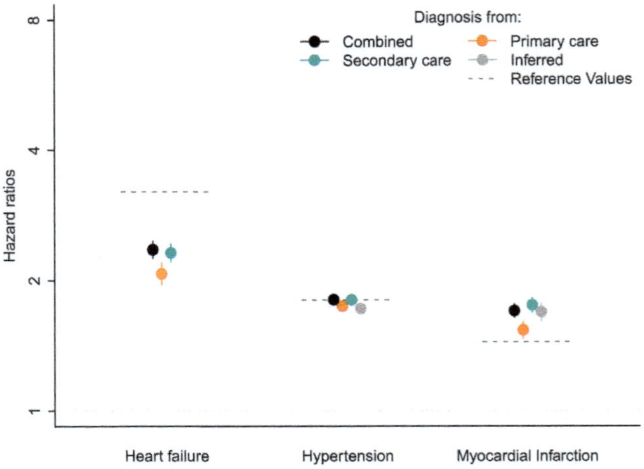

Figure 5. Hazard ratio estimates and 95% confidence intervals for pre-specified risk factors of interest. Results are shown separately for associations between each risk factor and incident AF, defined according to each source of cases and for a composite using all sources. All analyses were adjusted for age, sex, and practice ID. Note that the use of heart failure diagnosis in the algorithm for inferred AF precludes estimation of the hazard ratio. The dashed lines are point estimates of hazard ratios from the Framingham Heart Study for the same risk factors, adjusted for age and sex (see reference [58]).

understanding the EHR; a phenotype algorithm for AF based only on clinical guidelines could have required pulse palpation prior to diagnosis and would have excluded the vast majority of cases drawn from primary care data. However, Nicholson *et al.*, [2] found that "indicator markers" for rheumatoid arthritis in primary care, such as joint signs and symptoms or non-steroidal anti-inflammatory drug prescriptions, were potentially informative so the utility of "indicator markers" and screening tests should be evaluated on a disease-by-disease basis, and may inform further quality of care research as well as EHR research.

Integrating data from multiple sources identified more AF cases than examining any single source, as has been demonstrated for other cardiovascular conditions [7,59]. This was primarily due to the fact that a substantial percentage of cases were unique to each data source (13.8% from primary care, 41.0% from secondary care), but integrating data from both sources to infer diagnoses also identified unique cases (9.3%). This demonstrates that clinically informed combinations of treatment records and diagnoses of other conditions can be useful for interrogating EHR datasets, although this may not be true for all conditions in all contexts. For example, Pascoe *et al.* [60] found that procedure codes (such as mastectomy) and prescriptions (such as tamoxifen) could be combined to improve identification of cancer cases in UK EHR data, but we found that procedure codes (such as direct current cardioversion) did not improve AF case detection because they were almost exclusively recorded in patients with a pre-existing AF diagnosis. Additionally, coding combinations could be so complex for some conditions that this approach is infeasible; the inferred AF diagnosis incorporated not only medications but also whether diagnoses were recorded for another condition for which these medications might be used, namely HF, DVT, and PE. The CALIBER programme facilitated this as case definitions and associated EHR phenotypes had already been developed for these conditions; without access to a resource such as this, use of treatment and/or comorbidity information could be substantially more onerous.

The AF patients we identified differed by data source in regard to age, sex, and comorbid conditions, and also over time. Patients identified in secondary care were comparatively older than those identified in primary care, and in many cases AF was a secondary diagnosis made when the patient was admitted for another condition. These patients were also more likely to have a comorbid diagnosis for another condition such as HF, renal failure, or diabetes. Focusing on only one source of data could, therefore, give misleading results about the age distribution and relative health of the AF patient population; integrating data from multiple sources is important for obtaining a representative sample. Ignoring the temporal context of EHR data could also misrepresent the sample and present challenges for phenotyping. We found, as have others (e.g. [61]), that the impact of clinical guidelines can be investigated using EHR data. In our sample, the proportion of inferred AF cases decreased over the study period, as did the time between meeting the inferred criteria and receiving an AF diagnosis code. This gradual change in diagnostic and coding practices may be due to increasing awareness of AF as a condition warranting specific treatment, and potentially the inclusion in the QOF from 2004, although we did not observe a sharp alteration around this time point. This has broader implications for identification of disease cases in EHR data, particularly where treatment information is incorporated; case definitions and phenotype algorithms may need to allow for temporal changes in clinical practice and recording, and not rely on a single strategy being equally effective for all time points.

Limitations

The work described here has three major limitations relating to the data sources available for use, the strategy used for the AF case definition, and the capacity for external validation. Currently our phenotype algorithm does not use natural language processing (NLP) or imaging data. Use of non-coded data via NLP has been shown to improve detection of other cardiovascular conditions that are difficult to diagnose, such as angina pectoris [62], but although work in this area for application to CALIBER data is ongoing [63,64], it is not currently ready for general use. Ideally, AF cases identified in EHR data would be confirmed by electrocardiogram readings that displayed variability in the R-R intervals [14], but this source of data is also not currently available on a national scale.

As our aim was to develop an AF phenotype that was of use to all researchers using EHR data, regardless of computational resources, we did not employ some of the more sophisticated techniques used in some other EHR phenotyping studies. We interpreted the first diagnosis code in a patient record as a confirmed diagnosis, but in other EHR phenotypes researchers have required multiple diagnosis codes (e.g. [65]), or used more complex analytical methods (e.g. [66]). These strategies are undoubtedly useful for EHR phenotyping, particularly if the probability of false diagnoses is high, but this will be disease- and context-specific. In the case of AF in the UK during the time period considered, under-diagnosis is the more likely clinical scenario [16,17], and thus we deemed one AF diagnosis code sufficient. The inferred AF case definition was developed to capture some patients without a recorded diagnosis, but of course this cannot capture patients for whom no AF-related codes were recorded.

An important aspect of EHR phenotype development is validation, preferably against a "gold standard" (such as a manual review of case notes). We could not validate the AF phenotype in this manner as for the CALIBER programme, the initiation and funding of a separate study is required for re-contacting participants or clinicians to confirm diagnoses or review records. However, previous research has shown that AF diagnoses recorded in NHS primary care have a high degree of reliability even when relying on a single diagnosis code [24], although similar information is not available for secondary care (particularly when AF is not the primary diagnosis). The inferred diagnosis category also requires further validation work, particularly as it incorporates information on multiple diagnoses which may have their own limitations (for example, some HF patients will inadvertently be classified as AF patients if the sensitivity of HF diagnoses is less than perfect). In the near future we will apply CALIBER phenotype algorithms to data from the UK Biobank resource, which provides scope for validation of EHR phenotypes against self-reported data and clinical notes [67]. In the absence of external confirmation of AF diagnoses, we evaluated our phenotype definition by conducting epidemiological analyses of the association between known risk factors for AF onset and disease diagnosis in the CALIBER data set, and comparing our estimates to those from other studies. Our point estimates for the hazard ratios for AF and HF, hypertension, and MI were in the same direction as those obtained from comparable analyses in both traditional cohort [58,68] and EHR studies [26,31], which suggests that our AF identification strategy indexes a similar AF patient population.

Future research

The AF phenotype we have developed has been primarily informed by clinical understanding and interpretation of the EHR data. However, research on EHR phenotypes for other conditions has shown that data-driven approaches, such as using lagged linear correlations, can inform the EHR phenotyping process and facilitate the identification of patient subgroupings [4,69]. Once more sources of data, such as electrocardiogram results and clinical notes, are available on a national scale such approaches may prove useful for improved identification (especially refining the inferred diagnosis category) and further classification of AF patients.

Conclusion

Overall, we have developed a transparent and reproducible method for identifying AF cases in data from linked EHR sources that detects more cases than using a single data source. We have also highlighted the importance of exploring the patient record prior to developing EHR phenotype algorithms, including a number of challenges that may be encountered and potential strategies for overcoming them. Development of CALIBER phenotype algorithms is an ongoing, iterative process involving researchers within, and outside, the CALIBER network. To facilitate this, the code lists, case definitions, and algorithm for AF are freely available via from the CALIBER website (www.caliberresearch.org), and we encourage feedback from those who make use of this, and other, CALIBER phenotype algorithms.

Supporting Information

Table S1 Hazard ratio point estimates and 95% confidence intervals for selected risk factors and incident atrial fibrillation.

Acknowledgments

The authors would like to thank the reviewers, S. L. Kristensen and D. Albers, for helpful comments that improved the manuscript.

Author Contributions

Conceived and designed the experiments: KIM JW SCD HH. Performed the experiments: KIM JW SCD RJH RSP PP ADS ADT RJS HH. Analyzed the data: KIM JW. Contributed reagents/materials/analysis tools: KIM JW SCD RJH RSP PP ADS ADT RJS HH. Wrote the paper: KIM JW SCD RJH RSP PP ADS ADT RJS HH.

References

1. Newton KM, Peissig PL, Kho AN, Bielinski SJ, Berg RL, et al. (2013) Validation of electronic medical record-based phenotyping algorithms: results and lessons learned from the eMERGE network. Journal of the American Medical Informatics Association. pp. e147–e154.
2. Nicholson A, Ford E, Davies KA, Smith HE, Rait G, et al. (2013) Optimising Use of Electronic Health Records to Describe the Presentation of Rheumatoid Arthritis in Primary Care: A Strategy for Developing Code Lists. PLoS ONE. pp. e54878.
3. Richesson RL, Hammond WE, Nahm M, Wixted D, Simon GE, et al. (2013) Electronic health records based phenotyping in next-generation clinical trials: a perspective from the NIH Health Care Systems Collaboratory. Journal of the American Medical Informatics Association. pp. 1–7.
4. Hripcsak G, Albers DJ (2013) Correlating electronic health record concepts with healthcare process events. Journal of the American Medical Informatics Association 20: e311–e318.
5. Hripcsak G, Albers DJ (2013) Next-generation phenotyping of electronic health records. Journal of the American Medical Informatics Association: JAMIA 20: 117–121.
6. Weber GM, Mandl KD, Kohane IS (2014) Finding the Missing Link for Big Biomedical Data. JAMA: the journal of the … 311: 2479–2480.
7. Rapsomaniki E, Timmis A, George J, Pujades-Rodriguez M, Shah AD, et al. (2014) Blood pressure and incidence of twelve cardiovascular diseases: lifetime risks, healthy life-years lost, and age-specific associations in 1.25 million people. Lancet 383: 1899–1911.
8. Albers DJ, Hripcsak G (2010) A statistical dynamics approach to the study of human health data: resolving population scale diurnal variation in laboratory data. Physics Letters A 374: 1159–1164.
9. Albers DJ, Hripcsak G (2012) Using time-delayed mutual information to discover and interpret temporal correlation structure in complex populations. Chaos (Woodbury, NY) 22: 013111–013111.
10. Conen D, Chae CU, Glynn RJ, Tedrow UB, Everett BM, et al. (2011) Risk of death and cardiovascular events in initially healthy women with new-onset atrial fibrillation. JAMA. pp. 2080–2087.
11. Lip GYH, Tse HF, Lane DA (2012) Atrial fibrillation. Lancet. pp. 648–661.
12. Denaxas SC, George J, Herrett E, Shah AD, Kalra D, et al. (2012) Data Resource Profile: Cardiovascular disease research using linked bespoke studies and electronic health records (CALIBER). International Journal of Epidemiology. pp. 1625–1638.
13. Camm AJ, Lip GYH, De Caterina R, Savelieva I, Atar D, et al. (2012) 2012 focused update of the ESC Guidelines for the management of atrial fibrillation: an update of the 2010 ESC Guidelines for the management of atrial fibrillation. Developed with the special contribution of the European Heart Rhythm Association. European heart journal 33: 2719–2747.
14. National Collaborating Centre for Chronic Conditions (2007) Atrial fibrillation: national clinical guidline for management in primary and secondary care. London: Royal College of Physicians. 1–171 p.
15. Kirchhof P, Curtis AB, Skanes AC, Gillis AM, Samuel Wann L, et al. (2013) Atrial fibrillation guidelines across the Atlantic: a comparison of the current recommendations of the European Society of Cardiology/European Heart Rhythm Association/European Association of Cardiothoracic Surgeons, the American College of Cardiology Foundation/American Heart Association/ Heart Rhythm Society, and the Canadian Cardiovascular Society. European heart journal 34: 1471–1474.
16. Fitzmaurice DA, Hobbs FDR, Jowett S, Mant J, Murray ET, et al. (2007) Screening versus routine practice in detection of atrial fibrillation in patients aged 65 or over: cluster randomised controlled trial. BMJ (Clinical research ed) 335: 383–383.
17. Scowcroft ACE, Cowie MR (2014) Atrial fibrillation: improvement in identification and stroke preventive therapy - data from the UK Clinical Practice Research Datalink, 2000–2012. International journal of cardiology 171: 169–173.
18. Gillam S, Steel N (2013) The Quality and Outcomes Framework–where next? BMJ (Clinical research ed) 346: f659–f659.
19. National Institute for Health and Care Excellence (2006) Atrial fibrillation: The management of atrial fibrillation. Available: http://www.nice.org.uk/guidance/cg36/resources/guidance-atrial-fibrillation-the-management-of-atrial-fibrillation-pdf. Accessed 2014 Oct 2.

20. De Caterina R, Ruigómez A, Rodríguez LAG (2010) Long-term use of anti-inflammatory drugs and risk of atrial fibrillation. Arch Intern Med. pp. 1450–1455.
21. Gallagher AM, Setakis E, Plumb JM, Clemens A, Van Staa T-P (2011) Risks of stroke and mortality associated with suboptimal anticoagulation in atrial fibrillation patients. Thromb Haemost. pp. 968–977.
22. Grosso A, Douglas I, Hingorani A, MacAllister R, Smeeth L (2009) Oral Bisphosphonates and Risk of Atrial Fibrillation and Flutter in Women: A Self-Controlled Case-Series Safety Analysis. PLoS ONE. pp. e4720.
23. Van Staa TP, Setakis E, Di Tanna GL, Lane DA, Lip GYH (2011) A comparison of risk stratification schemes for stroke in 79884 atrial fibrillation patients in general practice. Journal of Thrombosis and Haemostasis. pp. 39–48.
24. Ruigómez A, Johansson S, Wallander MA, Rodríguez LAG (2002) Incidence of chronic atrial fibrillation in general practice and its treatment pattern. Journal of clinical epidemiology 55: 358–363.
25. Watanabe H, Tanabe N, Makiyama Y, Chopra SS, Okura Y, et al. (2006) ST-segment abnormalities and premature complexes are predictors of new-onset atrial fibrillation: the Niigata preventive medicine study. Am Heart J 152: 731–735.
26. Ahlehoff O, Gislason GH, Jørgensen CH, Lindhardsen J, Charlot M, et al. (2012) Psoriasis and risk of atrial fibrillation and ischaemic stroke: a Danish Nationwide Cohort Study. European heart journal 33: 2054–2064.
27. Alonso A, Agarwal SK, Soliman EZ, Ambrose M, Chamberlain AM, et al. (2009) Incidence of atrial fibrillation in whites and African-Americans: the Atherosclerosis Risk in Communities (ARIC) study. American Heart Journal 158: 111–117.
28. Chiang C-H, Huang C-C, Chan W-L, Huang P-H, Chen Y-C, et al. (2013) Herpes simplex virus infection and risk of atrial fibrillation: A nationwide study. International journal of cardiology 164: 201–204.
29. Emilsson L, Smith JG, West J, Melander O, Ludvigsson JF (2011) Increased risk of atrial fibrillation in patients with coeliac disease: a nationwide cohort study. European heart journal 32: 2430–2437.
30. Fedorowski A, Hedblad B, Engström G, Gustav Smith J, Melander O (2010) Orthostatic hypotension and long-term incidence of atrial fibrillation: the Malmö Preventive Project. Journal of internal medicine 268: 383–389.
31. Friberg J, Buch P, Scharling H, Gadsbphioll N, Jensen GB (2003) Rising rates of hospital admissions for atrial fibrillation. Epidemiology (Cambridge, Mass) 14: 666–672.
32. Frost L, Vestergaard P (2004) Alcohol and risk of atrial fibrillation or flutter: a cohort study. Archives of internal medicine 164: 1993–1998.
33. Grundvold I, Skretteberg PT, Liestøl K, Gjesdal K, Erikssen G, et al. (2012) Importance of physical fitness on predictive effect of body mass index and weight gain on incident atrial fibrillation in healthy middle-age men. The American journal of cardiology 110: 425–432.
34. Nyrnes A, Mathiesen EB, Njølstad I, Wilsgaard T, Løchen M-L (2012) Palpitations are predictive of future atrial fibrillation. An 11-year follow-up of 22,815 men and women: the Tromso Study. European journal of preventive cardiology.
35. Perez MV, Dewey FE, Marcus R, Ashley EA, Al-Ahmad AA, et al. (2009) Electrocardiographic predictors of atrial fibrillation. American heart journal 158: 622–628.
36. Psaty BM, Manolio TA, Kuller LH, Kronmal RA, Cushman M, et al. (1997) Incidence of and risk factors for atrial fibrillation in older adults. Circulation 96: 2455–2461.
37. Schnabel RB, Aspelund T, Li G, Sullivan LM, Suchy-Dicey A, et al. (2010) Validation of an atrial fibrillation risk algorithm in whites and African Americans. Archives of internal medicine 170: 1909–1917.
38. Selmer C, Olesen JB, Hansen ML, Lindhardsen J, Olsen A-MS, et al. (2012) The spectrum of thyroid disease and risk of new onset atrial fibrillation: a large population cohort study. BMJ (Clinical research ed) 345: e7895–e7895.
39. Stewart S, Hart CL, Hole DJ, McMurray JJ (2001) Population prevalence, incidence, and predictors of atrial fibrillation in the Renfrew/Paisley study. Heart (British Cardiac Society) 86: 516–521.
40. Tsang TSM, Gersh BJ, Appleton CP, Tajik AJ, Barnes ME, et al. (2002) Left ventricular diastolic dysfunction as a predictor of the first diagnosed nonvalvular atrial fibrillation in 840 elderly men and women. Journal of the American College of Cardiology 40: 1636–1644.
41. Djoussé L, Levy D, Benjamin EJ, Blease SJ, Russ A, et al. (2004) Long-term alcohol consumption and the risk of atrial fibrillation in the Framingham Study. The American journal of cardiology 93: 710–713.
42. Heeringa J, Kors JA, Hofman A, van Rooij FJA, Witteman JCM (2008) Cigarette smoking and risk of atrial fibrillation: the Rotterdam Study. American heart journal 156: 1163–1169.
43. Lipworth L, Okafor H, Mumma MT, Edwards TL, Roden DM, et al. (2012) Race-specific impact of atrial fibrillation risk factors in blacks and whites in the southern community cohort study. The American journal of cardiology 110: 1637–1642.
44. Maddox TM, Ross C, Ho PM, Magid D, Rumsfeld JS (2009) Impaired heart rate recovery is associated with new-onset atrial fibrillation: a prospective cohort study. BMC cardiovascular disorders 9: 11–11.
45. Gottesman O, Kuivaniemi H, Tromp G, Faucett WA, Li R, et al. (2013) The Electronic Medical Records and Genomics (eMERGE) Network: past, present, and future. Genetics in medicine: official journal of the American College of Medical Genetics 15: 761–771.
46. Kho AN, Pacheco Ja, Peissig PL, Rasmussen L, Newton KM, et al. (2011) Electronic medical records for genetic research: results of the eMERGE consortium. Science translational medicine 3: 79re71–79re71.
47. Köhler S, Doelken SC, Mungall CJ, Bauer S, Firth HV, et al. (2014) The Human Phenotype Ontology project: linking molecular biology and disease through phenotype data. Nucleic acids research 42: D966–974.
48. McCarty Ca, Chisholm RL, Chute CG, Kullo IJ, Jarvik GP, et al. (2011) The eMERGE Network: a consortium of biorepositories linked to electronic medical records data for conducting genomic studies. BMC medical genomics 4: 13–13.
49. Overby CL, Pathak J, Gottesman O, Haerian K, Perotte A, et al. (2013) A collaborative approach to developing an electronic health record phenotyping algorithm for drug-induced liver injury. Journal of the American Medical Informatics Association. pp. 1–11.
50. Perlis RH, Iosifescu DV, Castro VM, Murphy SN, Gainer VS, et al. (2012) Using electronic medical records to enable large-scale studies in psychiatry: treatment resistant depression as a model. Psychol Med. pp. 41–50.
51. Rea S, Pathak J, Savova G, Oniki TA, Westberg L, et al. (2012) Building a robust, scalable and standards-driven infrastructure for secondary use of EHR data: The SHARPn project. Journal of Biomedical Informatics. pp. 763–771.
52. Ritchie MD, Denny JC, Crawford DC, Ramirez AH, Weiner JB, et al. (2010) Robust replication of genotype-phenotype associations across multiple diseases in an electronic medical record. American journal of human genetics 86: 560–572.
53. Hodgkinson JA, Taylor CJ, Hobbs FDR (2011) Treatment pathways for patients with atrial fibrillation. International Journal of Clinical Practice. pp. 44–52.
54. Cox DR (1972) Regression models and life-tables. J R Stat Soc Ser B 34.
55. Andersen PK, Abildstrøm SZ, Rosthøj S (2002) Competing risks as a multi-state model. Statist Med 26: 2389–2430.
56. R Core Team (2013) R: A language and environment for statistical computing. Vienna, Austria: R Foundation for Statistical Computing.
57. Davis RC, Hobbs FDR, Kenkre JE, Roalfe AK, Iles R, et al. (2012) Prevalence of atrial fibrillation in the general population and in high-risk groups: the ECHOES study. Europace 14: 1553–1559.
58. Schnabel RB, Sullivan LM, Levy D, Pencina MJ, Massaro JM, et al. (2009) Development of a risk score for atrial fibrillation (Framingham Heart Study): a community-based cohort study. Lancet 373: 739–745.
59. Herrett E, Shah AD, Boggon R, Denaxas S, Smeeth L, et al. (2013) Completeness and diagnostic validity of recording acute myocardial infarction events in primary care, hospital care, disease registry, and national mortality records: cohort study. BMJ. pp. f2350.
60. Pascoe SW, Neal RD, Heywood PL, Allgar VL, Miles JN, et al. (2008) Identifying patients with a cancer diagnosis using general practice medical records and Cancer Registry data. Family practice 25: 215–220.
61. Pivovarov R, Albers DJ, Hripcsak G, Sepulveda JL, Elhadad N (2014) Temporal trends of hemoglobin A1c testing. Journal of the American Medical Informatics Association: JAMIA: 1–7.
62. Pakhomov SS, Hemingway H, Weston SA, Jacobsen SJ, Rodeheffer R, et al. (2007) Epidemiology of angina pectoris: role of natural language processing of the medical record. Am Heart J 153: 666–673.
63. Shah AD, Martinez C, Hemingway H (2012) The freetext matching algorithm: a computer program to extract diagnoses and causes of death from unstructured text in electronic health records. BMC Medical Informatics & Decision Making 12.
64. Wang Z, Shah AD, Tate AR, Denaxas S, Shawe-Taylor J, et al. (2012) Extracting diagnoses and investigation results from unstructured text in electronic health records by semi-supervised machine learning. PLoS One 7: e30412.
65. Peissig PL, Rasmussen LV, Berg RL, Linneman JG, Mccarty CA, et al. (2012) Importance of multi-modal approaches to effectively identify cataract cases from electronic health records. Journal of the American Medical Informatics Association. pp. 225–234.
66. Perotte A, Hripcsak G (2013) Temporal properties of diagnosis code time series in aggregate. IEEE Journal Biomed Health Inform 17: 477–483.
67. Collins R (2012) What makes UK Biobank special? Lancet 379: 1173–1174.
68. Smith JG, Platonov PG, Hedblad B, Engstrom G, Melander O (2010) Atrial fibrillation in the Malmo Diet and Cancer study: a study of occurrence, risk factors and diagnostic validity. Eur J Epidemiol 25: 95–102.
69. Hripcsak G, Albers DJ, Perotte A (2011) Exploiting time in electronic health record correlations. Journal of the American Medical Informatics Association: JAMIA 18 Suppl 1: i109–115.

Permissions

All chapters in this book were first published in PLOS ONE, by The Public Library of Science; hereby published with permission under the Creative Commons Attribution License or equivalent. Every chapter published in this book has been scrutinized by our experts. Their significance has been extensively debated. The topics covered herein carry significant findings which will fuel the growth of the discipline. They may even be implemented as practical applications or may be referred to as a beginning point for another development.

The contributors of this book come from diverse backgrounds, making this book a truly international effort. This book will bring forth new frontiers with its revolutionizing research information and detailed analysis of the nascent developments around the world.

We would like to thank all the contributing authors for lending their expertise to make the book truly unique. They have played a crucial role in the development of this book. Without their invaluable contributions this book wouldn't have been possible. They have made vital efforts to compile up to date information on the varied aspects of this subject to make this book a valuable addition to the collection of many professionals and students.

This book was conceptualized with the vision of imparting up-to-date information and advanced data in this field. To ensure the same, a matchless editorial board was set up. Every individual on the board went through rigorous rounds of assessment to prove their worth. After which they invested a large part of their time researching and compiling the most relevant data for our readers.

The editorial board has been involved in producing this book since its inception. They have spent rigorous hours researching and exploring the diverse topics which have resulted in the successful publishing of this book. They have passed on their knowledge of decades through this book. To expedite this challenging task, the publisher supported the team at every step. A small team of assistant editors was also appointed to further simplify the editing procedure and attain best results for the readers.

Apart from the editorial board, the designing team has also invested a significant amount of their time in understanding the subject and creating the most relevant covers. They scrutinized every image to scout for the most suitable representation of the subject and create an appropriate cover for the book.

The publishing team has been an ardent support to the editorial, designing and production team. Their endless efforts to recruit the best for this project, has resulted in the accomplishment of this book. They are a veteran in the field of academics and their pool of knowledge is as vast as their experience in printing. Their expertise and guidance has proved useful at every step. Their uncompromising quality standards have made this book an exceptional effort. Their encouragement from time to time has been an inspiration for everyone.

The publisher and the editorial board hope that this book will prove to be a valuable piece of knowledge for researchers, students, practitioners and scholars across the globe.

List of Contributors

Fuminori Odagiri, Masami Sugihara and Takeshi Suzuki
Department of Cellular and Molecular Pharmacology, Juntendo University Graduate School of Medicine, Tokyo, Japan
Department of Cardiovascular Medicine, Juntendo University Graduate School of Medicine, Tokyo, Japan

Hana Inoue and Masato Konishi
Department of Physiology, Tokyo Medical University, Tokyo, Japan

Takashi Murayama, Takashi Sakurai and Nagomi Kurebayashi
Department of Cellular and Molecular Pharmacology, Juntendo University Graduate School of Medicine, Tokyo, Japan

Takao Shioya
Department of Physiology, Faculty of Medicine, Saga University, Saga, Japan

Yuji Nakazato and Hiroyuki Daida
Department of Cardiovascular Medicine, Juntendo University Graduate School of Medicine, Tokyo, Japan

Sachio Morimoto
Department of Clinical Pharmacology, Graduate School of Medical Sciences, Kyushu University, Fukuoka, Japan

Shin Watanabe, Takahiro Horie, Kazuya Nagao, Yasuhide Kuwabara, Osamu Baba, Hitoo Nishi,
Naoya Sowa, Takeshi Kimura and Koh Ono
Department of Cardiovascular Medicine, Graduate School of Medicine, Kyoto University, Kyoto, Japan

Michiko Narazaki and Tetsuya Matsuda
Department of Systems Science, Graduate School of Informatics, Kyoto University, Kyoto, Japan

Genzou Takemura
Department of Internal Medicine, Asahi University, Gifu, Japan

Hiromichi Wada and Koji Hasegawa
Division of Translational Research, Kyoto Medical Center, National Hospital Organization, Kyoto, Japan

David Williams, Melissa Byrne, Mandar Joshi, Duncan Horlock and Nicholas T. Lam
Heart Failure Research Group, Baker IDI Heart & Diabetes Institute, Melbourne, Australia

Kylie M. Venardos and David M. Kaye
Heart Failure Research Group, Baker IDI Heart & Diabetes Institute, Melbourne, Australia
Department of Medicine, Monash University, Melbourne, Australia

Paul Gregorevic
Muscle Research & Therapeutics Laboratory, Baker IDI Heart & Diabetes Institute, Melbourne, Australia

Sean L. McGee
Metabolic Research Unit, Deakin University, Geelong, Australia

Jeffrey A. Bakal and Finlay A. McAlister
Patient Health Outcomes Research and Clinical Effectiveness Unit, University of Alberta, Edmonton, Alberta, Canada
Division of General Internal Medicine, University of Alberta, Edmonton, Alberta, Canada

Wei Liu and Justin A. Ezekowitz
Division of Cardiology, University of Alberta, Edmonton, Alberta, Canada

Li-na Hou
State Key Laboratory of Organ Failure Research, Department of Cardiology, Nanfang Hospital, Southern Medical University, Guangzhou, Guangdong, P.R.China
Department of healthy management, Nanfang Hospital, Southern Medical University, Guangzhou, Guangdong, P.R.China

Fei Li
Department of Urology, Nanfang Hospital, Southern Medical University, Guangzhou, Guangdong, P.R.China

Qing-chun Zeng, Liang Su, Ping-an Chen, Zhi-hao Xu, Din-ji Zhu, Chang-hua Liu and Ding-li Xu
State Key Laboratory of Organ Failure Research, Department of Cardiology, Nanfang Hospital, Southern Medical University, Guangzhou, Guangdong, P.R.China

Nicole Nigro and Mirjam Christ-Crain
Department of Endocrinology, University Hospital Basel, Basel, Switzerland
Department of Clinical Research, University Hospital Basel, Basel, Switzerland

Karin Wildi and Christian Mueller
Department of Cardiology, University Hospital Basel, Basel, Switzerland
Department of Clinical Research, University Hospital Basel, Basel, Switzerland

Philipp Schuetz and Beat Mueller
Medical University Clinic and Division of Endocrinology, Diabetology and Metabolism, Kantonsspital Aarau, Aarau, Switzerland
Department of Clinical Research, University Hospital Basel, Basel, Switzerland

Felix Fluri
Department of Neurology, University Hospital Basel, Basel, Switzerland
Department of Clinical Research, University Hospital Basel, Basel, Switzerland

Mira Katan
Department of Endocrinology, University Hospital Basel, Basel, Switzerland
Department of Neurology, University Hospital Zurich, Zurich, Switzerland
Department of Clinical Research, University Hospital Basel, Basel, Switzerland

Sangita Choudhury, Soochan Bae, Qingen Ke, Ji Yoo Lee, Sylvia S. Singh, Federica del Monte, Peter M. Kang
Cardiovascular Institute, Beth Israel Deaconess Medical Center and Harvard Medical School, Boston, Massachusetts, United States of America

René St-Arnaud
Shriners Hospital and Departments of Surgery and Human Genetics, McGill University, Montreal, Canada

Juan F. Gomez, Karen Cardona, Lucia Romero, Jose M. Ferrero Jr. and Beatriz Trenor
Instituto de Investigación en Ingeniería Biomédica, Universitat Politècnica de València, Valencia, Spain

Johannes T. Kowallick, Jan M. Sohns, Martin Fasshauer, Wieland Staab and Joachim Lotz
Institute for Diagnostic and Interventional Radiology, Georg-August-University Göttingen, Göttingen, Germany
DZHK (German Centre for Cardiovascular Research), partner site Göttingen, Göttingen, Germany

Pablo Lamata
Department of Computer Science, University of Oxford, Oxford, United Kingdom
Division of Imaging Sciences and Biomedical Engineering, The Rayne Institute, St. Thomas' Hospital, King's College London, London, United Kingdom

Shazia T. Hussain
Papworth Hospital NHS Trust, Papworth Everard, Cambridgeshire, United Kingdom

Shelby Kutty
Children's Hospital and Medical Center, University of Nebraska College of Medicine, Omaha, Nebraska, United States of America

Michael Steinmetz
Department of Pediatric Cardiology and Intensive Care Medicine, Georg- August-University Göttingen, Göttingen, Germany
DZHK (German Centre for Cardiovascular Research), partner site Göttingen, Göttingen, Germany

Christina Unterberg-Buchwald and Gerd Hasenfuß
Department of Cardiology and Pneumology, Georg-August-University Göttingen, Göttingen, Germany
DZHK (German Centre for Cardiovascular Research), partner site Göttingen, Göttingen, Germany

Boris Bigalke
Division of Imaging Sciences and Biomedical Engineering, The Rayne Institute, St. Thomas' Hospital, King's College London, London, United Kingdom
Medizinische Klinik III, Kardiologie und Kreislauferkrankungen, Eberhard-Karls-Universität Tübingen, Tübingen, Germany

Andreas Schuster
Department of Cardiology and Pneumology, Georg-August-University Göttingen, Göttingen, Germany, Division of Imaging Sciences and Biomedical Engineering, The Rayne Institute, St. Thomas' Hospital, King's College London, London, United Kingdom
DZHK (German Centre for Cardiovascular Research), partner site Göttingen, Göttingen, Germany

Michael A. McDonald, Juarez R. Braga and Heather J. Ross
Division of Cardiology, Peter Munk Cardiac Centre, University of Toronto, Toronto, Canada

Jing Li, Cedric Manlhiot and Andrew N. Redington
Division of Cardiology, Hospital for Sick Children, University of Toronto, Toronto, Canada

Xiao Lu, Zhen-Du Zhang, Xiaomei Guo, Jenny Susana Choy, Junrong Yang and Mark Svendsen
Department of Biomedical Engineering, Indiana University Purdue University Indianapolis, Indianapolis, Indiana, United States of America

Ghassan Kassab
Department of Biomedical Engineering, Indiana University Purdue University Indianapolis, Indianapolis, Indiana, United States of America
Department of Surgery, Indiana University Purdue University Indianapolis, Indianapolis, Indiana, United States of America
Cellular and Integrative Physiology, Indiana University Purdue University Indianapolis, Indianapolis, Indiana, United States of America

Mohsen Bayati
Stanford University, Stanford, California, United States of America

Mark Braverman
Princeton University, Princeton, New Jersey, United States of America

Michael Gillam, Karen M. Mack, George Ruiz and Mark S. Smith
MedStar Health and Washington Hospital Center, Washington, D. C., United States of America

Eric Horvitz
Microsoft Research and University of Washington School of Medicine, Redmond, Washington, United States of America

Jun-qing Yang, Peng Ran, Ji-yan Chen, Li-wen Li, Ning Tan, Guang Li, Shuo Sun, Yong Liu, Jia-xin Zhan, Jian-yi Zheng and Ying-ling Zhou
Department of Cardiology, Guangdong Cardiovascular Institute, Guangdong General Hospital, Guangdong Academy of Medical Sciences, Guangzhou, Guangdong, China

Yi-ting He
Department of Cardiology, Shunde first hospital, Foshan, Guangdong, China

Jenny S. Choy and Zhen-Du Zhang
Department of Biomedical Engineering, Indiana University Purdue University Indianapolis, Indianapolis, Indiana, United States of America

Koullis Pitsillides
Transonic EndoGear Inc., Davis, California, United States of America

Margo Sosa
Transonic Systems Inc., Ithaca, New York, United States of America

Ghassan S. Kassab
Department of Biomedical Engineering, Indiana University Purdue University Indianapolis, Indianapolis, Indiana, United States of America
Department of Surgery, Indiana University, Indianapolis, Indiana, United States of America, 5 Department of Cellular and Integrative Physiology, Indiana University, Indianapolis, Indiana, United States of America

Ana Ortega, Esther Roselló -Lletí, Estefanía Tarazón, Maria Micaela Molina-Navarro, Jose David Montoro-Mateos, Miguel Rivera, Manuel Portolés
Cardiocirculatory Unit, Health Research Institute of La Fe University Hospital, Valencia, Spain

Luis Martínez-Dolz and Antonio Salvador
Heart Failure and Transplantation Unit, Cardiology Department, La Fe University Hospital, Valencia, Spain

José Ramón Gonzá lez-Juanatey, Francisca Lago
Cellular and Molecular Cardiology Research Unit, Department of Cardiology and Institute of Biomedical Research, University Clinical Hospital, Santiago de Compostela, Spain

Natalie McCormick
Faculty of Pharmaceutical Sciences, University of British Columbia, Vancouver, British Columbia, Canada
Arthritis Research Centre of Canada, Richmond, British Columbia, Canada
Diane Lacaille and J. Antonio Avina-Zubieta
Arthritis Research Centre of Canada, Richmond, British Columbia, Canada
Division of Rheumatology, Department of Medicine, University of British Columbia, Vancouver, British Columbia, Canada
Cardiovascular Committee of the Canadian Rheumatology Administrative Data Network, Richmond, British Columbia, Canada

Vidula Bhole
Arthritis Research Centre of Canada, Richmond, British Columbia, Canada
EpiSolutions Consultancy Services, Thane, India

Terri R. Fried
Clinical Epidemiology Research Center, VA Connecticut Healthcare System, West Haven, Connecticut, United States of America
Department of Medicine, Yale School of Medicine, New Haven, Connecticut, United States of America

John O'Leary and Deanna K. Martin
Clinical Epidemiology Research Center, VA Connecticut Healthcare System, West Haven, Connecticut, United States of America
Program on Aging, Yale School of Medicine, New Haven, Connecticut, United States of America

Virginia Towle and Mark Trentelange
Program on Aging, Yale School of Medicine, New Haven, Connecticut, United States of America

Mary K. Goldstein
Palo Alto Geriatrics Research Education and Clinical Center (GRECC), VA Palo Alto Health Care System, Palo Alto, Connecticut, 94304, United States of America
Center for Primary Care and Outcomes Research, Stanford University School of Medicine, Stanford, California, 94305, United States of America

Natasha A. Loghmanpour and James F. Antaki
Department of Biomedical Engineering, Carnegie Mellon University, Pittsburgh, Pennsylvania, United States of America

Marek J. Druzdzel
Decision Systems Laboratory, School of Information Sciences, University of Pittsburgh, Pittsburgh, Pennsylvania, United States of America
Faculty of Computer Science, Bialystok University of Technology, Bialystok, Poland

Rodrigo W. A. Souza, Warlen P. Piedade, Luana C. Soares, Paula A. T. Souza, Ivan J. Vechetti-Júnior, Robson F. Carvalho and Maeli Dal-Pai-Silva
Department of Morphology, São Paulo State University, Botucatu, São Paulo, Brazil

Andreo F. Aguiar
Centre of Biological and Health Sciences, North University of Paraná, Londrina, Paraná, Brazil

Dijon H. S. Campos and Katashi Okoshi
Department of Internal Medicine, São Paulo State University, Botucatu, São Paulo, Brazil

Ana A. H. Fernandes and Antonio C. Cicogna
Department of Biochemistry, São Paulo State University, Botucatu, São Paulo, Brazil

Katherine I. Morley
Farr Institute of Health Informatics Research, University College London, London, United Kingdom, and Clinical Epidemiology, Department of Epidemiology and Public Health, University College London, London, United Kingdom
Institute of Psychiatry, Psychology and Neuroscience, King's College London, London, United Kingdom
Melbourne School of Global and Population Health, The University of Melbourne, Melbourne, Australia

Joshua Wallace, Spiros C. Denaxas, Anoop D. Shah and Harry Hemingway
Farr Institute of Health Informatics Research, University College London, London, United Kingdom, and Clinical Epidemiology, Department of Epidemiology and Public Health, University College London, London, United Kingdom

Ross J. Hunter, Adam D. Timmis and Richard J. Schilling
Barts NIHR Biomedical Research Unit, Queen Mary University London, London, United Kingdom

Riyaz S. Patel
Farr Institute of Health Informatics Research, University College London, London, United Kingdom
The Heart Hospital, University College London NHS Trust, London, United Kingdom

Pablo Perel
Farr Institute of Health Informatics Research, University College London, London, United Kingdom, and London School of Hygiene and Tropical Medicine, London, United Kingdom

Index